Operative Techniques in
Facial Aesthetic
Surgery

Operative Techniques in Facial Aesthetic Surgery

EDITORS

Charles H. Thorne, MD
Chairman
Department of Plastic Surgery
Lenox Hill Hospital
New York, New York

Sammy Sinno, MD
Private Practice
Chicago, Illinois

Kevin C. Chung, MD, MS
EDITOR-IN-CHIEF

Chief of Hand Surgery, Michigan Medicine
Director, University of Michigan Comprehensive Hand Center
Charles B. G. de Nancrede Professor of Surgery
Professor of Plastic Surgery and Orthopaedic Surgery
Assistant Dean for Faculty Affairs
Associate Director of Global REACH
University of Michigan Medical School
Ann Arbor, Michigan

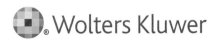

Philadelphia • Baltimore • New York • London
Buenos Aires • Hong Kong • Sydney • Tokyo

Executive Editor: Brian Brown
Development Editor: Ashley Fischer
Editorial Coordinator: John Larkin
Marketing Manager: Julie Sikora
Senior Production Project Manager: Alicia Jackson
Senior Designer: Joan Wendt
Artist/Illustrator: Body Scientific International
Senior Manufacturing Coordinator: Beth Welsh
Prepress Vendor: SPi Global

Cataloging-in-Publication Data available on request from the Publisher.
ISBN 978-1-4963-4923-1

Dedicated to my daughter, Wells Thorne—my standard for beauty, harmony, and ethics.

—CHT

To my wonderful and patient wife, Rosa—without her support this book would not be possible, I love you. To Genoa and Giovanni—thank you for being the best kids I could ask for and completing my life. To my parents for their lifetime of support and love and being the best role models. To my great plastic surgery mentors who have inspired me, including Charlie Thorne, whom working with on this book with has been a tremendous joy.

—SS

To Chin-Yin and William.

—KCC

Contributors

Jamil Ahmad, MD
Director of Research and Education
The Plastic Surgery Clinic
Mississauga, Ontario, Canada
Assistant Professor
Department of Surgery
University of Toronto
Toronto, Ontario, Canada

Mithat Akan, MD
Professor
Department of Plastic Surgery
Istanbul Medipol University
Istanbul, Turkey

Amir Allak, MD, MBA
Facial Plastic/Reconstructive Surgery
Fellow
Division of Facial Plastic Surgery
Department of Otolaryngology—Head
and Neck Surgery
University of California, Davis
Sacramento, California

Stephen B. Baker, MD, DDS
Professor and Program Director
Director, Center for Facial Restoration
Department of Plastic Surgery
MedStar Georgetown University
Hospital
Washington, District of Columbia
Medical Director, Craniofacial
Program
Inova Children's Hospital
Falls Church, Virginia

Lawrence S. Bass, MD, FACS
Clinical Assistant Professor of Plastic
Surgery
Zucker School of Medicine at Hofstra
Northwell
New York, New York

Daniel A. Belkin, MD
Clinical Assistant Professor
Ronald O. Perelman Department of
Dermatology
NYU Langone Medical Center
Associate
Laser & Skin Surgery Center of
New York
New York, New York

Francisco G. Bravo, MD, PhD
Clinica Gomez Bravo
Madrid, Spain

Barış Çakir, MD
Plastic Reconstructive and Aesthetic
Surgery Specialist
Visiting Staff of American Hospital
(Sisli/İstanbul)
Istanbul, Turkey

Ashley A. Campbell, MD
Assistant Professor of Ophthalmology
Wilmer Eye Institute
Johns Hopkins University School of
Medicine
Baltimore, Maryland

Nuri A. Celik, MD
Private Practice
Istanbul, Turkey

Jong-Woo Choi, MD, PhD, MMM
Professor
Department of Plastic Surgery
Asian Medical Center
Seoul, South Korea

Jeffrey R. Claiborne, MD
Private Practice Plastic Surgeon
Sieveking and Claiborne Plastic Surgery
Nashville, Tennessee

C. Spencer Cochran, MD
Dallas Rhinoplasty Center
Assistant Professor
Department of Plastic Surgery
Clinical Assistant Professor
Department of Otolaryngology
UT Southwestern Medical Center
Dallas, Texas

Mark B. Constantian, MD, FACS
Traveling Professor, American Society
for Aesthetic Plastic Surgery
Clinical Adjunct Professor of Surgery
(Plastic Surgery)
University of Wisconsin
Madison, Wisconsin
Visiting Professor
Department of Plastic Surgery
University of Virginia
Charlottesville, Virginia

Sebastian Cotofana, MD, PhD
Associate Professor
Albany Medical College
Albany, New York

Clayton Crantford, MD
Private Practice
Charleston, South Carolina

Eric J. Culbertson, MD
Body and Breast Cosmetic
Surgeon
The Jacobs Center for Cosmetic
Surgery
Healdsburg, California

Daniel A. Cuzzone, MD
Craniofacial Fellow
Children's Healthcare of Atlanta
Atlanta, Georgia

Rollin K. Daniel, MD
Clinical Professor
Department of Plastic Surgery
Irvine Medical Center
University of California
Orange, California
Private Practice
Newport Beach, California

Erez Dayan, MD
Plastic & Reconstructive Surgery
Massachusetts General Hospital/
Harvard Medical School
Boston, Massachusetts

Gehaan D'Souza, MD
Editor-in-Chief
CEO Iconic Plastic Surgery
Carlsbad, California

Nguyen Phan Tu Dung, MD, PhD
Chief of Rhinoplasty and Maxillofacial
Department
Director of Vietnam JW Anesthetic
Hospital
Ho Chi Minh City, Vietnam

Dino Elyassnia, MD, FACS
Marten Clinic of Plastic
Surgery
San Francisco, California

Julius W. Few, MD
Director, The Few Institute for
    Aesthetic Plastic Surgery
Clinical Professor, Division of Plastic
    Surgery
University of Chicago Pritzker School
    of Medicine
Health Science Clinician
Feinberg School of Medicine
Northwestern University
Chicago, Illinois

Roy G. Geronemus, MD
Director, Laser & Skin Surgery Center
    of New York
Clinical Professor of Dermatology
New York University Medical Center
Attending Surgeon
Department of Plastic Surgery
New York Eye and Ear Infirmary
Mt Sinai School of Medicine
New York, New York

Ashkan Ghavami, MD
Assistant Clinical Professor
David Geffen School of Medicine
UCLA
Los Angeles, California
Private Practice
Beverly Hills, California

Jacob Nathaniel Grow, MD
Integrated Plastic Surgery Resident
University of Kansas Medical Center
Kansas City, Missouri

Bahman Guyuron, MD, FACS
Editor-In-Chief, Aesthetic Plastic
    Surgery Journal
Emeritus Professor, Department of
    Plastic Surgery
Case Western Reserve University
    School of Medicine
Cleveland, Ohio

David A. Hidalgo, MD
Clinical Professor of Surgery
Weill-Cornell Medical College
New York-Presbyterian Hospital
New York, New York

Clyde H. Ishii, MD
Immediate Past President
American Society for Aesthetic Plastic
    Surgery
Assistant Clinical Professor of Surgery
John Burns School of Medicine
University of Hawaii
Chief of Plastic Surgery
Shriners Hospital
Honolulu, Hawaii

Elizabeth B. Jelks, MD
Adjunct Staff
Department of Plastic Surgery
Lenox Hill Hospital
New York, New York

Glenn W. Jelks, MD, FACS
Associate Professor
Hansjorg Wyss
Department of Plastic Surgery
Associate Professor
Department of Ophthalmology
New York University School of
    Medicine
New York, New York

Woo Shik Jeong, MD
Clinical Assistant Professor
Department of Plastic Surgery
Asan Medical Center
University of Ulsan College of
    Medicine
Seoul, South Korea

Yumiko Kadota, BSc, MBBS
Surgical Assistant
Private Practice
Chatswood, New South Wales,
    Australia

George N. Kamel, MD
Division of Plastic Surgery
Department of Surgery
Montefiore Medical Center
Albert Einstein College of Medicine
Bronx, New York

Jeffrey M. Kenkel, MD, FACS
Professor and Chairman
Betty and Warren Woodward Chair
    in Plastic and Reconstructive Surgery
Director, Clinical Center for Cosmetic
    Laser Treatment
Department of Plastic Surgery
Dallas, Texas

Aaron M. Kosins, MD
Clinical Assistant Professor
Department of Plastic Surgery
University of California, Irvine Medical
    Center
Orange, California
Private Practice
Newport Beach, California

T. Jonathan Kurkjian, MD
Clinical Assistant Professor
Department of Plastic Surgery
University of Texas Southwestern
    Medical Center
Dallas, Texas

Nicholas Lahar, MD
Sherman Oaks, California

Val Lambros, MD
Clinical Professor of Plastic Surgery
University of California, Irvine
Irvine, California

Johnson C. Lee, MD
Private Practice
Beverly Hills, California

Michael R. Lee, MD, FACS
Assistant Professor
Department of Plastic Surgery
University of Texas Southwestern
Dallas, Texas

Benjamin T. Lemelman, MD
Section of Plastic Surgery
Department of Surgery
University of Chicago Medical
    Center
Chicago, Illinois

Steven M. Levine, MD
Aesthetic and Reconstructive Plastic
    Surgeon
Private Practice
New York, New York

Richard D. Lisman, MD, FACS
Professor
Department of Ophthalmology
New York University School of
    Medicine
Director of Ophthalmic Plastic
    Surgery—Hans Wyss
Department of Plastic Surgery
NYU Medical Center
Manhattan Eye and Ear Hospital
New York, New York

Christopher C. Lo, MD
Fellow
Division of Orbital and Ophthalmic
    Plastic Surgery
Stein and Doheny Eye Institutes
University of California, Los
    Angeles
Los Angeles, California

Z. Paul Lorenc, MD, FACS
Lorenc Aesthetic Plastic Surgery
    Center
Department of Plastic Surgery
Lenox Hill Hospital
New York, New York

Timothy Marten, MD, FACS
Marten Clinic of Plastic Surgery
San Francisco, California

Alan Matarasso, MD, FACS
Clinical Professor of Surgery
Hofstra University/Northwell School of
    Medicine
President-Elect
American Society of Plastic Surgeons,
    Executive Committee & Board of
    Directors
Past President, The Rhinoplasty Society
    & Chair Board of Trustees, & 2016-
    2017 Traveling Professor
Past President, New York Regional
    Society of Plastic Surgeons & Chair
    Board of Trustees
New York, New York

Thomas A. Mustoe, MD
Stuteville Professor of Plastic Surgery
Chief of Plastic Surgery
Division of Plastic Surgery
Feinberg School of Medicine
Northwestern University
Chicago, Illinois

Foad Nahai, MD, FACS
The Maurice J. Jurkiewicz Chair in Plastic
   Surgery and Professor of Surgery
Department of Surgery
Emory University
Atlanta, Georgia

Warwick J. S. Nettle, MBBS, FRACS
Private Practice
Sydney, Australia

Mustafa Özgön, MD
Staff Anaesthesiologist
Amerikan Hospital
Istanbul, Turkey

Peter Palhazi, MD
Clinical Anatomist at the Department
   of Anatomy, Histology and
   Embryology
Semmelweis University
Budapest, Hungary
Plastic Surgery Resident at the
   Department of Plastic and
   Reconstructive Surgery
University of Pecs
Pecs, Hungary

Ximena A. Pinell-White, MD
Division of Plastic Surgery
Emory University
Atlanta, Georgia

Navid Pourtaheri, MD, PhD
Chief Resident
Department of Plastic Surgery
School of Medicine
Case Western Reserve University
Cleveland, Ohio

Allen Putterman, MD
Professor of Ophthalmology
Co-director of Oculofacial Plastic Surgery
College of Medicine
Chicago, Illinois

Rod J. Rohrich, MD
Clinical Professor and Founding Chair
Department of Plastic Surgery
Distinguished Teaching Professor
UT Southwestern Medical Center
Founding Partner
Dallas Plastic Surgery Institute
Dallas, Texas

Jason Roostaeian, MD
Assistant Clinical Professor
Division of Plastic Surgery
David Geffen School of Medicine at UCLA
Los Angeles, California

Saoussen Salhi, MD, CM, FRCSC
Attending Pediatric Plastic,
   Reconstructive and Craniofacial
   Surgeon
Nicklaus Children's Hospital
Miami, Florida

Jillian Schreiber, MD
Plastic Surgery Resident
Division of Plastic and Reconstructive
   Surgery
Montefiore Medical Center
New York, New York

David A. Sieber, MD
Private Practice
Sieber Plastic Surgery
San Francisco, California

Sammy Sinno, MD
Private Practice
Chicago, Illinois

Ji H. Son, MD, MS
Resident Physician
Department of Plastic and
   Reconstructive Surgery
Case Western School of Medicine
Cleveland, Ohio

Jeffrey T. Steitz, MD
Division of Facial Plastic and
   Reconstructive Surgery
Department of Otolaryngology—Head
   & Neck Surgery
University of Illinois at Chicago
Chicago, Illinois

James M. Stuzin, MD
Division of Plastic Surgery
Leonard M. Miller School of
   Medicine
University of Miami
Miami, Florida
Department of Plastic Surgery
Cleveland Clinic Florida
Weston, Florida

Man-Koon Suh, MD
Director
JW Plastic Surgery Center
Seoul, Korea

Christopher C. Surek, DO
Plastic Surgeon
Private Practice
Overland Park, Kansas
Clinical Assistant Professor of Plastic
   Surgery
Department of Plastic Surgery
University of Kansas Health
   System
Assistant Professor of Anatomy
Department of Anatomy
Kansas City University of Medicine and
   Biosciences
Kansas City, Missouri

Jonathan Sykes, MD
Professor Emeritus
UC Davis Medical Center
Granite Bay, California

Geo N. Tabbal, MD
Assistant Professor
Department of Plastic Surgery
UT Southwestern Medical Center
Dallas, Texas

Nicolas Tabbal, MD
Clinical Associate Professor
Plastic Surgery
New York University
New York, New York

Shruti C. Tannan, MD
Plastic Surgeon
Tannan Plastic Surgery
Raleigh, North Carolina

Ali Teoman Tellioğlu, MD
Dışkapı Yıldırım Beyazıt Eğitim ve
   Araştırma Hastanesi
İrfan Baştuğ Cad
Dışkapı/Ankara
Turkey

Oren M. Tepper, MD
Director of Craniofacial Surgery
Director of Aesthetic Surgery
Co-Director 3D Printing & Innovation
   Laboratory
Assistant Professor of Surgery
Montefiore Medical Center
Albert Einstein College of Medicine
Bronx, New York

Dean M. Toriumi, MD
Professor
Division of Facial Plastic and
   Reconstructive Surgery
Department of Otolaryngology—Head
   & Neck Surgery
University of Illinois at Chicago
Chicago, Illinois

Ali Totonchi, MD
Associate Professor, Case Western
   Reserve University
Associate Director of the Plastic
   Surgery Residency Program
MetroHealth Medical Center
Cleveland, Ohio

Jacob G. Unger, MD
Assistant Clinical Professor of Plastic
   Surgery
Vanderbilt University
Private Practice
Maxwell Aesthetics Suite
Nashville, Tennessee

Robin Unger, MD
Assistant Professor
Department of Dermatology
Mount Sinai Hospital
New York, New York

Walter Unger, MD
Clinical Professor
Department of Dermatology
Mt. Sinai Hospital
New York, New York

Dev Vibhakar, DO
Fellow, Adult Reconstructive &
  Aesthetic Craniomaxillofacial
  Surgery
Division of Plastic & Reconstructive
  Surgery
Massachusetts General Hospital
Boston, Massachusetts

S. Anthony Wolfe, MD, FACS, FAAP
Chief of Plastic Surgery
Nicklaus Children's Hospital
Miami, Florida

Michael J. Yaremchuk, MD
Clinical Professor of Surgery
Director–Residency Training
  Program
Harvard Medical School
Chief of Craniofacial Surgery
Massachusetts General Hospital
Boston, Massachusetts

Barry M. Zide, MD, DMD
Professor of Plastic Surgery
Hansjorg Wyss Department of Plastic
  Surgery
NYU Langone Health
New York, New York

James E. Zins, MD, FACS
Chair, Department of Plastic Surgery
Head, Section of Cosmetic Surgery
Professor of Surgery
Cleveland Clinic Lerner College of
  Medicine at Case Western Reserve
Cleveland Clinic
Cleveland, Ohio

Preface

Illuminating the face and changing facial anatomy are considered art rather than science. This textbook on facial aesthetic surgery strives to share the collective experience of many authorities in this field to help enhance outcomes in an illustrated format. Under the guidance of Drs. Thorne and Sinno, this outstanding textbook is organized based on a carefully crafted template so that you can follow the sequence of the operation in an efficient fashion. I congratulate all the authors of this textbook for their care in imparting their career-long experience. Rather than presenting a number of choices for a particular problem, we asked the authors to present their preferred surgical technique that has been proven to be successful in their hands. The passion of the authors is palpable by presenting each chapter in a grand rounds fashion to filter the voluminous amount of information in a conceptual framework format.

I have enjoyed editing every chapter, and I can attest that this book is one of the best textbooks on facial aesthetics in the publishing world. I hope you will cherish this book in your care of your patients.

Kevin C. Chung, MD, MS
Chief of Hand Surgery, Michigan Medicine
Director, University of Michigan Comprehensive Hand Center
Charles B. G. de Nancrede Professor of Surgery
Professor of Plastic Surgery and Orthopaedic Surgery
Assistant Dean for Faculty Affairs
Associate Director of Global REACH
University of Michigan Medical School
Ann Arbor, Michigan

Contents

Video Clips

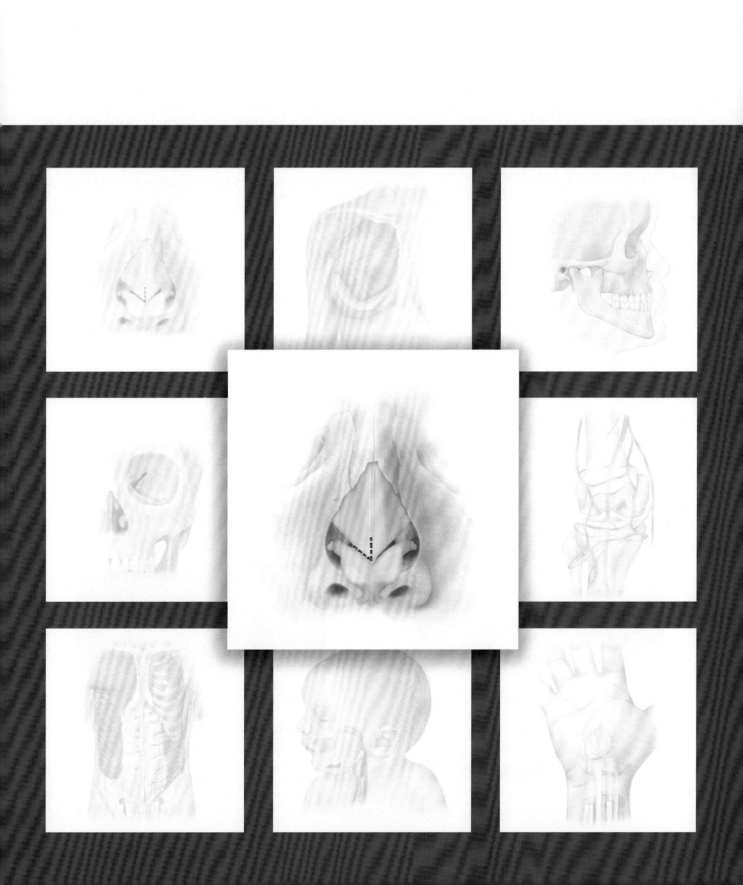

Section I: Techniques for Botulinum Toxins in the Face

Injection of Botulinum Toxin to the Glabellar Region

CHAPTER 1

Jonathan Sykes, Peter Palhazi, and Amir Allak

DEFINITION

- Hyperfunctioning of muscles in the periorbital region results in a tired, aged appearance and increased rhytids.
- Hyperdynamic glabellar musculature can create an angry appearance, whereas overuse of the lateral eyelid muscles can narrow the eyelid aperture.
- The position and orientation of the eyebrow is related to the relative strength and contraction of the brow depressors vs the brow elevators.
- The only elevators of the eyebrow are the paired frontalis muscles, whereas depression of the eyebrow is accomplished by contraction of the midline procerus muscles, the paired corrugator, and orbicularis oculi muscles.
- Treatment with botulinum toxin can lessen the contraction of hyperdynamic periorbital muscles and can improve the eyelid aperture, improve brow position, and decrease periorbital rhytids.[1]

ANATOMY

- The corrugator supercilii (CS) are paired, obliquely oriented muscles located in the inferomedial brow deep to the inferior portion of the frontalis muscles.
- The CS muscle originates from the bony superomedial orbital rim and passes in a superior and lateral direction to insert onto the fascia of the frontalis muscle and into the overlying skin (**FIG 1**).
- In addition to coursing superiorly and laterally from its insertion, the CS becomes more superficial as it travels laterally.

- The CS muscle body is pierced by the supraorbital and supratrochlear neurovascular bundles carrying sensory input to the trigeminal nerve (V1). The nerves then pierce the frontalis muscles approximately 2 to 3 cm above the supraorbital rim to travel subcutaneously to the forehead and scalp (**FIG 2**).
- The medial head of the CS has motor innervation from the zygomatic branch of the facial nerve, whereas the lateral portion is supplied by the temporal branch of the nerve.
- Contraction of the muscle causes vertical grooves in the glabellar skin and imparts an angry expression. Contraction also causes an inferomedial descent of the medial clubhead of the brow.
- The procerus is a midline flat and pyramidally shaped muscle located at the root of the nose contributing to upper nasal contour.
- The procerus originates from the periosteum and perichondrium of the nasal bones and upper lateral cartilages and from the fascia of the nasal superficial musculoaponeurotic system (SMAS) (see **FIG 2**).
- Procerus inserts into the midline skin overlying the nasal root and interdigitates superiorly with the frontalis muscle (see **FIG 2**).
- The motor innervation to the procerus is supplied by the zygomatic branch of the facial nerve.
- Contraction of the midline muscle is responsible for horizontal glabellar rhytids, transverse rhytids on the nasal dorsum, and descent of the medial brow.

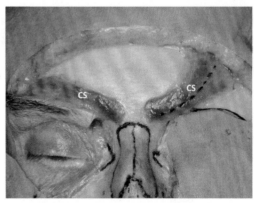

FIG 1 • Cadaveric dissection of the relationship of the corrugator muscle to the nasal root and frontalis. CS, corrugator supercilii.

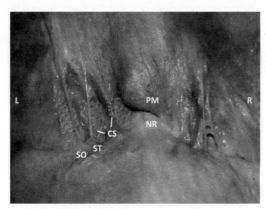

FIG 2 • Cadaveric dissection with coronal forehead flap elevated viewed from the superior aspect of the head. L, patient's left; R, patient's right; SO, supraorbital neurovascular bundle; ST, supratrochlear neurovascular bundle; NR, nasal root (indicating midline); PM, procerus muscle.

PATIENT HISTORY AND PHYSICAL FINDINGS

- It is important to evaluate the eyebrow and eyelid margin position prior to any injection of botulinum toxin in the periorbital region.
- The position of the eyebrow is related to the relative contraction of the brow elevator (the frontalis muscle) vs the brow depressors (the CS and procerus muscles medially and the orbicularis oculi muscle laterally).
- In patients who are brow depressor dominant, the brow will assume a relatively inferior position and appear ptotic; chemodenervation will elevate the brow and enhance periorbital appearance.
- The position of the upper eyelid margin in relation to the globe is also important to evaluate prior to any botulinum toxin injection in the periorbital region. The amount of ptosis is related to the amount of globe coverage by the upper eyelid.
- The distance from the superior to the inferior limbus of the globe is 11 mm in most adults with the upper eyelid typically covering the superior limbus by 1 mm. If the upper eyelid position is inferior to this level, the lid is considered ptotic.
- It is important to diagnose any upper eyelid ptosis preinjection as any injection into the periorbital musculature will affect brow position and injection into the frontalis muscle in patients with eyelid ptosis may cause a decrease in the visual field.
- Any asymmetries in eyebrow and/or upper eyelid position should be noted, documented, and discussed with the patient before injection of botulinum toxin.
- Hypercontraction of the corrugator muscles produces an angry, scowling appearance. Muscular contraction depresses the medial clubhead of the brow and causes a vertical fold that appears at right angles to the muscular axis.

- The brow clubhead is moved both medially and inferiorly with contraction of the corrugator. This is important in patients who have cosmetically removed medial brow hairs, as injection of botulinum toxin will cause elevation and lateralization of the brow clubhead.
- Hypercontraction of the procerus muscle draws the medial brow inferiorly and causes a horizontal furrow at the root of the nose.
- Injection of botulinum toxin of the procerus causes elevation of the medial brow and lessens the horizontal deep rhytid at the nasal root.

SURGICAL MANAGEMENT

Preoperative Planning

- Patients should be screened for neuromuscular disorders including amyotrophic lateral sclerosis, myasthenia gravis, and Eaton-Lambert syndrome because these are contraindications for the use of the product.
- Use in pregnant or nursing mothers is not advised, though no studies have shown teratogenic damage to fetus or adverse effects to breast-feeding infants.
- Patient medications should be screened for aminoglycoside antibiotics because these affect the pharmacokinetics of the toxin and can potentiate the effects.

Positioning

- The patient is examined in an upright position along with full facial analysis. The treatment position is surgeon preference, upright, slightly recumbent, or supine.

Approach

- Delivery of the product is performed uniformly with percutaneous injection.

■ Injection of Botulinum Toxin Into the Glabellar Region

- Topical anesthetic cream, commonly containing lidocaine, is applied and left in place for a minimum of 15 to 20 minutes and sometimes longer for maximal anesthetic effect.
- Botox is reconstituted into sterile injectable saline to the concentration of 2.5 to 4 units/0.1 mL. This is drawn up into a 1-cc syringe, and a 30-gauge short Luer Lock needle is prepared for injection.
- To avoid any spread of toxin into the extraocular muscles, or the upper eyelid retractors (levator aponeurosis and Müller muscle), the needle is usually directed away from the globe.

- Injection of the glabellar muscles should be performed with a no. 30- to no. 32-gauge needle.
- Approximately 20 to 25 units of botulinum toxin (or equivalent) are typically sufficient to treat the glabellar musculature including both the CS and procerus. This is usually distributed in a V-shaped pattern with the apex at the nasal root.
- The medial corrugator/depressor (clubhead) injection should be deep (just superficial to bone), and the tail of the muscle should be injected closer to the skin with the needle tangential to the skin.
- Injection of toxin into the procerus should be at moderate depth over the midline of the nasal root, with the needle being placed perpendicular to the skin at the nasion.

TECHNIQUES

PEARLS AND PITFALLS

Avoidance of denervation and ptosis of eyelid and brow	▪ To avoid diffusion of toxin into eyelid elevator muscles and ptosis, injection should be directed superiorly and obliquely. ▪ If injection is performed too far superiorly above the region of the corrugator, the medial inferior frontalis muscle can be affected causing medial brow ptosis.
Dosing	▪ A total of 20–25 units of Botox (or equivalent) is typically used for treatment of the glabellar muscles. ▪ A higher dosage may be necessary in males for optimal results.

POSTOPERATIVE CARE

- Ice packs should be provided to the patient and placed immediately after injection.
- Some patients may bruise post procedure, especially if anti-coagulated. This can be expected to resolve in several days.
- Avoidance of topical massage for 24 hours postinjection is suggested. Although some injectors suggest exercising injected facial muscles for 24 hours after a botulinum toxin injection, there is no evidence to prove that this affects outcomes.

OUTCOMES

- Onset of effect usually become apparent in 1 week.
- The neuromodulation is commonly effective for 12 to 20 weeks wherein it would need to be redosed for continued effect. This can vary from patient to patient.
- The outcome of botulinum toxin injection into the glabellar musculature is to decrease or alleviate the glabellar frown lines and elevate the medial brow. The cumulative effect is to eliminate the frowning or scowling appearance.[2]
- Satisfaction after injection of glabellar botulinum toxin is usually high. The procedure is simple, is fast, and causes no to very minimal downtime.
- If all of the musculature is not denervated after an injection and the patient requests additional toxin, it is simple to add toxin during a follow-up office visit.

COMPLICATIONS

- Inadvertent spread of the toxin into the upper eyelid retractor muscles can cause ptosis of the upper eyelid via diminished contraction of the levator aponeurosis/Müller muscle complex, allowing the eyelid protractors (orbicularis oculi muscles) to dominate the eyelid position.[3]

- If upper eyelid ptosis occurs, treatments exist to elevate the ptotic upper eyelid. These treatments are designed to strengthen the eyelid retractors or to slightly weaken the upper lid protractors. Either of these treatments changes the protractor/retractor muscle balance, thereby elevating the ptotic eyelid.
- Initial treatment in patients with toxin-induced ptosis is to instill topical sympathomimetic eye drops. Topical drops, such as apraclonidine, stimulate the sympathetic nervous system causing contraction of Müller muscle, resulting in 1 to 3 mm of upper eyelid elevation. The drops are placed every 6 to 8 hours as needed to alleviate the ptosis.
- The other means to treat inadvertent upper eyelid ptosis is to inject small amounts of additional botulinum toxin into the pretarsal fibers of the orbicularis oculi muscles. Diminishing the tone and contraction of the upper eyelid protractor (orbicularis oculi muscle) also can result in upper eyelid elevation and treatment of the ptotic eyelid.

ACKNOWLEDGMENT

The authors thank Sebastian Cotofana, MD, PhD, for his contribution to the preparation of this chapter.

REFERENCES

1. Monheit G. Neurotoxins: current concepts in cosmetic use on the face and neck—upper face (glabella, forehead, and crow's feet). *Plast Reconstr Surg.* 2015;136(5 Suppl):72S-75S.
2. Prager W, Bee EK, Havermann I, Zschocke I. Onset, longevity, and patient satisfaction with incobotulinumtoxinA for the treatment of glabellar frown lines: a single-arm, prospective clinical study. *Clin Interv Aging.* 2013;8:449-456.
3. Jia Z, Lu H, Yang X, et al. Adverse events of botulinum toxin type A in facial rejuvenation: a systematic review and meta-analysis. *Aesthetic Plast Surg.* 2016;40(5):769-777.

Injection of Botulinum Toxin to the Forehead

David A. Sieber and Jeffrey M. Kenkel

DEFINITION

- *Static rhytids*: wrinkles in the skin present at rest
- *Dynamic rhytids*: wrinkles in the skin present with muscle activation/animation

ANATOMY

- Frontalis muscle: broad, fan-shaped muscle originating from the galea aponeurotica below the coronal suture with insertions interdigitating into the procerus, corrugator supercilii, depressor supercilii, and orbicularis oculi[1,2] (**FIG 1**).

PATIENT HISTORY AND PHYSICAL FINDINGS

- Patients will present complaining of static and/or dynamic rhytids on their forehead.
- Have the patients contract their frontalis muscles by asking them to raise their brows and assess:
  - Muscle length and width
  - Strength of muscle (with stronger muscles having a few coarse rhytids and weaker muscles with many fine rhytids)
  - Whether muscle has a decussation in the midline
  - Activity beyond temporal fusion line
- Notice any superficial blood vessels, as injury of these during injection will cause unnecessary post-treatment bruising.

- Take note of brow position, depth, and strength of frontalis muscle as weakening the frontalis muscle may worsen an already low brow or one that is held in position with activation.

NONOPERATIVE MANAGEMENT

- Nonoperative management using any form of the currently available botulinum toxins (onabotulinumtoxinA, abobotulinumtoxinA, and incobotulinumtoxinA) is able to successfully treat forehead rhytids.

Positioning

- The patient should be comfortably seated in an upright position.

Approach

- The forehead may be injected either from the side of the patient or behind the patient's head.
- It is the author's preferred approach to inject standing to the side of the patient.
- When injecting from one side of the patient only, it is important to be cognizant that the contralateral side is treated as desired and directed by assessments done from the front of the patient.

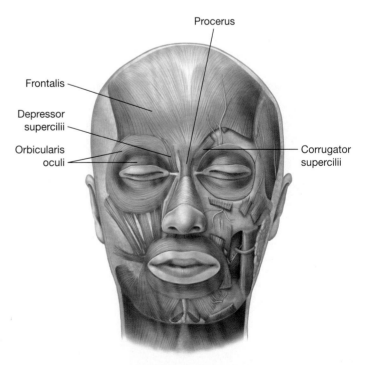

Procerus

Frontalis

Depressor
supercilii

Orbicularis
oculi

Corrugator
supercilii

FIG 1 • Shape of the frontalis muscle with insertions in the orbicularis oculi, corrugator supercilii, depressor supercilii, and procerus muscles.

■ Injection of Botulinum Toxin in the Forehead

- The botulinum is mixed according to manufacturer recommendations or physician preference.
- Skin is prepped using alcohol and ice may be applied for anesthetic and as a distractor.
- The patient is asked to animate to demonstrate muscular boundaries (see above).
- Injections start medially and proceed across the patient's forehead. The neurotoxin is placed superficially beneath the dermis and raises a small skin wheal. Additional rows of neurotoxin are placed above or below as needed.
- Care should be taken when injecting around the brows as diffusion of the product into the levator palpebrae superioris may cause the patient to have temporary upper lid ptosis.
- To prevent this, injections should not be performed beneath the lowest brow crease or less than 2 cm above the orbital rim.

PEARLS AND PITFALLS

Technique	■ To avoid upper lid ptosis, neurotoxin should not be placed below the lowest dynamic rhytid or less than 2 cm above the orbital rim.
Technique	■ Dosing and placement are determined by pretreatment assessment and often may include a dose of toxin lateral to the temporal crest and in the midline (in contrast to classic definitions of the frontalis).
Patient selection	■ Patients with severe brow ptosis and strong dynamic lines may need to be declined treatment with neurotoxins to avoid exacerbation of brow ptosis.

POSTOPERATIVE CARE

- Patients are sent home with small pack of ice and may apply as needed for swelling and/or bruising.

OUTCOME

- Excellent outcomes are achievable as demonstrated in **FIG 2** with preservation of natural brow position and shape (see **FIG 2**).

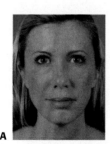 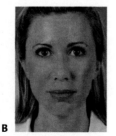

A   **B**

FIG 2 • A 44-year-old female before **(A)** and after **(B)** having 38 units of onabotulinumtoxinA placed into her forehead, glabella, and crow's feet. Note the preservation of brow shape and position after treatment as well as slight opening of orbital aperture.

COMPLICATIONS

- Patients should be counseled on possible risks of procedure including bleeding, bruising, brow and upper eyelid ptosis, and facial asymmetry.

REFERENCES

1. Choi YJ, Won SY, Lee JG, et al. Characterizing the lateral border of the frontalis for safe and effective injection of botulinum toxin. *Aesthet Surg J*. 2016;36:344-348.
2. Lorenc ZP, Smith S, Nestor M, et al. Understanding the functional anatomy of the frontalis and glabellar complex for optimal aesthetic botulinum toxin type A therapy. *Aesthetic Plast Surg*. 2013;37:975-983.

Injection of Botulinum Toxin to Soften Crow's Feet

Sammy Sinno

DEFINITION

- *Lateral canthal lines*, or *"crow's feet,"* are one or more radial lines extending laterally from the lateral canthus (**FIG 1**).

ANATOMY

- The orbicularis oculi muscle is responsible for the appearance of crow's feet. Chronic contraction of this muscle (during squinting and smiling) as well as thinning of the dermis with age accentuates these lines.

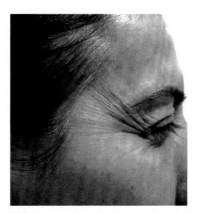

FIG 1 • Lateral canthal lines, or "crow's feet."

PATIENT HISTORY AND PHYSICAL FINDINGS

- Patients with crow's feet at rest commonly present initially in their 40s and 50s, though younger patients who desire softening of their crow's feet during animation may present earlier.

IMAGING

- No imaging is required for this procedure.

MANAGEMENT

Preoperative Planning

- The patient is asked to smile and squint repeatedly. The crow's feet radiating from the lateral canthus are noted.

Positioning

- The patient is seated in an upright position.

- After allowing 30 to 45 minutes for topical anesthetic to take effect, a cooling device is used to further desensitize the area of injection.
- 12 units of botulinum toxin are then injected on each side:
  - 4 units at 1 cm lateral to the lateral canthus
  - 4 units directly above
  - 4 units directly below (**TECH FIG 1**)
- Care is taken on the inferior injection to avoid the zygomaticus major muscle, which would cause unwanted smile abnormalities.

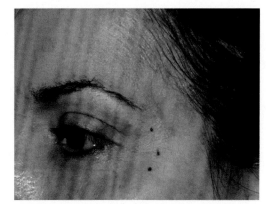

TECH FIG 1 • Target areas marked for injection into the orbicularis oculi muscle.

PEARLS AND PITFALLS

Anesthesia	▪ Allow adequate time for topical anesthesia to take effect.
Injection	▪ Inject 1 cm lateral to the lateral canthus. ▪ 12 units of botulinum toxin should be injected per side. ▪ Avoid injection into the zygomaticus major muscle.
Postoperative care	▪ Avoid strenuous exercise for 1–2 d. ▪ No tight goggles for 3 d. ▪ Sleep on back for 1–2 d postprocedure.

POSTOPERATIVE CARE

- Cold compresses are given following injection to minimize postprocedure bruising and edema.
- Patients are instructed to sleep on their backs for 1 to 2 days postprocedure and avoid wearing goggles for 3 days to avoid migration of toxin and unwanted effects.
- Strenuous exercise is permitted after 1 to 2 days.

OUTCOMES

- See pre- and postprocedure photos.

COMPLICATIONS

- Inadvertent injection into the zygomaticus major muscle can cause unwanted smile deformity.
- Migration of toxin postprocedure can also have unwanted effects including brow ptosis.

Injection of Botulinum Toxin for Treatment of the Gummy Smile

David A. Sieber and Jeffrey M. Kenkel

DEFINITION

- Gummy smile is the hyperactivity of the levator labii superioris alaeque nasi with animation causing excess upper lip elevation and exposure of the gums.

ANATOMY

- The levator labii superioris alequae nasi originates on the medial wall of the maxilla and then divides into two heads that insert into the nasal ala and medial orbicularis oris (**FIG 1**).

PATIENT HISTORY AND PHYSICAL FINDINGS

- Patients may present complaining of "too much teeth or gums showing while smiling" or may also state that their "upper lip is too short" with animation.

NONOPERATIVE MANAGEMENT

- Nonoperative management using any form of the currently available botulinum toxins (onabotulinumtoxinA, abobotulinumtoxinA, and incobotulinumtoxinA) can successfully treat a gummy smile. Typically, 2 to 4 units per side are selected as a starting dose, depending on degree of deformity and prior patient injection history.

Positioning

- The patient should be comfortably seated in an upright position.

Approach

- It is the authors' preferred approach to inject standing to the side of the patient.
- When injecting from one side of the patient only, it is important to ensure that both sides are treated in the same anatomical locations.

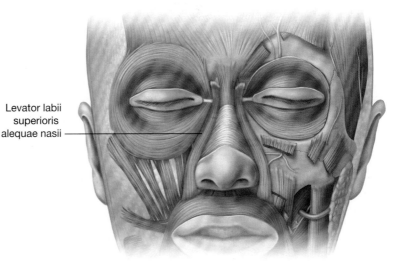

Levator labii superioris alequae nasii —

FIG 1 • Diagram illustrating orientation and length of levator labii superioris alaeque nasi muscle.

■ Injection of Botulinum Toxin for Treatment of the Gummy Smile

- The botulinum is mixed according to manufacturer recommendations or physician preference.
- Skin is prepped using alcohol, and ice may be applied for anesthetic and as a distractor.
- The needle should be inserted 1 cm above the lateral extent of the ala down to the supraperiosteal plane at the piriform aperture (**TECH FIG 1**).[1]

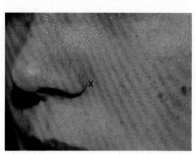

TECH FIG 1 • Location of injection site 1 cm above the lateral extent of the ala.

PEARLS AND PITFALLS

Patient selection	■ It is best to start with a low dose and have the patient come back for more. Overtreating initially can cause central lip ptosis on smiling.
Technique	■ Using a very dilute concentration may cause more neurotoxin to diffuse into the muscle of the orbicularis, causing muscular weakness. Start with 2–4 units per side.

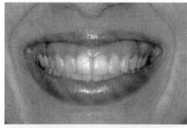

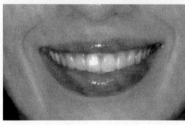

FIG 2 • Patient photo before **(A)** and after **(B)** Botox treatment for gummy smile.

POSTOPERATIVE CARE

- Patients are sent home with small pack of ice and may apply as needed for swelling and/or bruising.

OUTCOME

- Excellent outcomes are achievable as demonstrated in **FIG 2** with improvement in the gummy smile with animation.

COMPLICATIONS

- Patients should be counseled on possible risks of procedure including bleeding, bruising, lip ptosis, facial asymmetry, and weakness of the orbicularis oris.

REFERENCE

1. Mazzuco R, Hexsel D. Gummy smile and botulinum toxin: a new approach based on the gingival exposure area. *J Am Acad Dermatol.* 2010;63:1042-1051.

Injection of Botulinum Toxin for Treatment of Perioral Rhytids

Z. Paul Lorenc and Johnson C. Lee

5

CHAPTER

DEFINITION

- The orbicularis oris (OO) and depressor anguli oris (DAO) muscles produce raylike perioral lines and pull downward on the angle of the mouth, respectively.
- Small doses of botulinum toxin type A injection directly into the OO prevent perioral rhytids.
- Botulinum toxin injections into the DAO soften marionette lines and raise the corners of the mouth.

ANATOMY

- The OO muscles originate from both the maxilla and mandible, creating a ring with insertions into the upper lip, lower lip, and modiolus.
- The OO is innervated by both the buccal and the marginal mandibular branches of the facial nerve.
- Contraction of this ring of muscles closes the lips and creates a competent seal against intraoral pressure.
- The DAO is the most superficial muscle in the chin originating from the lower edge of the mandible and inserting into the modiolus at the angle of the mouth.
- The DAO is innervated by the marginal mandibular branch of the facial nerve and contraction pulls the corners of the mouth downward with assistance from the platysma, accentuating the marionette lines (**FIG 1**).

PATHOGENESIS

- Dermal atrophy due to aging, bony resorption, and environmental factors reveals vertical lines around the lips from OO contraction.

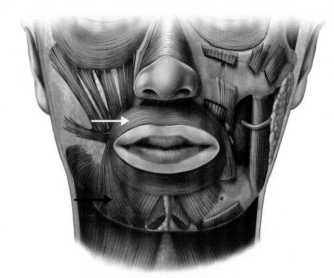

FIG 1 • The orbicularis oris (*white arrow*) creates a ring around the lips and contraction of this muscle creates a competent seal against intraoral pressure while producing vertical rhytids around the mouth. The depressor anguli oris (*black arrow*) inserts into the angle of the mouth, creating a downward pull, and accentuating the marionette lines.

- Marionette lines start from the corners of the mouth to the chin and are a combination of tissue descent, age-related volume loss, and DAO activity.

PATIENT HISTORY AND PHYSICAL FINDINGS

- Patients may report static or dynamic rhytids around the lips as well as prominent marionette lines or a "frownlike" appearance.

- The perioral and chin area is sterilely prepped with an alcohol pad.

Vertical Rhytids

- The patient is instructed to purse or tightly pucker the lips.
- Visible rhytids are injected along the base of each line at the vermillion border in the subcutaneous plane (**TECH FIG 1**).
- Inject 0.5 to 1 unit of Botox per site. A total of 2 units maximum are placed onto each side in the upper lip and 2 units into the lower lip for a total dose of 6 units (100 units/4 cc NaCl).
- For patients with significant dermal atrophy, a combination of hyaluronic acid filler can be combined with botulinum toxin type A for maximal effect.
  - After extruding 0.2 cc of material from a 1.0-cc syringe (Restylane Refyne), 0.2-cc solution of botulinum toxin type A containing 5 units(100 u/4 cc NaCl) is mixed using an accessory kit.
  - This homogenous HA/BTX material is then injected along the vermillion border in the potential space using a 27G 25-mm blunt tip cannula.
- For deep static rhytids, additional hyaluronic acid filler such as Restylane Refyne, Belotero, or Juvederm Volbella XC can be injected vertically or horizontally along each line for direct increase in volume.

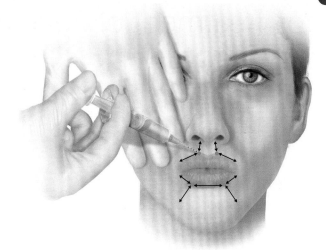

TECH FIG 1 • While the patient is pursing the lips, botulinum toxin is injected along at vermillion border in the subcutaneous plane (*dots*). For severe rhytids, this can be combined with hyaluronic acid filler injection (*arrows*) injected alone or perpendicular to the rhytids' direction.

Marionette Lines

- The patient is instructed to frown and pull the corners of the mouth downward.
- The injection point is marked with the patient animating and in the upright position.
  - The marking is halfway between the oral commissure and the jawline.
  - Because the DAO is a vertically oriented pyramidal muscle, injection in its midportion, where the DAO muscle mass is minimal, will have a more pronounced and longer lasting effect.
  - The marking is made lateral to the Marionette line.
- Inject 2.5 units of Botox into each DAO to elevate the corners of the mouth and reduce the shadowing of the Marionette lines (**TECH FIG 2**).
- Pronounced Marionette lines should also undergo concurrent augmentation with a hyaluronic acid filler such as Restylane Lyft, Juvederm Ultra Plus, or Juvederm VOLUMA or a CaHA agent such as Radiesse.

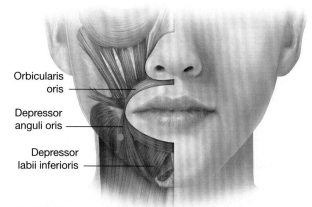

Orbicularis oris

Depressor anguli oris

Depressor labii inferioris

TECH FIG 2 • The DAO should be injected with 2.5 units of Botox, halfway between the oral commissure and the jawline where the DAO muscle mass is thinnest. Injection should be performed laterally to the marionette line to avoid weakening of the depressor labii inferioris muscle.

PEARLS AND PITFALLS

Equipment	▪ Use a 27G 25-mm cannula, 32G ½ in. needle.
Choice of botulinum toxin	▪ Botox and Xeomin—4–5 units the upper lip, 2 units the lower lip. ▪ Dysport—10–20 units the upper lip, 10 units the lower lip.
Technique	▪ Injection of the OO should occur closer to the midline/philtrum to reduce risk of oral incompetence from laterally placed injections. ▪ Maximum limit of 4 units of Botox each in the upper and lower lip to minimize risk of incompetence. ▪ Injection into the thinnest area of the DAO will allow for maximal effect with the lowest dose. ▪ Care must be taken to inject the lateral aspect of the DAO to avoid injection into the depressor labii inferioris. ▪ Marionette lines should also undergo concurrent augmentation, when appropriate, with a hyaluronic acid filler such as Restylane Lyft, Juvederm Ultra Plus, or Juvederm VOLUMA or CaHA agent such as Radiesse.

POSTPROCEDURAL CARE

- Patients ice the area immediately after the procedure (15 minutes).
- Avoid pressure, sweating, and alcohol for the remainder of the day to minimize swelling.

OUTCOMES

- Patient should expect additional treatments every 3 to 4 months (**FIG 2**).
- Because of use of conservative dosages to avoid oral incompetence, perioral retreatments may be needed even sooner.

COMPLICATIONS

- Slight bleeding, discomfort, or ecchymosis can occur after injection.
- Excessive injection of botulinum (8 units or greater) into the OO can result in oral incompetence, which can last for several weeks.

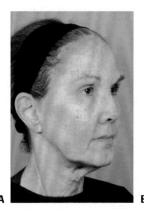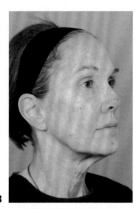

A   **B**

FIG 2 • Before **(A)** and after **(B)** botulinum toxin injection in the perioral area.

- Incorrect injection medial to the DAO will result in weakening or paralysis of the depressor labii inferioris and an asymmetric smile.

CHAPTER 6

Injection of Botulinum Toxin to the Depressor Anguli Oris

Amir Allak, Sebastian Cotofana, and Jonathan Sykes

DEFINITION

- Hyperfunction of the muscular depressor anguli oris (DAO) results in a scowling, aged appearance, and marionette lines.
- The position and orientation of the oral commissure is related to the relative strength and contraction of the DAO (and to a lesser extent the depressor labii inferioris [DLI]) vs the elevators of the oral commissure (levator anguli oris, levator labii superioris).
- Treatment with botulinum toxin can lessen the contraction of hyperdynamic DAO muscles and can elevate the downturned oral commissure, resulting in a more rejuvenated appearance.[1]

ANATOMY

- The depressor DAO is a paired bilateral muscle that originates from the soft tissue overlying the oblique line and the inferior border of the anterior body and parasymphysis of the mandible. DAO inserts onto the lateral aspect of the lower lip and oral modiolus (**FIG 1**).
- The DAO is innervated by the marginal mandibular branch of the facial nerve, and its activation moves the oral commissure inferolaterally.
- The shape of the DAO is roughly a triangle with its base inferiorly at its origin and its apex superiorly near the modiolus of the oral commissure.
- At its origin, the DAO muscular body is continuous with the platysma muscle inferiorly within the superficial musculoaponeurotic system.

- The DLI is a paired bilateral muscle that is directly medial to the DAO, which also originates from the inferior border of the parasymphysis of the mandible but inserts mostly on the body of the lower lip (see **FIG 1**). Its action, as its name implies, depresses one side of the lower lip.
- In the areas where the DAO and DLI overlap, the DLI lies deep to the DAO (see **FIG 1**).
- The facial artery runs superomedial from the mandibular notch, and the inferior labial artery arises inferior to the modiolus. The inferior labial artery, a branch of the facial artery, runs deep to the DAO fibers (**FIG 2**).

PATIENT HISTORY AND PHYSICAL FINDINGS

- Overactivation of the DAO contributes to an aged-appearing downturn of overall lip shape and rhytids that follow from the oral commissure inferolaterally (paralleling the course of the muscle), known commonly as marionette lines.[2]

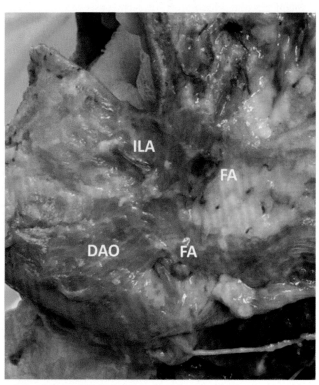

FIG 1 • Cadaveric dissection of muscles acting at the angle of the mouth. Mo, modiolus; DLI, depressor labii inferioris; DAO, depressor anguli oris; OO, orbicularis oculi; LAO, levator anguli oris; ZM, zygomaticus major; LLS, levator labii superioris.

FIG 2 • Cadaveric dissection demonstrating the relationship of the facial vasculature to the depressor anguli oris. FA, facial artery; DAO, depressor anguli oris; ILA, inferior labial artery.

- There is often an associated soft tissue depression just inferior to the oral commissure that is partially related to muscular activity and partially attributed to descent of the cheek fat pad relative to the lower lip subunit.

IMAGING

- No imaging is required for this procedure.

SURGICAL MANAGEMENT

Preoperative Planning

- Patients should be screened for neuromuscular disorders including amyotrophic lateral sclerosis, myasthenia gravis, and Eaton-Lambert syndrome because these are contraindications for the use of the product.

- Use in pregnant or nursing mothers is not advised, though no studies have shown teratogenic damage to fetus or adverse affects to breast-feeding infants.
- Patient medications should be screened for aminoglycoside antibiotics because these affect the pharmacokinetics of the toxin and can potentiate the effects.

Positioning

- The patient is examined in an upright position along with full facial analysis. The treatment position is surgeon preference, upright, slightly recumbent, or supine.

Approach

- Delivery of the product is performed uniformly with percutaneous injection.

■ Injection of Botulinum Toxin Into the DAO

- Topical anesthetic cream, commonly containing lidocaine, is applied and left in place for a minimum of 15 to 20 minutes (and sometimes longer) for maximal anesthetic effect.
- Botox is reconstituted into sterile injectable saline to the concentration of 2.5 to 4 units/0.1 mL. This is drawn up into a 1-cc syringe, and a 30-gauge short Luer Lock needle is prepared for injection.
- The patient is asked to grimace to reveal the area of maximal activation of the DAO and its distribution along the marionette line.
- The mandibular groove is palpated at the junction of the posterior body and angle on the inferior border of the mandible.

- This is the area where the facial artery and vein course from the deep neck to supply and drain the facial soft tissue.
- Injection in this area should be avoided.
- The product is typically injected in two to three locations, following the shape of the inverted triangle of the DAO: two at the inferior aspect and one superiorly for a total of 3 to 6 units per side.
- Injection should be posterior to the oral commissure to avoid the DLI and anterior to the mandibular groove to avoid the facial vascular structures.
- Injection should be delivered in a relatively superficial plane to avoid the DLI and the inferior labial artery running deep to the DAO.

TECHNIQUES

PEARLS AND PITFALLS

Location of injection	■ Injection should be anterior to the mandibular notch to avoid vascular structures and posterior to the oral commissure to avoid injection of the DLI and subsequent smile asymmetry. ■ The plane of injection should be relatively superficial because the DAO fibers run superficial to the DLI and inferior labial artery.
Dosing	■ 3–6 units are divided in 2–3 doses in a line or triangular orientation. ■ More product may be required in men.

POSTOPERATIVE CARE

- Ice packs should be provided to the patient and placed immediately after injection.
- Some patients may bruise post procedure, especially if anticoagulated. This can be expected to resolve in several days.

OUTCOMES

- Onset of effect usually become apparent in 1 week.
- Inactivation of the DAO should lead to less downturn of the oral commissures and some relief and softening of marionette lines.[3]

- The neuromodulation is commonly effective for 12 to 20 weeks wherein it would need to be redosed for continued effect. This can vary from patient to patient.

COMPLICATIONS

- Injection of the DLI or migration of product so as to chemically denervate this muscle will lead to asymmetry when smiling because the ipsilateral muscle will not activate the lower lip to depress. The effect of the product should wane over the normal metabolic period.
- Intravascular injection, though exceedingly rare, can cause systemic effect similar to botulism (generalized weakness, visual disturbance, dysarthria, etc.)

ACKNOWLEDGMENT

The authors thank Peter Palhazi, MBBS, for his contribution to the preparation of this chapter.

REFERENCES

1. Wu DC, Fabi SG, Goldman MP. Neurotoxins: current concepts in cosmetic use on the face and neck—lower face. *Plast Reconstr Surg.* 2015;136:76S-79S.
2. Choi YJ, Kim JS, Gil YC, et al. Anatomical considerations regarding the location and boundary of the depressor anguli oris muscle with reference to botulinum toxin injection. *Plast Reconstr Surg.* 2014;134(5):917-921.
3. Goldman A, Wollina U. Elevation of the corner of the mouth using botulinum toxin type A. *J Cutan Aesthet Surg.* 2010;3(3):145-150.

Injection of Botulinum Toxin to Platysma Bands

Z. Paul Lorenc and Johnson C. Lee

DEFINITION

- Platysma bands become more pronounced with age and activity.
- Botulinum toxin injection directly into the muscular cords relaxes the muscle, efface the vertical bands, and define the mandibular border.
- Treatment of the platysma muscle is routinely combined with treatment of the depressor anguli oris (DAO) to lessen the downward forces of the muscles of the neck and face.

ANATOMY

- The platysma originates along the fascia of the superior portions of the pectoralis major and deltoid muscles. The muscle fibers run superiorly and obliquely before inserting into the perioral muscles, dermis of the cheek and chin, and inferior mandibular symphysis posterior to the DAO origin (**FIG 1**).
- The platysma is innervated by the cervical branch of the cervicofacial trunk of the facial nerve with some superior coinnervation by the mandibular branch.
- Activation causes depression of the corners of the mouth and mandible, tightening the anterior neck skin, and blunting of the mandibular border.

PATHOGENESIS

- Contraction of the free anterior and posterior fibers in the submental and neck regions creates both vertical platysma bands and horizontal neck lines.
- Excess or lax skin can compound the appearance of platysma bands even at rest.
- With aging, loss of submental fat contributes to platysma bands prominence.

PATIENT HISTORY AND PHYSICAL FINDINGS

- Patients may report the appearance of bands when speaking or making facial expressions, which become more pronounced with age.
- Patients with significant skin laxity component may have suboptimal results.

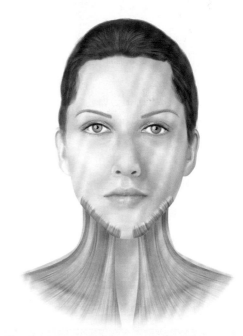

FIG 1 • The platysma originates along the pectoralis major and deltoid muscles and inserts into the anterior mandible and skin of the lower face. Activation causes the formation of vertical bands.

■ Preparation

- Choice of botulinum toxin
  - Botox (onabotulinum toxin type A)
  - Xeomin (incobotulinum toxin type A)
  - Dysport (abobotulinum toxin type A)

- Suggested dilution
  - Onabotulinum toxin type A—100 units/2.5 cc NaCl
  - Incobotulinum toxin type A—100 units/2.5 cc NaCl
  - Abobotulinum toxin type A—300 units/1.5 cc NaCl
- The neck area is sterilely prepped with an alcohol pad.
- The patient is in an upright sitting position.

TECHNIQUES

■ Botulinum Toxin Injection

- The patient is instructed to voluntarily contract the platysma by grimacing or pulling the corners of the mouth and lower lip downward and laterally while tightening the skin of the neck.
- Visible anterior and lateral platysma bands are marked using a marking pen with 1-cm spacing.
  - Platysma injection points at the mandibular border as well as the depressor anguli oris (DAO) injection sites are marked, if clinically necessary.
- Visible cords are held between the thumb and index finger during the injection (**TECH FIG 1**).

- Injections are given directly into the vertical muscular cords with a 32-gauge needle using a 1.0-cc Luer-Lok tip syringe.
- Dosage total depends on the choice of botulinum toxin:
  - 25 to 50 units of onabotulinum toxin type A
  - 25 to 50 units of incobotulinum toxin type A
  - 100 to 150 units of abobotulinum toxin type A
- Additional injections can be performed along the mandibular border, at the posterior platysma bands, and the DAO injection points for improved jawline.

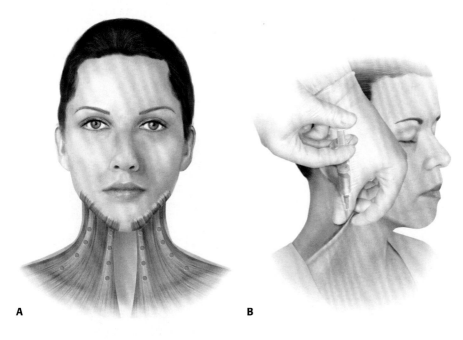

A   **B**

TECH FIG 1 • Visible cords **(A)** are held between the thumb and index finger **(B)**, and botulinum toxin is injected evenly spaced approximately 1 cm apart at the level of the deep dermis.

PEARLS AND PITFALLS

Equipment	■ Use a 32-gauge needle, 1.0-cc Luer-Lok tip syringe.
Technique	■ Retract the individual cord away from the deeper muscles. ■ Inject into the deep dermal layer to avoid deeper structures or the hypoglossal nerve.

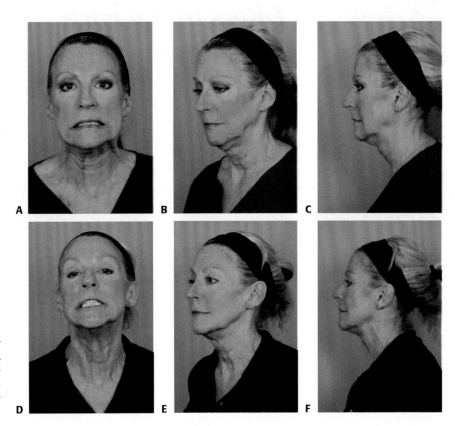

FIG 2 • Before **(A–C)** and 60 days **(D–F)** after treatment. Full animation, ¾ view, side view. A 62-year-old female, total dose: 80 units incobotulinum toxin type A (100 units/2.5 cc NaCl). Muscles injected: platysma, medial, lateral, mandibular border, depressor anguli oris.

POSTPROCEDURAL CARE

- Patients place ice over the area immediately after the procedure.
- Avoid pressure, sweating, alcohol for the remainder of the day to minimize postinjection sequelae.

OUTCOMES (FIG 2)

- Resolution of platysma banding may not occur for up to 3 to 5 days after treatment.
- Patient is seen 1 week post injection for additional therapy if necessary.

- Patient should expect additional treatments every 3 to 4 months.
- Horizontal banding, if necessary, may be addressed with injectable hyaluronic acid filler with low G′ characteristics.

COMPLICATIONS

- Slight bleeding, discomfort, or ecchymosis can occur after injection.
- Accidental botulinum toxin injection into the strap muscles, deeper muscles of the neck, or hypoglossal nerve injury can cause dysarthria, dysphagia, dysphonia, or breathing difficulties.

8 CHAPTER

Section II: Technique for Injection of Fillers in the Face
Injection of Fillers in the Glabella, Forehead, and Brow

David A. Sieber and Jeffrey M. Kenkel

DEFINITION

- Hyaluronic acid: a naturally found glucosaminoglycan polymer found in human tissue, which is reversible with hyaluronidase
- Tyndall effect: bluish hue created in the skin from light scattering off superficially injected particles of filler

ANATOMY

- The supratrochlear artery lies approximately 2 cm lateral to midline between the corrugator and frontalis/orbicularis, traversing the frontalis/orbicularis 1.5 to 2.5 cm above the orbital rim transitioning into the subcutaneous plane[1] (**FIG 1**).
- The supraorbital artery runs approximately 3 cm lateral to midline, piercing the frontalis between 2 and 4 cm above the orbital rim also transitioning to a subcutaneous plane.[1,2]
- The supraorbital nerve originates 2.1 to 3.5 cm from midline and divides into superficial and deep branches. The deep branch courses deep to the corrugator supercilii and frontalis muscles, traveling between the periosteum and galea superiorly and laterally toward the temporal fusion line.[3,4]

PATIENT HISTORY AND PHYSICAL FINDINGS

- Patients will often present complaining of static rhytids in the glabella and forehead that persist after adequate treatment with neurotoxins.
- Other patients will have hollowing of the inferior brow, complaining of an aged and gaunt appearance of the eyes.

NONOPERATIVE MANAGEMENT

- The senior author's preference is to use hyaluronic acid fillers due to their temporary nature and ability to be reversed through the use of hyaluronidase.

Positioning

- The patient should be comfortably seated in an upright position.

Approach

- The glabella, forehead, and brow may be injected from either side of the patient.
- It is the author's preferred approach to inject standing to the side of the patient.

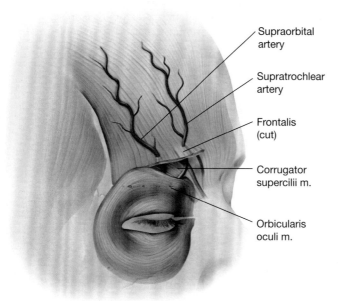

Supraorbital artery

Supratrochlear artery

Frontalis (cut)

Corrugator supercilii m.

Orbicularis oculi m.

FIG 1 • Location of the supratrochlear and supraorbital arteries. Notice the transition to a more superficial plane as they ascend in the forehead.

- For most hyaluronic acid products, the authors add 0.2 cc of 0.5% lidocaine with epinephrine using a Luer-lock to Luer-lock connector to help constrict local blood vessels, reducing the risk of postprocedural ecchymosis.
- When superficial/dermal injections are performed, the authors follow Dr. Fagien's recommendations regarding dilution, which reconstitutes the product 1:1 with 1% lidocaine.[5]

- Although injections may be performed with a 30-gauge needle, 27-gauge needle, 25-gauge cannula, or 27-gauge cannula, the authors' preference is to use a cannula for injections of the inferior brow along the orbital rim and a 30-gauge needle for treatment of superficial rhytids of the forehead.
- Skin is always prepped using a swab containing 4% chlorhexidine gluconate prior to injection.

■ Injection of Fillers in the Glabella and Forehead

- A 30-gauge needle is advanced into an intradermal plane parallel to the rhytids being treated.
- The filler is then deposited in a serial retrograde fashion along the course of the rhytid.
- This area is slightly overcorrected and then massaged to produce an even result.

- Additional cross-hatching may be necessary for complete correction of the rhytid, especially in treating deep vertical lines of the glabella.
- Care is taken to stay very superficial (intradermal) so as to not cannulate or injure the supratrochlear or supraorbital vessels.

■ Injection of Fillers in the Brow

- A common portal is made in the lateral tail of the brow with a needle.
- The cannula is advanced medially along the brow periosteum to just past the area needing correction. This is below the inferior border of the brow.

- Filler is gently injected along the inferior border of the superior orbital rim as the cannula is withdrawn laterally.
- Multiple passes may be necessary to achieve the desired effect.
- An additional portal may be needed medially to reach the more medial aspects of the orbital rim.
- After placement, the product is massaged into place along the orbital rim to produce an even, natural result.

PEARLS AND PITFALLS

Technique	■ The supratrochlear and supraorbital arteries lie in the subcutaneous plane starting 2 cm above the orbital rim; care must be taken to not cannulate or injure these during injection.
	■ When injecting the glabella and upper forehead, filler should be placed into a superficial/dermal plane to avoid injury to the supratrochlear and supraorbital vessels.
	■ Filler placed along the superior orbital rim can produce a subtle brow lift in patients with pre-existing brow ptosis.
	■ Filler placed along the superior orbital rim helps with orbital hollowing and correction of "A" frame deformities.

POSTOPERATIVE CARE

- Patients are sent home with small packs of ice and may apply as needed for swelling and/or bruising.
- Patients should keep their heads elevated for a few hours after injection and should abstain from exercise for 4 hours.

OUTCOMES

- Excellent outcomes are achievable as demonstrated in **FIG 2** with correction of the brow hollowing (see **FIG 2**) and superficial rhytids of the forehead (**FIG 3**).

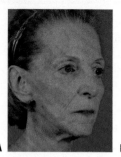 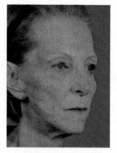 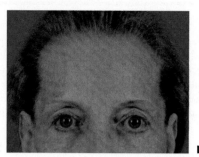 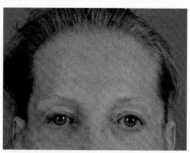

A   **B**   **C**   **D**

FIG 2 • A 66-year-old female pre **(A)** and post **(B)** injection of 0.5 cc Restylane Lyft into each temporal region/lateral brow, 1 cc total of Restylane Silk into the lips/perioral region, and 0.4 cc Restylane Lyft into each sub-brow region. Notice the more youthful appearance of the brow/periocular region **(C,D)**.

COMPLICATIONS

- Patients should be counseled on possible risks of procedure including bleeding, bruising, facial asymmetry, and intravascular injection leading to skin necrosis and/or blindness.

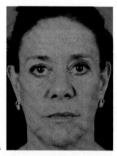 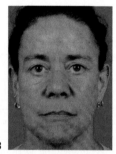

A   **B**

FIG 3 • A 50-year-old female pre **(A)** and post **(B)** treatment with a total of 2 cc Restylane Silk placed into static forehead rhytids as well as perioral lines.

REFERENCES

1. Kleintjes WG. Forehead anatomy: arterial variations and venous link of the midline forehead flap. *J Plast Reconstr Aesthet Surg.* 2007;60:593-606.
2. Erdogmus S, Govsa F. Anatomy of the supraorbital region and the evaluation of it for the reconstruction of facial defects. *J Craniofac Surg.* 2007;18:104-112.
3. Christensen KN, Lachman N, Pawlina W, Baum CL. Cutaneous depth of the supraorbital nerve: a cadaveric anatomic study with clinical applications to dermatology. *Dermatol Surg.* 2014;40:1342-1348.
4. Knize DM. A study of the supraorbital nerve. *Plast Reconstr Surg.* 1995;96:564-569.
5. Fagien S. Variable reconstitution of injectable hyaluronic acid with local anesthetic for expanded applications in facial aesthetic enhancement. *Dermatol Surg.* 2010;36:815-821.

Filler Injection Into the Upper Periorbital Area

Val Lambros

DEFINITION

- The upper periorbital area refers to the superior orbital rim inferiorly to roughly the height of the eyebrow, from the medial temple to medial-most orbit.
- The reason to fill the brows is that a certain population of patients looks better with fuller upper periorbital than hollow.

ANATOMY

- The anatomy of the brow is well known. The pertinent anatomy is aesthetic and vascular.
- The supraorbital and supratrochlear arteries arise from the bone and rise to the level of the frontalis muscle.
- The superior orbital rim in most young persons is characterized by skin that most clinicians characterize as "tight" as well as generalized fullness of subcutaneous fat. The overall look in many of these eyes is a full orbital rim and upper lid, which describes a low and horizontal path across the orbit. These young eyes tend to look longer from medial to lateral than the does old eye. Part of this phenomenon is secondary to the stretch of the lateral canthal tendon, and part is from the height versus width ratio: the visual height of the orbit is low in relation to its length.

PATIENT HISTORY AND PHYSICAL FINDINGS

- In patients whose faces age by thinning, it is very common for the orbit to hollow. Therefore, eyes that fit the description above become eyes that look larger vertically (less fat volume) and round (greater height for width, as well as a shorter lid aperture). This look when extreme is sometimes descriptively called a nursing home eye (**FIG 1**).

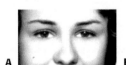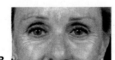

FIG 1 • Contrast of youthful (**A**) versus aged (**B**) periorbita.

- Older eyes tend to have greater eyelid show and room for makeup. Some patients like this look. In young eyes that have had surgery with a great deal of fat removal, the loss of fat can in time accelerate the natural aging of the eyelid.
- The thesis of this chapter is simply that some upper lids and superior orbital rims look better when fuller than not.

Preoperative Planning

- Though the criteria above give a hint as to who may be good candidates for filling the supraorbital area, some patients with configurations described above may look better with fill and some not.
- Though most patients would understand the effect of filling in a wrinkle, filling certain areas of the face is not intuitive, for example, the temples, brows, and anterior jawline, where a small amount of filler may make a huge change visually.
- Because cosmetic alterations of the face are visual by definition, there is an easy way to show patients the visual alternatives before the final injections and get their understanding and approval of the procedure before it is actually done. Though one may use preoperative computer imaging, I prefer the use of a small amount of local anesthesia to duplicate the effect of the filler.

Positioning

- Injections are performed with the patient seated upright.

Approach

- I prefer to block all filler injection with local anesthesia with epinephrine before placing the filler. The primary reasons are for pain control and vasoconstriction. The least common but most feared complication of filler injections is intra-arterial injection of product. Injecting into a vasoconstricted environment would logically be expected to reduce its incidence. If one is going to inject local anesthetic anyway, one may as well get additional benefit from doing so, and that is to show the patient the intended outcome of the final result.

■ Filler Injection Into the Upper Periorbital Area

- In my experience, patients uniformly like the idea of visualizing the result before committing to the injection; it tilts the balance of power from the doctor to the patients, and all patients are familiar with the idea of trying on clothes before buying them.
- Most patients like the preview with local anesthesia, and the filler injection is performed immediately afterward.
  - The patients who do not like the preview do not have to find out after spending money and experiencing a result that they do not like.
  - The extra 5 minutes that this takes is well worth the effort in my opinion. No one has told me that they did not like an injection that was previewed and approved.
- Placing the local anesthetic is more difficult than doing the final injection. It is all too easy to place a blob of fluid in the tissues that demonstrates nothing but lack of injection ability; with some practice, one learns to place the local anesthetic in even threads, which are quite convincing.
  - The local is massaged and the patient is shown the result, and the area is now numb and vasoconstricted.
  - The presence of the local does not complicate the injection at all as one knows both the dose and distribution already and the smoothness is confirmed by feel.
- Either a cannula or a needle is used for the final injection.
  - From long experience, I use a 30 G ½ in. needle.
  - The presence of the local helps with the distribution of the product.
  - Most commonly, the dose is ½ cc per side.
- The injection of product itself begins laterally at about the tail of the brow. It is in the middle level, below the

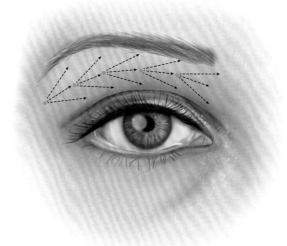

TECH FIG 1 • Injection into the upper periorbital.

orbicularis oculi, but not subdermal or adjacent to the bone. There are two reasons not to be deep here:
  - In some patients, the globe is immediately adjacent to the bone, increasing the possibility of injury.
  - The supraorbital and supratrochlear as well as other forehead arteries arise from the bone or adjacent to it and may be more easily injured with the needle (**TECH FIG 1**).
- The injection is done in a fanning manner with an injection headed superiorly straight ahead and inferiorly to the injection path.
  - Usually about 5 needle placements are necessary, making a total of about 15 passes.
  - As the dose is typically ½ cc per side, that makes about 0.03 cc per pass.

PEARLS AND PITFALLS

Patient selection	■ The first and most important criterion for patient and doctor satisfaction is patient selection.
	■ In the currently popular volume-centric approach to facial cosmetic surgery, patients may be treated by rote or by principle that faces should be made fuller regardless of the face. Though some faces may deflate with age, many do not in the American population. Volume treatments across the face and specifically around the eye may look ridiculous and be permanent.
	■ When one is changing as visually important a part of the face as the periorbital area, one wants to know that the patient will like it and that complications can be treated.
Filler selection	■ I invariably use HA fillers around the eyes. Fillers in this class, which, at the time of this writing, include Restylane and Juvederm, have unique properties that make them invaluable in the periorbital area.
	■ The longevity in the periorbita (as well as the temple and tip of the nose) is much greater than in the lips and nasolabial fold. I tell patients that it will last 2 years, but it is common to see 3 or 4 years of persistence. In addition, HA filers can be dissolved with hyaluronidase, thus making it easy to erase lumps and most complications. These luxuries are simply not available when using calcium- or lactic acid–based fillers.

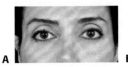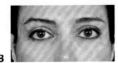

FIG 2 • Pre **(A)** and post **(B)** injection.

POSTOPERATIVE CARE

- Postprocedure care is minimal. Ice usually suffices. Using a needle has a higher incidence of bruising, which takes the usual course. Cannulas have less bruising but are less maneuverable and precise.

OUTCOMES

- **FIGS 2** to **5** show before and after photos in four patients.

COMPLICATIONS

- Complications specific to the periorbital area are similar to other parts of the face. Occasional irregularities may be supplemented with more product or sometimes dissolved with a low dose of hyaluronidase.
- Arterial injection injuries are rare but most serious. It is thought that some lesions from arterial injection are embolic

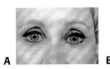

FIG 4 • Pre **(A)** and post **(B)** injection.

by virtue of distal arterial flow, whereas some occur from flow proximal to the injection point.

- Severe injuries include duskiness of the skin to full-thickness necrosis of the skin or even blindness. Suggestions for prevention include using a cannula, vasoconstriction, and low-pressure injection with a moving needle.
- Cannulas would be expected to generate less arterial perforations than needles though arterial injections have been generated with cannulas as well. Aspiration of the syringe before injection, though traditionally recommended, does not seem to be reliable, as HA fillers injected through a small needle are too viscous to allow product to backflow into the syringe. The only article that characterized the incidence of "severe complications" gave an incidence of close to 1 in 1 000 000,[1] though the incidence is probably higher than that.

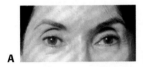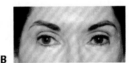

FIG 3 • Pre **(A)** and post **(B)** injection.

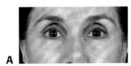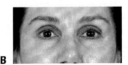

FIG 5 • Pre **(A)** and post **(B)** injection.

REFERENCE

1. Ozturk CN, Li Y, Tung R, et al. Complications following injection of soft-tissue fillers. *Aesthet Surg J*. 2013;33(6):862-877.

10

CHAPTER

Tear Trough and the Lid-Cheek Junction

Z. Paul Lorenc and Johnson C. Lee

DEFINITION

- The tear trough and lid-cheek junction are natural anatomical structures that become accentuated with time due to changes in the skin and periorbital structures.
- Proper placement of injectable fillers restores volume and support to these structures for periorbital rejuvenation.

ANATOMY[1,2]

- The tear trough or nasojugal groove is the natural depression 4 to 6 mm caudal to the arcus marginalis at the orbital rim and extends inferolaterally from the medial canthus to the midpupillary line.
- The lid-cheek junction extends from the tear trough at the midpupillary line and lies below and parallel to the infraorbital rim.
- In the subcutaneous plane, both the tear trough and the lid-cheek junction correlate with a junctional cleft between the palpebral and orbital portions of the orbicularis muscle.
The lid-cheek junction has an additional deep submuscular plane at the orbitomalar ligament (**FIGS 1** and **2**).

PATHOGENESIS

- The tear trough and lid-cheek junction are normal anatomic features that can be seen in many youthful individuals.

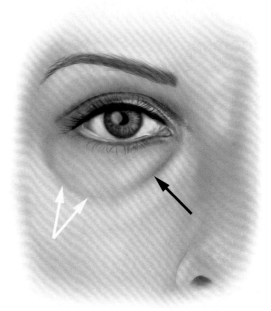

FIG 1 • The tear trough deformity (*arrow*) is the natural groove extending inferolaterally from the medial canthus to the midpupillary line. The lid-cheek junction (*white arrow*) extends laterally.

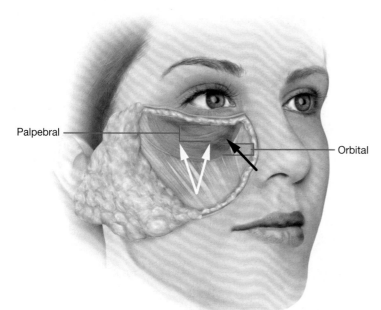

Palpebral

Orbital

FIG 2 • The underlying anatomy is shown with the malar fat pad reflected. The tear trough deformity (*black arrow*) lies at the junction of the palpebral and orbital components of the orbicularis oculi muscle. This continues laterally with the lid-cheek deformity (*white arrows*).

- With age, there is skin and fat atrophy and attenuation of the periorbital structures allowing orbital fat herniation and increasing shadows.
- The tear trough and lid-cheek junction become more visible and accentuated by overlying pigment, texture, and shadow changes.

PATIENT HISTORY AND PHYSICAL FINDINGS

- Patients may report a "tired" or "aged" under-eye appearance which is not relieved with rest, hydration, or topical therapies.
- A depression can be seen starting at the medial canthus and parallel to the orbital rim.

The tear trough and lid-cheek junction deformity can be accentuated by actively increasing orbital fat herniation with upward gaze or globe pressure (**FIG 3A**).

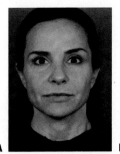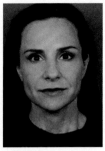

FIG 3 • Patient photos before **(A)** and after **(B)** injection.

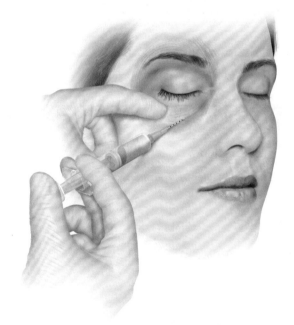

TECH FIG 1 • Injection technique—The orbital rim is palpated, and the cannula is inserted between the two portions of orbicularis muscle of the tear trough and onto the supraperiosteal plane. Filler is then injected in a medial to lateral and retrograde fashion.

■ Preparation

- The area is cleansed and sterilized with a sterile alcohol pad.
- Marking of the areas for filler injection of the tear trough and the lid-cheek junction is made with the patient in an upright position with the orbicularis oculi muscle in a completely relaxed state. Cannula access port is marked in the midpupillary line 0.5 cm inferior to the border of the orbital rim.
- Topical anesthetic (benzocaine 20%, lidocaine 6%, tetracaine 4%) is carefully applied to the area with cotton-tipped applicators for 30 to 45 minutes prior to injection.
- Cannula access port is injected with 0.1 cc of 1% lidocaine solution and epinephrine 1:100 000.
- Just prior to cannula insertion, a 25G 5/8″ needle is used to puncture the skin and create the cannula access port.

Tear Trough

- Restylane-L (Galderma Laboratories, L.P.) is diluted with 2% lidocaine 1:1 (off-label use). When reconstituting an agent, make sure there is a homogenous distribution of the material throughout the syringe.
- After insertion of the cannula, injections begin medially to laterally with a 27G 25-mm cannula in a retrograde fashion at the supraperiosteal level.
- Using the free hand, the orbital rim is palpated.
- Care is made to inject below the orbital rim, deep to the muscle, and onto the periosteum between the palpebral and orbital portions of the orbicularis oculi muscle.
- Injection of small aliquots (0.01–0.05 cc) is made in a retrograde fashion.
- Average reconstituted volume delivered is 0.6 cc.
- Minimal massage, if any, can be used to blend (**TECH FIG 1**).

Lid-Cheek Junction

- The 27G 25-mm cannula is advanced from the access port laterally at the supraperiosteal plane toward the lateral canthus.
- Injections are made directly onto the periosteum with a 27G 25-mm cannula in a retrograde fashion similar to the tear trough but now laterally to medially stopping short of the access port.

- Average reconstituted volume delivered is 0.4 cc.
- Minimal massage, if any, can be used to blend (**TECH FIG 2**).

Additional Agents

- Belotero Balance (Merz, Inc. Frankfurt, Germany)—short-lived HA filler (6 months or more) can also be placed intra- or subdermally.
- Juvederm Ultra XC (Allergan, Inc., Santa Barbara, Calif.)—hydrophilic HA filler if used, should be injected conservatively.
- Restylane Refyne (Galderma Laboratories, L.P.)—a flexible HA recently cleared in the United States, as all agents, is recommended to be injected in the supraperiosteal plane.

TECHNIQUES

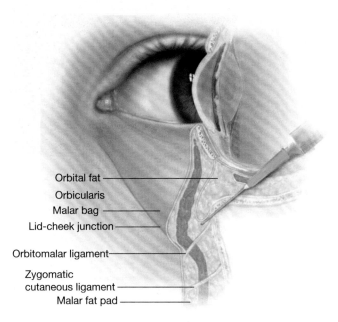

Orbital fat
Orbicularis
Malar bag
Lid-cheek junction
Orbitomalar ligament
Zygomatic cutaneous ligament
Malar fat pad

TECH FIG 2 • Injection technique—The lid-cheek junction is injected in a similar fashion to the tear trough in the supraperiosteal plane below the orbicularis oculi muscle at the level of the orbitomalar ligament from lateral to medial toward the cannula insertion point located at the midpupillary line.

PEARLS AND PITFALLS

Equipment	■ A 30G 13-mm needle may be used. Multiple punctures routinely result in increased ecchymosis. Injections are performed at 90 degrees to the skin surface at the supraperiosteal plane.
Choice of injectable filler	■ Hydrophilic or fillers with higher lifting capacity should be used conservatively and injected in the deepest plane possible to minimize complications. ■ Fillers with a high elastic modulus (G′) and lifting capacity can be more safely placed laterally along the lid-cheek junction with caution.
Technique	■ Be aware of the orbital rim at all times. ■ Inject conservative amounts in a retroactive manner, and avoid overcorrection. ■ Slow injection should be performed at all times.

POSTPROCEDURAL CARE

■ Makeup and other under-eye products should not be used until the following day.
■ Patients may ice the area immediately after the procedure and should remain with their head elevated for the next 24 hours to minimize swelling.
■ Gentle digital pressure can be used to blend areas of edema or irregularity. Massage is not recommended.

OUTCOMES

■ Patients may expect edema, ecchymosis, and injection site tenderness for the first 24 to 48 hours lasting up to 7 to 10 days.
■ Patient should expect additional treatments every 6 to 12 months depending on the filler used and or associated use of botulinum toxin type A in the periorbital area.
■ See **FIG 3** for before and after patient photos.

COMPLICATIONS

■ Irregularities and nodules occur rarely and are secondary to poor technique and/or overcorrection.
■ A gray-bluish hue of the skin caused by the Tyndall effect can be seen if a hyaluronic acid (HA) product is placed too superficially or undiluted.
■ Injection of material above the rim or posterior to the orbital septum can cause prolonged edema or contour abnormalities.
■ Excessive volume, malposition of filler material, or contour abnormalities can be resolved with hyaluronidase (10 units of hyaluronidase/0.1 cc of HA filler) for HA products. Allow swelling to subside for evaluation prior to attempting reversal.

REFERENCES

1. Flowers RS. Tear trough implants for correction of tear trough deformity. *Clin Plast Surg*. 1993;20:403-415.
2. Haddock NT, Saadeh PB, Boutros S, Thorne CH. The tear trough and lid/cheek junction: anatomy and implications for surgical correction. *Plast Reconstr Surg*. 2009;123(4):1332-1340.

Injection of Fillers in the Malar Region

Benjamin T. Lemelman and Julius W. Few

DEFINITION

- Injection of filler in the malar region addresses the aesthetic concerns of the aging patient without the need for surgery.
- The primary filler is hyaluronic acid (HA) gel due to its many properties and U.S. Food and Drug Administration approval.[1]
  - Replaces lost midfacial soft tissue volume due to aging.
  - Increases tissue's capacity to bind water.
- The authors use a combination of U.S. Food and Drug Administration (FDA)–approved fillers including Juvéderm Voluma XC (Allergan, Inc., Irvine, CA) and Restylane Lyft (Galderma Laboratories, Fort Worth, TX).
- Various rheologic properties contribute to the ability of the HA filler to enhance volume and lift the midface:
  - One of these factors is the G′ (G-prime). This describes the firmness or elasticity of the HA product. A product with higher G′ has an increased firmness or density.
  - Restylane Lyft has a reported higher G′ than that of Voluma.
  - Despite the differences in G′, both are considered "high density" and have shown success in midface rejuvenation.[1-3]
  - Cross-linking of the HA particles during production also contributes to the product characteristics.

ANATOMY

- The midface extends from the lower eyelid-cheek junction to the nasolabial fold.
- The three target regions for midface enhancement include (**FIG 1A**)[1]:
  - Zygomaticomalar region
  - Anteromedial cheek region
  - Submalar region

- Additionally, the midface can be divided into four regions V1 to V4 (**FIG 1B**)[4]:
  - V1—zygomatic arch
  - V2—zygomatic eminence
  - V3—anteromedial cheek
  - V4—submalar
- In the V3 region, knowledge of the location of the infra-orbital nerve and neuromuscular bundle is essential. The authors use a blunt cannula technique to minimize risk of intravascular injection of HA, when injection is anywhere other than on the periosteum.

PATHOGENESIS

- Midface aging is a result of many contributing factors including volume loss and tissue descent.
- Changes in underlying bony anatomy, soft tissue volume, and skin thinning all contribute to the aging mid face.[1-3]

PATIENT HISTORY AND PHYSICAL FINDINGS

- A detailed history and physical examination is required prior to any intervention.
- The main reasons for patients to seek aesthetic procedures are to appear younger and more attractive, and feel more confident.[1]
- History of allergies, tobacco use, autoimmune disorders, connective tissue diseases, anticoagulation therapy, and herbal therapies are important issues to discuss with patients.
- Note any prior surgeries on the midface or history of filler use; discuss the type of filler and the number of previous treatments.
- Examination of the face must be performed with the patient in the upright position, as gravity is a major component of tissue descent.

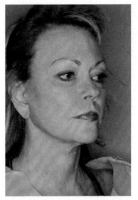 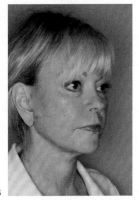 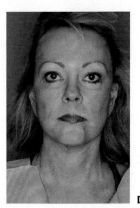 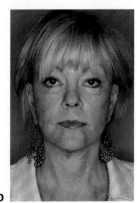

A   B   C   D

FIG 1 • A–D. Before and after results following a total of 3 mL of HA filler to the three regions of bilateral midface of a 65-year-old woman with history of a facelift 5 years prior to presentation. The results shown are after 12 months.

- Examine for facial symmetry, midface firmness, function, sensation and presence of rhytids, skin lesions, or masses.
- A standardized informed consent is obtained from each patient, ensuring they understand the risks, benefits, and alternatives.

IMAGING

- Use of photographic documentation is essential for both the patient and surgeon to examine the effectiveness of the procedures.
- Many computer programs and imaging modalities have the ability to create 3D images to allow the surgeon to digitally modify the patient's midface features, showing the desired outcomes prior to injection.
- Surgeons must obtain standardized before and after photographs for each patient undergoing midface rejuvenation.

NONOPERATIVE MANAGEMENT

- Injection of HA gel is a good option for patients desiring midface rejuvenation. The technique is detailed in this chapter.
- Off-label use of calcium hydroxyapatite is an effective filler substance for the midface but lacks the reversibility seen with HA injection and is not currently approved by the U.S. Food and Drug Administration.

SURGICAL MANAGEMENT

- Autologous fat transfer to augment the aging midface is one surgical option.
- One disadvantage of fat transfer is the requirement for a surgical procedure and the associated donor-site morbidity.
- Other surgical interventions to address the midface include the transconjunctival midface lift or standard facelift.

- Following informed consent, the patient is positioned in the upright position to mark the midface zones and highlight the areas of concern (**TECH FIG 1A**).
- No anesthesia is required for midface injections with Voluma XC or Restylane Lyft, as each product contains lidocaine.
  - Optional topical lidocaine or related anesthetic gel may be used prior to injection.
- Clean the entry site on the midface with betadine or chlorhexidine prep.
- Using a 25 (for a 27G cannula) gauge needle, make a hole in the skin at the desired entry point.
- Focus on targeting the three main regions of the midface: zygomaticomalar, anteromedial cheek, and submalar regions (**TECH FIG 1B**).
- Target the injection in the subcutaneous space.
- The periosteal plane may also be targeted, and we prefer the use of included 27- or 30-gauge needles for the injection of Juvederm Voluma and Restylane Lyft, respectively.
- Thread the product in retrograde fashion to create the desired effect when using the cannula technique; 0.2- to

0.3-mL sequential bolus injections are preferred for needle-based periosteal placement.
- Fanning or cross-hatching of the product may also be employed.
- Take note to avoid the V2 neurovascular bundle in the anteromedial cheek region.
- Cross-hatching, with or without fanning, may be employed.
- Massage of the injection sites can help manipulate the tissues to the desired result.
- Each therapy should be tailored to the patient's desired effect.
- When finished, reassess the patient in the upright position to evaluate any areas needing further therapy.
- On average, approximately 2.5 mL of HA filler is used per side during the initial procedure for Voluma.[1]
- About 1 month later, patients may undergo reinjection with an average of approximately 1 mL per side, to achieve optimal correction.[1]
- Patients with a history of oral herpes simplex virus are placed on prophylactic antiviral therapy 2 days before and 5 days after injection.

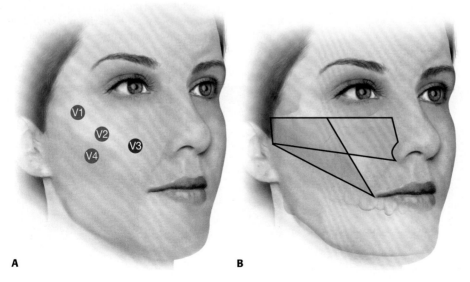

A   **B**

TECH FIG 1 • A. Midface zones. **B.** Midface regions.

PEARLS AND PITFALLS

Techniques	■ The authors prefer a blunt cannula technique to avoid intravascular injection.
	■ Moderate manual massage by the surgeon helps to mold the filler.
	■ Layering of the product in microaliquots can help achieve the desired aesthetic result.
Complications	■ Hyaluronidase must be immediately available.

POSTOPERATIVE CARE

- There are no activity restrictions for patients following the procedure.
- Ice packs are provided for pain relief and/or edema.
- Patients with history of bruising are provided Arnica Montana, a natural remedy, and/or vascular-based nonablative laser.

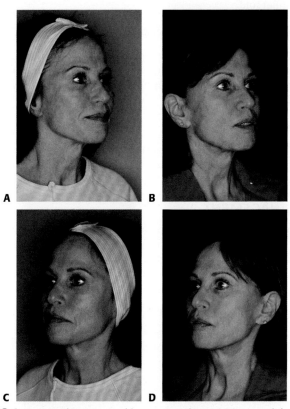

FIG 2 • A–D. This 63-year-old woman underwent injection of three syringes of HA filler to the three regions of the midface.

OUTCOMES

- Studies reveal results can last up to 2 years.
- Most patients require an initial touch-up (approximately 1 mL per side) 1 month after the initial injection.
- **FIGS 1** and **2** are examples of patient results.

COMPLICATIONS

- Potential complications are listed on all consent forms and must be discussed prior to injection.
- The most common complications include tenderness, swelling, firmness, lumps, or bumps. Most issues resolve at 2 weeks.
- Other complications include bruising, pain, redness, discoloration, and itching. Most of these symptoms also resolve within 2 weeks.[1]
- The most devastating complication is intravascular injection of HA filler, which can result in tissue damage.
- Hyaluronidase must be readily available in any office of clinical setting providing HA fillers.
- A standardized clinical protocol must exist for treatment of accidental intra-arterial injection.
- Idiopathic HA-based nodules have been reported and appear to respond to anti-inflammatory agents combined with strategic hyaluronidase injection.

REFERENCES

1. Few J, Cox SE, Paradkar-Mitragotri D, Murphy DK. A multicenter, single-blind randomized, controlled study of a volumizing hyaluronic acid filler for midface volume deficit: patient-reported outcomes at 2 years. *Aesthet Surg J.* 2015;35(5):589-599.
2. Jones D, Murphy DK. Volumizing hyaluronic acid filler for midface volume deficit: 2-year results from a pivotal single-blind randomized controlled study. *Dermatol Surg.* 2013;39(11):1602-1612.
3. Weiss RA, Moradi A, Bank D, et al. Effectiveness and safety of large gel particle hyaluronic acid with lidocaine for correction of midface volume deficit or contour deficiency. *Dermatol Surg.* 2016;42(6): 699-709.
4. Cotofana S, Schenck TL, Trevidic P, et al. Midface: clinical anatomy and regional approaches with injectable fillers. *Plast Reconstr Surg.* 2015;136(5 suppl):219S-234S.

12 CHAPTER

Nasolabial Fold With Hyaluronic Acid Filler Injection

Christopher C. Surek and Jacob Nathaniel Grow

DEFINITION

Deepening of nasolabial fold is one of the most common complaints in patients with an aging face. A deep nasolabial shadow is the result of bony and soft tissue changes that occur with aging and can be addressed with both operative and nonoperative techniques. The purpose of this chapter is to discuss augmentation of the nasolabial fold with filler injection.[1-17]

ANATOMY

- The nasolabial fold represents a musculofibrous septation supporting the malar soft tissues superiorly.
- The intimate relationship of the facial artery to the nasolabial fold *must* be respected, although the course is highly variable (**FIGS 1** and **2**).
  - The facial artery most commonly travels medial to the fold, starting 1.7 mm inferomedially and crossing beneath the fold at a depth of 5 mm at the superior third, eventually reaching a point 3.2 cm lateral to the nasal ala.[17]
  - The levator labii superioris, levator labii superioris alaeque nasi, and zygomaticus minor muscle fibers encase the facial artery as it traverses the fold and also distribute select muscle fibers that insert into the fold.
- The deep pyriform space is a concavity just adjacent to the pyriform aperture. As the bony pyriform recesses, there is decreased support of the lateral nasal ala and increased prominence of peripyriform shadowing. Adding volume to the deep pyriform space can help restore support and shape in the peripyriform region (**FIG 3**).

NATURAL HISTORY

- In the aging face, bony recession in the anterior maxilla and pyriform aperture coupled with deflation and descent of the midface soft tissue leads to deepening of the nasolabial fold.

PATIENT HISTORY AND PHYSICAL FINDINGS

- Physical findings often include midfacial soft tissue descent, shadowing in the pyriform region adjacent to the lateral nasal base, deepening of the nasolabial fold, and evidence of associated perioral aging.

IMAGING

- We recommend obtaining standardized 2D or 3D photography for preinjection planning and to assess postinjection results.

MANAGEMENT

Nonoperative management of the nasolabial fold is performed through volume augmentation with various fillers and in some cases autologous fat. The most common material used is hyaluronic acid filler through needle or blunt cannula injection technique.

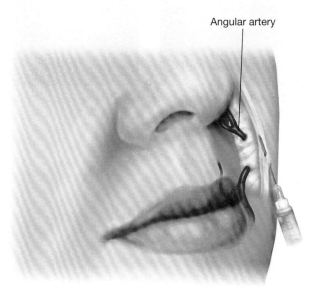

Angular artery

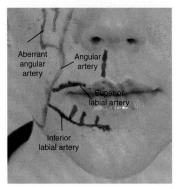

Aberrant angular artery

Angular artery

Superior labial artery

Inferior labial artery

FIG 1 • Demonstration of vasculature location and pathways relative to the nasolabial fold.

FIG 2 • The depth relationship between the angular artery and the targeted depth for needle placement in nasolabial fold injection.

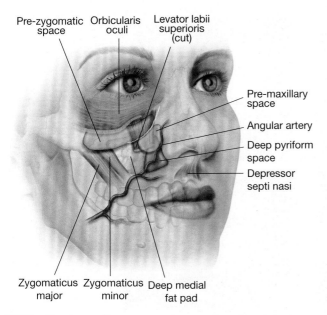

FIG 3 • The deep pyriform space and surrounding adjacent structures.

Preoperative Planning

- Preprocedure photographs should be obtained.
- Complete history and physical exam along with documentation of drug allergies and current medications should be recorded.
- Written informed consent should be obtained to document discussing the indications, risks, and benefits of the injection. Most importantly, patients should be educated on the risk of intravascular injections and counseled on the potential sequelae and treatment following vascular compromise during filler injection.
- The skin involved in the area of injection should be cleaned with an alcohol wipe or antiseptic prep swab.
- Topical anesthetic can be applied to the nasolabial fold skin and allowed to sit for 15 to 20 minutes for the anesthetic to take effect.

- We do not routinely perform infraorbital nerve blocks in our patients. However, it is certainly a reasonable option in select cases if the injector deems necessary.

Positioning

- The patient should be marked sitting up in the chair at 90 degrees.
- For the injection procedure, we recommend reclining the chair to 45 degrees at a height comfortable for the injector.

Approach

- For needle injection, specific entry points along the nasolabial fold are selected. Typically, we use three needle insertion sites for our linear injections. The distance between each insertion point often depends on the length of the needle being used. When using a cross-hatching method, additional needle sites may be required.
- For blunt cannula injection, one or two port sites are selected for skin insertion. The distance between the ports often depends on the length of cannula being used (**FIG 4**).

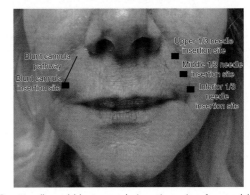

FIG 4 • Needle and blunt cannula insertions sites for nasolabial fold enhancement.

▪ Traditional Needle Injection

- Needle insertion sites at the upper one-third, middle one-third, and inferior one-third are selected.
- Once the needle is inserted into the skin at the desired location, the injector can elevate the needle against the overlying tissues and should see a gentle "white" blanching of the skin (**TECH FIG 1A**). If the gray color of the needle is visible through the skin, then the needle is too superficial and the injector is at risk of creating a Tyndall effect if the filler is deposited at this level.
- The injector will perform a gentle subcision release with the needle and then perform retrograde injection with the bevel facing down (**TECH FIG 1B**).

- Sequential linear injections in the reticular dermis or immediate subcutis are performed in a cranial to caudal direction (**TECH FIG 1C**).
- Once the liner injections are completed, the injector can perform cross-hatching injections horizontally across the fold to smooth out any contour irregularities. These are performed in a cranial to caudal direction (**TECH FIG 1D**).
- To guide proper depth placement with the needle during the cross-hatching injections, the injector can use their noninjecting hand to spread the cheek tissue. This provides tension and creates a taut fold.

T E C H N I Q U E S

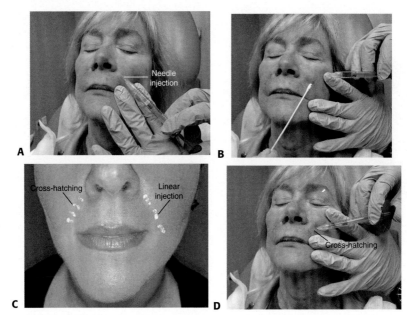

TECH FIG 1 • **A.** Needle injection into the nasolabial fold. Note the gentle blanching of the skin underneath the needle during subcision. The injector wants to see a slight white blanching of the skin but does not want to see the gray color of the needle, which would indicate a too superficial of a plane. **B.** The injector's assistant can clean blood spotting with a cotton tip applicator. **C.** Demonstration of preferred location of filler placement during nasolabial fold enhancement with needle injection. **D.** Demonstration of cross-hatching technique for nasolabial fold enhancement.

■ Blunt Cannula Injection

- A common alternative to the traditional needle injection technique is to thread a blunt cannula immediately subcutaneous in the nasolabial crease.

- Insertion ports are created with a needle stick, then the blunt cannula is inserted and passed deep to the reticular dermis in line with desired area of volume augmentation.
- Retrograde injection is performed with the blunt cannula until desired result is achieved.

■ Adding Volume to the Peripyriform Region

- Recession of the bony pyriform coupled with changes in peripyriform soft tissues results in a deep pyriform shadow at the superior apex of the nasolabial fold. A augmentation bolus on the bone within the deep pyriform

space re-establishes support to the peripyriform region and can soften the skin shadowing.
- Upon completion of deep pyriform volume augmentation, the injector can inject intradermal in the peripyriform shadow. We recommend injecting either intradermally or on the deep bone as the angular artery will travel in a tissue plane between the dermis and the sub-SMAS (**TECH FIG 2**).

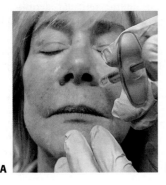
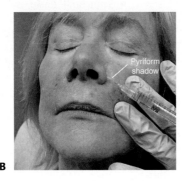

TECH FIG 2 • **A.** Demonstration of deep injection into the deep pyriform space for re-establishing support of the peripyriform region. **B.** Demonstration of superficial injection into the peripyriform shadow for softening the pyriform shadow.

■ Threading Subcision of the Nasolabial Fold

- Various methods have been described to perform a threading subcision of the fold attachments using a wire scalpel or suture threading technique (**TECH FIG 3**).

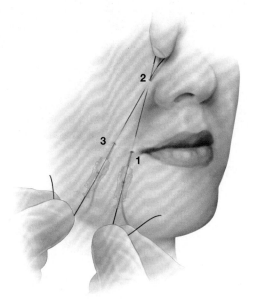

TECH FIG 3 • Medical illustration of the suture threading technique for nasolabial fold treatment.

■ Additional Methods of Nasolabial Fold Treatment

- Some surgeons advocate for botulinum toxin injections into the nasolabial fold as alternative means for fold effacement.

- Release of the dermal attachments of the mimetic muscles in the nasolabial fold is also a well-established tenant in rhytidectomy.

PEARLS AND PITFALLS

Needle placement	■ Needle placement should be within the reticular dermis or immediate subcutis.
	■ The injector can perform a linear retrograde injection technique along the vertical axis of the fold or "cross-hatch" with small horizontal injections across the fold.
	■ Blunt cannula injection should occur in the subcutaneous plane just beneath the reticular dermis.
Depth of injection	■ Be cognizant of the depth of the angular artery (approximately 5 mm deep to the skin).
	■ Be aware of the level at which the angular artery crosses underneath the nasolabial fold (junction of the proximal third) in a medial to lateral direction.
	■ To confirm depth, the injector should see the white color of blanching skin but not the gray color of the needle when placing the needle in the skin. If the injector sees the gray of the needle, the needle location is too superficial and should be readjusted.
	■ We recommend a gentle needle subcision of the fold followed by retrograde injection of medium-sized hyaluronic acid filler.

POSTOPERATIVE CARE

- We recommend placing a ice pack on the injected areas following injection and monitoring the patient in the clinic for 10 to 15 minutes to ensure that there is no evidence of vascular injury.
- If performing perioral injections in conjunction with nasolabial fold filler, we recommend a short course of postinjection antiherpetic prophylaxis.

OUTCOMES

- The primary goal is softening of the nasolabial fold to improve the shadows and contour reflections along the fold. The objective is not to completely efface the fold because this will distort the natural transition between the cheek and perioral aperture (**FIG 5**).

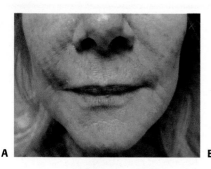 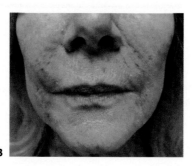

FIG 5 • **A.** Preprocedure photograph in nasolabial fold enhancement with needle injection technique. **B.** Postprocedure photograph in nasolabial fold enhancement with needle injection technique. The patient also underwent injections of the marionette lines.

COMPLICATIONS

- Postinjection bruising is not an uncommon occurrence. Anecdotally we have found adjuncts such as Arnica and ice packs help expedite the resolution of the bruising. Most bruising should resolve within 3 to 5 days.
- Tyndall effect is a bluish hue within dermis following an injection that was too superficial. This is the result of light reflection off the deposited hyaluronic acid filler. The injector can attempt massage to soften the area or dissolve the filler with a hyaluronidase injection.
- If you suspect vascular compromise following injection, immediate hyaluronidase injection is recommended. Doses ranging from 40 to 200 units are recommended depending on the amount of filler injected and the particle size of the filler. Inject immediately and repeat as many times as needed until manifested skin changes improve. Watch the patient very carefully and monitor them in your office until you feel the problem is resolved.

REFERENCES

1. Arlette JP, Trotter MJ. Anatomic location of hyaluronic acid filler material injected into nasolabial fold: a histologic study. *Dermatol Surg.* 2008;34:S56-S63.
2. Braz A, Humphrey S, Weinkle S, et al. Lower face: clinical anatomy and regional approaches with injectable fillers. *Plast Reconstr Surg.* 2015;136:235-257.
3. Cohen JL, Biesman BS, Dayan SH, et al. Treatment of hyaluronic acid filler–induced impending necrosis with hyaluronidase: consensus recommendations. *Aesthet Surg J.* 2015;35:844-849.
4. Costa CR, Kordestani R, Small KH, Rohrich RJ. Advances and refinement in hyaluronic acid facial fillers. *Plast Reconstr Surg.* 2016;138:233-236.
5. Goodier M, Elm K, Wallander I, et al. A randomized comparison of the efficacy of low volume deep placement cheek injection vs. mid- to deep dermal nasolabial fold injection technique for the correction of nasolabial folds. *J Cosmet Dermatol.* 2014;13:91-98.
6. Lee S, Sung K. Subcision using a spinal needle cannula and a thread for prominent nasolabial fold correction. *Arch Plast Surg.* 2013;40(3):256-258.
7. Lupo MP, Smith SR, Thomas JA, et al. Effectiveness of juvéderm ultra plus dermal filler in the treatment of severe nasolabial folds. *Plast Reconstr Surg.* 2008;121:289-297.
8. Nguyen AT, Ahmad J, Fagien S, Rohrich RJ. Cosmetic medicine: facial resurfacing and injectables. *Plast Reconstr Surg.* 2012;129:142-153.
9. Ozturk CN, Li Y, Tung R, et al. Complications following injection of soft-tissue fillers. *Aesthet Surg J.* 2013;33:862-877.
10. Pinsky MA, Thomas JA, Murphy DK, Walker PS. Juvéderm injectable gel: a multicenter, double-blind, randomized study of safety and effectiveness. *Aesthet Surg J.* 2008;28:17-23.
11. Prager W, Wissmueller E, Havermann E, et al. A prospective, split-face, randomized, comparative study of safety and 12-month longevity of three formulations of hyaluronic acid dermal filler for treatment of nasolabial folds. *Dermatol Surg.* 2012;38(7):1143-1150.
12. Rzany B, DeLorenzi C. Understanding, avoiding, and managing severe filler complications. *Plast Reconstr Surg.* 2015;136:196-203.
13. Rubin MG. Treatment of nasolabial folds with fillers. *Aesthet Surg J.* 2004;24:489-493.
14. Scheuer JF, Sieber DA, Pezeshk RA, et al. Anatomy of the facial danger zones: maximizing safety during soft-tissue filler injections. *Plast Reconstr Surg.* 2017;139:50-58.
15. Sun ZS, Zhu GZ, Wang HB, et al. Clinical outcomes of impending nasal skin necrosis related to nose and nasolabial fold augmentation with hyaluronic acid fillers. *Plast Reconstr Surg.* 2015;136:434-441.
16. Wilson AJ, Taglienti AJ, Chang CS, et al. Current applications of facial volumization with fillers. *Plast Reconstr Surg.* 2016;137:872-889.
17. Yang HM, Lee JG, Hu KS, et al. New anatomical insights on the course and branching patterns of the facial artery: clinical implications of injectable treatments to the nasolabial fold and nasojugal groove. *Plast Reconstr Surg.* 2014;133:1077-1082.

Injection of Fillers to the Lips, Oral Commissures, Marionette Lines, Prejowl Area, and Temporal Region

David A. Sieber and Jeffrey M. Kenkel

DEFINITION

- Hyaluronic acid is a naturally found glycosaminoglycan polymer found in human tissue that is reversible with hyaluronidase.

ANATOMY

- The takeoff of the superior labial artery (SLA) from the facial artery is approximately 1 to 1.2 cm lateral to the superior corner of the mouth (**FIG 1A**).[1,2]
  - The SLA then runs superior to the vermilion border, coursing inferiorly across the border just before reaching the Cupid's bow.
  - In the upper lip, the SLA is 3 to 8 mm deep to the skin, running in a plane between the oral mucosa and the orbicularis oris at the junction between the dry and wet vermilion.
  - The course and location of the inferior labial artery (ILA) are more varied than those of the SLA; however, the depth of the ILA remains greater than 3 mm beneath the skin.[3,4]
- The mental foramen is most commonly situated inferior to the second premolar and gives way to the mental nerve and artery (**FIG 1B**).[5]

- The frontal branch of the superficial temporal artery (STA) runs within the temporoparietal fascia (TPF) 2 cm above the zygomatic arch, transitioning to a completely subcutaneous plane just superior to the brow and lateral to the lateral border of the frontalis (**FIG 1C**).[6,7]
  - The middle temporal vein runs 2 cm above and parallel to the zygomatic arch within the superficial temporal fat pad.[8]

PATIENT HISTORY AND PHYSICAL FINDINGS

- There are three components that define attractive and youthful lip aesthetics[9]:
  - Shape and definition of the white roll
  - Shape and projection of vermilion
  - Shape and volume of red roll
- Younger patients typically present desiring enhancement (volume and/or projection) of their existing lip shape.
- Older patients often have lost definition of their white roll and Cupid's bow as they age. There is also significant volume loss in the lips, contributing to the appearance of perioral rhytids.
- Patients also present complaining of down-turned commissures saying they have a "sad" or "angry" appearance to their mouth.

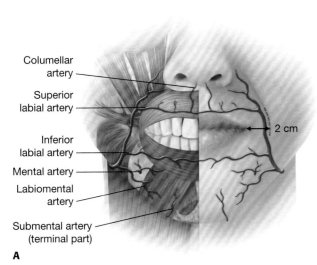

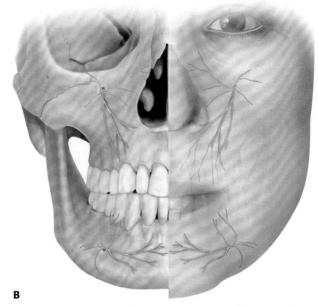

Columellar artery

Superior labial artery

Inferior labial artery

Mental artery

Labiomental artery

Submental artery (terminal part)

2 cm

A

B

FIG 1 • A. Location of the facial, superficial labial, and inferior labial arteries as they relate to anatomical landmarks. **B.** Location of the mental foramen along the mandibular border.

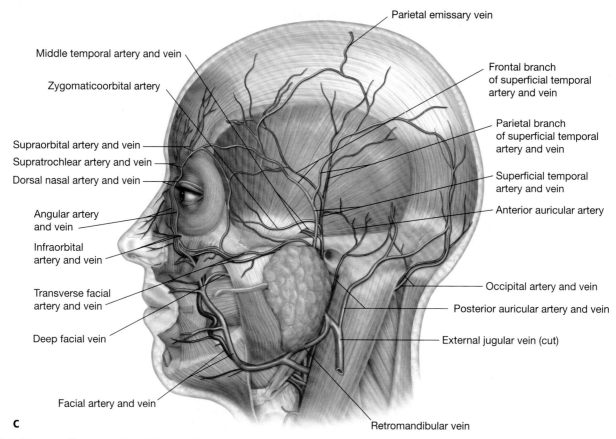

FIG 1 (Continued) • **C.** Location of the superficial temporal artery, transverse branch of superficial temporal artery, and middle temporal vein.

- Other common patient complaints are jowling or excess skin and soft tissue hanging from their mandibular border and temporal hollowing with aging.

NONOPERATIVE MANAGEMENT

- The senior author's preference is to use hyaluronic acid fillers owing to their temporary nature and ability to be reversed through the use of hyaluronidase.
- A topical anesthetic may be used along with ice prior to injection to make the patient more comfortable.

- The skin is always prepped using a swab containing 4% chlorhexidine gluconate prior to injection.
- Injections can be performed with a 30-gauge needle, 27-gauge needle, 25-gauge cannula, or 27-gauge cannula.
- The patient should be comfortably seated in an upright position.
  - Injections are made from a standing position beside the patient.

■ Injection of Filler Into the Lips, Oral Commissures, or Marionette Lines

Preparation

- For most hyaluronic acid products, the authors add 0.2 cc of 0.5% lidocaine with epinephrine using a Luer-lok-to-Luer-Lok connector to constrict local blood vessels, reducing the incidence of postprocedural ecchymosis.
- The authors' preference is to use a 30-gauge needle for injections of the lips and marionette lines, which allows for better control in their hands.

Lips

- If the patient needs further enhancement of the white roll, injections are typically started at the lateral border of the lip.
  - The needle is advanced into a precise location beneath the white roll, filling the area using an antegrade or retrograde linear threading technique.
  - Serial injections are continued until the midline portion of the white roll has been treated, reestablishing an aesthetically pleasing lip shape.
  - Very small amounts are needed and seldom greater than 0.2 mL per side.

- Next, lip volume and projection are addressed again using a linear threading technique.
  - For lip volume, the product is placed at or just posterior to the red line.
  - For lip projection, the product is placed 2 mm beneath the white roll, at the dry vermilion.
- A single vertical injection is done in the center of Cupid's bow for better definition of the tubercle.
- Dermal injections along the lateral borders of Cupid's bow may help better delineate the lateral borders of Cupid's bow.

Oral Commissures

- A triangle-shaped injection is performed at the inferior commissure to help lift the corners of the mouth and refill areas of soft tissue deflation.
  - Cross-hatching of the product is often necessary and may be more efficacious when placed in the deeper dermis.
- A retrograde serial puncture technique is used to place a small amount of product within the fine radial, vertical lines around the lips in an intradermal plane.

- Care is taken to manually massage product in the lips, and the commissures as this area can be palpable to the patient.
- Overly aggressive massage in the perioral region may lead to exaggerated and prolonged lip edema.

Marionette Lines

- Marionette lines are approached starting near the oral commissure.
- Using a linear technique, the needle is inserted into the deep dermis or subdermal location parallel to the marionette line, and filler is placed fairly superficially until the desire result is achieved.
- Additional cross-hatching may be necessary depending on the degree of reinflation required.
- The deformity may extend down to the mandibular border in some patients requiring more volume.
- Some areas may need to be gently massaged to ensure there are no palpable nodules.

■ Injection of Fillers in the Prejowl Area

- For most hyaluronic acid injections in the prejowl region, the authors add 0.2 cc of 0.5% lidocaine with epinephrine using a Luer-Lok-to-Luer-Lok connector to constrict local blood vessels, reducing the incidence of postprocedural ecchymosis.
- A serial puncture technique may be done with a needle, but it is the authors' preference to treat the prejowl area with a cannula.
- A filler with a higher G' is preferred for use in this area
- The index finger or thumb of the nondominant hand is placed below the inferior border of the mandible to

ensure no product is placed below this point, which would give the illusion of lengthening the mandible in the vertical plane.
- A common portal is created using a needle just lateral to the jowl area needing correction.
- The cannula is then used to place product in a subcutaneous plane along the mandible.
- At all times, the index finger or thumb of the nondominant hand is checking to ensure the cannula remains superior to the inferior border of the mandible.
- After correction, product is very gently massaged to ensure there are no palpable areas.

■ Injection of Fillers in the Temporal Region

- For temporal injections, the hyaluronic acid being injected is diluted with 0.5 cc of 0.5% lidocaine with epinephrine 1:100 000 using a Luer-Lok-to-Luer-Lok connector.
- The addition of epinephrine to the filler helps to constrict local blood vessels and prevent postprocedural ecchymosis.
- Injections can be performed with a 27-gauge needle, 25-gauge cannula, or 27-gauge cannula. The authors' preference is to use a 27-gauge needle for injection of the temporal area.

- A superficial or deep injection may be used in this area. It is the authors' preferred approach to perform a deep injection for correction.
- The needle should be inserted 1 cm above and 1 cm lateral to the temporal crest.
- The needle is inserted directly down to the bone, and product is injected onto the periosteum until desired correction is achieved.
- Slight compression at the hairline may help keep the product more anterior, where its impact is seen.
- The product can be gently massaged to create an even appearance.

PEARLS AND PITFALLS

Lips, oral commissures, and marionette lines	▪ Knowledge of the location of the labial artery between the oral mucosa and orbicularis oris helps to prevent ecchymosis and intravascular injections. ▪ The superior labial artery commonly crosses the white roll at the lateral third of the upper lip. Injections should be very superficial at this location to avoid injury. ▪ Proper product placement can effectively improve projection, volume, and definition of the lips. ▪ Volume loss at the commissures is common and benefits from correction with product. ▪ The patients should be reassured that the product may be palpable for up to 7–10 days.
Prejowl area	▪ This area can be fibrous and difficult to pass a cannula. If serial puncture is performed, the product must be massaged so a homogenous result may be achieved. ▪ Care must be taken to avoid inadvertent injury to the mental nerve, which lies in this area.
Temporal region	▪ Be cautious of any superficial veins while injecting as these may lead to unnecessary bleeding and bruising.

POSTOPERATIVE CARE

▪ Patients are sent home with small packs of ice and may apply as needed for swelling and/or bruising.
▪ Patients should keep their heads elevated for a few hours after injection and should abstain from exercise for 24 hours.

OUTCOMES

▪ Excellent outcomes are achievable through replacement of lost lip volume, enhancement of lip shape, improvement in the appearance of radial perioral rhytids, restoration of lost volume around the oral commissures, and correction of the prejowl area and temporal hallowing (**FIGS 2** to **5**).
▪ Restoration of lost lip/perioral volume also reduces the prominence of the nasolabial folds and marionette lines (see **FIG 3**).

COMPLICATIONS

▪ Patients should be counseled on possible risks of procedure, including bleeding, bruising, facial asymmetry, and intravascular injection leading to skin necrosis and/or blindness.

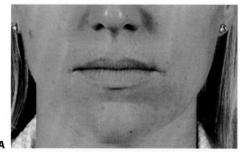 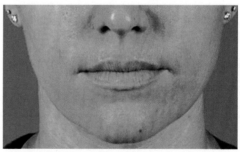

FIG 2 • A 34-year-old woman before **(A)** and after **(B)** injection of 1 cc Juvaderm Ultra Plus into her perioral lip lines.

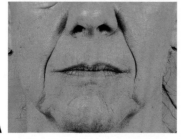 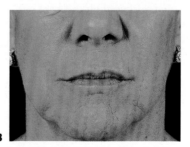

FIG 3 • A 50-year-old woman before **(A)** and after **(B)** treatment with a total of 2 cc Restylane Silk placed into her lips, nasolabial folds, and marionette lines.

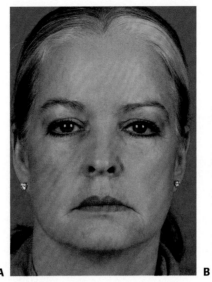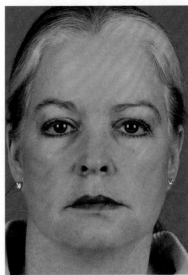

FIG 4 • A 62-year-old woman before **(A)** and after **(B)** treatment with 0.5 cc Restylane placed into each prejowl region.

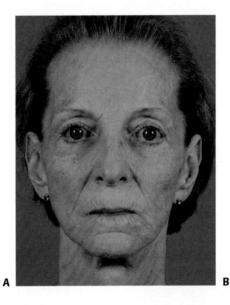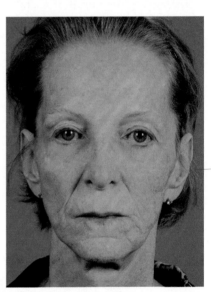

FIG 5 • A 66-year-old woman before **(A)** and after **(B)** injection of 0.5 cc Restylane Lyft into each temporal region/lateral brow, 1 cc total of Restylane Silk into the lips/perioral region, and 0.4 cc Restylane Lyft into each prejowl region.

REFERENCES

1. Magden O, Edizer M, Atabey A, et al. Cadaveric study of the arterial anatomy of the upper lip. *Plast Reconstr Surg.* 2004;114:355-359.
2. Tansatit T, Apinuntrum P, Phetudom T. A typical pattern of the labial arteries with implication for lip augmentation with injectable fillers. *Aesthetic Plast Surg.* 2014;38:1083-1089.
3. Al-Hoqail RA, Meguid EM. Anatomic dissection of the arterial supply of the lips: an anatomical and analytical approach. *J Craniofac Surg.* 2008;19:785-794.
4. Pinar YA, Bilge O, Govsa F. Anatomic study of the blood supply of perioral region. *Clin Anat.* 2005;18:330-339.
5. von Arx T, Friedli M, Sendi P, et al. Location and dimensions of the mental foramen: a radiographic analysis by using cone-beam computed tomography. *J Endod.* 2013;39:1522-1528.
6. Lee JG, Yang HM, Hu KS, et al. Frontal branch of the superficial temporal artery: anatomical study and clinical implications regarding injectable treatments. *Surg Radiol Anat.* 2015;37:61-68.
7. Trussler AP, Stephan P, Hatef D, et al. The frontal branch of the facial nerve across the zygomatic arch: anatomical relevance of the high-SMAS technique. *Plast Reconstr Surg.* 2010;125:1221-1229.
8. Jung W, Youn KH, Won SY, et al. Clinical implications of the middle temporal vein with regard to temporal fossa augmentation. *Dermatol Surg.* 2014;40:618-623.
9. Surek CC, Guisantes E, Schnarr K, et al. "No-touch" technique for lip enhancement. *Plast Reconstr Surg.* 2016;138:603e-613e.

14
CHAPTER

Injection of Filler to the Nose

T. Jonathan Kurkjian, Jamil Ahmad, and Rod J. Rohrich

DEFINITION

- Volume deficiencies of the nose including both congenital and postoperative deformities
- Contour irregularities of the postoperative nose

ANATOMY

- The nose is constituted of multiple layers. From deep to superficial, these layers consist of the mucosal lining, osteo-cartilaginous framework, musculoaponeurotic tissue, subcutaneous fat, and skin.
- The aesthetic subunits of the external nose include the nasal tip, dorsum, sidewalls, columella, soft tissue triangles, and paired alae (**FIG 1**).[1]
- The vasculature of the nose has contributions from both the internal and external carotid systems by way of the ophthalmic and facial artery, respectively. The arterial arcades are located superficial to the musculoaponeurotic layer. The subdermal plexus is located in a more superficial location deep to the dermis.

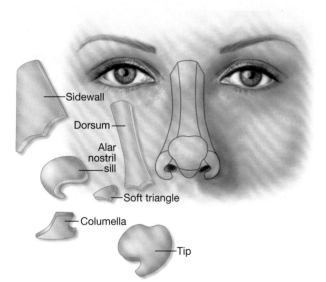

FIG 1 • Aesthetic subunits of the nose include the nasal dorsum, sidewall, tip, soft tissue triangle, ala, and columella.

PATIENT HISTORY AND PHYSICAL FINDINGS

- The patient history and physical findings are fundamental components to determine if soft tissue filler injection to the nose is an appropriate option.
- Careful understanding of the patient's aesthetic complaints is critical to formulating the treatment plan.
- Physical examination must include a detailed nasal aesthetic analysis to determine the specific nasal deformities. An internal nasal examination should always be a part of the complete nasal examination.
- The patient's history of previous nasal trauma, surgery, and soft tissue filler injections should be documented. Careful examination for surgical scars is also warranted to confirm the provided history.
- Assessment of skin thickness and cicatrix is absolutely critical to planning safe soft tissue filler injections.

IMAGING

- High-resolution digital photography should be used to obtain standard nasal views. These views include frontal, lateral (left and right), oblique (left and right), and basal views.
- Preinjection computer imaging can be used to simulate results prior to injection.
  - Preinjection imaging is particularly useful for the patient who has a preconceived treatment plan.
  - Although computer imaging enables involvement of the patient in the planning process, great care should be taken to communicate that there is no implied guarantee of results.

SURGICAL MANAGEMENT

Preoperative Planning

- Review of the patient's history is important to ensure that patients do not take any medications that may make them more prone to bleeding as this may increase the propensity for postinjection bruising.
- Photographs should be available for preinjection planning and reassessment during treatment.
- Only hyaluronic acid gel fillers are used (ie, Restylane [Medicis, Scottsdale, AZ], Juvederm [Allergan, Irvine, CA]). Particulate-based fillers (ie, Sculptra [Valeant, Bridgewater, NJ], Radiesse [Merz, San Mateo, CA), are not used to avoid long-term palpability.[2]

- Soft tissue filler choice is determined by the aesthetic subunit that is to be injected.
  - Restylane has a higher level of cross-linking and lower hydrophilicity; thus, it is used for the nasal dorsum and sidewalls.
  - Juvederm Ultra or Juvederm Ultra Plus tends to be more malleable several days after injection. This ability to mold Juvederm proves to be helpful for the aesthetically sensitive nasal tip and ala.[2]

Positioning

- The patient should be positioned in an exam chair so that he or she is comfortable and thus less likely to require a change of position during the procedure. Typically, the patient is positioned with the feet slightly elevated and the chair back slightly reclined.

Approach

- Transcutaneous syringe injection approach is preferred as a more sterile route than a transmucosal injection.

- Some patients may require the skin to be anesthetized with topical anesthetic. The injector may also use 1% lidocaine with epinephrine to perform a nerve block to bilateral maxillary divisions of the trigeminal nerve. The resulting vasoconstriction can theoretically help minimize the risk for intravascular injection. However, vasoconstriction may prevent recognition of vascular compromise of the skin.
- Proper cleansing of the skin prior to injection can help avoid infectious complications. All makeup should be removed, and the skin should be cleansed with chlorhexidine.
- Aspiration prior to each injection is critical to help prevent intravascular injection and associated sequelae including tissue necrosis and blindness.

- All injections should be completed with small volumes and with minimal pressure to avoid contour deformities and intravascular injection. It is critical that all injections are deep to avoid palpability and intravascular injection.
- Gentle massage of the hyaluronic acid can assist with even distribution of the product.
- The injector should allow 15 minutes to pass prior to assessing the final contour. This gives sufficient time for the product to diffuse fully.
- Skin color and turgor should be assessed continuously throughout the procedure as an indication of proper soft tissue perfusion.
- Injection volumes must be monitored closely to help avoid pressure necrosis.
- The technique of nasal injection depends significantly on the aesthetic subunit that is being injected.

■ Injection of the Nasal Dorsum

- The threading injection technique is preferred to maintain the linear conformation of the dorsum. The needle is inserted along the long axis of the nose, thus respecting the dorsal aesthetic lines while pursuing a more pleasing profile. Careful injection deep along the nasal bone and midvault cartilages will help prevent visibility and palpability of product (**TECH FIG 1**).[2]

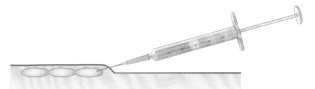

TECH FIG 1 • Linear threading injection technique. The needle is inserted to its full length along a distance and the filler is then injected uniformly with removal of the needle.

TECHNIQUES

■ Injection of the Nasal Sidewall

- Injection of the nasal sidewall should be avoided due to the inherent risk of intravascular injection. If sidewall injection is necessary, a cross-hatching technique is the preferred method of injection to assist with uniform volume augmentation of the relatively flat nasal sidewall. The needle is inserted parallel to the sidewall thus maintaining a deep supraperiosteal plane during injection (**TECH FIG 2**).[1,2]

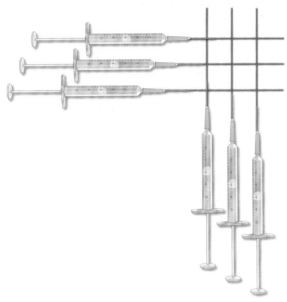

TECH FIG 2 • Cross-hatching injection technique. The needle is inserted in a grid pattern to achieve a smooth contour over a flat plane.

■ Injection of the Nasal Tip/ala

- The nasal tip and ala are injected with a serial injection technique using small aliquots of hyaluronic acid. It is particularly important to continuously monitor the skin of the nasal tip during injection for any blanching, which may indicate hypoperfusion due to excessive pressure (**TECH FIG 3**).[2]
  - Soft tissue filler should never be injected along the alar groove to avoid intravascular injection into the lateral nasal artery.
  - In order to avoid contour deformities, the filler should be injected deep and never along the alar rim.

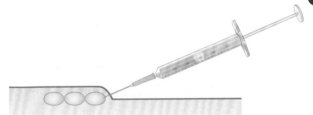

TECH FIG 3 • Serial puncture injection technique. The needle is inserted to a shallow depth, and a small aliquot of filler is injected to maximize accuracy and precision.

PEARLS AND PITFALLS

Clinical assessment	■ Accurate clinical assessment is absolutely necessary to achieve optimal aesthetic results.
Filler choice	■ Hyaluronic acids are the safest and most forgiving products to use for soft tissue filler injection of the nose. ■ Restylane is the preferred soft tissue filler for the nasal dorsum and sidewalls. ■ Juvederm is preferred for the nasal tip and ala.
Technique	■ Each anatomic subunit of the nose is best treated with a specific injection technique, thus enabling accurate and reproducible volume augmentation. ■ Aspiration is recommended prior to each injection to minimize the risk for intravascular injection.
Necrosis	■ The skin should be continuously monitored for any signs of hypoperfusion that may occur as a result of intravascular injection or pressure necrosis. ■ Injection into the previously operated nose should be performed by those with significant injection experience and understanding of the altered blood supply.

POSTOPERATIVE CARE

- Patients are advised to avoid pressure to the injected areas for 2 weeks because it may impact the aesthetic outcome.
- For 24 hours after injection, patients are instructed to avoid exercise, alcohol, and aspirin to minimize the risk of bruising.

OUTCOMES

- The aesthetic outcomes depend greatly on the clinical analysis of the nose prior to injection.
- Clinical experience indicates that Juvederm Ultra/Ultra Plus or Restylane can persist in the nose for 2 to 3 years as opposed to the shorter durations seen with injection to other locations in the face (**FIGS 2** and **3**).[3]

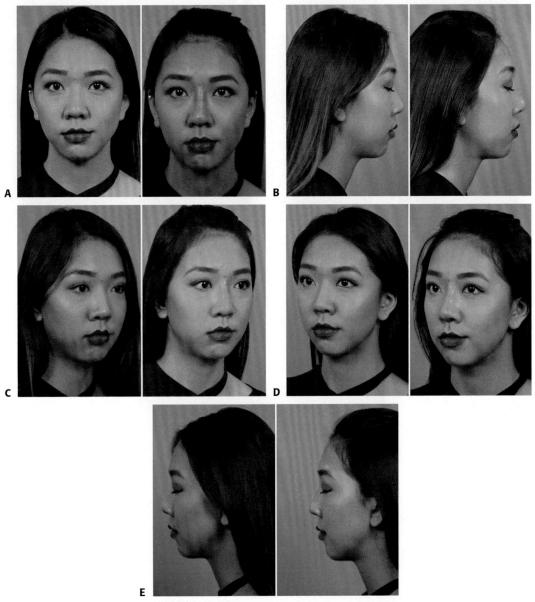

FIG 2 • Low radix and inadequate dorsal and tip projection. Preprocedure (*left*) and postprocedure (*right*) views of a 19-year-old woman with a low radix and inadequate dorsal projection. She was treated with 0.8 mL of Restylane to the dorsum and radix and 0.1 mL of Juvederm to the nasal tip.

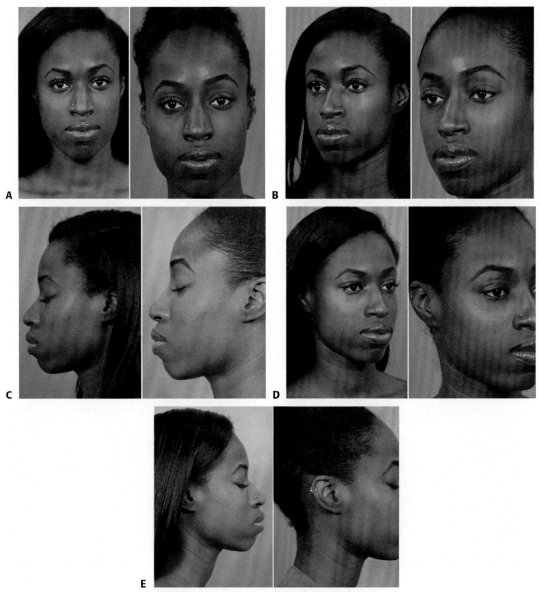

FIG 3 • Asymmetric dorsal aesthetic lines and low radix. Preprocedure (*left*) and postprocedure (*right*) views of a 26-year-old woman with asymmetric dorsal aesthetic lines, narrow midvault, and low radix. She was treated with 0.3 mL of Restylane to the left nasal sidewall and 0.2 mL of Restylane to the right nasal sidewall and 0.5 mL of Restylane to the radix and nasal dorsum.

COMPLICATIONS

- Intravascular injection of hyaluronic acid may cause local tissue necrosis and even blindness. To avoid this complication, aspiration should always be attempted prior to each injection. Small needles (27 g or smaller) are preferred with careful attention to minimize pressure of injection.
- Pressure necrosis can result from volume injected in excess to the compliance of the overlying soft tissue and skin. This complication is more common in the previously operated nose where cicatrix can greatly reduce the pliability of the skin.
- If skin blanching is observed, the injection should be stopped immediately. If the blanching does not improve, hyaluronidase should be injected into the area. If the skin still appears to be hypoperfused, the patient should be started on oral aspirin and topical nitropaste. If a wound results, hyperbaric oxygen may assist with wound healing (**FIG 4**).[2]

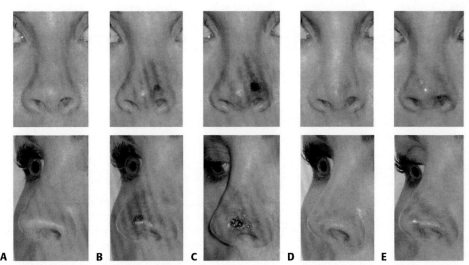

FIG 4 • Management of tissue necrosis. **A.** Preprocedure view of a 36-year-old woman with asymmetry of the nasal tip including an irregularity of right tip-alar junction and an over-reduced nasal tip after eight previous rhinoplasty surgeries. She was injected with 0.1 mL of Juvederm Voluma to the right tip-alar junction and 0.2 mL to the supratip and left tip-alar junction. **B.** At 6 days postprocedure, she began to show signs of tissue necrosis. Three separate injections at 10-minute intervals delivering a total of 30 units of hyaluronidase in 1.5 mL of 2% lidocaine were injected to the nasal tip, alae, dorsum, and sidewalls. The patient was started on 81 mg aspirin daily, and nitropaste was applied topically every 8 hours. Hyperbaric oxygen treatment was started and she had a total of 12 sessions. **C.** At 8 days postprocedure with the maximum amount of tissue necrosis that she experienced. **D.** At 6 months after the initial injection. **E.** After injection of 0.1 mL of Juvederm Refine to the right tip-alar junction and 0.05 mL to the left tip-alar junction over two treatment sessions at 4-week intervals. Both the type of product and the volume injected during the session may have contributed to this complication. (From Kurkjian TJ, Ahmad J, Rohrich RJ. Soft-tissue fillers in rhinoplasty. *Plast Reconstr Surg.* 2014;133:121e-126e, with permission.)

REFERENCES

1. Millard DR Jr. Aesthetic reconstructive rhinoplasty. *Clin Plast Surg.* 1981;8(2):169-175.
2. Kurkjian TJ, Ahmad J, Rohrich RJ. Soft tissue fillers in rhinoplasty. *Plast Reconstr Surg.* 2014;133(2):121e.
3. Rohrich RJ, Ghavami A, Crosby MA. The role of hyaluronic acid fillers (Restylane) in facial cosmetic surgery: review and technical considerations. *Plast Reconstr Surg.* 2007;120(Suppl 6):41S-54S.

Section III: Fat Grafting of the Face

Fat Grafting at the Time of Face-Lifting

CHAPTER 15

Sammy Sinno and James M. Stuzin

DEFINITION

- The aging face is characterized by complex problems that evolve over time.
- Fat descent, deflation, and radial expansion of fat away from the central face contribute to some of the changes seen with aging.
- The goal of a facelift is to surgically reposition fat to create a more youthful facial contour. Surgery alone, however, cannot treat deflation of fat that occurs with age.
- Autologous fat grafting has become a common technique utilized by most surgeons today performing facial rejuvenation.[1] In addition to treating volume deflation, fat can make smooth the noticeable demarcations between aesthetic regions in the face that occur with aging.

ANATOMY

- Studies have identified precise anatomic compartments of the face where fat should ideally be placed.[2,3]
- The anatomy of the deep malar compartment has only been recently elucidated, clarifying that there is deep volumetric support that exists in the plane deep to the mimetic muscles and superficial to the periosteum of the orbit and anterior cheek.[4] This deep fat system provides volumetric support between the lower eyelid and anterior cheek in youth.
- The medial deep malar compartment is situated along the pyriform aperture and blends the anterior cheek with the perioral region in youth. Similarly, the central aspect of the deep malar fat pad abuts the buccal extension of the buccal fat pad, allowing for a smooth blending of contour between the lateral cheek and the anterior cheek. Augmenting this compartment is critical to correct the deep deflation that occurs with aging.[1]

PATIENT HISTORY AND PHYSICAL FINDINGS

- In aging, typically both deep and superficial malar compartment deflation develops, leading to demarcation lines between aesthetic subunits of the midface. Visually, the lower lid sinks into the cheek, developing the infraorbital V deformity.

- Similarly, the nasolabial fold deepens, and, in many patients, an abrupt transition is noted between the lateral cheek and the anterior cheek over time. All of these characteristics are hallmarks of deep malar deflation.[1]
- Other areas that should be assessed for potential volume augmentation include the perioral region, temples, tear trough, and prejowl sulcus.

IMAGING

- No imaging is needed for this procedure other than routine preoperative testing.

SURGICAL MANAGEMENT

Preoperative Planning

- Patients are asked to bring pictures from their youth. Patients who have sustained volume loss with age in various compartments of the face are candidates for fat grafting.
- Particular attention is paid to patients who have deep compartment deflation.
- The amount of fat needed for facial fat grafting is estimated.
- A donor site (abdomen, thighs, or hips) is selected with adequate fat for harvesting.
- Importantly, patients should be counseled that not all fat survives, and repeat fat grafting procedures may be necessary 6 to 12 months postoperatively to adequately augment the areas of interest.

Positioning

- The patient is in a supine position for this procedure.

Approach

- Fat grafting can be performed immediately prior to the facelift or immediately after. Advantages to fat grafting before the facelift include minimized tissue trauma and swelling prior to placement. Advantages to fat grafting after facelift include the ability to visualize the effect of surgical repositioning prior to grafting and also avoid displacing the grafted fat during surgical dissection.

■ Fat Grafting at the Time of Facelifting

Fat Harvest

- The goal of fat harvest is to acquire fat as gently as possible.
- The Coleman technique is utilized for fat grafting procedures.[5]
- Possible donor sites include the abdomen, thighs, or hip area.
- The area is infiltrated with a solution of dilute lidocaine and 1:200 000 epinephrine.
- Stab incisions are made with an 11-blade scalpel.
- Fat is collected using a harvesting cannula attached to a 10-cc syringe (**TECH FIG 1**).

Fat Processing

- A Luer Lock plug is attached to the end of the syringe and the syringe spun in a balanced centrifuge for 3 minutes at 3000 rpm (**TECH FIG 2A**).
- The oil layer (ruptured adipocytes) is removed with a neuropad whereas the aqueous layer (blood and local anesthesia) is evacuated, leaving intact adipocytes (**TECH FIG 2B**).
- Fat is transferred to a 1-cc syringe in preparation for grafting (**TECH FIG 2C**).

Fat Placement

- An 18-gauge needle is used for access.
- Fat is injected using a 1-cc syringe and a 27-gauge Tulip blunt tip side-port cannula (**TECH FIG 3**).
- All fat should be placed in small aliquots in multiple passes with the cannula in constant motion under low pressure.

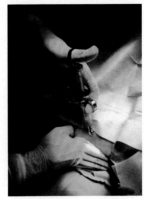

TECH FIG 1 • Fat harvest.

Injection by Anatomic Location

- Deep malar compartment
  - Although facelift techniques can be successful in repositioning superficial malar facial fat into areas of deflation, it is technically difficult to reposition fat into the deep compartment.
  - For this reason, deep compartment augmentation requires volumetric addition for correction. Volumetric addition to the deeper compartments is technically straightforward,[6] and our preference is to approach this injection via the alar base.
  - Approximately 1 to 3 cc is placed depending on the severity of deflation deep onto the periosteum (**TECH FIG 4**).

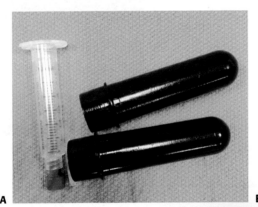

A

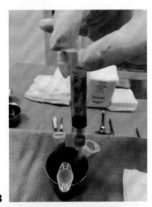

B

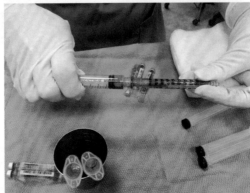

C

TECH FIG 2 • **A.** Luer Lock plugged syringe and centrifuge carriers. **B.** Centrifuged syringes with ruptured adipocytes in the top layer and an aqueous layer at the bottom; fat to be injected is in the middle and then **(C)** transferred to 1-cc syringes.

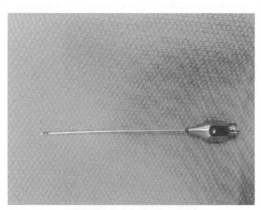

TECH FIG 3 • Injection cannula.

- Superficial and lateral malar compartments
  - Though typically addressed with surgical repositioning, 1 to 3 cc of fat can be injected directly into these compartments to accentuate malar convexity.
- Nasolabial folds
  - The nasolabial folds are injected directly with 1 to 2 cc of fat depending on fold depth in the subcutaneous and preperiosteal layers.
  - Care is taken to avoid injection into the angular vessels.
- Temples
  - Significant temporal hollowing can result with aging.

- Often a significant amount of fat, 3 to 5 cc or more, injected onto the periosteum is required for correction.
- Tear trough and eyelid-cheek junction
  - The tear trough is anatomically a very challenging area to inject.
  - Aesthetic goals in this area are to restore smooth transitions between topographic compartments in the face, overcoming sharp demarcations that become evident with aging.
  - If injected, less than 0.5 cc of fat should be injected cautiously directly into the tear trough with care to avoid causing any irregularities.
  - 1 cc of fat can be injected to blend the eyelid-cheek junction.
- Prejowl sulcus
  - To create a well-defined mandibular border, 1 to 2 cc of fat can be injected preperiosteally into the prejowl sulcus (**TECH FIG 5**).
- Lips
  - Significant perioral rejuvenation can be achieved with fat injection into the lips.
  - 1 or 2 cc of fat is injected with access from the commissure.

Completion

- Following injection, all access sites are closed with a 4-0 plain gut suture.

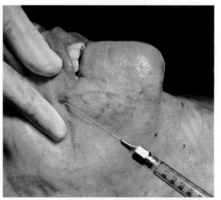

TECH FIG 4 • Fat injection into the deep malar compartment.

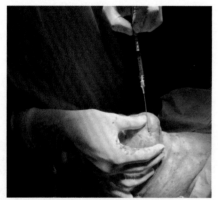

TECH FIG 5 • Fat injection into the prejowl sulcus.

PEARLS AND PITFALLS

Aesthetic considerations	▪ Surgery alone cannot correct deep compartment deflation that occurs with age. ▪ Fat augmentation at the time of facelifting should be considered into areas of volume deflation (ie, deep malar compartment) and into areas where volume will help blend demarcations between anatomic regions that occur with age.
Harvest	▪ Fat can be harvested from the abdomen, thighs, or hip area.
Processing	▪ Fat is prepared using the Coleman technique of centrifugation followed by removal of the oil and aqueous layers.
Injection	▪ All fat should be placed in small aliquots in multiple passes with the cannula in constant motion under low pressure. ▪ Avoid superficial injections that can cause contour irregularities. ▪ Exercise extreme caution when injecting into the tear trough. ▪ Pay close attention to the anatomy of vasculature in the areas of injection to avoid intravascular complications.
Revisions	▪ Typically, 5%–60% of the injected fat is viable at 1 year. ▪ Augmentation with additional fat can be performed at 3 months, but it is advisable to wait 6–12 months if possible.

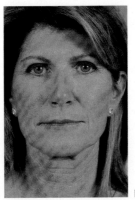 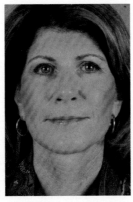 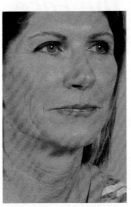 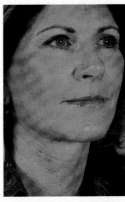

FIG 1 • A–D. A 54-year-old female seen prior to and following an extended SMAS facelift. Autologous fat (3 cc) was injected into the central deep malar compartment, and 2 cc of autologous fat were injected into the lateral aspect of the deep malar compartment. Note the blending between the lower eyelid, anterior cheek, and lateral cheek as superficial fat repositioning is combined with deep compartment augmentation.

POSTOPERATIVE CARE

- Head of bed elevation is encouraged to minimize swelling.
- Patients will also follow instructions for postoperative face-lift care.
- Deep massage is discouraged to avoid displacing injected fat.

OUTCOMES

- The combination of facial fat repositioning, which alters shape by shifting volumetric highlights, in conjunction with volume addition, which further corrects deflation, provides greater aesthetic control in surgical outcome (**FIG 1**).
- Additional fat grafting, or supplementation with off the shelf fillers, can be performed at 3 to 6 months.
- Additional fat grafting is typically performed under sedation.

COMPLICATIONS

- Contour deformity (most common)
- Fat necrosis
- Infection
- Unnatural growth of fat
- Tissue necrosis (rare)
- Intravascular injection

REFERENCES

1. Sinno S, Mehta K, Reavey PL, et al. Current trends in facial rejuvenation: an assessment of ASPS members' use of fat grafting during face lifting. *Plast Reconstr Surg.* 2015;136(1):20e-30e.
2. Rohrich RJ, Pessa JE. The retaining system of the face: histologic evaluation of the septal boundaries of the subcutaneous fat compartments. *Plast Reconstr Surg.* 2008;121(5):1804-1809.
3. Rohrich RJ, Pessa JE. The fat compartments of the face: anatomy and clinical implications for cosmetic surgery. *Plast Reconstr Surg.* 2007;119(7):2219-2227.
4. Gierloff M, Stohring C, Buder T, et al. Aging changes of the midfacial fat compartments: a computed tomographic study. *Plast Reconstr Surg.* 2012;129(1):263-273.
5. Coleman SR. Structural fat grafting. *Aesthetic Surg J.* 1998;18(5): 386, 388.
6. Rohrich RJ, Arbique GM, Wong C, et al. The anatomy of suborbicularis fat: implications for periorbital rejuvenation. *Plast Reconstr Surg.* 2009;124(3):946-951.

16
CHAPTER

Section IV: Laser Resurfacing of the Face
Techniques for Laser Resurfacing of the Face

Daniel A. Belkin and Roy G. Geronemus

DEFINITION

- With age, there is a loss of the supporting frame of the skin: collagen, elastin, and hyaluronic acid. Skin laxity results, with increased redundancy, accentuated skin folds, and uneven texture. Skin aging is expedited by exogenous factors, most importantly chronic sun exposure and cigarette smoking, resulting in further wrinkling and dyspigmentation.
- Resurfacing of the skin of the face can be achieved with dermabrasion, chemical peels, energy devices (radiofrequency and plasma energy), and laser surgery, which is the focus of this chapter. Laser resurfacing stimulates collagen synthesis and improves rhytides, dyspigmentation, and the overall quality of the skin.

ANATOMY

- The histology of skin treated with laser resurfacing has been well studied and varies based on the specific laser or device used.
- Resurfacing lasers are either ablative or nonablative and either fractionated or nonfractionated.
  - Ablative lasers vaporize treated zones of skin with surrounding heat injury and coagulation, whereas nonablative lasers produce heat injury without vaporization.
  - Fractionated lasers create small columns of injury within treated areas, leaving large zones of unaffected skin between them, rather than injuring the entire treated area at once (**FIG 1**).

PATHOGENESIS

- Resurfacing lasers tend to use wavelengths in the near- and mid-infrared range and target water as their chromophore. Destruction can therefore be achieved to any thickness through the skin. The depth and extent of injury are determined by the wavelength of the laser source (nm) and the power delivered, known as fluence (J/cm^2).
- Once injury is produced, new collagen is formed via the wound healing response of dermal fibroblasts, and the epidermis is repopulated from stem cells found in skin appendages.

PATIENT HISTORY AND PHYSICAL FINDINGS

- Patient expectation, skin quality including Fitzpatrick skin type, and relevant medical history should be assessed before treatment.
- Patient history
  - An appropriate patient has reasonable expectations for cosmetic outcome, and the primary concern is related to the indications described above. Patients should understand the side effect profile and be able to manage the necessary downtime following treatment (depends on modality—see Table 1).
  - Topical and oral medications and medication allergies should be reviewed.
  - History of herpes simplex virus, connective tissue disease, local inflammatory skin disease, and other conditions that may affect wound healing should be elicited.
- Physical examination
  - For most laser resurfacing techniques, it is best if the patient is Fitzpatrick skin types I to IV. Caution is advised in patients of skin types V and VI as they are at risk for dyspigmentation.
  - The aesthetic issue to be addressed will determine the type of resurfacing. Subtle fine lines, sun damage, mottled pigmentation, and hypopigmented scars are some conditions that will respond to noninvasive fractional nonablative resurfacing. Moderate to severe rhytides and atrophic scars will respond to more invasive fractional ablative resurfacing. Elevated lesions, such as fibrous papules or papular scars, may require the localized use of a nonfractionated ablative laser (see Table 1).

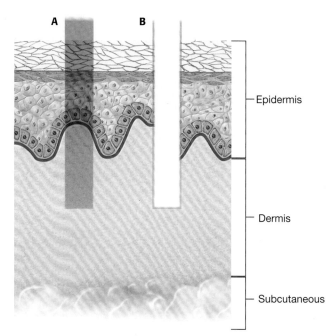

FIG 1 • A schematic of fractional treatment. Healing occurs via stem cells within zones of viable tissue amidst columns of injury, either coagulation (**A**) or ablation (**B**).

Table 1 Representative Resurfacing Devices and Our Protocols for Their Use

Selected Representative Devices	Category	Medium	Wavelength (nm)	FST	Preoperative Preparation	Preoperative Medications (for full face)	Indications	Downtime	Postoperative Care	Risks and Complications
Fraxel dual (Solta)	Fractional nonablative	Thulium/erbium glass	1927/1550	I–III	1 hour topical lidocaine/prilocaine	Anti-HSV antiviral, prednisone	Actinic damage, fine lines, enlarged pores, dyschromia, dull tone and texture, acne scars	3–7 days erythema, dryness, and bronzing	Nonocclusive emollient q8h	HSV, hyperpigmentation, acneiform eruption
Clear and brilliant Perméa (Solta)	Fractional nonablative (low energy)	Diode	1927	I–VI	1 hour topical lidocaine/prilocaine (optional)	Anti-HSV antiviral (optional)	Dull tone and texture, melasma/hyperpigmentation	1–2 days erythema and dryness	None necessary	Multiple treatments required
Fraxel repair (Solta) Halo profractional (Sciton)	Fractional ablative	Carbon dioxide Erbium-YAG	10 600 2940	I–III I–IV	1 hour topical lidocaine/prilocaine, nerve blocks (mental, infraorbital, supraorbital), local lidocaine infiltration	Anti-HSV antiviral, prophylactic antibiotics, prednisone	Surgical, traumatic, or acne scars, moderate to severe rhytides, skin laxity	7- to 10-day wound	Distilled water soaks and healing ointment QID, gentle face wash after 24 h	Hypopigmentation, prolonged erythema, HSV, bacterial infection, scarring
Burane (Alma)	Nonfractional ablative	Erbium-YAG	2940	I–VI	Local lidocaine infiltration, nerve blocks (mental, infraorbital, supraorbital)	Not recommended for full face; targeted areas only	Resurfacing of elevated scars, angiofibromas, syringomas, epidermal nevi	7- to 14-day wound	Healing ointment BID	Hypopigmentation, hypersensitivity, hyperpigmentation, scarring, infection

IMAGING

- No radiologic or diagnostic studies are necessary prior to routine laser resurfacing.

SURGICAL MANAGEMENT

Preoperative Planning

- Topical retinoids should generally be stopped a week before treatment and only restarted after complete healing has occurred.
- There is controversy over how long to wait to resurface after a course of oral isotretinoin; to be safe, it is reasonable to wait six months for ablative procedures until there is further data.
- Pre- and postoperative medication depends on provider preference, patient medical history, and device used.
  - Full-face nonablative fractional resurfacing, except for low-energy low-density treatment, may warrant immediate preoperative and postoperative treatment with corticosteroids (eg, prednisone 40 mg prior to procedure and then daily for 2 more days) and antiviral prophylaxis (eg, valacyclovir 500 mg prior to procedure and then BID for 3 more days).
  - Full-face ablative fractional resurfacing often warrants corticosteroids as above, antiviral prophylaxis extended to 7 days, and antibiotic prophylaxis for 7 days (eg, dicloxacillin 500 mg prior to procedure and then BID × 7 days).
- Localized treatment areas often need no pre- or postoperative treatment, including localized treatment with nonfractional ablative devices. Localized ablative fractional treatment around the eyes or mouth is an exception, and prophylaxis above should be considered.

Positioning

- Laser resurfacing requires the patient to recline on an exam table in the supine position with protective eyewear in place.
  - Eyewear may generally be opaque tanning goggles or sticky pads.
  - For ablative resurfacing (fractional or nonfractional) within the orbital rim, protective stainless steel corneal shields should be employed.

Approach

- Some devices require a stamping motion, whereas others require a scanning motion.
  - Fractional nonablative treatments and some fractional ablative devices employ the scanning technique whereby the practitioner paints the skin with a rolling handpiece.
    - The laser should be applied in multiple passes in different directions with attention paid to the total amount of energy (kJ) applied to each subunit of the face.
  - Nonfractional ablative devices and some fractional ablative devices employ the stamping technique whereby the practitioner applies a certain spot size to targeted areas.

T E C H N I Q U E S

- Please refer to Table 1 for further details of selected representative devices.

■ Nonablative Fractional Resurfacing

- These devices include the Fraxel Dual, Palomar LUX 1540, Affirm Multiplex, Clear + Brilliant, Clear + Brilliant Perméa, and Palomar Emerge.

- They have near-infrared wavelengths in the range of 1410 to 1927 nm and penetrate from 100 μm to 1.1 mm.
- They create columns of coagulation and leave zones of spared tissue between (**FIG 1A**).

■ Ablative Fractional Resurfacing

- These devices include the Fraxel Repair, Lumenis Active FX and Deep FX, Sciton Pro-Fractional, Sciton Core, Deka SmartXide, Alma Pixel, and MiXto SX.
- They have mid-infrared wavelengths of either 2940 nm or 10 600 nm and penetrate up to 1.6 mm.

- They create columns of ablation surrounded by coagulation and leave zones of spared tissue between (**FIG 1B**).
- In some cases, the zone of coagulation can be controlled; in general, coagulation improves skin tightening effect but may be counterproductive in darker skin types and hypertrophic scars.

■ Ablative Nonfractional Resurfacing

- Nonfractional resurfacing can often be done by setting the density on fractional devices to 100%.

- At our practice, we use the erbium-doped yttrium aluminum garnet (Er:YAG) laser for the purpose of localized full ablation. Fully ablative resurfacing of the entire face carries a higher risk of scarring and permanent pigmentary loss than does fractional treatment.

PEARLS AND PITFALLS

- Fractional ablative resurfacing produces much faster healing times and a lower rate of scarring and hypopigmentation than full-field ablative resurfacing
- In general, lower densities (of both ablative and nonablative resurfacing) should be used in darker skin types
- Ablative resurfacing off the face, including on the neck, must be done with caution (and generally with much lower energy and density) as fewer sebaceous glands increase likelihood of scarring
- Acneiform eruptions after nonablative resurfacing can be treated with a course of oral tetracyclines such as doxycycline and/or topical antibiotics such as clindamycin
- Postoperative healing should be largely painless; pain should prompt investigation and possible empiric treatment for herpetic or bacterial infection

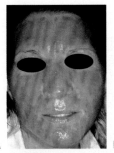 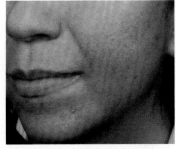

FIG 2 • One day post-treatment. Fractional ablative **(A)** and fractional nonablative **(B)**.

POSTOPERATIVE CARE

- Postoperative care differs among treatments, which produce different degrees of injury (**FIG 2**; Table 1).
- For all modalities, strict sun avoidance and generous emollients are important until healing is complete.

OUTCOMES

- Outcomes depend on indication, patient, and device (see Table 1). Some possible outcomes include
  - Improvement in fine lines (**FIG 3**)
  - Improvement of hypopigmentation (**FIG 4**)
  - Improvement of dyschromia (**FIG 5**)
  - Improvement of under-eye festooning (**FIG 6**)
  - Smoothing of moderate to severe rhytides (**FIG 7**)
  - Improvement in acne scarring (**FIG 8**)
  - Improvement in atrophic surgical scarring (**FIG 9**)

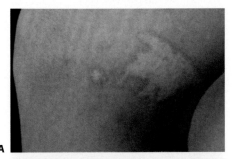

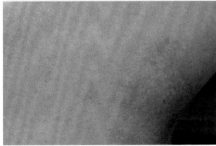

FIG 4 • Improvement of hypopigmentation. Fractional nonablative therapy with 1927 nm was used with 10 mJ fluence at 65% density. **A.** pretreatment and **(B)** post-treatment.

- Eyelid lift[1]
- Clearance of actinic damage[2]

COMPLICATIONS

- Complications are outlined in Table 1 for each modality.

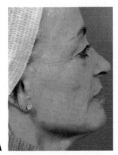 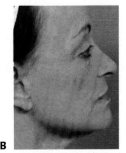

FIG 3 • Improvement in texture, dyschromia, and fine lines. Fractional nonablative therapy with 1550 nm was used with 70 mJ fluence at 40% density. **A.** pretreatment and **(B)** post-treatment.

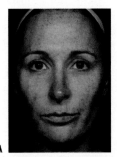 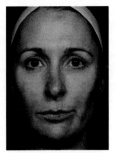

FIG 5 • Improvement of dyschromia. Fractional nonablative therapy with low energy low density 1927 nm was used with 7 mJ fluence at 10% density. **A.** pretreatment and **(B)** post-treatment.

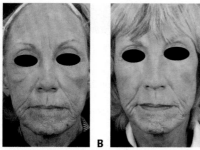

FIG 6 • Treatment of under-eye festoons. Fractional ablative therapy with 10600 nm carbon dioxide laser was used with 70 mJ at 50% density. **A.** pretreatment and **(B)** post-treatment.

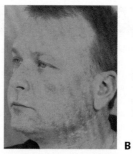
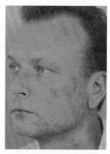

FIG 8 • Improvement in acne scars. Fractional ablative therapy with 10600-nm carbon dioxide laser was used with 70 mJ fluence at 50% density. Some neck retraction was also achieved. **A.** pretreatment and **(B)** post-treatment.

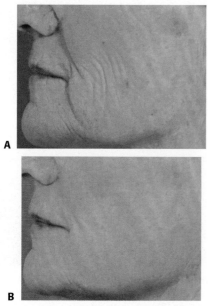

FIG 7 • Smoothing of moderate to severe rhytides. Fractional ablative therapy with 10600 nm carbon dioxide laser was used with 70 mJ at 50% density. **A.** pretreatment and **(B)** post-treatment.

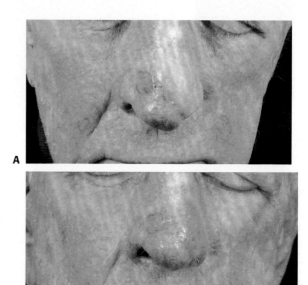

FIG 9 • Improvement in atrophic surgical scar. Fractional ablative therapy with 10600-nm carbon dioxide laser was used with 70 mJ fluence at 60% density. **A.** pretreatment and **(B)** post-treatment.

- Feared complications of ablative laser include permanent hypopigmentation and scarring; these are much less likely when energy is fractionated.
- Postinflammatory hyperpigmentation is an important complication and is avoided by careful sun protection post-treatment and caution with darker skin types.
- Acneiform reactions can occur following nonablative treatment and can be treated like acne vulgaris with oral tetracyclines and topical antibiotics.
- Wounding of the skin may predispose to herpes simplex reactivation and bacterial soft tissue infection warranting antiviral and antibacterial prophylaxis in certain cases.

ACKNOWLEDGMENT

We thank Julia Pettersen Neckman, MD, for her significant contributions to this chapter.

REFERENCES

1. Sukal SA, Chapas AM, Bernstein LJ, et al. Eyelid tightening and improved eyelid aperture through nonablative fractional resurfacing. *Dermatol Surg.* 2008;34(11):1454-1458.
2. Weiss ET, Brauer JA, Anolik R, et al. 1927-nm fractional resurfacing of facial actinic keratoses: a promising new therapeutic option. *J Am Acad Dermatol.* 2013;68(1):98-102.

TCA Peel to Face

17
CHAPTER

Steven M. Levine and Daniel C. Baker

DEFINITION

- The aging face changes in multiple facets.
- Surgery is the standard to address descent and laxity.
- Resurfacing is important to treat textural and other surface changes related to aging and environmental damage.
- Trichloro acetic acid (TCA) peel is one highly effective, reliable, and low-cost method to facial resurfacing.

ANATOMY

- Facial peeling can be performed on the entire face and neck or can be isolated to specific aesthetic units such as the lower lids or perioral region.
- The perimeter of any area being treated should be "feathered" to minimize the creation of a transition between peeled and nonpeeled tissue.

PATIENT HISTORY AND PHYSICAL FINDINGS

- Indications for peeling are broad and can include desire to improve skin texture, reduce visible fine lines, or ameliorate age spots (such as solar keratosis).
- It is important to elicit a history of oral herpes so that these patients can be pretreated with antiviral medication.
- Skin type is important to note.

SURGICAL MANAGEMENT

- TCA peeling can be performed as a stand-alone procedure or in combination with a face and necklift.

Preoperative Planning

- The primary consideration for preoperative planning is the patient's skin tone. The more pigmentation in the skin, the higher the chance for postpeel complications such as postinflammatory hyperpigmentation or areas of hypopigmentation.
- Some providers choose to pretreat patients with a retinol or bleaching agent for 4 to 6 weeks prior to TCA peel. Neither of the authors use pretreatment.
- TCA can be used in a variety of strengths. The authors prefer to keep only two strengths of TCA—25% and 35%.
  - 25% TCA is used for lighter peels and darker complexions (Fitzpatrick grade III).[1]
  - 35% TCA is used for heavier or more aggressive peels and lighter complexions (Fitzpatrick grades I and II).[1]

Positioning

- The patient is either supine if under sedation or full anesthesia or sitting upright in an exam chair while holding a fan if performing a peel on an awake patient.

Approach

- The approach to the peel can be accomplished using a variety of application techniques that yield a controlled, reproducible distribution of chemical to the skin.

■ Cotton Tip Applicator on Sedated Patient

- The patient is laid supine on the operating room table.
- The face is cleaned with alcohol to remove as much oil from the skin.
- A small amount of eye ointment is placed on the sclera to protect the eyes.
- An assistant should stand adjacent to the procedure table holding the TCA or the TCA should be kept on a Mayo stand away from the patient. An open bottle of TCA is NEVER placed over the patient or in any position where it can spill on the patient.
- For the majority of the face, two cotton tip applicator sticks are used to spread the TCA (**TECH FIG 1A**).

- Usually the forehead and nose are more keratinized and require a heavier coat of TCA.
- For the lower eyes, a single cotton tip applicator is used to apply the TCA. The skin beneath the lower lid is stretched with the nondominant hand for complete placement of the TCA to just before the lash line.
- Care is taken to "feather" the borders of any anatomic area that means lightening the amount of TCA applied to reduce the appearance of a transition zone.
- The skin will usually frost within 60 seconds (**TECH FIG 1B**).
- An area that does not frost or is not uniform can be retreated in the same manner.

TECHNIQUES

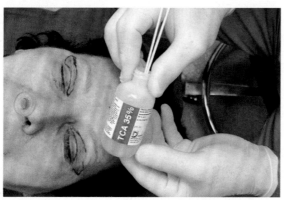
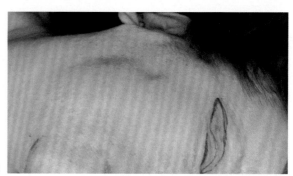

TECH FIG 1 • A. TCA peel is applied using cotton applicator sticks. **B.** TCA frost.

■ ## Cotton Tip Applicator on Awake Patient

- An identical technique is used on the awake patient with the addition of patient-held fan to increase comfort during the procedure.

- Usually, any burning or discomfort lasts less than 60 seconds as the TCA is neutralized by the skin.

PEARLS AND PITFALLS

Start low and light	■ Use 25% TCA and apply a thin coat until you get use to correlating the amount of frosting with the level of skin peel.
Avoid TCA spills	■ Never hold the bottle of TCA yourself while applying.
Safely combine procedures	■ TCA is a an excellent adjunct to a facial surgery procedure
Feathering	■ Always extend the treatment beyond the zone being treated (ie, beneath the jaw line if treating the full face).

POSTOPERATIVE CARE

- This procedure is often combined with a facelift in which traditional surgical preparation of the skin is not required in the setting of the TCA peel.
- If combined surgery is not planned, a petroleum-based ointment is applied to the patient's face immediately after the procedure.
- Cool packs are also used to reduce swelling.
- Patients are instructed to remain away from the sun during the acute peeling period (7–10 days postop).
- Sun avoidance should ideally be carried out for several months after TCA peel.
- Patients are instructed to use cool compressed at home for the first 24 to 48 hours.
- After 48 hours, patients are instructed to use warm compressed to speed the peeling process.
- Patients are instructed not to remove any peeled skin themselves (though if they are in the office, I will often do this for

them). The concern is the patient could be too aggressive and remove skin prematurely.
- Patients should apply a thin layer of petroleum-based ointment 3 times daily until the skin is re-epithelialized.

OUTCOMES

- TCA peel will predictably improve certain fine lines and reduce the appearance of certain superficial pigmentation issues.
- The provider needs to start using this technique in a metered fashion to gain comfort with expectations and limitations.

COMPLICATIONS

- The most feared complication is TCA entering the eye. If this happens, the eye should be irrigated with saline or water continuously and an ophthalmologist should be consulted immediately.

- Caution must be taken near hair-bearing areas such as the brow because they can trap TCA in the hair causing a deeper burn in that region than intended.
- Hyperpigmentation can occur which usually resolves on its own.
  - Sun avoidance is paramount.
  - Lightening agents such as hydroquinone 4% topical can be used if necessary.

- Hypopigmentation should not occur with 25% or 35% TCA peel in the patients who do not have dark skin.

REFERENCE

1. Reference to Fitzpatrick classification.

Indications and Technique for Phenol-Croton Oil Peels

Gehaan D'Souza and James E. Zins

DEFINITION

- Intermediate and deep chemical peeling imparts injury to the epidermis and varying depths of the dermis in a controlled manner in efforts to stimulate epidermal regrowth. Peeling has been shown to rejuvenate facial skin and has been used to treat acne, rhytides, and photodamage.[1]
- Chemical peels are available in a variety of formulas, which produce superficial, medium, and deep wounds.
  - Superficial peeling techniques are limited to epidermal injury only.[1,2] Intermediate and deep chemical peels most commonly involve trichloroacetic acid (TCA) and phenol-croton oil. Both TCA and phenol-croton oil depth can be varied by changing the concentration, number of applications, and the amount of peeling agent applied.
  - Deeper peels, such as the conventional phenol-croton oil formula, are the most effective in resurfacing skin but are also associated with more severe complications and may not be appropriate for certain patients.
- The use of phenol-based chemical peels declined with the advent of laser technologies.
  - There has been renewed interest in the use of this technique in recent years with the realization that reducing the concentration and application methods can reduce complications while maintaining results.[3,4]
  - The phenol-croton oil formulas use varying concentrations of phenol, croton oil, Septisol, and water.[3]
- Full facial phenol peels require deep sedation or general anesthesia and cardiac monitoring. Because of the potential for cardiac arrhythmias, full facial chemical peeling should be done based on anatomic units over a relatively prolonged period of time (1–1.5 hours).
- Additionally, these peels pose risk for renal failure and hepatotoxicity.[3,5]
- Adjusting croton oil concentration allows for variation in phenol-croton oil peel depth and achievement of more uniform results on different thicknesses of skin.[3]
  - Phenol-croton oil peels are increasingly being used as a medium-depth peeling modality and can be performed on a spectrum of ages and skin conditions.[4]

ANATOMY

- Phenol-croton oil, while most commonly recognized as a deep peeling technique, can also be used as a superficial or medium-depth peeling modality (**FIG 1**).[6]
- Chemical peels are divided into three categories based on the degree of injury caused by the treatment[7]:
  - Superficial peels—cause epidermal injury and do not penetrate below the basal layer

- Medium-depth peels—ablate the epidermis and varying degrees of the dermis
- Deep peels—remove the epidermis, papillary dermis, and generally extend to the midreticular dermis
- Indications for phenol-croton oil peels include[4,6,8]
  - Rhytides
  - Melasma
  - Acne

PATHOGENESIS

- Factors such as environmental damage, actinic damage, smoking, and radiation.[9–11]
- Rhytides form for a variety of reasons. The contraction of the musculature and attachments of the retinaculum cutis that attaches to the skin acts on the skin to create a wrinkle with animation.
- Strategies for preventing rhytides include sun avoidance, smoking cessation, and treatment of skin with retinoids.[11]
  - Once rhytides are present in the perioral area at rest, they are difficult to treat.

PATIENT HISTORY AND PHYSICAL FINDINGS

- Medical and surgical history, as well as physical examination should address general health or risks from current medications (eg, isotretinoin, birth control pills, or immunosuppressants), possibility of pregnancy, liver disease, history of herpes simplex virus, history of hypertrophic or keloid scars, history or risk of hepatitis or HIV, history of radiation exposure, and history of cutaneous disease at the peel site (eg, rosacea, seborrheic dermatitis, atopic dermatitis, psoriasis, and vitiligo).
- Previous injury to the reticular dermis including previous peeling, laser, or even electrolysis will affect how aggressive one is with peeling depth.
- Gender differences in perioral wrinkling have been described.
  - Women have a lower ratio of blood vessels to connective tissue than do men.[12] This can also be explained by the differences of follicles, sebaceous glands, and androgen-dependent hair.[13]
- The patient's skin type using a Fitzpatrick classification is important in determining the need for suppression of melanin and prevention of hyperpigmentation.
- The Glogau photoaging scale determines the depth of the peel.[14,15]
- Indications for chemical resurfacing:
  - Photoaging of the skin and rhytides
  - Preneoplastic or neoplastic lesions such as actinic keratosis and lentigines

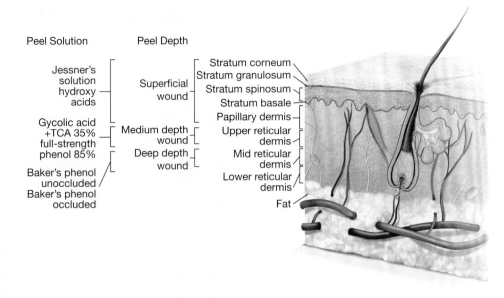

FIG 1 • Review of basic skin anatomy as it relates to peel depth.

- Acne or other underlying skin diseases
- Pigmentary dyschromias
- Demarcation lines secondary to other resurfacing procedures
- Contraindications to chemical resurfacing:
  - Absolute:
    - Isotretinoin therapy within the last 6 months or until pilosebaceous units begin functioning
    - Active infection or open wounds (eg, herpes, excoriations, or open acne cysts)
    - Lack of psychological stability and mental preparedness
    - Unrealistic expectations
    - Poor general health and nutritional status
    - Poor physician-patient relationship
    - History of abnormal scar formation or delayed wound healing and therapeutic radiation exposure
    - History of certain skin diseases (such as rosacea, seborrheic dermatitis, atopic dermatitis, psoriasis, and vitiligo) or active retinoid dermatitis; Fitzpatrick skin types IV, V, and VI are contraindications for medium and deep-depth peels.
  - Relative:
    - Need to proceed with caution with a history of medium-depth or deep resurfacing procedures within the previous 3 to 12 months
    - Chemical peeling at the time of rhytidectomy is practiced by some. This should not be done with phenol peels. Areas not undermined can be peeled with phenol peel. Patients must wait 3 months to peel undermined areas.

SURGICAL MANAGEMENT

- The goal of a phenol peel is to produce controlled partial-thickness skin injury. This leads to improving skin quality, reduction of fine lines, and coarse rhytides.
- Pretreatment (priming) with Retin-A and 4% hydroquinone is helpful to minimize post-treatment hyperpigmentation. In those with darker Fitzpatrick skin types, there should be a minimum of 6 weeks of treatment.

- Hypopigmentation and incidence of hypertrophic scarring are directly correlated with the depth of injury.
- In a phenol peel much like a TCA peel, the depth of injury can be controlled leading to peels from papillary dermis to midreticular dermis depending on the amount of facial aging. The depth of injury can be altered by changing the concentration and the number of applications of the peeling agent. The critical factor is the degree of frosting.
- Time to healing can vary from 5 days (superficial peel) to 10 to 14 days when a deep peeling technique is used.
- Hypopigmentation and hyperpigmentation are the most common complications.
- Damage to the melanocytes at the epidermal-dermal junction leads to hypopigmentation.
- Hypopigmentation is more noticeable in dark skin patients, so segmental applications should not be done in these patients.
- Hyperpigmentation usually results from peeling-induced inflammation with melanocyte overstimulation. Darker skin patients are more prone to this complication. This is exacerbated with premature sun exposure.

Preoperative Planning

- Consultation should be held with the patient to establish realistic goals and expectations.
- Peel depth should be determined by assessing and documenting patient's Fitzpatrick skin type and photoaging grouping, degree of actinic damage, sebaceous gland density, dyschromias, suspicious lesions, and scarring.
- The hands and neck have very few progenitor cells in the reticular dermis. The scarcity of these cells makes peeling in these areas risky.
- Gravitational changes can best be treated with facelift.
- Standard preoperative photographs should be taken for preoperative planning.
- Informed consent should be obtained and should include an overview of the healing process and phases, additional surgeries or procedures that may be necessary, complications,

explanations of what can and cannot be accomplished with the phenol-croton oil peel, and a description of financial responsibilities, including for revisions.

- Important considerations for ethnic skin[14]:
  - Ethnic skin, including that of Latino and Hispanics, may respond unpredictably to chemical peels and are more prone to melasma and postinflammatory hyperpigmentation than nonethnic skin types.

Preparation and Positioning

- Patient is pretreated with tretinoin and hydroquinone for 4 to 6 weeks to suppress melanin production.
- Patient is instructed to use acyclovir 400 mg TID 2 days before the procedure and continued until complete healing observed.
- Varying concentrations of phenol and croton oil have been used.[4]
  - Phenol-croton oil can be used as a superficial or medium to deep depth peel.
  - Technique is extremely important. By altering concentration and application technique (number of swipes or amount of solution applied), different depths can be achieved at different regions of the face. For example, a light peel, which uses a lower concentration of croton oil, can be used to peel the lower eyelids, while a higher concentration of croton oil may be used to peel more deeply wrinkled areas of the face, such as the perioral region.[6]
- Safety checks before peeling:
  - Mark the mandibular ramus, so that peel is not applied caudal to this line.
  - Begin an IV and run fluid.
    - Phenol is metabolized in the liver and excreted by the kidneys. Therefore, patients with liver disease should be treated with increased caution.
  - Monitor with cardiac monitoring equipment, pulse oximeter, and blood pressure monitoring.
  - Cardiac arrhythmias during chemical peeling have been reported; however, cause and effect relationship is controversial.
  - Ensure applicator and peeling agent never pass over the patient's eyes.

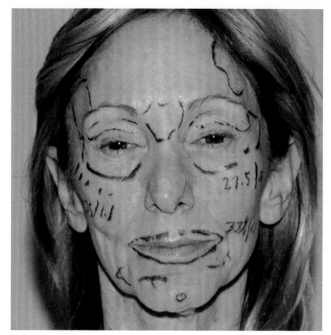

FIG 2 • Preoperative markings.

- Anesthesia:
  - Administer sedation and analgesia by performing facial nerve block and direct infiltration using a longer acting anesthetic.
  - Epinephrine should be avoided, as it can exacerbate cardiac arrhythmias.
  - Decadron (8–10 mg) or betamethasone (6 mg) may also be administered.
- Skin preparation:
  - Peel area should have been thoroughly washed the night before and morning of the surgery, with no residual makeup.
  - Clean peel area using Septisol (hexachlorophene with alcohol) to adequately degrease the skin. This step is essential for optimal results.
  - The patient's face is marked (**FIG 2**).
- Positioning:
  - The patient should be lying supine.

■ General Region Peel

- The phenol-croton oil wound agent should be applied using a moistened, wrung out cotton-tipped applicator, tending to the deep rhytides first.
- The peeling agent should be applied to aesthetic units over an extended period of time (1–1.5 hours).
- Because phenol does not affect hair growth, the agent should be spread into hair-containing areas.
- Apply swipes until a proper depth of injury is attained. Pink-white frost signifies a papillary dermal injury, and

dense white frost denotes a reticular dermal injury. Brown-white frost signifies a deep dermal injury.
- Allow 10 to 15 minutes between cosmetic units before applying a new coat to reduce renal and cardiovascular risk. The full procedure may last between 60 and 10 minutes.
- A thick layer of Vaseline and viscous Xylocaine solution should be applied to each region of the face as soon as it has been treated with the peeling agent, to prevent peeled areas from drying out. This acts as an occlusive dressing and as a pain reliever.

■ Periorbital Peel Technique

- Ensure that no agent drips into the patient's eye. Do not pass vials over the patient in case of spillage.
- Elevate the patient's head 30 to 45 degrees.
- Patient's tears should be wiped away using a cotton-tipped applicator at the medial and lateral canthus while holding the patient's eye open to prevent the peeling agent from entering the eye.
- For the lower eyelid, have the patient look up and apply the agent within millimeters of the eyelash margin by moving from the lateral crow's feet to the medial canthal area. For the upper eyelid, have the patient close her eyes and apply the agent from the lateral to inner canthal area. Avoid applying product below the superior tarsal plate, as it may lead to prolonged edema. Be certain to peel the orbital rims to avoid lines of demarcation.
- Apply an ice pack over the eyes for 6 to 8 hours after the peel to reduce swelling.

■ Perioral Peel[8]

- Applying peeling agent onto the vermilion border to avoid missing lipstick lines.
- Manually stretch the skin to create deeper and more even penetration.
- Use the wooden end of a cotton-tip applicator to apply peeling agent to individual rhytides (**TECH FIG 1**).
- Degreasing the skin by aggressive rubbing with alcohol swab until skin erythema has proven to be an effective method in treating especially perioral skin damage.
- If peeling the perioral area only, make sure to use to proper technique to avoid lines of demarcation. Apply the peeling agent just beyond the nasolabial fold, and then brush out the remaining regions of the face.

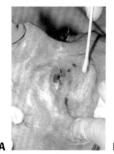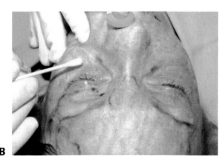

TECH FIG 1 • Intraoperative photos. **A.** Upper lid. Application of agent within millimeters of eyelash margin by moving from lateral crow's feet to the medial canthal area. **B.** Lower lid. The agent is applied with the patient looking upward.

■ Taping (for Occluded Peel)

- Taping increases the depth of injury.
- Apply precut, 1.5 to 4 cm strips of tape to each cosmetic unit after the completing the peel.
- Begin by applying the tape along the inferior border of the mandible in a saw tooth pattern, which produces a less discrete line. Continue taping outward, by placing strips 1 to 2 cm parallel to the inferior border of the mandible.
- The tape mask should be removed as a single unit, approximately 48 hours after the procedure, when the exudate has elevated the tape.

PEARLS AND PITFALLS

Intraoperative complications	■ Intraoperative complications may be the result of technical errors. Monitor for cardiac arrhythmias.
Pretreatment	■ Pretreatment with tretinoin and hydroquinone is helpful to minimize pigmentation problems in darker-skinned individuals.
Depth	■ Depth of peel is varied by pathology. Frosting is the key element to getting a good result.
Pigmentation	■ Secondary alternation of skin pigmentation is the most common complication and should be discussed with the patient.

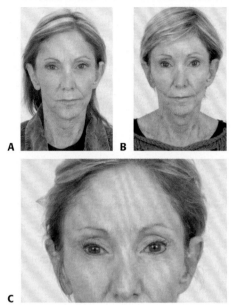

FIG 3 • A–C. Two years after phenol-croton oil peel of the perioral, periocular area, and temples. Phenol peel used 27.5% phenol, 0.105% croton oil for the periocular area, and 33% phenol and 1.1% croton oil for the perioral area. (Preoperative photos of the patient are shown in **FIG 2**.)

POSTOPERATIVE CARE

- Wound care: areas should be kept constantly moist with ointment. Discomfort is relieved with the use of Vaseline/Xylocaine mixture. This acts as a pain reliever and occlusive dressing. Expect considerable swelling and drainage. Erythema duration varies with the depth of injection and Fitzpatrick skin type. Patients are quite allergic in the early postoperative period. General pruritus can be decreased by steroid cream. Contact dermatitis should be similarly treated. Sign of infection is the development of significant pain in patients otherwise healing well. Infection can be bacterial, fungal, and viral.
  - Retouching of specific areas or repeeling may be necessary after 3 to 6 months for deeper wrinkles.
- Sleeping: While sleeping, head should be kept elevated using multiple pillows.
- Bathing/washing: Clean in the shower with unscented liquid soap. Perform a splashing action, and use fingers only. Do not use any type of exfoliating aide, such as a washcloth or sponge. Apply a thick coat of moisturizing ointment after each wash. Wash in the shower after 48 hours if no tape is present.
- Lifestyle: Avoid the sun completely. Sun exposure can lead to postoperative skin pigmentation. In addition to sun exposure, becoming pregnant or taking birth control pills before redness has subsided may cause blotching. Avoid contact of caps, shower caps, eyeglasses, or visors on peeled areas until the underlying skin has healed. Patients may return to work as early as 14 days postprocedure. Makeup and sunscreen may be applied on healed areas. Exercise should be avoided for 30 days postprocedure, as increased blood flow could cause microhemorrhaging or red blotching.

OUTCOMES

- The use of perioral phenol peel combined with facelifting has been found to add 5.3 years of reduction in apparent age after the combined facelift and peel[16] (**FIGS 3** to **6**).
- Using validated questionnaires, patient satisfaction was found to be high with the use of a combined phenol peel and facelift.
- Perioral phenol-croton oil peel resulted in a significant and objective wrinkle shown by the reduction in Glogau score.[16]
- When carefully assessed, some degree of hypopigmentation occurs with most patients, and hypopigmentation is subtly progressive. When peeling is confined to lower Fitzpatrick skin types, it is not disabling.

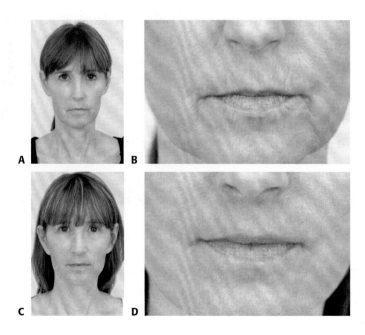

FIG 4 • A,B. Preoperative patient photos. **C,D.** Six months after bilateral rhytidectomy with extended SMAS and perioral phenol-croton oil peel and fat injections to the cheeks and nasolabial folds. Phenol peel to perioral area using 33% phenol and 1.1% croton oil.

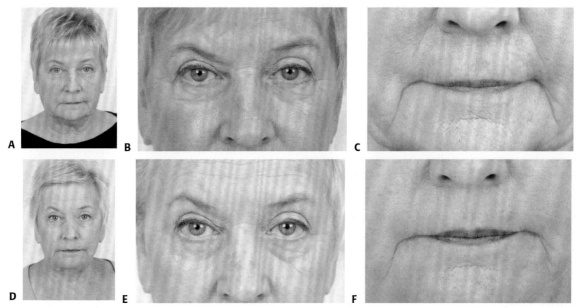

FIG 5 • A–C. Preoperative patient photos. **D–F.** Six months after bilateral rhytidectomy with extended SMAS and perioral phenol-croton oil peel and fat injections to the cheeks and nasolabial folds. Phenol peel to perioral area using 33% phenol and 1.1% croton oil.

COMPLICATIONS

- Complications following intermediate depth phenol-croton oil peeling are primarily of four types: preoperative, intraoperative, early postoperative, and late postoperative.[16]
- Preoperative:
  - Poor history—patients on Accutane, electrolysis, or previous peels
  - Lack of pretreatment of dark-skinned individuals
- Intraoperative:
  - Cardiac arrhythmias have been reported, but no cause and effect relationship has been established. Patient's cardiac status should be monitored during the procedure, and the peel duration needs to be extended over 1 to 1.5 hours.

- Peeling too deeply—failing to recognize the signs of the depth of peel.
- Segmental peeling in the area of the face results in splotchy appearance.
- Early postoperative:
  - Infection—bacterial, fungal, and viral: While bacterial infections from *Staphylococcus* and *Streptococcus* species are more common, infections from *Pseudomonas* species, mycobacteria, and fungi are rare. There has been no literature detailing the need for prophylaxis antibiotics. The characteristic of an infection is significant pain in the postoperative period.

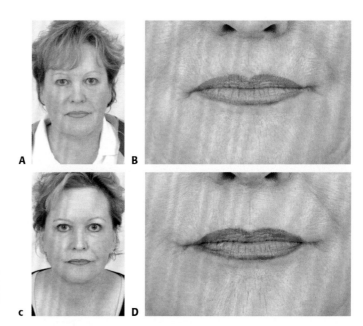

FIG 6 • A,B. Preoperative patient photos. **C,D.** Six months after bilateral rhytidectomy with extended SMAS and perioral phenol-croton oil peel and fat injections to the cheeks and nasolabial folds. Phenol peel to perioral area used 33% phenol and 1.1% croton oil.

- Late postoperative:
  - Milia, or benign, keratin-filled cysts that tend to occur around the periorbital area may occur 3 weeks after the peel. Milia can be physically extracted but also respond well to topical vitamin A derivatives, which also help to prevent future outbreaks.
  - Acneform eruptions, or tender, erythematous follicular popular, may occur as a result of the emollients or ointments being used for postoperative care. These can be treated with a topical antibiotic (eg, clindamycin, erythromycin, or systemic tetracycline and erythromycin therapy) and take approximately 5 to 10 days to clear.
  - Hyperpigmentation develops 4 weeks after the procedure. Hypopigmentation is a late complication and gets progressively worse. While hyperpigmentation can be treated with topical bleaching agents (eg, 4% hydroquinone) or topical steroids, there is no effective treatment for hypopigmentation.
  - Prolonged erythema may take between 3 to 6 months to resolve completely. This occurs most frequently in Fitzpatrick I patients.
  - Hypertrophic scars may result from delayed wound healing. Early postoperative redness, induration delineates an incipient hypertrophic scar. This is treated with dilute intralesional triamcinolone injections (5 mg/cc).

ACKNOWLEDGMENT

The authors thank Sonia Havale for her contribution to the preparation of this chapter.

REFERENCES

1. Fischer TC, Perosino E. Chemical peels in aesthetic dermatology: an update 2009. *J Eur Acad Dermatol Venereol*. 2010;24:281-292.
2. Larson DL, Karmo F. Phenol-croton oil peel: establishing an animal model for scientific investigation. *Aesthet Surg J*. 2009;29: 47-53.
3. Hetter GP. An examination of the phenol-croton oil peel. Part I. Dissecting the formula. *Plast Reconstr Surg*. 2000;105(1):227-239.
4. Hetter GP. An examination of the phenol-croton oil peel. Part IV. Face peel results with different concentrations of phenol and croton oil. *Plast Reconstr Surg*. 2000;105(3):1061-1083.
5. Landau M. Cardiac complications in deep chemical peels. *Dermatol Surg*. 2007;33:190-193.
6. Stone PA, Lefer LG. Modified phenol chemical face peels: recognizing the role of application technique. *Facial Plast Surg Clin North Am*. 2001;9(3):351-376.
7. Monheit GD, Chastain MA. Chemical peels. *Facial Plast Surg Clin North Am*. 2001;9(2):239-255.
8. Stuzin JM, Baker TJ, Gordon HL. Chemical peel: a change in the routine. *Ann Plast Surg*. 1989;23(2):166-169. http://www.ncbi.nlm.nih.gov/pubmed/2774443. Accessed August 1, 2016.
9. Caisey L, Gubanova E, Camus C, et al. Influence of age and hormone replacement therapy on the functional properties of the lips. *Skin Res Technol*. 2008;14(2):220-225.
10. Laporta R, Mercer N. Quid causit perioral wrinkles? *J Plast Reconstr Aesthet Surg*. 2013;66(4):579-581.
11. Kane M. The functional anatomy of the face as it applies to rejuvenation via chemodenervation. *Facial Plast Surg*. 2005;21(1): 55-64.
12. Paes EC, Teepen HJ, Koop WA, Kon M. Perioral wrinkles: histologic differences between men and women. *Aesthet Surg J*. 2009;29(6):467-472.
13. Chien AI, Cheng N. Perioral wrinkles are associated with female gender, aging, and smoking: development of a gender-specfic photonumeric scale. *J Am Acad Dermatol*. 2016;74(5):924-930.
14. Fitzpatrick TB. The validity and practicality of sun-reactive skin types I through VI. *Arch Dermatol*. 1988;124:869-871.
15. Glogau RG. Aesthetic and anatomic analysis of the aging skin. *Semin Cutan Med Surg*. 1996;15:134-138.
16. Ozturk CN, Huettner F. Outcomes assessment of combination of face and perioral phenol-croton oil peel. *Plast Reconstr Surg*. 2013;132:743e.

Techniques for Dermabrasion to the Face

Steven M. Levine and Daniel C. Baker

DEFINITION

- Surgery is the standard to address descent and laxity in the aging face.
- Resurfacing is important to treat textural and other surface changes related to aging and environmental damage.
- Dermabrasion is a highly effective, reliable, and low-cost method to facial resurfacing.
- It is particularly useful for vertical perioral rhytides.

ANATOMY

- Dermabrasion can be performed on the entire face and neck or can be isolated to specific aesthetic units such as the glabella or perioral region.
- The perimeter of any area being treated should be "feathered" to minimize the creation of a transition between dermabraded and nondermabraded tissue.

PATIENT HISTORY AND PHYSICAL FINDINGS

- Indications for dermabrasion are broad and can include desire to improve skin texture, reduce visible fine lines, or reduction in age spots (such as solar keratosis).
- It is important to elicit a history of oral herpes so that these patients can be pretreated with antiviral medication.
- Skin type is important to note.

SURGICAL MANAGEMENT

- Dermabrasion can be performed as a stand-alone procedure or in combination with a face and necklift.

Preoperative Planning

- The primary consideration for preoperative planning is the patient's skin tone. The more pigmentation in the skin, the higher the chance for postdermabrasion complications such as postinflammatory hyperpigmentation or areas of hypopigmentation.
- Some providers choose to pretreat patients with a retinol or bleaching agent for 4 to 6 weeks prior to dermabrasion.
  - The authors do not use pretreatment.
- A marker is used preoperatively to stain the fine lines for which the dermabrasion is targeting.

Positioning

- The patient is supine on the procedure table.
- Usually the head of bed is slightly elevated.
- The provider should be sitting for maximum stability.

Approach

- The approach can be accomplished using a variety of techniques that yield a controlled, reproducible distribution of mechanical resurfacing to the skin.

■ Mechanical Dermabrasion

- The patient's face is cleaned with alcohol.
- Marker was used to reinforce any marks that were removed during the prep. All rhytides to be addressed should be colored in marker.
- A small amount (0.1 cc for entire upper lip) of 1% lidocaine with epinephrine is injected into the dermis of the areas to be dermabraded.
- Eight minutes is allowed to pass to obtain full effect of the epinephrine.
- Choose the dermabrasion tip that you feel most comfortable within a specific area.
  - The authors use the bullet tip for areas above the lip and the barrel for larger areas like below the lip (**TECH FIG 1**).

- You can effectively dermabrade at a variety of speeds.
  - Start slow (5000–10 000 rpm and advance to 25 000 rpm).
- The key to dermabrasion is to keep the skin on tension and is accomplished with the nondominant hand.
  - Do not attempt to dermabrade an area that is not under tension.
- The end point is a combination of pinpoint bleeding and visualization of the rhytide effacement. The ideal goal is to completely efface the targeted rhytide before dermabrading too deep and damaging the melanocytes.
- Care is taken to "feather" the borders of any anatomic area that means reducing the depth of the dermabrasion to reduce the appearance of a transition zone.

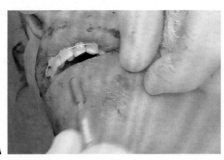 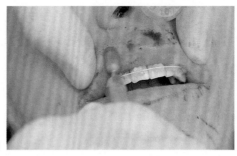

TECH FIG 1 • A. Dermabrasion tips include a barrel for larger areas. **B.** Note the nondominant hand applying tension to the skin under the dermabrasion tip.

PEARLS AND PITFALLS

Skin tension is paramount	■ Always place skin on tension prior to dermabrasion. This may include place a hand intraoral to accommodate tension around the mouth.
Keep moving	■ Keep the dermabrader moving to avoid getting too deep in any area.
Safely combine procedures	■ Dermabrasion is a an excellent adjunct to a facial surgery procedure.
Feathering	■ Always extend the treatment beyond the zone being treated (ie, beneath the jaw line if treating the full face).
Practice	■ Consider using an orange or grapefruit to practice your technique.

POSTOPERATIVE CARE

- This procedure is often combined with a facelift. In this case, the dermabrasion should be performed after the facelift.
- A petroleum impregnated gauze is applied to the dermabraded areas immediately after the procedure.
- Cool packs are also used to reduce swelling.
- Patients are instructed to remain away from the sun during the acute peeling period (7–10 days postop).
- Sun avoidance should ideally be carried out for several months after dermabrasion.
- Patients are instructed to use cool compressed at home for the first 24 hours.
- Patients should keep the gauze in place for several days. As the skin re-epithelializes, the gauze will fall off. When it does, patients should apply a thin layer of petroleum-based ointment 3 times daily until the skin is re-epithelialized.

OUTCOMES

- Dermabrasion will predictably improve certain fine lines and reduce the appearance of certain superficial pigmentation issues.

- The provider needs to start using this technique in a metered fashion to gain comfort with expectations and limitations.

COMPLICATIONS

- It is important to be aware of the entire surgical field.
  - Often a gauze is near the field to aid the provider in wiping blood from the operative field. This gauze can easily get caught in the dermabrader and whip around and hit the patient's face or eye.
- Overly aggressive dermabrasion can damage melanocytes and lead to areas of hyperpigmentation. Sometimes, this can reverse, but often it is permanent.
- Hyperpigmentation can occur which usually resolves on its own. Sun avoidance is paramount. Lightening agents such as hydroquinone 4% topical can be used if necessary.

Section VII: Brow Lifting

Indications and Techniques for Coronal Brow Lifting

Richard J. Warren

20

CHAPTER

DEFINITION

- Brow ptosis describes an abnormally low position of the eyebrow complex, either in whole or in part.
- Low lying or malpositioned eyebrows may be congenital or acquired through aging.
- Brow position and shape convey an impression of emotion. When the entire brow is low, the patient looks tired. When only the medial brow is low, the patient appears to be angry, and when only the lateral brow is low, the patient appears to be sad.[1]
- Brow ptosis encroaches on the upper lid sulcus, changing the dynamics of the upper lid/brow junction. Thus, brow ptosis will affect the assessment of patients presenting for blepharoplasty, periorbital fat grafting, or senile eyelid ptosis repair.

ANATOMY

- Underlying the forehead is the frontal bone. Laterally, the frontal bone is crossed by a curved ridge called the temporal crest (temporal ridge or temporal fusion line). This palpable landmark separates the forehead from the temporal fossa laterally (**FIG 1**). The temporalis muscle takes its origin from the temporal fossa.

- The surgical significance of the temporal crest line is that overlying fascial layers are tethered to bone in a band immediately medial to the palpable ridge. This has been called the zone of fixation or the zone of adhesion.[2,3] Inferiorly, where the ridge approaches the orbital rim, the fixation becomes broader and denser, forming the orbital ligament, also known as the temporal ligamentous adhesion. Regardless of the surgical technique used, when a full-thickness forehead flap is mobilized, all fascial attachments to bone must be released, including the zone of adhesion and the orbital ligament, plus attachments to the supraorbital rim and lateral orbital rim.[4]
- The temporal crest also marks a change in nomenclature as tissue planes transition from lateral to medial. The deep temporal fascia covers the temporalis muscle and is attached to bone along the temporal crest. It then continues medially as the periosteum of the frontal bone. Similarly, the superficial temporal fascia (also known as the temporal-parietal fascia) continues medially as the galea aponeurotica.
- The galea aponeurotica splits into a superficial and a deep layer to encompass the frontalis muscle. Inferiorly, the deep galea layer separates further into three separate layers: two layers encompass the galeal fat pad, and a third layer is adherent to periosteum.[2] Superficial to the deepest galeal

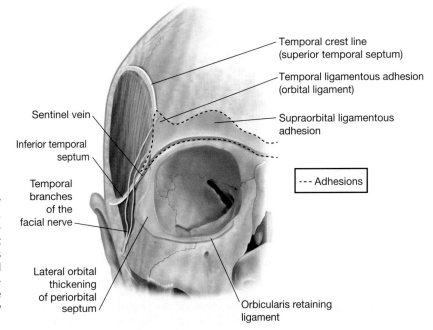

FIG 1 • Galeal attachments must be completely released to allow a forehead flap to move superiorly. The firmest attachment is at the temporal ligamentous adhesion (orbital ligament) but is also present along the supraorbital rim (supraorbital ligamentous adhesion), down the lateral orbital rim (lateral orbital thickening) and along the temporal crest line. In raising the flap, the temporal branches of the facial nerve will be in the roof of the dissection immediately above the medial zygomatic vein (sentinel vein).

Temporal crest line
(superior temporal septum)

Temporal ligamentous adhesion
(orbital ligament)

Supraorbital ligamentous
adhesion

Sentinel vein

Inferior temporal
septum

Temporal
branches
of the
facial nerve

Lateral orbital
thickening
of periorbital
septum

--- Adhesions

Orbicularis retaining
ligament

layer is the so-called glide plane space, which allows the scalp flap to shift superiorly.

- The galeal fat pad extends across the entire width of the lower 2 cm of the forehead; medially it encompasses the supratrochlear nerves and much of the corrugator musculature. The galeal fat pad is separated from the preseptal fat (retro-orbicularis oculi fat or ROOF) by one of the layers of galea (see above). Laterally, this galeal layer is thought to be inconsistent, with some individuals having continuity between the galeal fat pad and the preseptal fat (ROOF). Within the eyelid, the septum orbitale divides the preseptal fat (ROOF) from orbital fat.
- Muscle anatomy plays a significant role in determining eyebrow shape and position. In addition to the soft tissue attachments, the level of the eyebrow is the result of a balance between the muscular forces that elevate the brow, the muscular forces that depress the brow, and gravity.
- Brow depressors in the glabella originate from bone and insert into soft tissue. The procerus runs vertically near the midline, the depressor supercilii and supramedial orbicularis run obliquely, and the corrugator supercilii runs mostly transversely.
- The transverse corrugator supercilii is the largest and most significant of these muscles. Useful landmarks to locate the corrugator are as follows: the corrugator originates from the orbital rim at its most superomedial corner, right at the entrance to the orbit. The transverse head passes through galeal fat becoming more superficial until it interdigitates with the orbicularis and frontalis under a skin dimple that is visible when the patient frowns.
- The orbicularis encircles the orbit acting like a sphincter. Medially and laterally, the orbicularis fibers run vertically and act to depress brow level. Laterally, orbicularis is the only muscle that depresses brow position.
- The frontalis is the only elevator of the brow. It originates from the galea aponeurotica superiorly and interdigitates inferiorly with the orbicularis. Contraction raises this muscle mass and the overlying eyebrow, which is a cutaneous structure. The muscle is deficient laterally, so its primary lifting effect is on the medial and central portions of the eyebrow.

Sensory Nerves

- Innervation to the upper periorbita is supplied by the supraorbita and supratrochlear nerves, as well as two lesser nerves, the infratrochlear and zygomaticotemporal.
- The zygomaticotemporal nerve exits posterior to the lateral orbital rim piercing the deep temporal fascia just inferior to the sentinel vein. In coronal brow lifting, with complete release of the lateral orbital rim, it is often avulsed. Consequences of this are minimal and temporary.
- The supratrochlear nerve usually exits the orbit superomedially, although the exact location is variable. It immediately divides into four to six branches that usually pass through the substance of the corrugator. These branches then travel superiorly, on the superficial surface of the frontalis, innervating the central forehead and first few centimeters of the scalp.
- The supraorbital nerve exits the superior orbit through a notch in the rim, or about 10% of the time, through a foramen that is superior to the rim.
- The supraorbital nerve divides into two segments: superficial and deep. The superficial branch pierces orbicularis and frontalis, traveling as several small branches on the superficial surface of the frontalis to innervate the central forehead as far posteriorly as the first 2 cm of hair. The rest of the scalp, as far back as the vertex, is innervated by the

deep branch that runs between the periosteum and the deepest layer of galea and then pierces the frontalis near the hairline to innervate scalp skin.[5]

Motor Nerves

- The temporal branch of the facial nerve is the only motor nerve of surgical concern in this area. The temporal branch enters the temporal fossa as several (2–4) fine branches that lie on the periosteum of the zygomatic arch in its middle third. Between 1.5 and 3.0 cm above the arch, these branches become more superficial, traveling within the superficial temporal fascia (temporoparietal fascia) to innervate the frontalis, superior orbicularis, and glabellar muscles.[6] A number of different landmarks can be used to predict the course of the temporal branches. These include
  - The middle third of the palpable zygomatic arch
  - 1.5 cm lateral to the tail of the eyebrow
  - Parallel and adjacent to the inferior temporal septum
  - Immediately superior to the medial zygomaticotemporal vein (sentinel vein)
- In the coronal brow lift procedure, the dissection should be entirely deep to the temporal branches of the facial nerve.

PATHOGENESIS

- The periorbital region is the most expressive part of the human face. Subtle changes in eyebrow shape can profoundly affect facial appearance.[1]
- Because of the importance of periorbital expression, humans have historically resorted to any means at their disposal to alter their eyebrows. These have included eyebrow plucking and shaving, makeup, and tattoos.
- Aesthetically, the eyebrow is only one part of the puzzle in the periorbital zone. Other variables include the presence of senile eyelid ptosis, the loss of upper sulcus orbital fat, and the accumulation excess of upper eyelid soft tissue (skin, orbicularis muscle, and orbital fat).
- The preferred forehead will be devoid of vertical of transverse lines. It will be framed superiorly by a well-positioned aesthetically shaped hairline and inferiorly by well-positioned, attractively shaped eyebrows.
- The "ideal" eyebrow shape is affected by ethnicity, gender, and the era in which we live (**FIG 2**). There are certain themes that define aesthetically pleasing eyebrow in the 21st century:[7]
  - The medial eyebrow level should lie over the medial orbital rim.
  - The medial border of the eyebrow should be vertically in line with the medial canthus.
  - The eyebrow should rise gently, peaking slightly at least two-thirds of the way to its lateral end; typically, this peak lies vertically above or lateral to the lateral limbus.
  - The lateral tail of the brow should be higher than the medial end.
  - The male brow should be lower and less peaked.
- Abnormally low eyebrows can be congenital or acquired over time through aging.
- Age-related brow ptosis causes the forehead/eyebrow complex to encroach on the upper orbit, resulting in a pseudoexcess of upper eyelid skin. In response, patients subconsciously contract the frontalis to raise the eyebrows, leading to transverse forehead lines. This is accentuated with the presence of mild senile eyelid ptosis. Such patients will often present with a request for upper lid blepharoplasty.

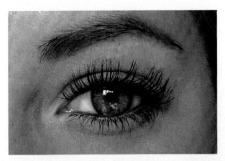

FIG 2 • The attractive eye exhibits a modest amount of visible upper lid ("tarsal show"); this dimension is about one-third of the distance from the lash line to the lower border of the eyebrow. The brow itself starts medially over the supraorbital rim and vertically in line with the medial canthus. It angles gently upward, peaking about two-thirds of the way along the brow toward its lateral extent. In females, this peak is at or lateral to the lateral limbus of the eye. In men, this peak is minimal or absent. Laterally, the "tail" of the brow should end at a higher point than the medial end of the brow.

- Other lines in the forehead are caused by the glabellar frown muscles. Vertical lines are caused by the transversely oriented corrugator, horizontal lines are caused the vertically running procerus, and oblique lines are caused by the depressor supercilii and orbicularis.
- Age-related brow ptosis is not universal. Up to 40% of people have relatively stable eyebrow position throughout life and are generally not candidates for brow lift surgery.[8]
- Frontalis is the only lifting force to counter balance the various muscles and gravity that depress the brow level. The lateral portion of the eyebrow is particularly sensitive to this interplay because frontalis action is attenuated laterally and also because the security of lateral brow fixation to bone is inconsistent.[9,10] Poor soft tissue attachment with no muscular lift will inevitably lead to ptosis of the lateral third of the eyebrow.

PATIENT HISTORY AND PHYSICAL FINDINGS

- Most patients will not be aware of the many factors involved in periorbital aging, and they may not want the multiple procedures required to treat all of these components. For that reason, identifying the main component of every patient's periorbital aging is important. Old photographs are very helpful in helping the surgeon determine which age-related changes predominate.
- Assessment is done with the patient awake and upright in the sitting or standing position. The following issues are evaluated: visual acuity, eyebrow and orbital symmetry, position of anterior hairline, thickness of scalp hair, transverse forehead lines, glabellar frown lines, thickness of eyebrow hair, eyebrow height, axis of the eyebrow (downward or upward lateral tilt), shape of the eyebrow (flat or peaked), passive and active eyebrow mobility, and the presence of old scars or tattoos. The upper eyelids should also be assessed for soft tissue redundancy, for upper sulcus hollowing, and for eyelid level (ptosis or lid retraction).
- To identify patients with chronic frontalis contraction, examination should be done with eyes open and eyes closed. When the eyes are closed, the frontalis can be made to relax, revealing the true position and shape of the eyebrows. If the eyebrows are forcibly held in this position when the patient opens their eyes, the eyebrow-eyelid relationship without frontalis effect will be revealed.

- A patient may be a candidate to have the entire brow complex lifted or more commonly to have only part of the eyebrow raised, thus improving eyebrow shape. Occasionally, in a patient who chronically looks angry, this may involve raising the medial brow only, but most commonly, it is the lateral third to one-half of the eyebrow that requires repositioning with little or no lift of the medial portion.
- Weakening or eliminating the glabellar frown musculature is a useful parallel objective.
- If brow lifting is contemplated, the effect on the upper eyelid complex must be considered. Previous upper lid blepharoplasty may have left a patient tissue deficient, so that brow lifting could impair eyelid closure. Also, brow lifting may reveal the previously unappreciated hollowing of the upper lid sulcus.

NONOPERATIVE MANAGEMENT

- Numerous nonoperative strategies are available to change eyebrow shape and/or position.
- Nonmedical: eyebrow plucking, cosmetic makeup, tattooing
- Medical, nonsurgical: botulinum toxin injection, synthetic filler injection, thread lifting
- Surgical, non-brow lift: transpalpebral frown muscle ablation

SURGICAL MANAGEMENT

Preoperative Planning

- There are many surgical techniques available to elevate or to reshape the eyebrow. The coronal approach is a traditional method with a long track record of proven results.[11,12]
- The preoperative discussion is an excellent time for the surgeon to teach the patient about periorbital aging. To achieve the patient's objectives, some concepts that are new to the patient may be introduced. A patient requesting brow rejuvenation surgery may also be a candidate for blepharoplasty, upper sulcus fat grafting, or eyelid ptosis repair.
- This procedure provides maximum visibility and flexibility. Therefore, during the planning process, the surgeon should develop a mental image of what portion of the eyebrows are to be lifted, how much lift is required, and if there is any brow asymmetry to be corrected.
- With the patient awake and in the upright position, with the forehead in repose, the desired amount and direction of eyebrow elevation are assessed by manually elevating the brow complex (**FIG 3**). Specific vectors have been described, but more artistic decision-making is preferred.

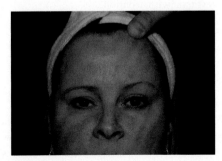

FIG 3 • With the frontalis muscle in repose, the desired amount and direction of eyebrow elevation are estimated by manually elevating the brow complex. The desired vector of lift can also be determined using this method.

- Essential preoperative markings include the incision and the vectors for flap mobilization.
- Ancillary markings that are useful include the expected course of the temporal branch of the facial nerve, the expected location of the supraorbital and supratrochlear nerves, and the location of the frown muscles (determined with the patient awake and frowning).

Positioning

- The patient is placed on the operating table in the supine position with the head on a small pillow or soft donut.
- The head of the bead is raised slightly to help reduce venous engorgement in the surgical area.
- Intermittent compression devices are applied to the legs, and a heating device covers the patient.

Approach

- Possible approaches for an open brow lift are
  - Coronal incision
  - Anterior hairline incision
  - Combination of these two (modified coronal) (**FIG 4**)
- Possible planes of dissection are
  - Subcutaneous
  - Subgaleal
  - Subperiosteal
- The coronal incision is well hidden in the hair of the scalp. There are two options for the dissection plane: subgaleal or subperiosteal. Of the two, the subgaleal approach is most often used because it provides a rapid bloodless plane of dissection with excellent exposure of the frown musculature.
- The anterior hairline incision puts the surgeon closer to the eyebrows and also provides excellent visibility. The main disadvantage of the anterior hairline incision is a potentially visible scar along the anterior hairline. Thoughtful incision techniques and careful suture techniques will mitigate this problem. There are three potential planes of dissection: subcutaneous, subgaleal, and subperiosteal. The subcutaneous plane offers some unique advantages: no transection of sensory nerves, the separation of skin from underlying frontalis,

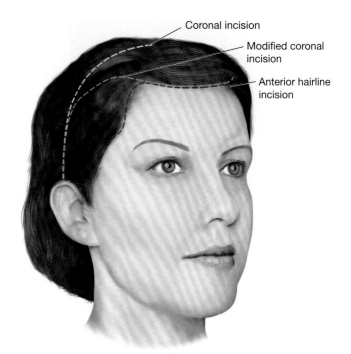

Coronal incision
Modified coronal incision
Anterior hairline incision

FIG 4 • Approaches for an open brow lift include the classic coronal incision, made about 6 cm behind the hairline, the anterior hairline incision, and a combination of the two—a modified version with an anterior hairline incision combined with a coronal-type approach laterally.

thus effacing transverse forehead lines and the direct shifting of the eyebrow, which is a cutaneous structure.[13]
- The modified coronal approach (anterior hairline approach with lateral incision placement like a coronal incision) is much like a coronal procedure but with a hairline incision used to avoid elevating the anterior hairline in patients with a high forehead. Like the coronal, this approach lends itself to the subgaleal plane, although it is technically straightforward to change planes at the anterior hairline, creating a subcutaneous plane deep to the forehead skin and a subgaleal plane laterally.

■ Coronal Brow Lift (Subgaleal Plane)

- Preoperative surgical marking will have been done (see above).
- The procedure is done under general anesthetic or local anesthetic with sedation.
- The head and neck area is prepped and draped with exposure of the entire face.
- A local anesthetic mixture composed of 1% lidocaine with 1:100 000 epinephrine and 0.25% bupivacaine with 1:200 000 epinephrine is infiltrated into the incision line, along the supra- and lateral orbital rims plus some injection under the scalp flap.
- After waiting for the epinephrine effect, the incision is made full thickness through the scalp down to periosteum over the skull centrally and laterally down to the deep temporal fascia. The scalpel is beveled parallel to the hair follicles. If an anterior hairline incision is planned, the scalpel is beveled in such a way that the hair follicles

will be partially transected, utilizing the Camirand principle[14] (**TECH FIG 1A**).
- The standard coronal incision is designed to be about 6 cm behind the hairline although this is variable, depending on the height of the forehead. Laterally, the marking extends to the ear and, in some cases, may be made in continuity with a facelift incision. The incision can be taken across the top of the head in a gentle curve, or it can peak slightly in the midline to allow for some flap rotation.
- With all coronal brow lift approaches, the superficial and deep branches of the supraorbital nerve will be transected, as will the anterior branch of the temporal artery, which will require hemostasis.
- The flap is easily raised in the subgaleal plane. This can be done with blunt dissection or with a scalpel blade beveled away from the periosteum (**TECH FIG 1B**). Lateral to the temporal crest, the superficial temporal fascia (temporoparietal fascia) is separated from the deep temporal

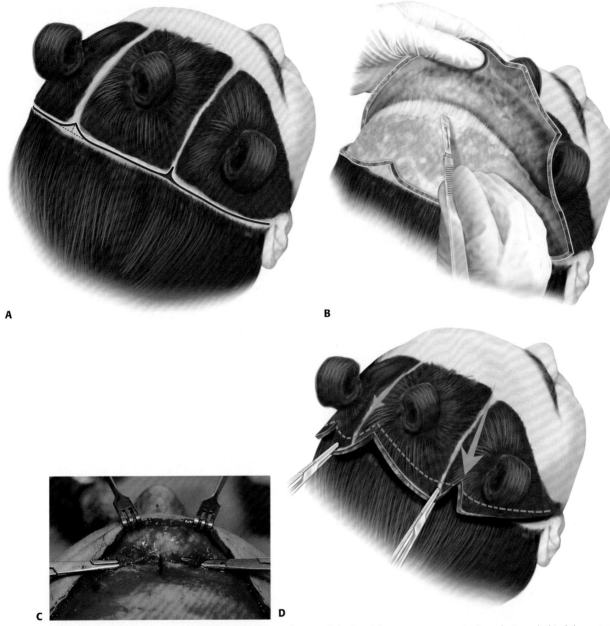

TECH FIG 1 • A. The standard coronal incision extends across the top of the head from ear to ear, approximately 6 cm behind the anterior hairline. Laterally, on either side, it can be curved forward to allow for greater flap mobility. It can also be designed to be contiguous with a facelift incision. **B.** The coronal flap is raised in the avascular subgaleal plane down to the orbital rim. Temporal facial nerve branches course within the flap laterally; cautery and traction in that area should be done cautiously. **C.** The corrugator muscles are demonstrated, taking their origin from the edge of the supramedial orbital rim. They can be seen coursing obliquely through galeal fat and become more superficial until they insert into the orbicularis/frontalis muscle mass at a skin dimple that can be seen when a patient frowns. The *purple line* marks the midline. The two procerus muscles can be seen coursing vertically from the origin on the nasal bones. Behind the tips of the clamps are vertically running fibers—the depressor supercilii muscles. **D.** Once the flap has been released from its deep attachments, it is mobilized along preplanned vectors. Normally, most of the flap advancement is done laterally, with typically 2 to 3 cm of scalp being excised. Centrally, the excision will be less than half that. After ablation of frown musculature, in the presence of an intact frontalis muscle, the medial brow will rise naturally without the need for tension on the scalp flap.

fascia. Along the zone of adhesion, just medial to the temporal crest line, soft tissue attachment to bone is released.

- In approaching the supraorbital rim, care is taken to look for the supraorbital nerve, which in 10% of cases will exit the skull through a foramen above (superior to) the supraorbital rim. Traction on the flap with skin

hooks and elevation with L-shaped retractors are useful maneuvers, but care should be taken to avoid traction damage to the temporal branches of the facial nerve that travel laterally within the flap.

- Complete release of the galeal attachment to the supraorbital and lateral orbital rims is necessary to achieve enough flap mobilization to create lasting brow elevation.

The most adherent zone is the region of the orbital ligament (temporal ligamentous adhesion). Adequate galeal release along the supraorbital rim is confirmed when retro-orbicularis fat (ROOF) is observed.

- Release of attachments to the lateral orbital rim should continue inferiorly as far as the level of the lateral canthus. When this dissection is done as an extension of the subgaleal plane, the periosteum will remain intact. The medial zygomaticotemporal vein (sentinel vein) is routinely encountered and can either be preserved or, to ensure better access, cauterized. Cautery should be done carefully due to the presence of the temporal facial nerve branches running in the flap above this vein.
- In the midline, in most cases, it is prudent to leave some attachment of the deepest galea to the periosteum. This will guard against excessive medial brow elevation. Conversely, in those cases where medial brow elevation is desired, this area should be released.
- Once the flap has been freed from the orbital rims, the corrugator supercilii is identified within the galeal fat (**TECH FIG 1C**). The muscle is removed in a piecemeal fashion from its medial origin to the supraorbital nerve laterally. In removing this muscle, branches of the supratrochlear nerve are encountered coursing through the substance of the corrugator. These are small branches accompanied by small vessels that may require cauterization; loupe magnification is therefore helpful.
- Depending on the preoperative findings, the paired procerus muscles and the vertically running depressor supercilii can also be removed, although this will be a partial, not a complete, removal.
- Removal of a large corrugator muscle can create a soft tissue deficiency; if so, a small fat graft is harvested elsewhere and sutured into the soft tissue defect.

- After muscle modification and flap mobilization are complete, the flap is then drawn superiorly along the pre-planned vectors. In most cases, the primary objective is to elevate the lateral half of the eyebrow with less (or no) elevation of the medial half. The desired flap overlap is normally maximal in a vector along the temporal crest line. Every case is individualized. Internal fixation may be done by suturing the advancing superficial temporal fascia down to the underlying deep temporal fascia at a higher level than it previously had been. This suturing should be done superior to the expected course of the temporal facial nerve branches. Typically, 3-0 PDS suture is used for this fixation.
- The scalp flap is advanced superiorly over the cut edge of the original scalp incision. To line up the flap, three short radial incisions made, and temporary key sutures are placed—centrally and along the temporal crest line bilaterally. Excess full-thickness flap is removed: typically about 2 cm of scalp flap laterally and 1 cm or less centrally (**TECH FIG 1D**).
- Repair of the scalp incision is done with absorbing stitches (3-0 Vicryl) in the galea and staples or interrupted sutures in the scalp. In the coronal brow lift technique, brow elevation depends on flap advancement and scalp removal. Consequently, some tension on the closure is inevitable, and the galeal sutures should bear the brunt of this. If scalp sutures or staples are excessively tight, hair follicles will be permanently damaged.
- In more vascular cases, a suction drain is put in place prior to suturing of the flap.
- A bupicaine block is done across the supraorbital rim, targeting the supratrochlear and supraorbital nerves.
- The head may be treated by exposing it with ointment along the suture line or be wrapping the head with a light head dressing.

■ Anterior Hairline Brow Lift (Subcutaneous Plane)

- Preoperative surgical marking will have been done (see above).
- The procedure is done under general anesthetic or local anesthetic with sedation.
- The head and neck area is prepped and draped with exposure of the entire face.
- A local anesthetic mixture composed of 1% lidocaine with 1:100 000 epinephrine and 0.25% bupivacaine with 1:200 000 epinephrine is infiltrated along the anterior hairline, and in an effort to hydro dissect the skin flap, the skin is infiltrated over the entire forehead in the subcutaneous plane, down to the eyebrows.
- After waiting for the epinephrine effect, the incision is made through the scalp skin, down to the frontalis muscle, taking care to preserve the sensory nerves, which will be seen running on the superficial surface of the frontalis.
- In making the anterior hairline incision, the scalpel is beveled in such a way that the hair follicles will be partially transected.[14]
- The skin flap is raised off the underlying frontalis muscle as far as the eyebrows and one-third of the way down the

lateral orbital rim. Hemostasis is an important aspect of dealing with this somewhat vascular plane of dissection.

- When the eyebrow is approached, under direct vision, the transverse running fibers of the orbicularis are identified.
- A 5-0 Vicryl or similar suture can be used to pexy the orbicularis to a higher point on the frontalis muscle, using two or three sutures for this purpose. Others have described progressive tension sutures from the underside of the flap down to the frontalis muscle.[15]
- The subcutaneous scalp flap is then advanced superiorly over cut edge of the original scalp incision. This is done with minimal tension but still with enough tension to cause the undermined flap to advance superiorly over cut edge of the scalp incision.
- The degree of overlap is marked, and excess forehead skin is removed from the inferior (undermined) side of the incision.
- Repair of the scalp incision is meticulously done with 5-0 nylon sutures.
- A bupivacaine block is done across the supraorbital rim, targeting the supratrochlear and supraorbital nerves.
- A light forehead dressing can be applied, or alternatively the incision is open with ointment applied along the suture line.

◼ Brow Lowering Procedure (Subgaleal Plane)

- The high hairline in conjunction with a long forehead can be a congenital condition, or it may be acquired through hair loss in the frontal hairline.
- The high hairline can be lowered and the long forehead shorted by advancing the hair-baring scalp and excising a portion of the upper forehead skin.[16]
- Preoperative markings delineate an incision at the anterior hairline and then coursing laterally into the temple and then into the temple (see **FIG 4** above).
- Anterior hairline incisions create less visible scars if the incision is wavy, not linear (**TECH FIG 2A**). Also, when very thin hair is present at the hairline, it is preferable to place the incision a few millimeters behind, into the zone of denser hair to hide the ultimate scar.
- The incision is made with a scalpel beveled in such a way as to transect some hair follicles, causing new hairs to grow through the resulting scar.
- Like the open coronal, the incision is carried down full thickness through scalp down to periosteum.
- Using blunt dissection or with a scalpel beveled away from the periosteum, a posterior dissection is done, raising the scalp flap as far posteriorly as the occiput.

- In order to advance the scalp flap anteriorly, shallow transverse releasing incisions are made into the galea, taking great care to not cut further into the flap. Clinical experience is that for every galeal releasing incision, expect about 1 mm of additional scalp advancement (**TECH FIG 2B**).
- Once the flap has been mobilized, gentle traction is applied for several minutes to allow for soft tissue creep.
- The anterior forehead flap is raised far enough to allow for the advancement of the posterior flap.
- After anterior advancement of the posterior scalp flap, it is fixed to bone, using 3-0 PDS (or equivalent) to some form of bony fixation such as LactoSorb bone tacks (**TECH FIG 2C**).
- The excess portion of the anterior forehead flap is excised (**TECH FIG 2D**).
- The incision is closed with absorbing sutures in the galea/frontalis plane (3-0 Vicryl) and fine sutures in the skin (running 5-0 nylon).
- Occasionally a patient may present with a high hairline in conjunction with low eyebrows. In such a case, through the anterior hairline incision, two procedures can be done at once: posterior scalp advancement (to lower the hairline) and an open brow lift (to raise and reshape the eyebrows).

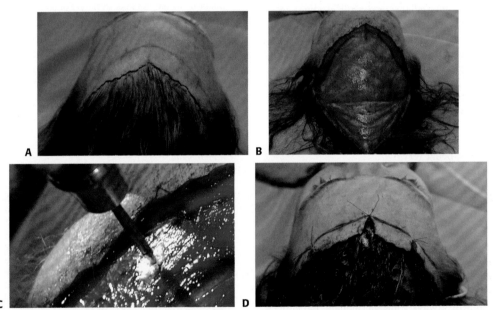

TECH FIG 2 • **A.** A slightly wavy line is used for the anterior hairline incision. It is placed a few hairs behind the hairline, and hair follicles are transected to encourage new hair growth through the scar. **B.** The scalp has been raised posteriorly to the occiput, and to improve its anterior mobility, multiple transverse releasing incisions have been made in the galea. **C.** To hold the advancing flap as far forward as possible, two points of bony fixation are used on either side of the midline at the leading edge of the flap. In this case, a dissolving bone tack is being used and is placed just posterior to the anticipated new location of the new hairline in order that the device will be hidden under hair-bearing scalp. **D.** After the scalp flap has been advanced anteriorly and fixed to bone, the excess forehead skin is excised.

PEARLS AND PITFALLS

Diagnosis	■ A preoperative aesthetic diagnosis is a vital step embarking on brow lift surgery. Variables that affect aesthetic decision-making include eyelid ptosis, excess upper lid soft tissue, or, conversely, deficient upper sulcus fat.
Eyebrow shape and height	■ Many patients have stable brow position throughout their lives and never develop brow ptosis. In patients whose brows become ptotic, it is lateral brow ptosis that usually predominates.
Technique	■ The elevated forehead through the coronal approach provides maximum visibility. Frown muscle ablation is easily accomplished, and the results of brow elevation are relatively predictable. ■ Sensory nerve transection during the coronal approach is inevitable. Patients should be warned of this in advance.
Closure	■ Excess suture tension on the scalp skin along the incision line can cause scar alopecia. Tension should be taken by the galeal sutures. ■ In most cases lateral brow elevation should exceed medial brow elevation.

POSTOPERATIVE CARE

■ Cold packs are applied to the upper third of the face, as required for comfort.

■ The patient is encouraged to keep the head elevated for the first week to decrease swelling.

■ A light dressing consisting of a head wrap is put in place.

■ Sutures are removed at 1 week postop.

OUTCOMES

■ An open coronal brow lift is relatively predictable. Complete relapse is uncommon, and the surgical result is long lasting.

■ This procedure affords unparalleled access for modification of frown musculature.

■ Unavoidable side effects are a long scar in the scalp, sensory nerve transection, and a posterior shift of the anterior hairline that lengthens the height of the forehead.

■ Unaesthetic overlifting of the central brow has historically been a problem, but with improved knowledge of forehead anatomy and the physiology of aging, this issue can be avoided.

■ In the end, after assessment at 18 to 24 months, patient satisfaction is reported as being very high.[11]

COMPLICATIONS

■ Unsatisfactory scar formation with scar alopecia can occur due to suture tension along the incision line. A systematic review identified this problem in 3.6% of cases.[17] Scar revision is usually successful.

■ Sensory nerve damage routinely occurs leading to dense scalp numbness initially. This recovers over time, but on testing, there is almost always some permanent paresthesia to part of the scalp. This is generally not a concern to patients after 18 to 24 months have passed.[12]

■ Hematoma is an uncommon complication at 0.5%.

■ Infection is uncommon at 0.2%

■ Motor nerve damage (temporal branch of the facial nerve) has rarely been reported with subgaleal coronal dissections.

■ The anterior hairline subcutaneous approach, when done in smokers, has led to a small incidence of partial skin necrosis in the forehead flap.[18]

REFERENCES

1. Knoll BI, Attkiss KJ, Persing JA. The influence of forehead, brow, and periorbital aesthetics of perceived expression in the youthful face. *Plast Reconstr Surg.* 2008;121:1793-1802.
2. Knize DM. An anatomically based study of the mechanism of eyebrow ptosis. *Plast Reconstr Surg.* 1996;97(7):1321-1333.
3. Warren RJ. The modified lateral brow lift. *Aesthet Surg J.* 2009;29(2):158-166.
4. O'Brien JX, Ashton MW, Rozen WM, et al. New perspectives on the surgical anatomy and nomenclature of the temporal region: literature review and dissection study. *Plast Reconstr Surg.* 2013;131(3):510-522.
5. Knize DM. A study of the supraorbital nerve. *Plast Reconstr Surg.* 1995;96:564.
6. Agarwa CA, Mendenhall MS, Foreman KB, et al. The course of the frontal branch of the facial nerve in relation to fascial planes: an anatomic study. *Plast Reconstr Surg.* 2010;125:532.
7. Gunter J, Antrobus S. Aesthetic analysis of the eyebrows. *Plast Reconstr Surg.* 1997;99:1808-1816.
8. Lambros V. Observations on periorbital and midface aging. *Plast Reconstr Surg.* 2007;120:1367-1376.
9. Lemke BN, Stasior OG. The anatomy of eyebrow optosis. *Arch Ophthalmol.* 1982;100:981.
10. Knize DM. Anatomic concepts for brow lift procedures. *Plast Reconstr Surg.* 2009;124(6):2118-2126.
11. Friedland JA, Jacobsen WM, TerKonda S. Safety and efficacy of combined upper blepharoplasties and open coronal browlift: a consecutive series of 600 patients. *Aesthetic Plast Surg.* 1996;20(6):453-462.
12. Cilento BW, Johnson CM Jr. The case for open forehead rejuvenation: a review of 1004 procedures. *Arch Facial Plast Surg.* 2009;11:13-17.
13. Ullmann Y, Levy Y. In favor of the subcutaneous forehead lift using the anterior hairline incision. *Aestheic Plast Surg.* 1998;22(5):332-337.
14. Camirand A, Doucet J. A comparison between parallel hairline incisions and perpendicular incisions when performing a face lift. *Plast Reconstr Surg.* 1997;99(1):10-15.
15. Pollock H, Pollock TA. Subcutaneous brow lift with precise suture fixation and advancement. *Aesthet Surg J.* 2007;27(4):388-395.
16. Guyuron B, Behmand RA, Green R. Shortening of the long forehead. *Plast Reconstr Surg.* 1999;103:218.
17. Byun S, Mukovozzov I, Farrokhyar F, Thoma A. Complications of brow-lift techniques: a systematic review. *Aesthet Surg J.* 2013;33(2):189-200.
18. Guyuron B, Davies B. Subcutaneous anterior hairline forehead rhytidectomy. *Aesthetic Plast Surg.* 1988;12:77-83.

Indications and Technique for Endoscopic Brow Lifting

Navid Pourtaheri, Ali Totonchi, and Bahman Guyuron

DEFINITION

- Age-related changes of the forehead include elongation of the forehead from a receding hairline and eyebrow ptosis, static and dynamic rhytides or frown lines, frontal bossing, glabellar flattening, and a misshapen eyebrow arch.
- An elongated forehead is defined as having an upper third of the face, hairline down to the glabella that is greater than approximately one-third of the vertical height of the face.

ANATOMY

- The forehead is the continuation of the scalp from the hairline to the eyebrows.
- The glabella, frontal sinuses, and frontal bone give the forehead its underlying contour.
- Overlying the bone, the soft tissue layers of the forehead, from deep to superficial, include the pericranium, loose areolar tissue, muscular layer (ie, frontalis muscle and galea aponeurosis), subcutaneous connective tissue and fat, dermis, and epidermis.
- Sensory nerves are supplied from supratrochlear and supraorbital nerves, emerging from the supraorbital rim at 1.7 and 2.5 cm from the midline, respectively, via a foramen or notch along with associated arteries.
- The paired frontalis muscles are brow elevators with vertically oriented fibers, and their attachments with the dermis give rise to horizontal rhytides of the forehead.
- Medial, intermediate, and lateral fibers of the frontalis are continuous with the procerus muscle, corrugator supercilii, and orbicularis oculi muscles, respectively.
- The procerus muscle is a brow depressor vertically oriented, originates from the periosteum over the nasal bones, and inserts into the frontalis muscle and the glabellar dermis which is responsible for rhytides at the root of the nose.
- The corrugator supercilii muscles are brow depressors obliquely oriented originating from the medial superciliary arch and passing through the orbicularis oculi muscle superolaterally inserting into the dermis of the brow and are responsible for vertical frown lines in the glabella.
- The paired depressor supercilii muscles are brow depressors originating from the medial orbital rim and inserting into the glabellar dermis and are responsible for oblique rhytides in the medial eyebrow area.
- The orbital portion of the orbicularis oculi muscle is a brow depressor (**FIG 1**).

PATHOGENESIS

- Recession of the upper hairline and temporal hairline increases the length and width of the forehead, respectively.
- Eyebrow ptosis occurs with age secondary to involutional changes of the facial soft tissues from thinning fat and dermis, collagen laxity, and aging. It is usually first seen in the lateral forehead and eyebrows because the frontalis muscle may compensate by elevating the medial two-thirds of the eyebrows. Brow ptosis may also occur due to blepharospasm from hyperactivity of the orbicularis oculi muscle or weakness of the facial nerve and frontalis muscle.
- Frontal bossing is typically due to hyperaeration of the frontal sinuses and less commonly due to soft tissue excess.

PATIENT HISTORY AND PHYSICAL FINDINGS

- A comprehensive analysis is recommended of the face, hairline, brow position and arch, forehead length, width, contour, soft tissue quality, and rhytides. A significantly elongated forehead is best rejuvenated with an open approach via a pretrichial incision to remove excess skin (discussed in another chapter). A useful method to analyze the brow position is to eliminate the compensation from the frontalis muscle by asking the patient to smile or close their eyes tightly and then open them just enough to see the examiner. The uncompensated position of the eyebrows is at the supraorbital rim in males or slightly above in females, with its apex at the lateral limbus of the eye.
- Then, rhytide evaluation is recommended in repose, smiling, and frowning. Deep static forehead rhytides are best treated with a subcutaneous approach rather than the endoscopic approach, whereas the fine rhytides are treated with laser resurfacing after endoscopic brow lift.

IMAGING

- Imaging is only warranted if there are contour abnormalities due to a soft tissue mass or underlying bony defect that must be evaluated and addressed prior to forehead rejuvenation.

NONOPERATIVE MANAGEMENT

- A combination of botulinum toxin injection, fillers, and fat grafting may be used to perform forehead rejuvenation nonoperatively.

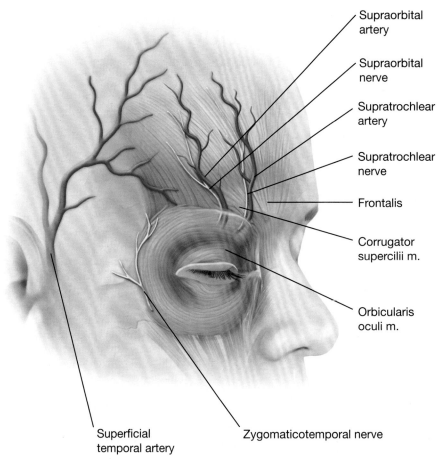

Supraorbital artery

Supraorbital nerve

Supratrochlear artery

Supratrochlear nerve

Frontalis

Corrugator supercilii m.

Orbicularis oculi m.

Superficial temporal artery

Zygomaticotemporal nerve

FIG 1 • Forehead anatomy. (Reprinted from Guyuron B. Forehead rejuvenation. In: Guyuron B, Eriksson E, Persing J, eds. *Plastic Surgery: Indications and Practice*. Philadelphia, PA: Saunders Elsevier, 2009:1409-1426, with permission from Elsevier.)

SURGICAL MANAGEMENT

- Endoscopic brow lift is indicated in patients with eyebrow ptosis and hyperactive forehead muscles without static deep horizontal forehead wrinkles or excess forehead length. This is done on an outpatient basis under intravenous sedation or general anesthesia. Compared to open technique, there is a smaller chance of hair loss or forehead elongation (commonly observed after a coronal incision), as well as improved visualization with magnification.
- Disadvantages of endoscopic rejuvenation include the need for specialized instruments and a learning curve due to operating while looking at a monitor with a two-dimensional view.

Preoperative Planning

- An AP photograph of the patient's forehead in repose and while furrowing the brow in a standardized fashion is recommended for analysis and postoperative comparison; any eyebrow asymmetry needs to be noted and addressed using differential eyebrow suspension during surgery.
- General medical conditions including hypertension and hyperglycemia, as well as smoking cessation, are best addressed prior to surgery to minimize wound-healing complications.

Positioning

- Surgery is done in supine position. After anesthesia/sedation and prepping and draping the patient, the marking is

started by marking a 1.2- to 1.5-cm incision on the midline from the hairline going posteriorly, followed by pairs of lateral incisions in the temple approximately 7 and 10 cm from the midline and 1.5 to 2 cm behind the hairline on either side. Each marking should be made vertically approximately 1.2 cm in length or 1.5 cm if the scalp is thick (**FIG 2**).

Approach

- This chapter explains the endoscopic approach of the brow lift. Open approaches are discussed in another chapter.

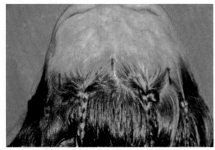

FIG 2 • Markings and hair braiding for endoscopic brow lift. (Reprinted from Guyuron B. Forehead rejuvenation. In: Guyuron B, Eriksson E, Persing J, eds. *Plastic Surgery: Indications and Practice*. Philadelphia, PA: Saunders Elsevier, 2009:1409-1426, with permission from Elsevier.)

■ Endoscopic Brow Dissection

- Following the positioning of the patient, the hair next to the incision line is either braided or clamped to prevent it from entering the incision.
- The non–hair-bearing forehead is injected with approximately 10 cc of 1% lidocaine with 1:100 000 units of epinephrine using a 27-gauge needle, and the hair-bearing scalp is injected caudally up to 7.5 cm behind the incision with approximately 10 cc of 1% lidocaine with only 1:200 000 units of epinephrine to minimize hair loss due to vasoconstriction.
- Five minutes after the injection, incisions are made using a no. 15 blade scalpel on the most lateral marking and then using a pair of baby Metzenbaum scissors, and the tissue is spread bluntly down to the deep temporal fascia.
- At this point, Obwegeser periosteal elevator is used to make a pocket above the deep and superficial temporal fascia to insert an endoscopic access device. To insert the access device, the inner shield is folded using a pair of large multitooth Adson forceps and with an assistant separating the wound margins using skin hooks, introducing the inner shield into the incision (**TECH FIG 1A**).
- A periosteal elevator is passed through the most lateral incision and advanced toward the adjacent temporal incision to dissect the tissues at the plane immediately superficial to the deep temporal fascia and frontal periosteum.
- Endoscopic access devices are inserted in the same fashion described before.
- Using a periosteal elevator, subperiosteal dissection is performed posterior to the incision in the hair-bearing area and lateral to the incision over the deep temporal fascia. Unlike posterior and lateral dissection that is performed blindly, the anterior dissection is performed with the assistance of an endoscope.

- A 30-degree 4-mm endoscope is used through the second access device on the right side, whereas the most lateral access device is used to control the dissector.
- Under endoscopic visualization, a periosteal elevator is introduced through the lateral temporal access device on the right, and dissection is continued inferiorly toward the supraorbital rim (**TECH FIG 1B**).
- To preserve the temporal branch of the facial nerve, it is important not to leave the plane of dissection from deep temporal fascia to more superficial layers. One practical point is to ensure that all fat cells over the deep temporal fascia are dissected off the deep temporal fascia and elevated with skin, subcutaneous, and deep layer of the deep temporal fascia until dissection reaches the zygomatic arch.
- At this point, using a longer periosteal elevator, soft tissue is separated from lateral orbital rim and zygomatic arch at subperiosteal plane (**TECH FIG 1C**).
  - Medial to the zone of adhesion of the temporal muscle, dissection is carried subperiosteally to the supraorbital rim where the supraorbital and supratrochlear nerves and vessels are identified after making a cut over the periosteum of the supraorbital rim.
  - The corrugator supercilii muscle is grasped and carefully avulsed using Daniel grasper or punch biopsy forceps.
  - Muscles need to be removed as thoroughly as possible to minimize the dynamic asymmetry and deformity of the area postoperatively. The corrugator muscle lies superficial to a communicating vein between the supratrochlear and supraorbital veins—this vein is cauterized using suction Bovie cautery. Bovie nerve hooks can be used to retract and prevent injury to the supraorbital and supratrochlear nerves during corrugator myectomy. The depressor supercilii can be

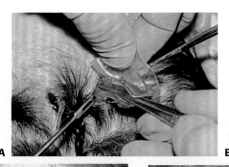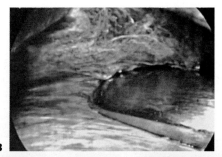
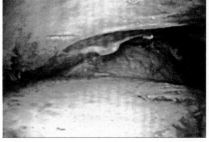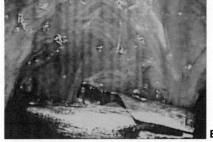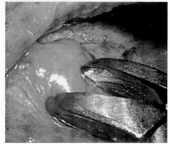

TECH FIG 1 • **A.** Endoscopic access device insertion into the temple. **B.** Endoscopic dissection is performed using a periosteal elevator in a plane superficial to the deep temporalis fascia in the temple and subperiosteal over the medial forehead. **C.** Release of the arcus marginalis and fibrous attachments of the eyebrow using a periosteal elevator. **D.** Resection of the corrugator supercilii using a grasper. **E.** A fat graft is harvested to replace the volume of the removed corrugator supercilii by making a small opening in the deep temporal fascia cephalad to the medial zygoma and then harvesting fat with biopsy forceps. (Reprinted from Guyuron B. Forehead rejuvenation. In: Guyuron B, Eriksson E, Persing J, eds. *Plastic Surgery: Indications and Practice*. Philadelphia, PA: Saunders Elsevier, 2009:1409-1426, with permission from Elsevier).

mistaken for the corrugator supercilii—it can be distinguished as the darker, more pliable muscle that lies deeper and more medial in its location (**TECH FIG 1D**).

- Elevation of the periosteum over the glabella and the central portion of the periosteum will cause the undesirable medial eyebrow elevation. Uncommonly, there may be significant medial eyebrow ptosis with skin folding over the radix. If so, dissection of the medial part is necessary. At this point, the process is repeated on the other side, and hemostasis is achieved with suction Bovie cautery.
- To prevent contour deformity, the removed corrugator muscle pieces are eyeballed to harvest and replace the similar-sized piece of fat at the corrugator site.

- Fat is usually harvested from deep temporal fat pad deep to the deep temporal fascia just above the zygomatic arch using the sharp end of the curved endoscopic periosteal elevator and grasper.
- If there is a second procedure to be performed in which there is access to fat for harvest, this alternate site may be used.
- Using a curved iris scissors, the harvested fat graft is trimmed to the size of the removed corrugator muscle. Then, using a periosteal elevator, the graft is delivered to the corrugator supercilii removal site (**TECH FIG 1E**).

■ Brow Resuspension

- Fascial suspension of the forehead is performed next. Usually, one lateral fascial suspension suture per side is sufficient.
  - Medial suspensions are avoided to prevent the elevation of the medial site.
  - Suspension is usually performed in the most lateral incision after removing the endoscopic access device, after placement of two single skin hooks at the junction of the caudal one-third and the cephalad two-thirds of the incision. While an assistant retracts the wound edges, a 3-0 polydioxanone suspension (PDS) suture is passed through the galea on two sides of the incision, and the forehead is suspended from deep temporal fascia after applying necessary tension. This is done while watching the eyebrow, and the suture

is tied down incrementally until the desired eyebrow position is reached (**TECH FIG 2A,B**).

- If additional fixation is needed to reposition the eyebrow or to correct asymmetry, a second suspension suture may be placed on the second port site.
  - A 3-0 PDS suspension suture is passed through the galea on two side of the incision, and the suture is pulled along the desired vector to confirm the position where it will be suspended cephalically from the frontal bone after making a bone tunnel.
  - Skin hooks are placed in the cranial half of the incision by retracting the scalp laterally and cephalically along the intended vector.
  - A narrow malleable retractor is placed at the posterior edge of the wound to protect the soft tissue.
  - A 1.1-mm drill bur with a safety guard length of 5 mm is connected to an office dermabrader.

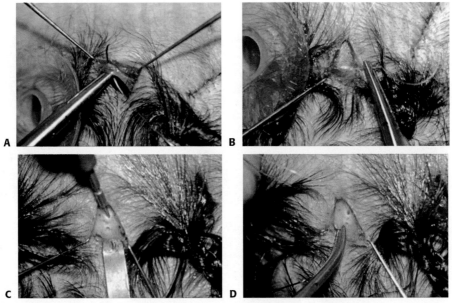

TECH FIG 2 • A. A 3-0 PDS suture being passed through the anterocaudal third of the lateral-most incision. **B.** The suspension suture passed through the anterior superficial temporal fascia of the incision is passed through the deep temporal fascia and then tied down incrementally to achieve the proper eyebrow position. **C.** A bone tunnel is made for suspension suture anchoring by drilling two 1.1-mm bur holes 3 to 4 mm apart opposing one another drilled at 45 degrees to the bone to meet at a depth of 3 to 4 mm. **D.** The suspension suture is bent to facilitate its passing through the bone tunnel. (Reprinted from Guyuron B. Forehead rejuvenation. In: Guyuron B, Eriksson E, Persing J, eds. *Plastic Surgery: Indications and Practice*. Philadelphia, PA: Saunders Elsevier, 2009:1409-1426, with permission from Elsevier).

- A Zimmer-Hall drill may be used to bur two opposing holes. Each hole should be drilled in at a 45-degree angle to the bone approximately 3 to 4 mm apart to meet at a depth of 3 to 4 mm (**TECH FIG 2C**).
- During drilling, the bone is irrigated with saline to minimize thermal damage. The free end of the PDS needle is bent using a pair of fine hemostat clamps. The needle is passed through the bony tunnel (**TECH FIG 2D**). The suture is tied down incrementally while watching the eyebrow to achieve the desired eyebrow position. The distance from the cranial border of the eyebrow to the eyelashes is measured while the eyes are closed—this distance should be approximately 2.5 cm. These steps are repeated for suspension on the contralateral side using one or two suspension sutures, beginning with the lateral most temporal incision.
- Screws or absorbable fixation devices such as the Endotine Forehead device can be used for fixation. Disadvantages of screw fixation over the proposed technique include the short length of the screws limiting penetration into the skull, the need for extraction of the screw, cost, short duration of fixation, and potential alopecia around the screw site.
- Drains are usually not necessary in this procedure. Skin closure is done by repairing the galea at each incision with buried 5-0 Monocryl suture and skin with simple interrupted 5-0 plain catgut sutures.

PEARLS AND PITFALLS

Periorbital release and corrugator resection	■ Complete release of the periorbita and adequate removal of the corrugator muscles is the most important factor in guaranteeing a smooth lift and aesthetically pleasing result.
Preserving the periosteum and fascia of the central glabella	■ Transection of the central glabellar attachments can result in excessive medial eyebrow elevation and a displeasing eyebrow curvature.
Pre-existing eyebrow asymmetry requires differential eyebrow elevation	■ Pre-existing eyebrow asymmetry will persist postoperatively and be a source of patient discontent. ■ This can be addressed by intraoperative differential eyebrow elevation with one to two suspension sutures per side. ■ Medial forehead suspension sutures are not recommended.
Hemostasis	■ Meticulous hemostasis with a suction Bovie is performed while the patient is at baseline preoperative blood pressure to prevent postoperative bleeding.

POSTOPERATIVE CARE

- Patients are typically allowed to shower on postoperative day 1 but instructed not to scrub their forehead or anterior hair-bearing scalp or submerge their head under water for 2 weeks.
- Patients are instructed to avoid strenuous activity and manage their blood pressure at home.

OUTCOMES

- With proper postoperative care, patients are usually pleased with the results of their forehead rejuvenation.
- Pre- and postoperative photographs of the patient's forehead in repose and while furrowing their brow can be used to highlight the outcomes of surgery to the patient at their postoperative visit.

COMPLICATIONS

- Inadequate, excessive, or asymmetric elevation of the eyebrows (may require corrective procedures)
- Dimpling upon animation
- Alopecia around the incision sites (usually temporary)
- Persistent paresthesia or temporary weakness due to injury to the temporal branch of the facial nerve (usually temporary)
- Persistent and intense itching of the forehead
  - No universally accepted treatment; antihistamines or antiserotonin-type compounds such as cyproheptadine, may provide some relief
- Infection
- Hematoma

22 CHAPTER

Indications and Techniques for Subcutaneous Lateral Brow Lifting

Richard J. Warren

DEFINITION

- Lateral brow ptosis describes an abnormally low position of the lateral third to one-half of the eyebrow complex.
- Brow position and shape convey an impression of emotion. When the lateral portion of the brow turns down, the patient appears sad or melancholy. It is also associated with aging.[1]
- Ptosis of the lateral eyebrow encroaches on the upper lid sulcus, changing the dynamics of the upper lid/brow junction. Thus, lateral brow ptosis will affect the assessment of patients who present for blepharoplasty, periorbital fat grafting, or senile eyelid ptosis repair.

ANATOMY

- Please refer to the anatomy section of the coronal brow lift chapter.
- The position of the lateral brow depends on two main issues: muscle anatomy and the firmness of soft tissue attachment.
- The level of the lateral eyebrow is the result of a balancing act between the muscular forces that elevate the brow and the muscular forces that depress the brow, along with the universal depressor, gravity (**FIG 1**).
- The frontalis is the only elevator of the eyebrow. It originates from the galea aponeurotica superiorly and interdigitates inferiorly with the upper orbicularis. Contraction

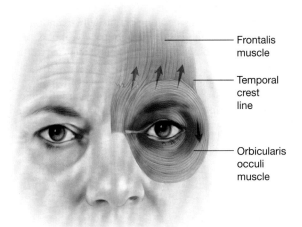

FIG 1 • The frontalis is the only muscle which lifts the eyebrow complex. On contraction, most of the movement occurs in the lower third of the muscle, and this action is strongest in the medial and central eyebrow. Laterally, frontalis action is weaker and is completely absent lateral to the temporal crest line. The orbicularis oculi acts like a sphincter surrounding the orbit. Laterally, it pulls the tail of the brow inferiorly.

Labels on figure: Frontalis muscle; Temporal crest line; Orbicularis occuli muscle

raises this muscle mass and the overlying eyebrow, which is a cutaneous structure. The muscle is deficient laterally and nonexistent lateral to the temporal crest line, so its primary lifting effect is exerted on the medial and central portions of the eyebrow.

- The primary muscular depressor of the lateral eyebrow is the orbicularis that encircles the orbit acting like a sphincter. Its action on the lateral brow can be temporarily reversed with botulinum toxin.

Sensory Nerves

- Innervation to the lateral brow and forehead is supplied by the supraorbital nerve that divides into two segments after it exits the orbit: the superficial and the deep branches.
- The superficial branches of the supraorbital nerve run on the superficial surface of the frontalis muscle and are visible when a subcutaneous flap is raised. These nerves innervate the forehead and the first 2 cm of the hair-bearing scalp. The rest of the scalp, back to the vertex, is innervated by the deep branch that courses laterally and is deep to the frontalis muscle.

Motor Nerves

- The temporal branch of the facial nerve crosses the middle third of the zygomatic arch as two or three branches. These branches are entirely deep to the frontalis muscle and are on the underside of the superficial temporal fascia. Therefore, they are completely safe during the raising of a subcutaneous forehead skin flap.

Vessels

- The anterior branch of the temporal artery and accompanying veins coursing superficial to the frontalis muscle and the superficial temporal fascia. These may require cauterization during the raising of a subcutaneous forehead flap.

PATHOGENESIS

- Please refer to the pathogenesis of eyebrow ptosis in the coronal brow chapter.
- The desired eyebrow shape and position vary with ethnicity, gender, and the era in which we live. In this era, the elevated lateral eyebrow is the preferred configuration with the lateral end of the eyebrow ideally being higher than the medial end.
- As mentioned, the lateral portion of the eyebrow has two causes for inferior displacement (lateral orbicularis contraction and gravity) balanced against the only force that

can lift: the frontalis. Despite this apparent imbalance, many patients (40% in one study) do not develop lateral brow ptosis over time.[2] The likely explanation for their brow stability is the strength of the underlying soft tissue attachments.

- Soft tissue fixation to bone is inconsistent in the lateral eyebrow. Laterally along the supraorbital rim, the galeal fat pad is separated from the preseptal fat (ROOF, retro orbicularis oculi fat) by one of the layers of galea. However, in the lateral brow, this galeal layer is thought to be variable, with some individuals having limited soft tissue attachment to bone. As a result, the galeal fat pad is contiguous with the preseptal fat (ROOF), and the lateral brow is relatively free to descend over time.[3]
- Many patients who develop lateral brow ptosis do so as a relatively early sign of facial aging.

PATIENT HISTORY AND PHYSICAL FINDINGS

- Please refer to the patient history and physical examination in the coronal brow chapter (Chapter 20).
- Patients with lateral brow ptosis may present with a request for upper eyelid blepharoplasty, or they may request a facelift procedure, hoping it will improve their brow position. Both scenarios provide the surgeon with an opportunity to teach the patient about the dynamics of eyebrow aging.
- The laxity of the lateral forehead skin is assessed by manually manipulating the tail of the brow. Patients best suited for a subcutaneous lateral brow lift are those with loose skin and a relatively lax attachment between their lateral forehead skin and the underlying frontalis and superficial temporal fascia.
- The eyebrow itself is a cutaneous structure, and shifting the deep plane tissues with a deeper procedure may not translate well to the overlying skin if that skin is loose. Conversely, a successful procedure to shift the skin will directly shift the eyebrow.
- The ptotic lateral eyebrow is a common physical finding in the patient demographic who seek facial rejuvenation surgery. Consequently, a subcutaneous lateral brow lift can be an excellent adjunctive procedure for the patient who is a candidate for a facelift or blepharoplasty (**FIG 2**).

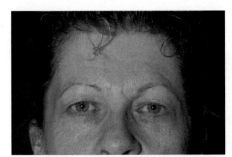

FIG 2 • This 56-year-old woman presents for blepharoplasty and facelift surgery. She has downturned lateral eyebrows that were not present in youth. The position of her medial and central brow is well maintained. In conjunction with the procedures she is requesting, a repositioning of the lateral eyebrows will be a useful adjunctive procedure.

- An examination of the temporal hairline will often demonstrate a triangular widow's peak where the hair is thin; this can be an ideal area to extend a hairline incision into the peak laterally.

NONOPERATIVE MANAGEMENT

- Nonoperative strategies to elevate the lateral eyebrow include the following:
  - Nonmedical: eyebrow plucking, cosmetic makeup, tattooing
  - Medical: botulinum toxin injection to the lateral orbicularis and the medial brow depressors, thread lifting

SURGICAL MANAGEMENT

Preoperative Planning

- The planned repositioning and degree of eyebrow elevation are reviewed with the patient who may have specific requests regarding eyebrow position and shape.
- The location of the hairline will affect the incision planning. The normal hairline will lend itself to an incision along the anterior hairline in the widow's peak area. Patients with a low hairline may benefit from an incision behind the hairline, which will shift the anterior hairline posteriorly. Patients in whom the temple hairline is positioned above (superior to) the lateral eyebrow may benefit from an incision placed in the temple hair.
- The presence of transverse forehead lines and the quality of forehead skin is assessed. The patient with thick corrugated skin may benefit from an incision made in a transverse forehead crease. This is often the case with middle age or older men.
- With the patient awake in the upright position and the forehead in repose, the desired amount and direction of lateral eyebrow elevation are assessed by manually elevating the lateral eyebrow. A mark is made on the skin, and the eyebrow is allowed to drop, thus determining the degree of elevation required.
- The most effective vector for eyebrow advancement is determined when the examiner manually repositions the brow. Most commonly, the desired vector runs along the axis of the temporal crest line.

Positioning

- The patient is placed on the operating table in the supine position with the head on a small pillow or soft donut.
- The head of the bead is raised slightly to help reduce venous engorgement.

Approach

- As described for preoperative planning, possible locations for subcutaneous lateral brow lifting are
  - At the hairline
  - Just behind the hairline
  - Lateral extension of a transverse forehead line
  - Directly adjacent to the eyebrow (**FIG 3**)
- All of these approaches are "skin deep" with varying degrees of subcutaneous dissection. For the first three incisions (hairline, behind the hairline, transverse forehead line), the dissection plane is subcutaneous, immediately superficial to the frontalis muscle. In the fourth option (adjacent to eyebrow), there is no skin undermining.

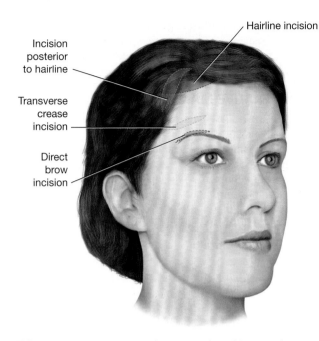

Hairline incision

Incision posterior to hairline

Transverse crease incision

Direct brow incision

FIG 3 • Incision options for subcutaneous brow lifting are shown. An incision posterior to the hairline involves the removal of hair-bearing skin posterior to the incision. An incision at the hairline involves the removal of forehead skin inferior to the incision. The transverse crease incision involves subcutaneous dissection on the eyebrow side of the incision, with skin excision on the inferior side of the crease. The direct brow incision does not involve undermining. The ideal vector for lateral eyebrow lifting is shown. This will be slightly different in every case but typically will follow the temporal crest line.

- The farther away from the eyebrow the incision is made, the less effective a subcutaneous lift will be.
- In planning the skin resection, the author's clinical experience has determined a "rule of thumb": at the time of surgery, an incision directly adjacent to the eyebrow will initially raise the eyebrow in a 1:1 ratio to the width of skin excised. An incision in the mid forehead will raise it in a 1:2 ratio, and an incision at the hairline will raise the eyebrow in a 1:3 ratio, or even 1:4, depending on the height of the forehead and the elasticity of the skin. In addition, over the first few months, there is always some relapse of lateral brow height that in some cases approaches 50% of the lift achieved at the time of surgery. Firm, thick forehead skin provides a more durable result than thin aged skin.
- Incisions posterior to the hairline are potentially the least visible but introduce the possibility of damaging hair follicles. Also, they will result in a slightly raised hairline.
- Incisions at the hairline are potentially visible but will not shift the hairline.
- Incisions in deep forehead lines provide a powerful lift and are potentially very well hidden, depending on the depth of the existing fold.
- Incisions adjacent to the eyebrow provide the most powerful lift of the various subcutaneous options. The scar can be well hidden when eyebrows are full or when there is an adjacent transverse fold in which to hide the scar.

T E C H N I Q U E S

■ Anterior Hairline Approach

Markings and Anesthesia

- The preoperative markings are done prior to surgery with the patient awake and in the upright position.
- The essential preoperative markings include the planned incisions and the desired vector for flap movement (**TECH FIG 1**).
- The incision length is determined by the length of the eyebrow and the amount of eyebrow to be lifted. This maybe just the tail or, possibly, the entire lateral half of the brow.
- Because of variability in desired lifting vectors as well as hairline variability, there is variability in the incision location. Every case is customized. Normally, the

incision starts medially at the mid pupillary line and extends laterally from there over a distance of 3 to 6 cm in length, entering the temporal scalp. If a widow's peak is present, the incision follows the hairline into the peak.

- The procedure is done under local anesthetic with or without sedation.
- The head and neck area is prepped and draped with exposure of the entire face.
- A local anesthetic mixture composed of 1% lidocaine with 1:100 000 epinephrine and 0.25% bupivacaine with 1:200 000 epinephrine is infiltrated into the superior incision line, along the supralateral orbital rim and in a hydrodissection manner, into the subcutaneous space between these two zones.

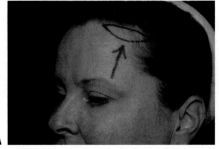

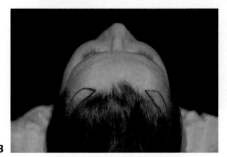

A   B

TECH FIG 1 • **A.** Preoperative marking is done with the patient upright and with the frontalis in repose. The planned incision is marked. In this case, the incision location is the anterior hairline, with a planned skin ellipse inferior to that. The vector for the lateral brow lift is marked. As in this case, the preferred vector is often along the temporal crest line. **B.** The planned incisions and skin removal as seen from above.

Incision and Dissection

- After waiting for the epinephrine effect, the incision is made a few hairs posterior to the hairline. The scalpel is beveled in such a way that the hair follicles will be partially transected, utilizing the Camirand principle.[4]
- The incision stops when the frontalis is visualized. Dissection then turns inferiorly, following the superficial surface of the frontalis (**TECH FIG 2A**).
- Initially, dissection is sharp, using fine scissors, but after 1 to 2 cm, Metzenbaum scissors can be used with a gentle spreading motion, with tips up toward the skin (**TECH FIG 2B**). Blunt finger dissection deeper in the dissection pocket is a useful adjunct (**TECH FIG 2C**).
- Care is taken to identify and protect the superficial branches of the supraorbital nerve that will be running on the superficial surface of the frontalis muscle.
- Subcutaneous veins may require cauterization, and the anterior branch of the temporal artery may be protected or, if necessary, cauterized.
- Laterally, dissection is taken down the upper third of the lateral orbital rim.

Suturing and Completion

- The transverse running fibers of the orbicularis oculi will normally be visualized. A 5-0 or 4-0 Vicryl or similar suture is then used to pexy the orbicularis to a higher point on the frontalis muscle, using two or three sutures (**TECH FIG 3**).
- Another option is to place similar sutures from the underside of the skin flap to the frontalis muscle, shifting the skin flap superiorly with progressive tension sutures.[5]
- Once internal suturing is done, the undermined flap is advanced superiorly over the cut edge of the scalp incision.
- The degree of overlap is marked and excess skin is removed from the inferior (undermined) side of the

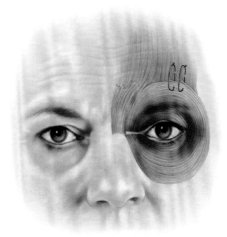

TECH FIG 3 • The placement of internal pexy sutures is an optional maneuver, especially in those cases where the eyebrow is very mobile. Two sutures (5-0 Vicryl, 4-0 Vicryl or equivalent) are placed from the transverse running fibers of the orbicularis to a higher level on the frontalis. Similar sutures can be used from the underside of the skin flap in a progressive tension fashion.

incision. Normally, the width of skin excision is in the range of 1.5 to 2.5 cm, depending on the age of the patient and the laxity of their skin.
- Repair of the scalp incision is done with 5-0 nylon sutures.
- A bupivacaine block is done across the supraorbital rim, targeting the supratrochlear and supraorbital nerves.
- The incision is left open with ointment applied along the suture line.
- In vascular cases, a light pressure dressing can be placed over the forehead, and an elastic head wrap can be put in place for 1 hour.

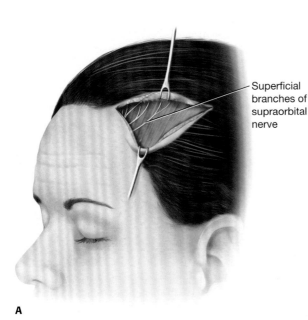

Superficial branches of supraorbital nerve

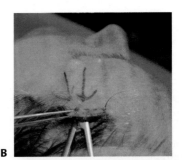

B

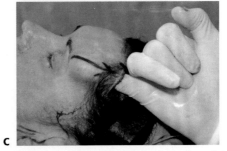

C

TECH FIG 2 • **A.** After carefully beginning the dissection, branches of the supraorbital nerve will be seen lying on the surface of the frontalis muscle. Dissection continues inferiorly as far as the eyebrow. **B.** Metzenbaum scissor dissection. **C.** Finger dissection.

■ Posterior to the Hairline Approach

Incisions and Dissection

- This procedure is identical to the hairline approach, except that the incision is placed in hair-bearing scalp, 1 cm posterior to the anterior hairline.
  - Consequently, the incision will follow the hairline and will usually be a gentle S-shaped incision following the hairline (**TECH FIG 4**).
- This incision is well suited for the patient with a hairline close to the tail of the eyebrow, where a modest shift of the hairline is not a problem and where a scar within the hair will be less visible than one at the leading edge of a low hairline.
- This incision is also helpful when the natural nap of hair lies in such a way that the anterior hairline incision scar would not be well hidden by the hair.
- The incision is made with the scalpel blade kept parallel to the hair follicles in order to preserve the hairs in the flap.
- Flap dissection toward the eyebrow is done on the superficial surface of the frontalis (or if the incision is lateral, on the superficial temporal fascia).

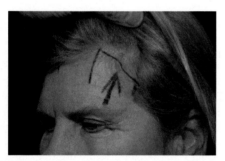

TECH FIG 4 • Markings designate an incision within the hairs of the temple behind the hairline. Following the hairline down into the temple, the inferior dissection will be done deep to the hair follicles and will then proceed subcutaneously the short distance to the eyebrow. After flap advancement along the planned vector, hair-bearing skin will be removed posterior to the planned incision. This marking designates the desired vector of lift and the planned incision. In this case, the incision is being placed within the fine hairs of the temple and skin excision will be done posterior to the incision.

- For the first 1 cm of dissection, care is taken to stay deep, directly on the frontalis and/or superficial fascia, to protect the hair follicles. Dissection is done with a scalpel or fine dissecting scissors
- After the first 1 cm, the hair follicles are no longer at risk, and dissection can continue inferiorly in the subcutaneous plane, in the same fashion as with the anterior hairline approach.

Suturing and Completion

- As with the anterior hairline approach, deep sutures may be placed to help with flap advancement superiorly.
- At the incision line, the overlapping flap is placed against the scalp, and the amount of overlap is marked.
- Excess scalp skin is then removed from the posterior (cranial) side of the incision.
- Scalp resection is done with the blade beveled to partially transect hair follicles. On closing the incision, the anterior hairline will be preserved but will be shifted slightly posteriorly.
- Occasionally, because of variations in a patient's hairline, this incision can be broken up into two separate incisions behind different parts of the hairline.
  - This provides excellent exposure and two different lifting vectors for the lateral brow (**TECH FIG 5**).

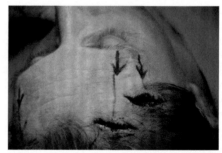

TECH FIG 5 • In this case, due to the shape of the hairline, two shorter incisions placed behind the hairline, each 2.5 cm in length, have been used for access. The subcutaneous flap has been raised, and the skin will be advanced superiorly and obliquely along two different vectors. Skin excision will be superior to the incision.

■ Transverse Forehead Line Approach

- Preoperative surgical markings are done in the upright position (**TECH FIG 6**).
- The procedure is done under local anesthetic with or without sedation.
- The head and neck area is prepped and draped with exposure of the entire face.
- A local anesthetic mixture composed of 1% lidocaine with 1:100 000 epinephrine and 0.25% bupivacaine with 1:200 000 epinephrine is infiltrated into the planned incision site and 1 to 2 cm inferior to that.
- After waiting for the epinephrine effect, the initial incision is made and the planned ellipse of skin is removed.

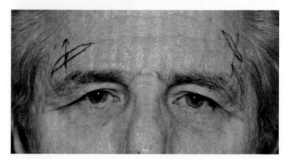

TECH FIG 6 • This 68-year-old man has deep transverse forehead lines. Preoperative markings designate three locations for transverse crease incisions with elliptical skin excisions inferior to the crease incisions.

- The inferior skin is then undermined for several millimeters, using a scalpel in the subcutaneous plane, freeing it from its attachment to the underlying frontalis.

- This incision is closed meticulously, using interrupted 6-0 or 5-0 permanent sutures.
- The incision is left open with ointment applied along the suture line.

■ Direct Eyebrow Incision

- Preoperative surgical markings are done.
- There are two possible incision locations for a direct eyebrow lift.
  - Directly adjacent to the eyebrow, cutting parallel to the hairs, and excising an ellipse of skin above (superior) to that
  - Within the lowest transverse fold which is near the eyebrow, excising an ellipse of skin below (inferior) to that
- The procedure is done under local anesthetic with or without sedation.
- The head and neck area is prepped and draped.
- A local anesthetic mixture composed of 1% lidocaine with 1:100 000 epinephrine and 0.25% bupivacaine with

1:200 000 epinephrine is infiltrated into the planned incision site.
- After waiting for the epinephrine effect, the inferior incision is made directly adjacent to eyebrow hair follicles, taking care to bevel the blade accurately along the axis of these hairs.
- No flap undermining is done.
- The planned ellipse of full-thickness skin is excised.
- The incision is closed meticulously, using 5-0 Vicryl (or similar) in the deep dermal layer and a fine suture in the skin, either a running subcuticular 5-0 nylon or interrupted 6-0 Prolene sutures.
- The incision is left open with ointment applied along the suture line.

PEARLS AND PITFALLS

Incision choice	■ Choose the anterior hairline approach when the forehead skin is mobile and the anterior hairline is high.
	■ Choose an incision behind the hairline when the hairline is low and the patient is averse to a potentially visible scar.
	■ Choose the transverse fold incision when forehead skin is thick and deep transverse folds are present.
	■ Choose the direct brow lift when there is a bushy eyebrow or when there is a deep nearby fold in which to hide the scar.
Suturing	■ All these procedures require very careful suture closure to minimize the chance of a visible scar.
Tension	■ For an incision in the vicinity of the anterior hairline, excess tension can create a widened scar and can lead to skin necrosis, especially in smokers.
Predictability	■ The longevity of a subcutaneous brow lift is somewhat unpredictable due to the inherent elasticity of skin.

POSTOPERATIVE CARE

- The patient is encouraged to keep the head elevated for the first week to decrease swelling.
- Sutures are removed 5 to 6 days postoperatively.
- At 7 to 10 days postoperatively, botulinum toxin can be injected into the lateral orbicularis to reduce the brow depressing effect of the lateral orbicularis during the healing phase.

OUTCOMES

- These subcutaneous procedures are all relatively simple. The operative time is short, and they can be done under local anesthetic in the day surgery setting. In appropriately selected cases, they accomplish the same objective as much more involved procedures such as open brow lifts or endoscopic brow lifts.
- Overall patient satisfaction is very high, and serious complications are rare.[6–10]

- Clinical experience does demonstrate a degree of unpredictability with respect to the magnitude of brow lift achieved and longevity of the surgical result. However, this issue is common to all brow elevation procedures.

COMPLICATIONS

- Subcutaneous procedures are truly "skin deep, and therefore they avoid potential damage to deeper anatomic structures. The biggest concern with subcutaneous brow lift procedures is the potential of visible scarring, but multiple series have demonstrated that this is not a problem reported by patients.[6,7]
- A recent series of subcutaneous lateral brow lifts report no cases with seromas, hematomas, infection, or nerve damage, either sensory or motor.[5]
- Accurately predicting the amount of relapse is a problem with subcutaneous brow lifting as it is with all brow lift procedures. Relapse is more likely to occur in patients with lax tissues and when the incision is relatively far removed from the eyebrow.

▪ Scar alopecia can occur along the incision line when sutures are placed in hair-bearing skin with excessive tightness.

REFERENCES

1. Knoll BI, Attkiss KJ, Persing JA. The influence of forehead, brow, and periorbital aesthetics of perceived expression in the youthful face. *Plast Reconstr Surg.* 2008;121:1793-1802.
2. Lambros V. Observations on periorbital and midface aging. *Plast Reconstr Surg.* 2007;120:1367-1376.
3. Knize DM. An anatomically based study of the mechanism of eyebrow ptosis. *Plast Reconstr Surg.* 1996;97(7):1321-1333.
4. Camirand A, Doucet J. A comparison between parallel hairline incisions and perpendicular incisions when performing a face lift. *Plast Reconstr Surg.* 1997;99(1):10-15.
5. Pollock H, Pollock TA. Subcutaneous brow lift with precise suture fixation and advancement. *Aesthet Surg J.* 2007;27(4):388-395.
6. Bidros RS, Salazar-Reyes H, Friedman JD. Subcutaneous temporal browlift under local anesthesia: a useful technique for periorbital rejuvenation. *Aesthet Surg J.* 2010;30(6):783-788.
7. Miller TA, Rudkin G, Honig M, et al. Lateral subcutaneous brow lift and interbrow muscle resection: clinical experience and anatomic studies. *Plast Reconstr Surg.* 2000;105(3):1120-1127.
8. Miller TA. Lateral subcutaneous brow lift. *Aesthet Surg J.* 2003; 23(3):205-210.
9. Mahmood U, Baker JL. Lateral subcutaneous brow lift: updated technique. *Aesthet Surg J.* 2015;35(5):621-624.
10. Bernard RW, Greenwald JA, Beran SJ, Morello DC. Enhancing upper lid aesthetics with the lateral subcutaneous brow lift. *Aesthet Surg J.* 2006;26(1):19-23.

Lowering the Overelevated Brow

Michael J. Yaremchuk, Erez Dayan, and Dev Vibhakar

DEFINITION

- Brow lift procedures can create brows with positions much higher and configurations much different than those seen in youth. This results in an older appearance, with hollowed upper lids and a raised hairline (**FIG 1**).[1,2]
- Brow lifts that preferentially elevate the medial brow and increase the distance between the medial brows create an unnatural, surprised, and unintelligent look.[1–3]

ANATOMY

- The ideal youthful eyebrow in women has been described as an arch where the brow apex terminates above the lateral limbus of the iris. The medial and lateral ends of the brow should be at the same horizontal, located at or below the supraorbital rim, not above it.
- Men have a flatter-shaped, lower-placed brow.[4]
- With aging, the gravitational descent of the medial two-thirds of the brow is often camouflaged by the reflexive action of the frontalis muscle to counteract upper lid descent. This lid descent results from the senile dehiscence of the levator muscle. Because the lateral aspect of the brow extends beyond the frontalis territory, it descends. As a result, brows often elevate with aging. As described by Garcia and Matros, brow shape may change from an apex lateral slant to an apex neutral position[1] (**FIG 2**).

PATHOGENESIS

- Brow lift procedures can raise the brow to positions higher than they existed in youth. Because the medial brow often elevates with aging, exaggerated brow lifts often have an aging effect due to this brow position.[1,2]

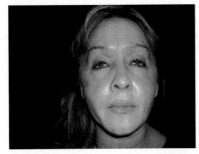

FIG 1 • Patient after brow lift with overelevated, flattened, and widened brow. Also, note elevated hairline and hollow upper lids.

- Over elevation of the brows also tends to decrease upper lid redundancy by exaggerating the hollow eyes of senility and accentuating lid ptosis.[2]
- Removal of the corrugator muscles in an attempt to eliminate glabellar frown lines allows the medial brows to separate and elevate.
- Overelevation of the brows may result in an unacceptably high hairline. This may disrupt the proportional balance of the horizontal zones of the face. Hairline elevation can also reflect senility.[1,2]

PATIENT HISTORY AND PHYSICAL FINDINGS

- Physical examination should focus on the forehead and periorbital area and its relation to the balance of the face. Analysis should document the height of the forehead, shape and position of the brows, depth of the upper lid sulcus, upper lid position, and levator function.
- History should focus on elements related to the periorbital area, including method and date of the brow lift surgery; periorbital surgeries or procedures including neurotoxins, fillers, and fat injections; and ocular health.

IMAGING

- Photographs documenting pre–brow lift appearance should be obtained.

SURGICAL MANAGEMENT

Preoperative Planning

- Informed consent should include intrinsic risks related to brow and hairline repositioning. These include infection, asymmetry, alopecia, and motor/sensory nerve injury.
- Preoperatively, with the patient both in the upright and supine position, the distance of the medial brow and the central hairline is measured in relation to the intercanthal line. The distance change to accomplish the desired locations is recorded.
- The authors' preference is to use general endotracheal or nasotracheal anesthesia. This allows optimal preparation of the operative site and control of the airway.[2]

Positioning

- Patients are placed supine on the operating room table at a 90-degree perpendicular position relative to the anesthesiologist for maximal exposure.

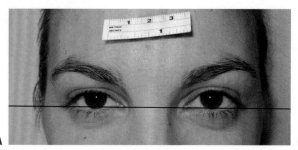 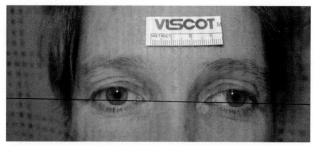

FIG 2 • A. In young patients, the medial brow is the lowest point or apex lateral slant. **B.** In older patients, the medial brow elevates, creating an apex neutral brow. This levels the brow in older patients, generating a flat appearance compared to the peaked brow of younger patients.

Preparation

- Prior to antiseptic preparation and draping, a dilute solution of lidocaine and epinephrine (1:200 000) is infiltrated into the operative site for postoperative pain control and intraoperative hemostasis.

- Intravenous cephalosporin or ciprofloxacin antibiotic prophylaxis is administered approximately 30 minutes preoperatively.

Incisions

- Bicoronal incisions are used for both previously performed open or closed (endoscopic) brow lift procedures. The incision is made to re-elevate the anterior scalp flap in a subperiosteal plane down to the supraorbital rim and just beyond the nasofrontal suture.
- If in the preoperative evaluation it was determined that the frontal hairline was high prior to the brow lift, a hairline incision may be used.
- After scalp incision and before flap elevation, the skull is scored with a drill directly beneath the scalp incision. The position of the anterior hairline is similarly marked. These marks serve as reference points during hairline and scalp repositioning (**TECH FIG 1**).

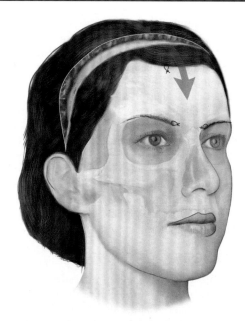

TECH FIG 1 • Coronal incision with register for hairline and Mitek anchors for medial brow positioning.

Brow Repositioning

- The anterior scalp flap is freed by subperiosteal dissection well onto the nasal root medially and the supraorbital rims laterally.
- The brow is repositioned relative to the medial canthus with Mitek anchoring system.
- The Mitek anchor is secured in the frontal bone at the desired distance (usually 15–18 mm) directly above each medial canthus. This places the anchors near the level of the nasofrontal suture. The inevitable penetration of the frontal sinus by this anchor is of no clinical significance.

- The nasofrontal suture is easily palpable through the skin and clearly visible when the scalp flap is reflected, and it is a useful reference when positioning the Mitek anchor.
- A 19-gauge needle is positioned at the most inferomedial aspect of the brow and passed through the scalp flap. This marks the area for Mitek anchor suture purchase (**TECH FIG 2**).
- The sutures are then tied, securing the posterior aspect of the flap and, hence, the medial aspect of the brow on its anterior surface to the desired position.
- Depending on the plan, this technique repositions the medial brow 3 to 8 mm inferiorly and 1 to 3 mm medially.

TECHNIQUES

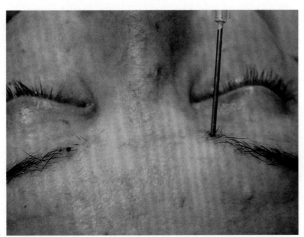 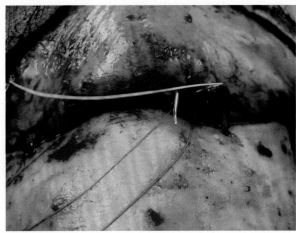

TECH FIG 2 • Anchoring the medial brow using transcutaneous needle **(A)** and Mitek anchor **(B)**.

- The midbrow and lateral brows are repositioned as determined by patient preference. Most often, an "apex lateral slant" appearance is created through manipulation of the lateral aspect of the scalp flap. This position is secured by suturing the galea beneath the hair-bearing skin over the tail of the brow to the deep temporal fascia.

- With the incision and hairline registration marks placed earlier as a reference, the anterior hairline is repositioned. This position is secured with Mitek anchor scalp fixation to the skull positioned just off the midline to avoid possible sagittal sinus penetration. Cortical tunnels are an alternative to anchors in providing a stable fixation point for suturing to the skull.

■ Posterior Scalp Flap Advancement

- Brow and hairline lowering inevitably leaves a gap between the anterior and posterior scalp flaps.
- In patients who have had their brow lift surgery performed endoscopically, no scalp is removed and the gap reflects tissue repositioned posteriorly.
- Sufficient tissue can be recruited from the posterior flap by widely undermining it back to the occiput and advancing it anteriorly.

- In patients who have had their brow lift surgery performed through an open approach, the gap reflects scalp that has been excised. Filling this defect requires serial scoring of the galea to expand the scalp surface area, as well as wide undermining and posterior scalp advancement.
- It is sometimes necessary to elevate the posterior scalp flap beyond the occiput to obtain sufficient posterior scalp flap length and forward movement.

■ Closure

- Prior to closure, a thin suction drain is placed immediately above the supraorbital rim.
- Closure is achieved in two layers with inverted dermal sutures and nylon skin sutures.

- Using the nasal dorsum as a point of fixation, the medial brow is taped in the desired position prior to initiating the suction apparatus. These measures are intended to control scalp flap adherence and, hence, desired brow position.

PEARLS AND PITFALLS

Apex lateral vs apex neutral slant	■ Younger patients have a medial brow that is low with the apex of the brow positioned lateral (at the lateral limbus). Older patients have an elevated medial and middle brow, which contributes to a flattened or apex neutral appearance.
Hairline repositioning	■ Scoring the calvarium at the scalp incision and hairline provides useful landmarks for subsequent hairline repositioning.
Medial brow positioning	■ The nasofrontal suture is a useful landmark for medial brow repositioning.
Brow and scalp fixation	■ Mitek anchoring sutures and cortical tunnels are valuable fixation methods to maintain the desired reposition of the scalp flap.

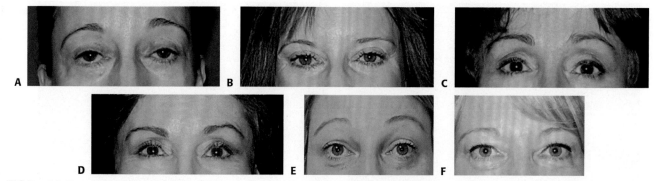

FIG 3 • A,B. Brow lift reversal was performed using a hairline incision in this patient who preoperatively had a high forehead. The patient also underwent infraorbital rim augmentation, subperiosteal midface lift, and lateral canthopexy. **C,D.** This patient underwent brow lift reversal and subperiosteal midface lift. **E,F.** This patient underwent brow lift reversal.

POSTOPERATIVE CARE

- The drain is removed the morning after surgery.
- Oral antibiotics are prescribed for 3 to 5 days after surgery.
- Patients are instructed to refrain from strenuous exercise for 2 to 3 weeks postoperatively.
- Sutures are removed at 7 to 10 days after surgery.

OUTCOMES

- In the senior author's experience of reversing brow lifts, the medial brow is typically lowered 4 to 10 mm (average 5 mm) relative to the intercanthal line and the anterior hairline is lowered 5 to 18 mm (average 10 mm). Repositioning of the brow has remained clinically stable during follow-up, and no revisional surgery to reposition the brow or hairline has been requested (**FIG 3**).

COMPLICATIONS

- Postoperative complications are rare following lowering of the over elevated brow and tend to involve concerns over asymmetry and temporary sensory nerve dysfunction.

- Areas of temporary and rarely permanent alopecia in the posterior scalp flap after galeal scoring are a potential complication after using this technique. Rogaine may be helpful in stimulating regrowth in these instances.
- Soft tissue redundancy may develop in the glabellar area after flap lowering, particularly in those patients who have had extensive corrugator resection during their brow lift surgery.
- Brow asymmetry may result with animation when corrugator resection was uneven during the initial brow lift surgery.

REFERENCES

1. Matros E, Jesus G, Yaremchuk MJ. Changes in eyebrow position and shape with aging. *Plast Reconstr Surg.* 2009;124:1296-1301.
2. Yaremchuk MJ, O'Sullivan N, Benslimane F. Reversing brow lifts. *Aesthet Surg J.* 2007;27:367-375.
3. Gunter JP, Antrobus SD. Aesthetic analysis of the eyebrows. *Plast Reconstr Surg.* 1997;99:1808-1816.
4. Freund RM, Nolan WB III. Correlation between brow lift outcomes and aesthetic ideals for eyebrow height and shape in females. *Plast Reconstr Surg.* 1996;97:1343-1348.

Indications and Techniques for Transpalpebral Corrugator Resection

Ximena A. Pinell-White and Foad Nahai

DEFINITION

- Horizontal glabellar frown lines result from contraction and hypertrophy of the corrugator supercilii and transverse lines from procerus muscle activity. Commonly, these central glabellar changes are also associated with lateral brow ptosis.

ANATOMY

- The paired corrugator supercilii muscles originate from the superomedial brow, traverse the galeal fat pad, and insert on the skin of the central brow. The corrugator muscles lie deep to the procerus and frontalis muscles. Contraction depresses the central brow, creating vertical and oblique glabellar rhytids (**FIG 1**).
- The procerus muscle takes its origin in the lower nasal bone and inserts into the skin overlying the nasal root. Contraction depresses the central brow and creates a transverse line at the nasal bridge.

PATIENT HISTORY AND PHYSICAL FINDINGS

- The procerus and corrugator muscles can be identified by asking the patient to frown.
- It is important to distinguish between dynamic lines, which are evident only on animation, and static rhytids, which are uniformly present and are more challenging to correct. The Glogau classification of photoaging describes the severity of actinic changes based on the degree of skin wrinkling.
  - Dynamic lines represent early to moderate photoaging (Glogau class II) and generally respond to less invasive procedures such as injection of neurotoxins.
  - Static wrinkles, on the other hand, indicate more advanced photodamage (Glogau class III) that will often require surgery.

NONOPERATIVE MANAGEMENT

- Injection of neurotoxins is most effective in relaxing the muscles to temporarily eliminate glabellar rhytids. Etched or deep lines may also be improved with resurfacing or injections of fillers.

SURGICAL MANAGEMENT

- Glabellar frown lines can be addressed through an upper eyelid blepharoplasty incision in patients with little or no medial brow ptosis and no excess skin above the nasal radix. In patients with significant lateral brow ptosis, the procedure can be paired with a lateral temporal brow lift.

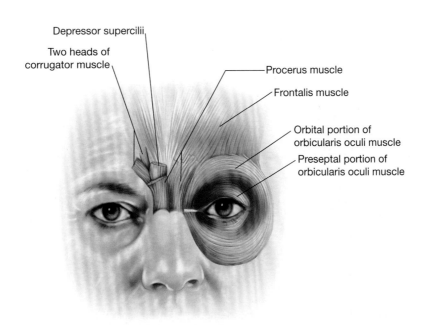

Depressor supercilii

Two heads of corrugator muscle

Procerus muscle

Frontalis muscle

Orbital portion of orbicularis oculi muscle

Preseptal portion of orbicularis oculi muscle

FIG 1 • Anatomy of the glabellar muscles.

Preoperative Planning

- The patient is marked preoperatively for an upper lid blepharoplasty. He or she is asked to frown to identify and mark the glabellar muscles. Note is made if the procerus should be divided.

Positioning

- The patient is positioned supine with slight elevation of the head.

Approach

- A transpalpebral approach to the glabellar muscles is employed at the time of upper lid blepharoplasty.

■ Transblepharoplasty Excision of Corrugator and Procerus Muscles

Incision and Dissection

- Upper lid blepharoplasty incisions are made, and the upper eyelid skin and, when indicated, muscle are excised.
- Any planned fat removal is deferred until after the glabellar muscles are excised so as to facilitate dissection of the orbicularis off of the orbital septum.
- The dissection is then continued superiorly, deep to the orbicularis muscle.
- The depressor supercilii portion of the orbicularis is divided to expose the diagonal and more deeply colored fibers of the corrugator muscle at the superior orbital rim (**TECH FIG 1A**).
- Our preference is to dissect with the cutting current of a Colorado tip needle.
- The supraorbital and supratrochlear nerves are visualized at this stage (**TECH FIG 1B**). The supraorbital nerve is more lateral and tends to be singular, larger, and in front of the muscle, whereas the supratrochlear nerve arborizes early and interdigitates with the fibers of the corrugator medially.

Muscle and Fat Excision

- After the nerves are identified and protected, a mosquito clamp is passed around the corrugator muscle to elevate it centrally (**TECH FIG 2A**).

- A portion of the muscle is resected using electrocautery so as to leave a central gap. More muscle is taken from the lateral cut edge when the corrugators are particularly hypertrophied (**TECH FIG 2B**).
  - There are often veins coursing with the nerves that should be avoided but when necessary can be cauterized with bipolar forceps. The trochlea of the superior oblique muscle tendon can theoretically be injured during dissection in the superomedial corner of the orbit, but this is rare and can be avoided by limiting dissection behind the origin of the corrugator.
- Patients with transverse dorsal nasal lines benefit from division of the procerus muscle.
  - This is accomplished by elevating the orbicularis muscle medially, directing a pair of scissors toward the nasal radix, and cutting the procerus muscle fibers just beneath the skin (**TECH FIG 3**).
  - This is a blind procedure and is often accompanied by some bleeding, which can easily be controlled with pressure.
- Fat removal from the upper lid can be performed if desired at this point, and the incision closed.
  - On occasion, I may place a small 5×5 mm piece of fat, harvested from the nasal fat pocket, in between the remaining edges of the corrugator. This would be to avoid a depression following removal of sections of the muscle.

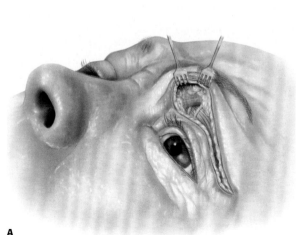

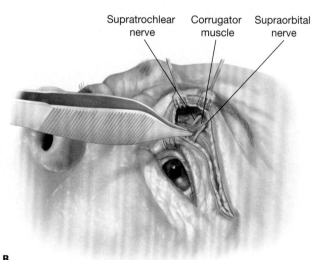

A　　　　　　　　　　　　　　　　　　**B**

TECH FIG 1 • **A.** Identification of the corrugator supercilii muscle. **B.** Location of the supraorbital and supratrochlear nerves.

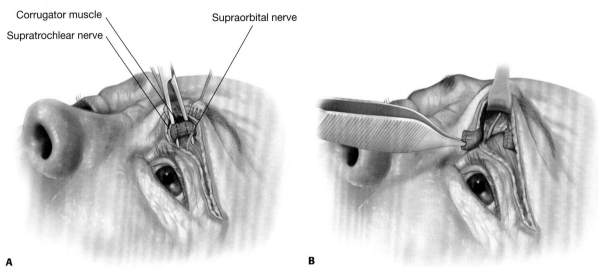

TECH FIG 2 • **A.** Division of the corrugator muscle. **B.** Appearance of corrugator after resection of central segment.

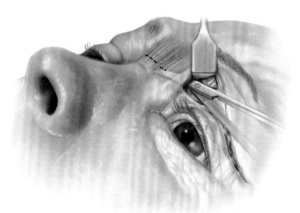

TECH FIG 3 • Division of the procerus muscle.

PEARLS AND PITFALLS

Incomplete muscle excision	▪ It is important that full-thickness portions of the muscle are removed. The muscle is wider than it may seem, and incomplete removal results in suboptimal results.
Bleeding	▪ We infiltrate with vasoconstrictors so the dissection is performed in a relatively bloodless field.
Nerve injuries	▪ The branches of the supratrochlear nerve are intertwined with the muscle and are at risk. The supraorbital nerve is much larger and lateral to the area of dissection and is therefore less at risk.

POSTOPERATIVE CARE

▪ Postoperative swelling after this procedure may be prolonged and more noticeable than following a standard blepharoplasty. This can be minimized by keeping the head elevated, applying ice packs to the eyelids, and in some cases, administering diuretics and a short course of steroids.

OUTCOMES

▪ This technique has proved very effective for treatment of glabellar frown lines (**FIG 2**).

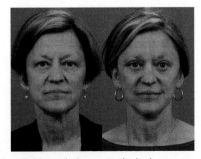

FIG 2 • Patient before and after transpalpebral corrugator resection.

COMPLICATIONS

- Injury to the supraorbital or supratrochlear nerves can produce anesthesia or paresthesias of the forehead and, in the case of the supraorbital nerve, the scalp behind the hairline.
- Contour defects following corrugator excision or procerus division are rare, but these can be filled with periorbital fat when necessary.

REFERENCE

1. Guyuron B, Michelow BJ, Thomas T. Corrugator supercilii muscle resection through blepharoplasty incision. *Plast Reconstr Surg.* 1995;95(4):691-696.

Indications and Techniques for Hairline Lowering

Warwick J. S. Nettle and Yumiko Kadota

CHAPTER 25

DEFINITION

- The ideal length of the female forehead should be approximately one-third of the length of the face (**FIG 1**).[1-4]
  - Forehead length should typically be 5.5 to 6 cm from the eyebrows to the anterior hairline.[2,4,5] This varies depending on eyebrow position and overall facial size.
- The forehead may be elongated congenitally, due to hairline recession with aging or iatrogenic causes, such as coronal incision brow lift.[1,4]
- A high hairline, or large forehead, causes the upper third of the face to be disproportionately larger than the middle and lower thirds.
- Young women find that a high hairline masculinizes their faces.[4]
- Hairline lowering utilizes a posterior scalp advancement flap.[1,3-6]

ANATOMY

- The hairline is an extended area consisting of various zones and borders that frame the face.[7]
- The frontal hairline has an irregular border that extends from temple to temple.
  - The transition zone is the anterior border of the frontal hairline where soft, small hairs are found.[7]
  - The defined zone is immediately behind the transition zone, where the hairs become coarser and denser.[7]
  - The midfrontal point is the midline, most anterior point of the hairline. This is where the "widow's peak" is, if it exists in the patient.
- The frontotemporal angle is the point where the frontal hairline meets the temporal hairline.[7] This angle is the angle of temporal hair recession, routinely found in males and sometimes found in females.
- The layers of the scalp from superficial to deep are
  - Skin: the thickest in the body and most hair-bearing
  - Dense connective tissue where the blood vessels run
  - Occipitofrontalis muscle
  - Galea aponeurotica between occipitalis and frontalis muscles. This aponeurosis blends with the temporalis fascia laterally, just above the zygomatic arch.
  - The subgaleal space of loose areolar tissue provides a plane for scalp mobility.
- Scalp blood supply
  - Blood supply to the scalp derives from external and internal carotid artery branches, which anastomose freely with each other.

- Scalping does not cause necrosis of the underlying skull, which receives blood supply from the middle meningeal artery.
- The external carotid artery gives rises to the occipital, posterior auricular, and superficial temporal arteries.
  - The occipital artery runs from the apex of the posterior triangle of the neck to supply the posterior scalp to the vertex.
  - The posterior auricular artery supplies the scalp behind the ear.
  - The superficial temporal artery is a terminal branch of the external carotid artery and supplies the skin over the temporalis fascia and scalp.
- The supraorbital and supratrochlear arteries derive from the internal carotid artery and supply the forehead and anterior scalp to the vertex.
- Scalp sensation
  - The greater occipital nerve (posterior ramus of C2) runs with the occipital artery and supplies the posterior scalp to the vertex.
  - The posterior scalp is also supplied by the third occipital nerve (posterior ramus of C3).
  - The lesser occipital nerve (anterior ramus of C2) runs with the posterior auricular artery and supplies sensation to the skin behind the ear.
  - The skin of the temple is supplied by the auriculotemporal and zygomaticotemporal nerves.
  - The forehead and anterior scalp are supplied by the supratrochlear and supraorbital nerves, which run with the corresponding arteries.

PATIENT HISTORY AND PHYSICAL FINDINGS

- Suitable candidates[3-5] have
  - High hairline
  - Good, healthy hair
  - Lack of cowlicks (posterior exiting hairs)
  - Good scalp mobility (measured by the ability of the scalp to rock back and forth on the skull)
  - Absence of scalp disease and previous scalp surgery
  - No history of stress-induced or unexplained hair loss
  - No family history of progressive hair loss

SURGICAL MANAGEMENT

- Hairline lowering is a day procedure, of about 2-hour duration.
- The major steps are as follows:

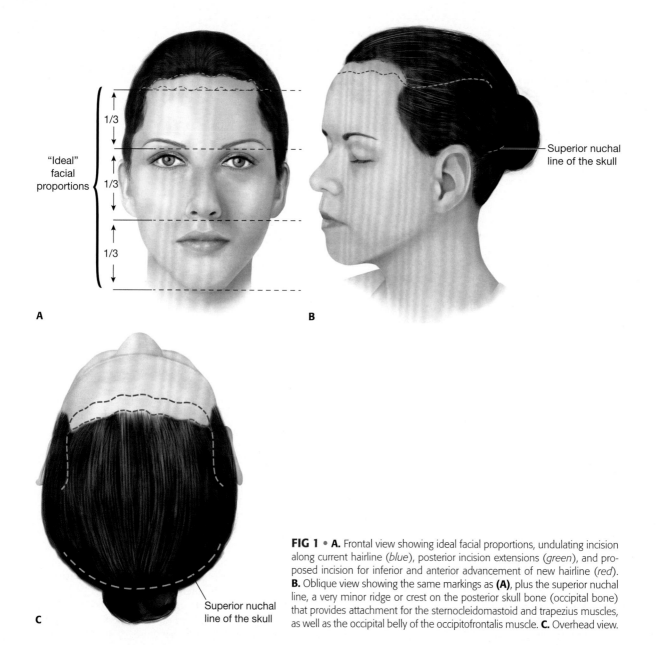

FIG 1 • **A.** Frontal view showing ideal facial proportions, undulating incision along current hairline (*blue*), posterior incision extensions (*green*), and proposed incision for inferior and anterior advancement of new hairline (*red*). **B.** Oblique view showing the same markings as **(A)**, plus the superior nuchal line, a very minor ridge or crest on the posterior skull bone (occipital bone) that provides attachment for the sternocleidomastoid and trapezius muscles, as well as the occipital belly of the occipitofrontalis muscle. **C.** Overhead view.

- The hairline is surgically advanced anteriorly using a posterior scalp advancement flap, to meet the proposed new hairline (**FIG 2A–D**).
  - It is easier to advance the central anterior hairline (narrow flap) than the whole frontal hairline (broad flap).
- The ellipse of the forehead skin between the pre-existing and new lower hairline is excised (**FIG 2C**).
- The scalp is secured in its advanced position to the underlying bone with sutures through converging outer cortical bone tunnels, Endotines, or other fixation devices (**FIG 2C**).

Preoperative Planning and Positioning

- Marking of the existing and new proposed hairlines is made preoperatively with the patient standing or sitting up.
  - The marking of the frontal hairline should be in an irregularly undulating fashion, which resembles the natural hairline and helps with camouflage of the incision (**FIG 3A**).[3–5]

- This marking is just posterior to the fine hairs of the anterior hairline but before the coarse hairs of the defined zone become denser.[3–5]
- If needed, the incision is made as lateral as possible, to allow for lateral as well as central advancement, and to avoid recession at the frontotemporal angle (temporal recession).
- The proposed new, lower hairline traces the superior marking (**FIG 3B**).
- The level is marked according to the patient's desires while taking into consideration the pre-existing scalp mobility.
- Usually 2.5 cm of scalp advancement is not difficult with a moderately mobile scalp.[5]
- The incision continues posteriorly bilaterally, in a shape similar to the arms of a pair of spectacles (**FIG 3C**).
- The patient is positioned supine, on a head ring at the superior most end of the table.
- Surgery is performed under general anesthesia or local anesthesia with sedation.[3–5]

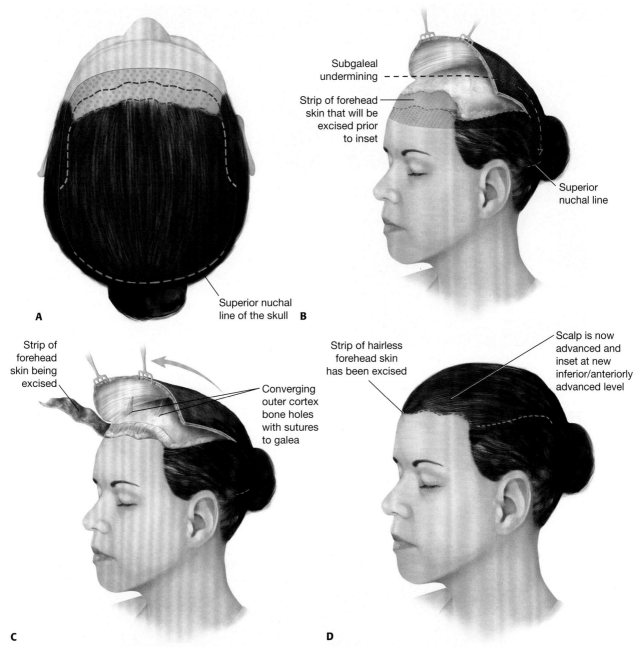

FIG 2 • A. The extent of subgaleal undermining, not only of the proposed scalp flap but also of the scalp and forehead 2 to 3 cm in addition to the scalp flap. The *blue line* is the undulating incision along the current hairline; the *green lines* are posterior incision extensions; the *red line* is the proposed new hairline, and the *pink area* is the limit of subgaleal scalp elevation. **B.** Elevation of the scalp away from the underlying skull. This occurs as far posteriorly as the superior nuchal line. Rake retractors are used to elevate the scalp flap. The scalp and forehead are undermined 2 to 3 cm lateral to the lateral incisions and anterior to the proposed new hairline. The strip of forehead skin to be excised remains in situ until the flap is advanced anteriorly. **C.** The undermined scalp is advanced anteriorly with the help of rake retractors. Bilateral bone holes (converging external cortical bone holes) that have been drilled are used with sutures to keep the scalp flap advanced. The undersurface of the scalp flap has galeotomies (incisions in the galea), which help it to stretch and reach further anteriorly. The strip of hairless forehead skin is excised and discarded prior to inset of the advanced flap. **D.** End result with hairline lowered by scalp flap. Insetting is accomplished with deep dissolvable sutures with staples laterally and sutures anteriorly. The undulating hairline is preserved.

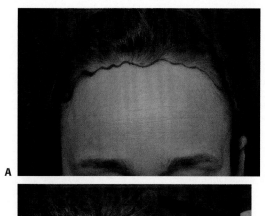

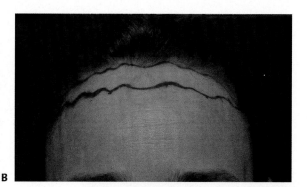

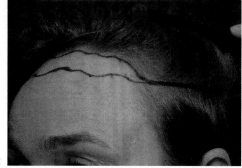

FIG 3 • A. Undulating irregularly irregular incision line marking at the existing hairline. The incision will be just posterior to this. **B.** Markings for the new proposed hairline are drawn on the forehead to match the undulating existing hairline marking. The two lines meet laterally to outline the ellipse of skin to be excised. **C.** Marking for the incision is extended posteriorly, in a shape similar to the arms of a pair of spectacles.

■ Local Anesthesia

- Local anesthesia (ropivacaine/marcaine/lignocaine) with epinephrine is used for both hemostatic and intraoperative and postoperative analgesic effects.
- The local anesthesia is injected at the brow to anesthetize the supraorbital and supratrochlear nerves (**TECH FIG 1A**).[3]

- Then it is injected along the existing and proposed new hairlines (**TECH FIG 1B**) and posteriorly in a circumferential manner, which produces a vasoconstrictive, pseudotourniquet effect (**TECH FIG 1C**).[3–6]

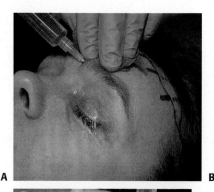

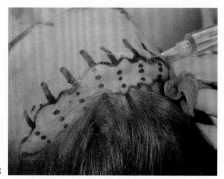

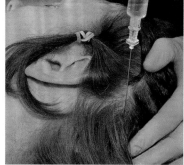

TECH FIG 1 • A. Local anesthetic is injected to block the supratrochlear and supraorbital nerves. **B.** Local anesthetic with epinephrine is injected along the incision lines. **C.** Local anesthetic with epinephrine is injected along the posterior incision line in a circumferential pattern toward the superior nuchal line using a spinal needle. Meeting the local anesthetic from the contralateral side produces a pseudotourniquet effect.

■ Incision and Dissection

- The incision anteriorly is made in a trichophytic beveled manner using a no. 15 blade.[1,3,4] This denudes or de-epithelializes hair follicles along the length of the anterior incision (**TECH FIG 2A,B**).
- It is just posterior to the forehead-scalp junction, posterior to the transition zone, just anterior to where the thicker hair of the defined zone starts.

- The incision is deepened to the subgaleal level with a no. 10 blade, in the same beveled manner (**TECH FIG 2C**), and transitions to become parallel to the hair follicles for the posterior extensions.[3]
- The incision is extended posteriorly parallel to the hair follicles (**TECH FIG 2D**).

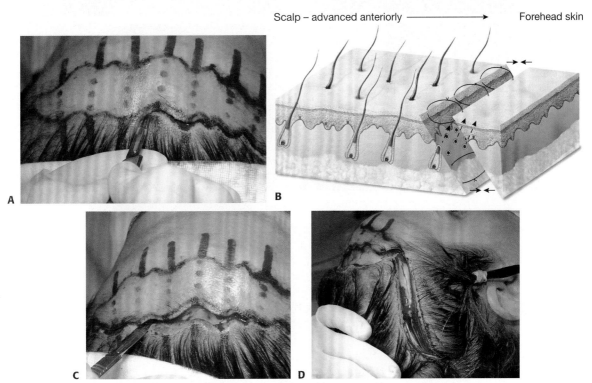

Scalp – advanced anteriorly ⟶ Forehead skin

TECH FIG 2 • **A.** The undulating existing hairline incision is made posterior to the markings, just posterior to the fine hairs of the transition zone. The incision is made in a beveled, trichophytic manner denuding follicles of the anterior scalp. **B.** Beveled incision causes the hairless forehead skin to overlap the denuded hair follicles of the anteriorly advanced scalp flap. Some of the denuded follicle hairs will exit the forehead skin anterior to the incision line, helping to camouflage the incision line. **C.** The initial incision is made with a no. 15 blade but deepened with the same bevel using a no. 10 blade. **D.** The incision is extended posteriorly parallel to the hair follicles.

■ Flap Elevation

- The scalp is raised posteriorly in a subgaleal plane using a no. 10 blade with the aid of multipronged rake retractors (**TECH FIG 3A**).
- Digital dissection is then used to further dissect this flap posteriorly (**TECH FIG 3B**).
- The Iconoclast helps to elevate this flap in the subgaleal plane in the difficult to reach portion, as far posteriorly as the superior nuchal line (**TECH FIG 3C,D**).
- The scalp laterally and forehead anteriorly are undermined in the subgaleal plane to facilitate tension-free closure.

- A sponge is placed in the recess between the skull and the raised flap for hemostasis (**TECH FIG 3E**).
  - Subgaleal undermining continues for 2 to 3 cm lateral to the posterior extension incisions and 4 to 5 cm anterior to the anterior incision line.
- The midline of both the skull and galea of the scalp flap is marked with a marking pen to ensure symmetry when the flap is advanced later (**TECH FIG 3F**).
- Outer cortical converging bone tunnels are made in the anterior skull, 4 to 5 cm from the midline, to attach the scalp once it has been advanced (**TECH FIG 3G,H**).[1,3,6]
  - Endotines or other fixation devices can be used if desired.[4,5]

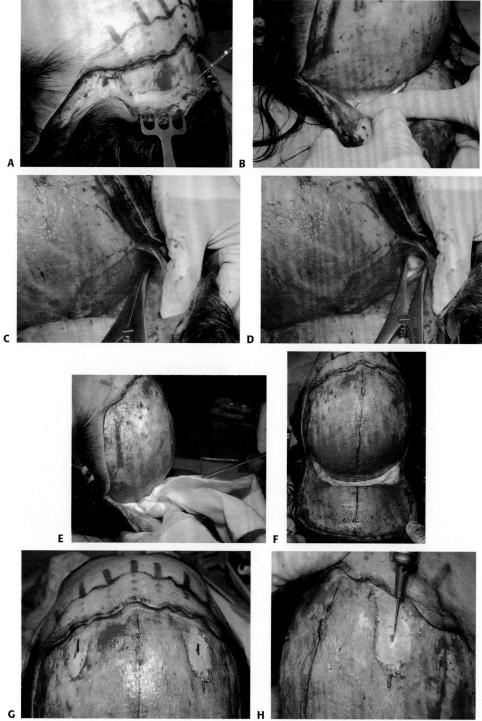

TECH FIG 3 • A. Initially the scalp is elevated in the subgaleal plane using a 10 blade with traction from rake retractors. **B.** Digital dissection in the subgaleal plane is used as the skull curves toward the neck. **C,D.** The Iconoclast is a spreading instrument used for subgaleal dissection posteriorly to the superior nuchal line. The instrument facilitates scalp flap elevation in the hard to reach posterior sections of the scalp. **E.** A sponge is placed in the scalp-skull recess to aid hemostasis. **F.** A marking pen is used to mark the midline of the skull and the scalp flap. This facilitates even and accurate scalp flap advancement. **G.** The periosteum of the scalp is elevated to expose the bone of the underlying skull, and markings for outer cortical bone holes are made on the anterior skull, equidistant from the midline. **H.** Converging external cortical bone holes are drilled.

■ Galeotomies

■ To achieve further advancement, galeotomies are made in the anterior to midscalp using an angled ophthalmic blade (**TECH FIG 4A,B**).[4,5]

■ Galeotomies must be made superficial to the underlying scalp vessels to preserve the scalp blood supply (**TECH FIG 4C**).[4,5]

■ Four or five galeotomies may be made, each of which generally advances the scalp a further 2 to 3 mm. They are generally made 1.5 to 2 cm apart.[3]

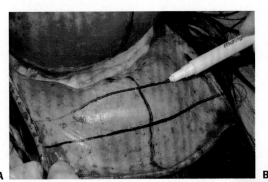
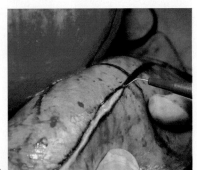
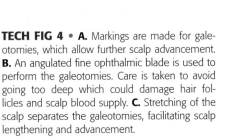
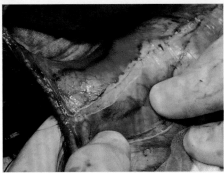

TECH FIG 4 • A. Markings are made for galeotomies, which allow further scalp advancement. **B.** An angulated fine ophthalmic blade is used to perform the galeotomies. Care is taken to avoid going too deep which could damage hair follicles and scalp blood supply. **C.** Stretching of the scalp separates the galeotomies, facilitating scalp lengthening and advancement.

■ Scalp Advancement

■ The sponge is removed, and the scalp is advanced (**TECH FIG 5A,B**).

■ The scalp is maintained in the advanced position by a suture through the bone tunnels, attached gently to the galea (**TECH FIG 5C–E**).

■ With the posterior scalp flap stabilized in the advanced position, excessive tension on the resulting incision closure is avoided.

■ Adjustments may now be made in the markings of the proposed new hairline (**TECH FIG 5F**).

■ The new hairline is incised in a similar beveled fashion to the original incision (**TECH FIG 5G**).

  ■ This beveled incision allows the forehead skin to slightly overlap the advanced scalp.

  ■ This facilitates growth of some hairs from the denuded scalp follicles through the forehead skin anterior to the incision line.[1,3,4,5]

■ The hairless forehead skin is removed (**TECH FIG 5H,I**).

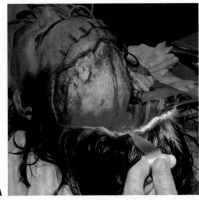
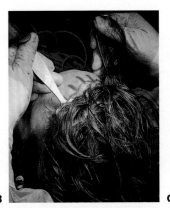
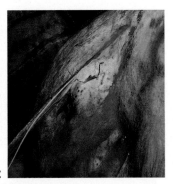

TECH FIG 5 • A,B. After the sponge is removed from the scalp-skull recess, rake retractors are used to advance the posteriorly based scalp flap. **C.** A suture is placed through the external cortical bone holes of the anterior skull.

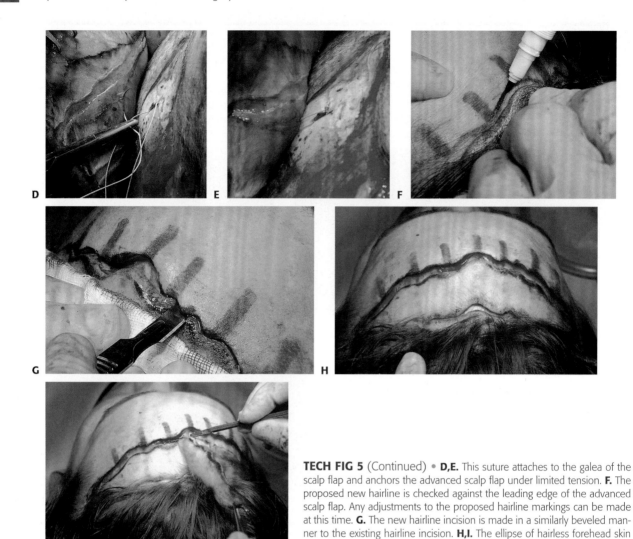

TECH FIG 5 (Continued) • **D,E.** This suture attaches to the galea of the scalp flap and anchors the advanced scalp flap under limited tension. **F.** The proposed new hairline is checked against the leading edge of the advanced scalp flap. Any adjustments to the proposed hairline markings can be made at this time. **G.** The new hairline incision is made in a similarly beveled manner to the existing hairline incision. **H,I.** The ellipse of hairless forehead skin is removed.

■ Scalp Fixation and Wound Closure

- The remainder of the procedure requires accurate insetting of the advanced scalp flap with dissolvable deep sutures (3-0 and 4-0 Monocryl). Tension is avoided (**TECH FIG 6A,C**).
- Interrupted or running 6-0 Prolene sutures are used anteriorly (**TECH FIG 6B**).

- Staples are used laterally (**TECH FIG 6D**).
- The patient's hair is washed with hydrogen peroxide and then saline or water (**TECH FIG 6E**).
- The hairline is covered with a light foam dressing, using a 10-cm conforming stretch bandage under minimal tension (**TECH FIG 6F**).

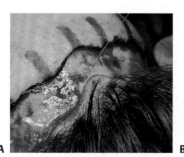
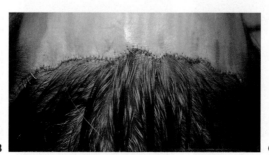
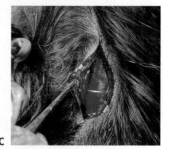

TECH FIG 6 • A. Dissolvable deep sutures under minimal tension are used to inset the advanced flap. **B.** The bevel used allows the denuded follicles of the scalp flap to slip deep to the hairless forehead skin. **C.** Interrupted or continuous Prolene sutures are used anteriorly. These will be removed between postoperative days 5 and 7.

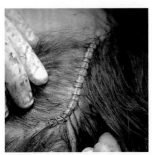 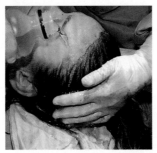 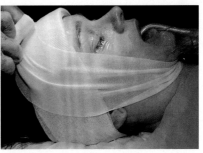

TECH FIG 6 (Continued) • **D.** Staples are used in the scalp. **E.** The hair is washed. **F.** A gentle foam dressing is applied.

PEARLS AND PITFALLS

Indications	▪ Follicular unit grafts are better for deep temporal recession. ▪ Cow licks (posterior exiting hairs) make incision camouflage more difficult. ▪ A two-stage procedure utilizing a scalp tissue expander may be necessary for patients with tight scalps or very high hairlines or where the desired anterior hairline advancement is more than 3 cm.
Flap elevation	▪ The Iconoclast is an instrument that allows subgaleal scalp elevation in the difficult to reach posterior scalp recesses.
Scalp advancement	▪ A narrow central scalp flap is easier to advance than a broad flap of the whole frontal hairline. However, most female patients desire a rounded hairline without temporal hairline recession. ▪ Broad flaps have a higher incidence of lateral incision line tension and minor incision line hair loss.
Scalp fixation	▪ Outer cortical converging bone holes allow stabilization and fixation of the scalp flap in an anterior position. ▪ Excessive tension must be avoided.
Wound closure	▪ Dissolving deep sutures allow tension-free closure of the incision lines. ▪ Overlap of the incision line denuded scalp follicles by hairless forehead skin is desired.

POSTOPERATIVE CARE

- The dressing is removed on postoperative day 1.
- Patients are able to shower and wash their hair from day 1 with warm water and a mild soap/shampoo.
- Patients are instructed not to blow-dry or brush their hair.
- Alternate staples and Prolene sutures may be removed at day 5 or 6.
- Remaining staples and Prolene sutures are removed on day 7 or 8.
- Most patients are back at work within a week or so.
- Patients are instructed to avoid the following:
  - Tasks that cause a Valsalva maneuver, such as heavy lifting or straining
  - Trips to the hairdresser/coloring hair for 6 weeks
  - Hot hairdryers/scalding hot showers
  - Tight caps and constricting helmets

OUTCOMES

- Reliable hairline advancement with immediate results[4]
- Good alternative to hair grafting—mobilizes many thousand follicular units[4]

COMPLICATIONS

- Visible scars
- Hyperpigmented or hypopigmented scars
- Scalp numbness and dysesthesia
- Hair loss
  - Telogen effluvium ("stress" or "shock" hair loss)[2,4,5]
  - Incision line alopecia (especially with broad scalp advancement)
  - Patchy scalp alopecia[2-6]
- Hairline aesthetic/shape issues
- Need for scar revision/need for hair grafts to finesse scars[4]
- Scalp necrosis[5]
- Future hair loss with progressive scar visibility

REFERENCES

1. Guyuron B, Rowe DJ. How to make a long forehead more aesthetic. *Aesthet Surg J.* 2008;28:46-50.
2. Guyuron B, Lee M. A reappraisal of surgical techniques and efficacy in forehead rejuvenation. *Plast Reconstr Surg.* 2014;134(3):426-435.
3. Marten TJ. Hairline lowering during foreheadplasty. *Plast Reconstr Surg.* 1999;103(1):224-236.
4. Ramirez AL, Ende KH, Kabaker SS. Correction of the high female hairline. *Arch Facial Plast Surg.* 2009;11:84-90.
5. Kabaker SS, Champagne JP. Hairline lowering. *Facial Plast Surg Clin North Am.* 2013;21:479-486.
6. Guyuron B, Behmand RA, Green R. Shortening of the long forehead. *Plast Reconstr Surg.* 1999;103:218-223.
7. Shapiro R, Shapiro P. Hairline design and frontal hairline restoration. *Facial Plast Surg Clin North Am.* 2009;21:351-361.

TECHNIQUES

26
CHAPTER

Section VIII: Upper Blepharoplasty

Techniques for Upper Blepharoplasty

Steven M. Levine

DEFINITION

- Surgery is the standard treatment to address the aging upper eye.
- The aging upper eye can be broken down into excess skin and excess fat.

ANATOMY

- Relevant anatomy pertains to the layers of the upper eyelid: notably, the skin, the orbicularis oculi muscle, and the preaponeurotic fat (central fat pad and medial/nasal fat pad).
- The lacrimal gland is located laterally and deep to the preaponeurotic fat pad. This gland can become ptotic and be confused as redundant fat.

PATIENT HISTORY AND PHYSICAL FINDINGS

- Beyond the usual history, to make sure a patient is an acceptable candidate for facial plastic surgery, certain physical findings should be noted.
- Ptosis should always be noted. Ptosis repair is not being addressed in this chapter.
- The eyes should be studied carefully to note the exact location of the excess or "hooded" skin.
- Ask for photographs of the patient when younger to note whether the upper lids were always "full."
  - This will avoid hollowing out a patient who is used to having full lids.
- The lateral extent of the excess should be noted and care taken to include that tissue in the resection (even if it falls beyond the lateral orbital rim).
- The tarsal insertion should be marked to represent, approximately, the inferior aspect of the surgical excision.

SURGICAL MANAGEMENT

- Surgery should be performed in an accredited operating room.
- An upper blepharoplasty can be performed under local anesthesia with or without sedation or general anesthesia.

Preoperative Planning

- The author requires all patients to be seen by an ophthalmologist and have a Schirmer tear test preoperatively.
- Consideration should be given as to whether the surgeon believes the patient will require fat to be removed.
  - If the operation is "skin only," it is easier to perform under local anesthesia.
- The patient should be marked while sitting upright.
- It is important to end the medial extent of resection prior to the medial canthus to avoid creation of a web.
- A "pinch test" should be performed on the estimated skin resection to ensure the surgery will not create a lagophthalmos.
- Use a ruler to ensure the markings are roughly equal on both sides.
  - Measure the distance from the lash line to the inferior aspect of resection and the distance from the lateral canthus to the lateral extent of the resection (**FIG 1**).
- The author rarely removes fat from the upper lid.
  - That said, the medial or nasal fat compartment is more commonly full and can benefit from fat removal.
- The globe is balloted to accentuate the excess fat, and a decision is made preoperatively as to where fat will be removed and how much.
  - Fat is not removed indiscriminately. The surgeon should know roughly how much fat he or she plans to excise.

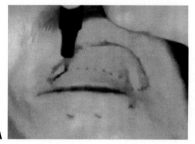 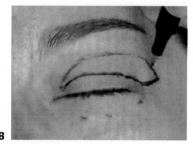

FIG 1 • **A** and **B.** The planned resection is marked in the standing position and then checked again on the operating table ensuring the accuracy of the markings.

- Discussion of scar placement, complications, and expected healing time should be reviewed with the patient.

Positioning

- The patient is supine on the procedure table.
- Usually, the head of bed is slightly elevated.
- The authors prefer to sit for maximum stability.

Approach

- Approach is dictated by the decision to remove skin, muscle, and/or fat.
  - If only fat is being removed, a small stab incision is made to access the fat. No further incision is required.
  - If skin is being removed, a small stab incision through the muscle and septum is made. The author does not favor an "open sky" technique.

■ Upper Blepharoplasty

- After 1% lidocaine with epinephrine 1:100 000 is infiltrated into a predesigned excision pattern, at least 8 minutes is allowed to pass to allow for vasoconstriction (**TECH FIG 1A**).
- The skin is excised using a no. 15 blade and the muscle is kept intact (**TECH FIG 1B**).
- If fat is to be removed, the globe is balloted to accentuate the excess fat, and sharp scissors are used to penetrate the muscle septum. The fat is then exposed through the small stab incision.

- Care is taken to remove only fat considered excess. Often, this is the size of an eraser head. (Note: this is where the surgeon's personal aesthetic sense comes into play. The key is to know how much fat you intent to remove before you do so.)
- A Bovie electrocautery is use to obtain hemostasis (**TECH FIG 1C**).
- The skin is closed from medial to lateral with a running 5-0 subcuticular nylon (**TECH FIG 1D**).
- If necessary, the closure is reinforced with either running or interrupted 6-0 nylon on the skin.

TECHNIQUES

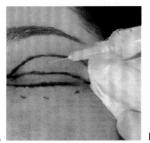 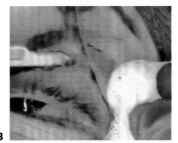 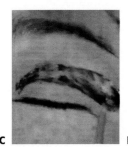 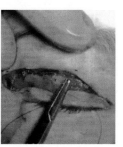

TECH FIG 1 • **A.** Administration of local anesthesia. **B.** Skin excision. **C.** Meticulous hemostasis is essential. **D.** Closure.

PEARLS AND PITFALLS

Markings	■ Mark the patient's tarsal crease preoperatively. This is more challenging when the patient is supine.
Lateral tissue removal	■ Do not leave excess lateral tissue. There is often a fear of extending the upper blepharoplasty incision beyond the orbital rim; however, this scar heals very well. This is also the area where patients are likely to complain of residual excess.
Fat removal	■ Do not over-resect fat. A surgeon can adversely change a person's appearance by converting the person from an individual with full upper lids to one with hollow upper lids.
Maintaining symmetry	■ Measure both eye markings to ensure symmetry. Scars at different heights on the lid need to be avoided.
Eye exam	■ A preoperative ophthalmologist exam may seem overly cautious, but in the event of a problem, it is very useful to have a consultation performed prior to surgery.

POSTOPERATIVE CARE

- Steri-Strips are placed over the incisions.
- Cool packs are also used to reduce swelling.
- Strict blood pressure control is enforced postoperatively.
- Patients are instructed no lifting or bending for 2 weeks.
- At 48 hours, the medial end of the running suture is trimmed to below the level of the skin to prevent inclusion cyst formation.
- If skin sutures were used, they are removed within 4 days.

- The author prefers to keep the running subcuticular suture in for 7 to 9 days.
- All patients are seen by the surgeon 48 hours after surgery.

OUTCOMES

- An upper blepharoplasty is a highly reliable and predictable operation.
- Scars are usually well concealed (including the extent beyond the lateral orbital rim).

COMPLICATIONS

- Bruising and bleeding are the most common complications.
- The surgeon must be cognizant of the creation of a retrobulbar hematoma. This is exceedingly rare if fat is not removed.
- On occasion, a second surgery is required to trim excess skin, but this is favored over removing too much tissue.

Transpalpebral Corrugator Resection

Ji H. Son, Ali Totonchi, and Bahman Guyuron

27 CHAPTER

DEFINITION

- Glabellar frown lines develop as a result of the contraction of the corrugator supercilii muscles and thinning of the overlying skin.
- Resection of these muscles corrects the deep furrowing and is usually accomplished through upper blepharoplasty incisions.

ANATOMY

- Frontalis muscle: elevates the eyebrows and causes transverse wrinkling of the forehead. Its contraction provides a constant, cranially directed force vector on the eyebrows.
- Orbicularis oculi muscle: depresses the eyebrows. The two main portions of this muscle are orbital and palpebral.
- Corrugator supercilii muscle: thin, long, hexagon-shaped muscle located at the medial end of the eyebrow, deep to frontalis and orbicularis oculi muscles. Corrugators pass between the orbicularis oculi and insert into the deep surface of the forehead skin.
- Depressor supercilii: a thin muscle that extends from the medial canthus area to the subcutaneous plane above the eyebrows.
- Procerus muscle: pulls the glabella area skin caudally. The procerus originates from the caudal portion of the nasal bones and inserts into the dermis between the eyebrows, which makes it a major stabilizer of the eyebrows. Hyperactivity of this muscle causes transverse lines in the glabellar area and the nasal root.
- Supraorbital nerve: exits the supraorbital notch or foramen 2.7 cm from the midline and runs with an associated artery.
- Supratrochlear nerve: located 1.7 cm from the midline and 0.8 cm anterior to the supraorbital nerve and runs with associated artery.

PATHOGENESIS

- Glabellar frown lines (vertical or oblique) develop due to the contraction/hyperactivity of the corrugator and depressor supercilii muscles and the thinning of the overlying skin.
- The overactive procerus muscle can result in horizontal lines in the radix area.

HISTORY

- Corrugator supercilii muscle resection is traditionally done using open or endoscopic forehead lift approaches. The senior author first introduced the transpalpebral approach in 1993.[1]

- This chapter will focus on the transpalpebral resection only. Other techniques are discussed in different chapters in this textbook.

PATIENT HISTORY AND PHYSICAL FINDINGS

- A comprehensive analysis of the face, hairline position, brow position and arch, forehead length, width, contour, soft tissue quality, and rhytids will aid in selection of the procedure that will best serve the patient.
- The upper face length is approximately one-third of the entire face.
  - Frontalis compensation is extremely common, and it is crucial to eliminate it for a more accurate judgment about the eyebrow position by asking the patient to smile or close the eyes tightly and then open them just enough to see the examiner, making every effort to avoid upward motion of the eyebrows.
  - The uncompensated position of the eyebrows is at the supraorbital rim in males and slightly above it in females, with its apex at the lateral limbus of the eye.
  - The evaluation of the forehead rhytids is recommended in repose, smiling, and frowning.
- The best candidates for transpalpebral corrugator resection are:
  - Patients who have proper lateral eyebrow position with hyperactive corrugator muscles[2-4]
  - Patients who are undergoing endoscopic forehead rejuvenation and blepharoplasty concomitantly
  - Patients with male pattern baldness, on whom incisions must be limited further laterally to avoid visible scars in the forehead area
  - Patients with long foreheads, who would not wish to have a forehead shortening procedure
  - Patients with proptosis and overactive glabellar muscle where elevation of the eyebrows needs to be avoided, which would otherwise expose the proptosis more and have an adverse effect on the patient's face
  - Similarly, patients with eyelid ptosis who decline eyelid ptosis correction whereby elevation of the eyebrows would enhance the ill effects of existing ptosis on the periorbital congruity[3,4]
  - Patients with documented frontal migraine headaches without the temporal component[5]

IMAGING

- Imaging is not indicated for transpalpebral corrugator resection, unless there is a clear reason such as mass or lesion in the area or frontal migraine headaches with the retrobulbar component.

NONOPERATIVE MANAGEMENT

- Botulinum toxin A or fillers injection: These would be appropriate for temporary reduction of corrugator hyperactivity or contour deformity for those who are not ready to undergo surgery.[6]
- Fat injection: Limited indication for the patient with permanent and static wrinkles, where the results are long lasting but less predictable than injectable fillers. Fat injection is indicated on patients who are not ready to undergo more invasive procedures.

SURGICAL MANAGEMENT

- The main objective of transpalpebral corrugator resection is to resect the hyperactive corrugator and depressor supercilii muscles through the upper blepharoplasty incisions as thoroughly as possible to correct the deep furrowing lines in a lasting manner.

Preoperative Planning

- An AP photograph of the patient's forehead in repose and while frowning in a standardized fashion is recommended for analysis and postoperative comparison. Any asymmetry needs to be noted and discussed with the patient.
- General medical conditions including hypertension and hyperglycemia, as well as smoking cessation, are imperative to be addressed prior to surgery to minimize wound healing complications.
- Risks, benefits, and expectations need to be clearly discussed with the patient prior to surgery, with specific attention to risk of anesthesia, asymmetry, incomplete resolution of glabellar frown lines, and paresthesia in the supraorbital and supratrochlear regions.

Approach

- The surgery can be done under general or monitored anesthesia care (MAC).
- After positioning the patient supine and prior to anesthesia, the supratarsal crease is marked as the incision line.
  - If a concomitant blepharoplasty is intended, the entire blepharoplasty incision is designed.
  - Otherwise, the medial half or third of a blepharoplasty incision is used.

■ Incision and Dissection

- The upper eyelids and the lower forehead area as well as glabellar area are injected with mixture of 1% lidocaine with 1:100 000 epinephrine mixed with 0.5% of Naropin using a 30-gauge needle generously.
- Incision is made on the upper eyelid in supratarsal crease (**TECH FIG 1A**) and taken through the orbicularis muscle (**TECH FIG 1B**).

- Skin hooks are placed at the skin edges to retract the skin and orbicularis muscle cephalically.
- Dissection is started in the plane between the orbicularis muscle and the orbital septum while staying immediately under the orbicularis muscle and aiming toward the supraorbital rim. Initially, the dissection is done with a cautery for an extent of 5 to 10 mm (**TECH FIG 1C**) and is then continued using Metzenbaum scissors (**TECH FIG 1D**).

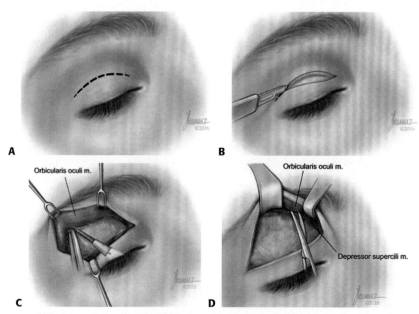

TECH FIG 1 • A. Upper eyelid incision using conventional blepharoplasty incision. **B.** Incision down to the orbicularis muscle. **C.** Dissection between the orbicularis muscle and the orbital septum. **D.** Continuation of dissection between the orbicularis muscle and the orbital septum until depressor supercilii is visualized. (From Guyuron B. Transpalpebral corrugator resection: 25-year experience, refinements and additional indications. *Aesth Plast Surg.* 2017;41:339-345.)

■ Removal of the Corrugator and Depressor Supercilii Muscle

- After elevation of the skin and the orbicularis muscle, a thin layer of the depressor supercilii muscle overlying the darker and more friable corrugator supercilii muscle comes into view; it is dissected (**TECH FIG 2A**) and removed (**TECH FIG 2B**).
- Upon removal of the depressor supercilii muscle, a branch of the supraorbital nerve piercing the corrugator supercilli muscle is identified and followed deep into the muscle using a mosquito hemostat (**TECH FIG 2C**).
- The supraorbital nerve is deeper and bigger than the supratrochlear nerve.
- The corrugator muscle is lifted to identify and protect the main nerve branches above the periosteum (**TECH FIG 2D**).

- The caudal portion of the muscle is isolated and removed first using coagulating cautery (**TECH FIG 2E**), followed by the cephalic segment.
- The remaining portion of a muscle is removed in a piecemeal fashion using the cautery as thoroughly as possible, including a lateral segment of the procerus muscle, the end point being the exposure of the fat in the subcutaneous plane.
- If the intention of the surgery is to treat frontal migraine headaches, the supratrochlear and supraorbital arteries are removed as well. If the nerve and vessels pass through a foramen, a foraminotomy is carried out using a 2-mm osteotome or a rongeur while protecting the orbital content (**TECH FIG 2F**).

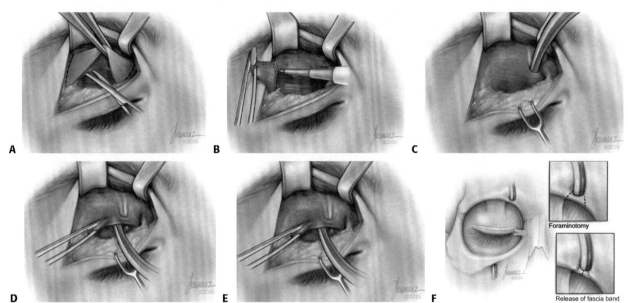

TECH FIG 2 • **A.** Corrugator supercilii is dissected. **B.** Corrugator supercilii is removed. **C.** Branch of the supraorbital nerve is identified and followed deep in the muscle using a hemostat. **D.** The same nerve branch is identified above the periosteum and protected. **E.** Corrugator supercilii caudal to the nerve is lifted and removed using cautery, medially and then laterally. **F.** If the intention of the surgery is to treat frontal migraine headaches, the supratrochlear and supraorbital arteries are removed due to their roles in compressing the nerve, and if the nerve and vessels pass through a foramen, a foraminotomy is carried out. (From Guyuron B. Transpalpebral corrugator resection: 25-year experience, refinements and additional indications. *Aesth Plast Surg.* 2017;41:339-345.)

■ Fat Grafting and Closure

- The upper eyelid nasal (medial) fat pad is gently isolated and injected with small amount of lidocaine with 1:100 000 epinephrine and removed with cautery (**TECH FIG 3A**).
- For the patient without protruding medial fat pads, 1 to 2 cc of fat is harvested from the abdomen and injected in the area.
- Fat graft or injection will prevent the depression resulting from a thorough removal of the muscles, minimize

the potential for the recurrence of the frown lines by avoiding the reattachment of the muscle to the skin, and rejuvenate the glabellar area by restoring the naturally lost volume because of aging.

- After fat harvest, it is flattened and placed in the corrugator site and fixed to the underlying periosteum using a 6-0 Vicryl suture to avoid any depression and to restore the lost glabellar volume to the site (**TECH FIG 3B**).
- The skin incision is closed using a 6-0 plain gut in a subcuticular fashion.

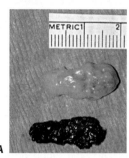
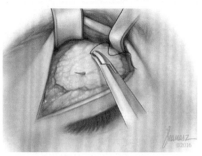

TECH FIG 3 • A. Isolated fat graft. **B.** The fat is flattened and placed in the corrugator site and fixed to the underlying periosteum using a 6-0 Vicryl suture. (From Guyuron B. Transpalpebral corrugator resection: 25-year experience, refinements and additional indications. *Aesth Plast Surg.* 2017;41:339-345.)

PEARLS AND PITFALLS

- Inadequate removal of the muscle will result in irregularities and flaws mostly during animation.
  - Only the lateral fibers of the procerus muscle are removed because complete or almost complete removal of the procerus muscle can cause excessive elevation of the medial eyebrows, resulting in an aesthetically displeasing outcome.
- The depressor supercilii muscle is commonly mistaken for the corrugator muscle. The latter is darker, more pliable, and located deeper and medial to the former. The goal of the surgery is complete or near complete removal of the muscles between the orbicularis muscle/skin and the periosteum.
- Some patients with established skin wrinkles may require fat injection or graft to the central portion of the glabella and laser surfacing to obtain optimal results.

POSTOPERATIVE CARE

- Head elevation for the first few days along with the use of a cold compress during the first 24 hours of surgery will help with edema and ecchymosis.
- Patients are instructed not to apply pressure on the glabellar area for a few days.

- Ophthalmic ointments help prevent dryness of the incisions, corneal abrasion, and exposure keratitis.

OUTCOMES

- Long-term satisfaction is usually very gratifying as long as the muscle is removed thoroughly (**FIG 1A,B**).

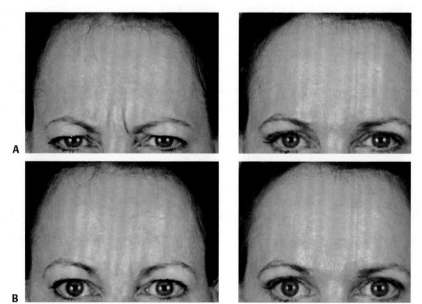

FIG 1 • Before (*left*) and 1 year after (*right*) transpalpebral corrugator resection. **A.** In repose. **B.** animated expression. (From Guyuron B. Transpalpebral corrugator resection: 25-year experience, refinements and additional indications. *Aesth Plast Surg.* 2017;41: 339-345.)

COMPLICATIONS

- The most common complication of transpalpebral corrugator resection is anesthesia/paresthesia of the forehead, which is often temporary.
- Early recurrence of glabellar furrowing may occur if the corrugator muscle is not adequately resected or is not replaced with fat graft. If the fat graft is not secured in place, it can migrate caudally causing excessive upper eyelid fullness.
- Patients who undergo transpalpebral corrugator resection with blepharoplasty experience more ecchymosis, compared with those who have blepharoplasty alone.

REFERENCES

1. Guyuron B. Corrugator supercilii muscle resection through blepharoplasty incision, ASPRS (ASPS) Annual Meeting, New Orleans, Louisiana, September 1993.
2. Knize DM. Transpalpebral approach to the corrugator supercilii and procerus muscles. *Plast Reconstr Surg.* 1995;95:52-60.
3. Guyuron B. Michelow BJ, Thomas T. Corrugator supercilii muscle resection through blepharoplasty incision. *Plast Reconstr Surg.* 1995;95:691-696.
4. Guyuron B. Corrugator supercilii resection through blepharoplasty incision. *Plast Reconstr Surg.* 2001;107:604-605.
5. Guyuron B, Varghai A, Michelow BJ, et al. Corrugator supercilii muscle resection and migraine headaches. *Plast Reconstr Surg.* 2000;106(2 suppl):429-434.

Technique for Ptosis Correction

Ashley A. Campbell, Christopher C. Lo, and Richard D. Lisman

DEFINITION

- Blepharoptosis, or ptosis, is the abnormally low position of the upper eyelid in primary gaze. Ptosis is classified by its etiology as congenital, involutional, neurogenic, myogenic, and mechanical.

ANATOMY (FIG 1)

- In normal eyelid anatomy, the upper eyelid retractors are the levator muscle (innervated by cranial nerve III) and the Mueller muscle (innervated by the sympathetic system).
- The levator muscle extends from the lesser wing of the sphenoid just above the annulus of Zinn to Whitnall ligament; at this point, it transitions to become the levator aponeurosis.
- The lid height is determined by the attachment of fine strands from the levator aponeurosis to the pretarsal skin and orbicularis muscle.
- The upper eyelid fold is subsequently created by the overhanging skin, fat, and orbicularis muscle superior to the crease.
- Mueller muscle originates from the undersurface of the levator aponeurosis to the superior tarsal margin. It provides about 2 mm of elevation to the upper lid.
- The upper eyelid tarsus is a dense plate of connective tissue that acts as structural support to the eyelids. It measures 10 to 12 mm in the vertical dimension.

PATHOGENESIS

- The most common type of ptosis is involutional (also referred to as aponeurotic).
- This occurs gradually with age and is thought to be related to dehiscence of the levator from its attachment to tarsus.
- Involutional ptosis may be related to contact lens use, prior eye or periocular surgery, eye rubbing, and chronic ocular allergy. These all produce a levator dehiscence.

NATURAL HISTORY

- Involutional ptosis typically presents as a gradual decrease in lid height over time.

PATIENT HISTORY AND PHYSICAL FINDINGS

- Patient's primary complaint is often eyelid height or crease asymmetry and/or a gradual decrease in the size of the palpebral aperture.
- This often produces the complaint of a tired appearance in patients presenting for aesthetic correction.
- Visual symptoms include superior visual field loss and even central loss of vision in severe cases.
- This often presents with highly elevated/arched eyebrows with deep frontalis contraction in an involuntary attempt to open each aperture. Less commonly, the patient may present with a chin-up posture in an involuntary attempt to look

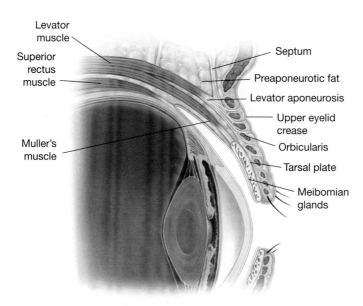

FIG 1 • Normal anatomy of the upper eyelids.

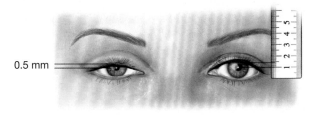

FIG 2 • Marginal reflex distance is measured from the central corneal light reflex to the upper eyelid while the patient sustains a neutral gaze in primary position.

0.5 mm

out from under the resultant "canopy effect." If long standing, neck pain or postural problems can result.

- Pertinent questions to ask in the patient's history include onset of ptosis, a history of trauma, a history of contact lens wear, prior surgery or botulinum toxin injections, fluctuations in the eyelid height, diplopia, and any associated systemic manifestations.
- Ocular history, especially including the history of dry eyes, should be obtained.
- Old photographs are useful in determining onset and degree of prior ptosis.
- Important aspects of the physical examination include the following:
  - Margin reflex distance (MRD): measured from the central corneal light reflex (usually the center of the pupil) to the upper eyelid margin. Normal measurement is 3 to 4 mm. In ptosis patients, this is reduced (**FIG 2**).
  - Palpebral fissure (PF): measured from the lower to upper eyelid margin in the midpupillary axis. Normal measurement is 8 to 10 mm. In ptosis patients, this is reduced.
  - Levator function (LF): measures the upper eyelid excursion from extreme downgaze to extreme upgaze while the brow is neutralized (**FIG 3**). This is critical in determining what ptosis repair technique is most appropriate. Normal measurement is 14 to 16 mm, and a value less than 5 mm indicates that either congenital blepharoptosis or acquired neurogenic etiologies need to be investigated prior to ptosis correction.
  - Lid crease height (LC): should evaluate shape and height. In the case of involutional ptosis, the LC is often elevated as the levator muscle is disinserted from its attachment to the tarsus.

- Bell phenomenon: the involuntary upward movement of the eye on lid closure. This needs to be assessed to determine the degree of corneal exposure should there be any lagophthalmos postoperatively.
- In asymmetric ptosis, Hering law should be evaluated by mechanically lifting one ptotic eyelid and observing the contralateral eyelid positional change.
- Pupillary examination should be performed to assess symmetry and reactivity in light and dark to rule out a Horner syndrome.
- Humphrey visual field testing performed with and without taping of the upper eyelid can be performed to demonstrate a superior visual field defect that is often present in patients with severe ptosis.

IMAGING

- Imaging is not typically required in the ptosis workup, unless there is any indication of a myogenic or neurologic etiology for ptosis.
- If the patient describes any variation in the amount of ptosis throughout the day or any double vision, a myogenic cause of ptosis (such as myasthenia gravis, chronic progressive external ophthalmoplegia, and myotonic dystrophy) should be considered. In this case, a referral to neuro-ophthalmology for further lab testing is indicated.
- If there is any evidence of unilateral ptosis in the context of a meiotic pupil (suggesting a Horner syndrome) or abnormal eye movements (suggesting a cranial nerve III palsy), a referral to neuro-ophthalmology for further workup is also indicated.

DIFFERENTIAL DIAGNOSIS

- Congenital ptosis
- Myogenic
  - Myasthenia gravis
  - Chronic progressive external ophthalmoplegia
  - Myotonic dystrophy
- Neurogenic
  - Horner syndrome
  - Cranial nerve III palsy
- Mechanical
  - Traumatic
  - Dermatochalasis/blepharochalasis

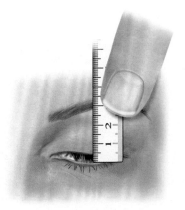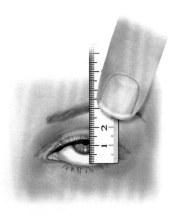

FIG 3 • To clinically evaluate levator function, measure the upper eyelid excursion in millimeters from extreme downgaze to upgaze with the brow relaxed or neutralized by the examiner's hand.

SURGICAL MANAGEMENT

- Many operative techniques have been described for the correction of involutional ptosis associated with moderate or good levator function. These include levator reinsertion, mullerectomy, and the Fasanella-Servat procedure.
- Here, we describe the modified Fasanella-Servat procedure, which is our procedure of choice out of many for aesthetic patients who obviously demand the most symmetry and have a good tear film and tear production. It is also possible to perform this ptosis correction in conjunction with other aesthetic procedures, and it does not require the patient's cooperation.

Preoperative Planning

- Prior to surgery, a careful ophthalmic examination should be performed particularly to assess for any evidence of dry eye disease, as there is a risk of increased early postoperative dry eye.
- If there is evidence of dry eye, history of laser in situ keratomileusis (LASIK), or a poor Bell phenomenon, a conservative ptosis correction should be considered. This is usually a conservative levator reattachment procedure.

- If there is asymmetric ptosis, Hering law of central and equal innervation to the levator muscles should be considered, as unilateral ptosis correction on the more ptotic-appearing side could then unmask ptosis on the normal-appearing eyelid.

Positioning

- A typical blepharoplasty incision site is marked in the preoperative holding area with the patient seated or in a semireclined position.
- Upon arrival to the operating room, the patient is placed in the supine position, and either monitored sedation or general anesthesia is used.
- Tetracaine ophthalmic drops are placed in each eye.
- Protective corneal shields covered with ophthalmic ointment are placed over both eyes.
- 2% lidocaine with 1:100 000 epinephrine is injected into both upper eyelids to achieve local anesthesia.

Approach

- The various approaches to consider in mild-moderate ptosis repair include levator reinsertion, mullerectomy, and the modified Fasanella-Servat. In this text, the modified Fasanella-Servat procedure will be further elaborated.

■ Modified Fasanella-Servat Procedure

- A no. 15 blade is used to incise the skin in the previously made blepharoplasty mark.
- The skin and orbicular oculi muscle are removed with curved Steven scissors.
- Hemostasis is obtained with unipolar cautery and epinephrine-soaked pledgets.
- The orbital septum is incised along the extent of the incision.
- Any excess central or medial fat is judiciously resected with the Colorado needle tip.
- The orbicularis muscle is contoured with the same device.
- Two symmetrically sized and shaped curved hemostat clamps are chosen for the tarsoconjunctival resection. The pair should be matched with care, as these will ultimately create the eyelid contour (**TECH FIG 1A,B**).
- The upper eyelid is everted, and a small (2 mm), medium (4 mm), or large (6 mm) tarsoconjunctival resection is

delineated with the clamps. It is anticipated that 1 mm of lift is achieved with a small resection, 2 mm for a medium resection, and 3 mm for a large resection.
- The clamps are placed so that the largest resection occurs over the medial aspect of the pupil in primary gaze.
- At least 4 mm of residual tarsus and conjunctiva on the upper eyelid is required to avoid lid destabilization and potential entropion.
- A 5-0 nylon suture on a P-3 needle is loaded backhand and passed from inside the upper eyelid wound centrally and directed laterally to exit at the posterior aspect of the clamp (**TECH FIG 1C**).
- The suture is passed in a running, buried fashion, just posterior to the clamps, medially to laterally (**TECH FIG 1D,E**). It is important that each suture pass begins in the previous suture hole, thereby burying the suture. If exposure of the suture occurs, the patient will experience foreign body sensation and may develop a corneal abrasion or ulcer.

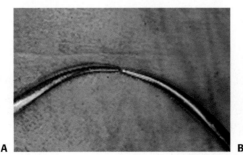 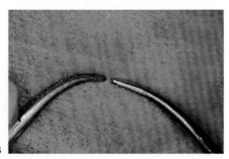

A   **B**

TECH FIG 1 • A. Symmetrically sized and shaped hemostat clamps with a smooth contour will result in a smooth upper eyelid contour. **B.** Poor clamp selection and positioning may result in eyelid peaking and contour abnormalities.

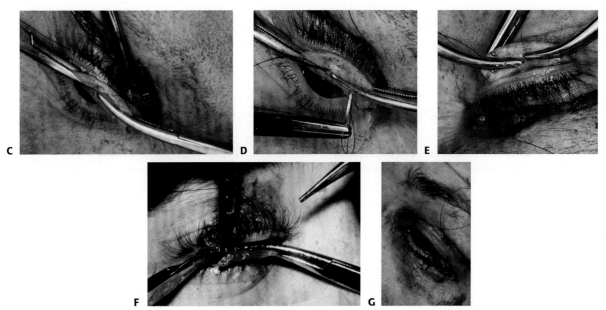

TECH FIG 1 (Continued) • **C.** A 5-0 nylon placed on a P-3 needle loaded backhand is passed from inside the upper eyelid wound centrally and directed laterally to exit at the posterior aspect of the clamp. **D,E.** The running 5-0 nylon suture is passed posterior to the hemostat clamps medially to laterally in a buried fashion. **F.** A tarsoconjunctival resection is performed with a no. 15 blade using the clamps as a guide to ensure a smooth contour. **G.** The ends of the 5-0 nylon suture are tied with multiple knots and left long for easy retrieval postoperatively. This suture is externalized through the upper eyelid blepharoplasty wound.

- The tarsoconjunctival resection is performed with a no. 15 blade using the clamps as a guide, ensuring a smooth contour (**TECH FIG 1F**).
- The lateral clamp is removed, and the suture is passed from the posterior aspect of the eyelid to exit in the upper eyelid wound just adjacent to the opposite arm of the suture. The medial clamp is then removed. Careful attention is given to ensure that the needle with its first and last pass traverse the entire eyelid thickness and pass through the levator as the procedure actually reattaches a levator disinsertion to a foreshortened tarsus. The release of the clamp adhesions with separation allows for later

readjustment, if needed, just prior to the dense scarring after postoperative days 8 to 10.
- The suture is tied with multiple knots and left long for easy retrieval at the time of suture removal. This suture is externalized through the upper eyelid wound (**TECH FIG G**).
- The contour of the upper eyelid should be smooth at this point. The eyelid height, however, should not be evaluated.
- The upper eyelid wound can be closed using whatever technique the surgeon prefers, as long as the 5-0 nylon Fasanella-Servat suture is externalized.

PEARLS AND PITFALLS

Curved clamp selection	■ Make sure each curved clamp is symmetric given that the curve of the clamp will ultimately determine the curvature of the eyelid. ■ Choice of two asymmetric clamps may result in significant lid peaking and contour abnormality.
Closure	■ Ensure that the knot is externalized through the blepharoplasty incision to facilitate suture removal at postoperative week 1.
Burying the suture	■ Failure to bury the suture through the previous suture hole when running nylon suture through the palpebral conjunctiva can result in foreign body sensation and a corneal abrasion. ■ If a corneal abrasion should develop, it is recommended to place a bandage contact lens until the suture is removed. ■ The antibiotic/steroid drop should be changed to an antibiotic drop alone if a bandage contact lens is placed.
Postoperative adjustment	■ At postoperative days 5 to 7, an adjustment can be made in the office if there is eyelid peaking, overcorrection on the surgical site, or undercorrection on the opposite side. This involves gentle downward tugging in the desired area of adjustment from the lashes or eyelid margin.

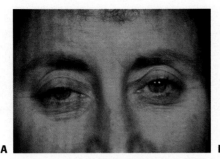 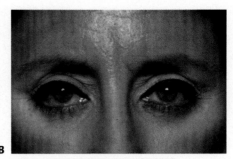

FIG 4 • Female with moderate, asymmetric, right-worse-than-left involutional ptosis, and dermatochalasis. **A.** Preoperative photos. **B.** A 2-month status post bilateral modified Fasanella-Servat procedure and quad blepharoplasty with symmetric eyelid height and contour.

POSTOPERATIVE CARE

- Postoperatively, a topical antibiotic/steroid eye drop is recommended four times a day for 1 week.
- For the first 72 hours postoperatively, patients should sleep with their head elevated and apply cold compresses.
- Patients should be instructed to avoid heavy lifting, bending, and straining for at least 2 weeks after surgery.
- If the patient should develop any foreign body sensation or evidence of a corneal abrasion, this could mean exposure of the nylon suture along the palpebral conjunctiva. This can be managed with placement of a bandage contact lens, which is removed at the time of suture removal. At this point, the antibiotic/steroid drop should be changed to an antibiotic drop alone.
- At postoperative week 1, the Fasanella suture can be removed. At this time, adjustments can be made as necessary (**FIG 4**).

OUTCOMES

- The Fasanella-Servat procedure is unique in that subtle correction of lid contour and height asymmetries can be made in the early postoperative period. Given that tarsus does not adhere until postoperative day 8 or 9, early adhesions can be broken around postoperative days 5 to 7 at the time of suture removal (**FIG 5**).
- Indications for adjustment include eyelid peaking, overcorrection on the surgical side, or undercorrection on the opposite side (**FIG 6**).
- Adjustment requires a gentle downward tugging in the desired area from the lashes or lid margins (**FIG 7**). Use of a cotton-tipped applicator to apply pressure at the superior border of the tarsus separates early tarsal adhesions. Local anesthesia or sedation is not needed.
- In the case of bilateral surgery, readjustment is aimed at lowering the higher lid given that the lower eyelid will secondarily elevate due to the phenomenon of Hering law.

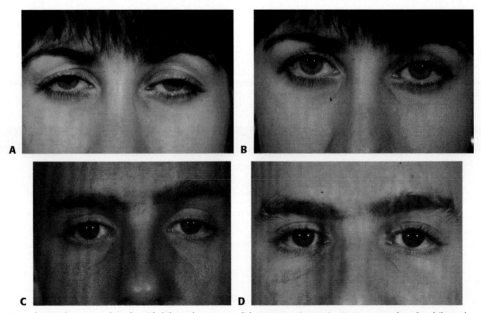

FIG 5 • **A.** Preoperative photo of a young female with bilateral upper eyelid aponeurotic ptosis. **B.** Two months after bilateral upper eyelid modified Fasanella-Servat procedure showing improved MRD, symmetry, and contour restoring a youthful appearance. **C.** Preoperative photo of a male with unilateral aponeurotic ptosis and compensatory left brow elevation. **D.** Postoperative photo 2 months after left modified Fasanella-Servat surgery with deviation of the left upper eyelid. Left brow drop further contirbutes to overall symmetry and balance of periorbital features.

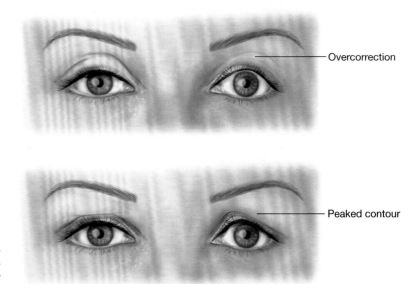

FIG 6 • Aberrant contour and eyelid height are complications of all methods of eyelid ptosis repair. With the modified Fasanella-Servat procedure, these pitfalls can be easily reversed with postoperative in-office adjustments.

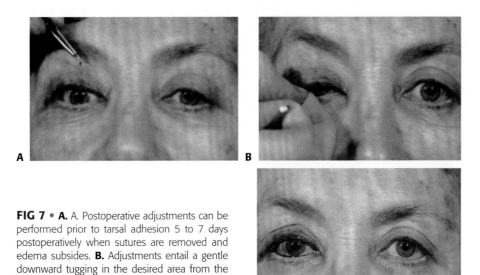

FIG 7 • **A.** A. Postoperative adjustments can be performed prior to tarsal adhesion 5 to 7 days postoperatively when sutures are removed and edema subsides. **B.** Adjustments entail a gentle downward tugging in the desired area from the lashes or lid margins. **C.** It is common to see some blood in the tear film after a successful adjustment.

- In general, approximately 20% of patients require a small postoperative adjustment. Once adjusted, nearly 100% of patients can attain a satisfactory result.[1]
- Final lid height is determined at about 14 to 21 days postoperatively or when all the edema has fully cleared.
- Although it is rare to need a reoperation, if an additional surgery is necessary, it is recommended to wait at least 3 months postoperatively.[2]

COMPLICATIONS

- Foreign body sensation or a corneal abrasion can occur immediately postoperatively if there is exposure of the nylon suture through the palpebral conjunctiva. This can be addressed by placement of a bandage contact lens that is kept in place until suture removal at postoperative days 5 to 7.

- Dry eye is a known complication after any ptosis surgery, especially if dry eye is a pre-existing condition. This can be treated with increased lubrication including antibiotic acutely and artificial tears chronically.
- Asymmetry between lids is a risk factor in ptosis surgery. In the Fasanella-Servat procedure, mild asymmetry can be consistently corrected postoperatively with a minor in-office adjustment (**FIG 7**).

REFERENCES

1. Rosenberg C, Lelli GJ, Lisman RD. Early postoperative adjustment of the Fasanella-Servat procedure: review of 102 consecutive cases. *Ophthalmic Plast Reconstr Surg.* 2009;25:19-26.
2. Buckman G, Jakobiec FA, Hyde K, et al. Success of the Fasanella-Servat operation independent of Muller's smooth muscle excision. *Ophthalmology.* 1989;96(4):413-418.

29
CHAPTER

Technique for Ptosis Correction

Nuri A. Celik

DEFINITION

- There have been many procedures advocated for the treatment of the upper eyelid ptosis. Some of the techniques in the literature use incisional/excisional methods to deal with the levator mechanism failures.[1]
- The technique described in this chapter relies solely on the preservation of the anatomical integrity of the levator system that is either stretched or detached because of various reasons. The key to using this technique is the presence of a good levator function. This is easily calculated by measuring the excursion of the upper eyelid during extreme upper and downward gaze (**FIG 1**).
- Practically, any measurement above 10 mm is proper to use this technique efficiently. Iatrogenic or senile levator detachment patients are a different group, because they present with decreased levator function; however, in most cases, the system is intact to perform this type of correction. Fatty degeneration of the levator muscle is also a possibility with aging.

ANATOMY

- The upper eyelid is a complex structure that consists of multiple tissue layers that seem to adhere to each other around the upper anterior tarsal surface. When the skin and muscle layers are incised and a skin muscle flap is elevated as a superiorly based flap, one notices a thin layer of adipose tissue on

top of the upper orbital septum that is more defined medially and somewhat less laterally (**FIG 2**). The increased convexity of the globe is possibly responsible from this uneven distribution of the fat layer. The underlying septum should always be incised laterally and higher than the upper tarsal border in order not to injure the levator mechanism inadvertently. There usually is a preaponeurotic fat pad present, if not previously excised or developmentally absent. Under the fat pad, toward the upper orbital rim, one can find the vertically oriented fibers of the levator muscle. The surgeon should always keep in mind that immediately under the levator aponeurosis, there is the vertically oriented arterial loop of the supratarsal arch that might resemble the fibers of the levator muscle, for untrained eyes, that might be difficult to differentiate.

PATHOGENESIS

- Periorbital aging is a very complex phenomenon. Twelve percent of the patients in Dr. Lambros' series had upper eyelid ptosis; however, there is no reference to frontalis activity in his patient population.[2] Increased frontal muscle activity is a common finding in the elderly population and usually is a compensation for a ptotic upper eyelid. The original percentages of upper eyelid ptosis should be higher in the aging population due to the weakening of the levator attachments or stretching of the aponeurosis.

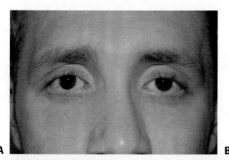
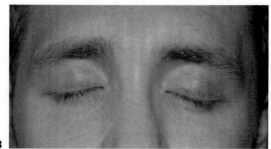
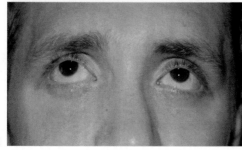

FIG 1 • This young patient presents with bilateral ptotic upper eyelids. **A.** He has empty upper sulci and an increased supratarsal fold distance. **B,C.** The upper eyelid excursion during the upper and lower gazes is 12 mm, and he has good levator function.

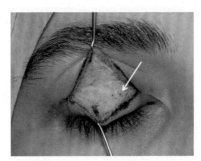

FIG 2 • Skin muscle flap elevated following upper blepharoplasty incision. There is a thin layer of adipose tissue medially and less laterally. This fatty layer is a landmark to be able to distinguish the upper orbital septum.

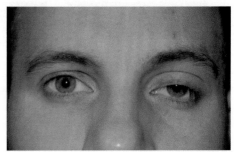

FIG 3 • This 28-year-old patient underwent two unsuccessful left ptosis repair attempts in the previous 2 years. The second surgery consisted of resection and shortening of the levator aponeurosis. The ptosis recurred a week after surgery. He has the typical symptoms of levator detachment with an increased supratarsal distance, upper eyelid ptosis, and slight elevation of the left eyebrow. The loss of the levator aponeurosis contribution to the lateral canthus resulted in relaxation of the lower eyelid on the left side causing a scleral show and distortion of the proper cant of the eye. Even the vertical orientation of the eyelashes is affected due to loss of the levator aponeurosis pull on the skin.

- There are still some centers that use incisional and excisional surgical methods on the levator mechanism. It is very important not to distort the anatomy of the levator system.
  - The most frequent complications happen with resection of the levator aponeurosis, because failure of the suture correction results in recurrence of ptosis and loss of levator function (**FIG 3**).
  - Another possible mechanism is inadvertent surgical damage to the aponeurosis (**FIG 4**).

PATIENT HISTORY AND PHYSICAL FINDINGS

- In younger patients, when present, ptosis is a significant complaint because a higher upper eyelid arch is the norm in early decades of life.
  - In severe cases, there might be significant visual field obstruction (**FIGS 5** and **6**).
  - Asymmetric cases are easily diagnosed.
  - In senile ptosis, most of the time, the patient is not aware of the problem if it is bilateral. Senile ptosis takes a long time to advance, and by that time, compensatory mechanisms such as frontalis hyperactivity develop (**FIG 7**).

- An occasional patient might complain about transverse wrinkles as a result of the long-standing frontalis muscle contraction.
- The anatomy of the brow-upper eyelid interface changes in ptosis patients. If there is no skin excess to camouflage the superior sulcus, this area appears hollow (**FIG 8**). The supratarsal crease-eyelash margin distance is increased, and the upper eyelid covers more than 2 mm of the upper limbus. In elderly cases, brow ptosis and skin excess disguise the deformity, and supratarsal crease might appear to be of proper dimension. In these cases, elevating the eyebrows will reveal the underlying pathology (**FIG 9**). A meticulous preoperative assessment and planning ensure symmetric eyelid levels and supratarsal crease distances.[3] The superior sulcus fullness should also be evaluated separately on both sides, and upper eyelid fat manipulation should be taken into account in order to achieve a satisfactory outcome (**FIG 10**).

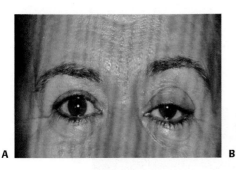

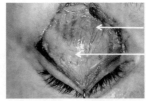

Levator muscle

Levator aponeurosis

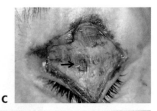

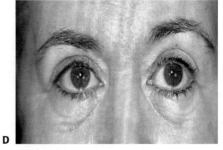

FIG 4 • **A.** A 64-year-old patient seen following a cyst removal from the left upper eyelid. She has left frontalis muscle hyperactivity due to left eyelid ptosis, an increased supratarsal distance. **B.** Intraoperative findings of the patient. The upper orbital septum is opened, and the preaponeurotic fat pad is retracted to expose the levator system. The right upper eyelid shows a normal anatomy of levator muscle and mechanism. **C.** The left upper eyelid levator aponeurosis has a significant injury medially, which possibly caused complete detachment of the system resulting in upper eyelid ptosis. **D.** One year after treatment with a levator advancement technique, she had bilateral blepharoplasty to equalize the supratarsal fold and correct the left ptosis. However, the frontalis muscle hyperactivity is not completely resolved.

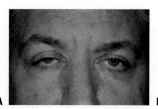 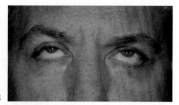 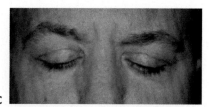

FIG 5 • A. A 52-year-old male patient with asymmetric ptosis—right side more droopy than the left. He has more frontalis muscle compensation on the right side due to obliteration of the pupil. The laxity of the lateral canthal tendon and the scleral show are possible signs for the levator system detachment from its insertion on the tarsus. The ptotic brows mask the supratarsal fold deformity. **B,C.** The patient demonstrates good levator muscle function that makes him an excellent candidate for levator advancement correction.

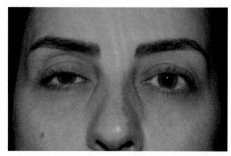

FIG 6 • A 39-year-old patient with unilateral right ptosis and the lack of frontalis muscle compensation. The superior orbital sulcus fat volume is significantly decreased. The left upper eyelid fat and excess skin are camouflaging the real location of the supratarsal fold. In these patients, skin excision should always be accompanied with upper sulcus fat grafting.

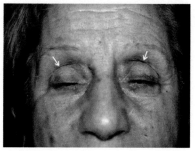

FIG 7 • A 73-year-old female patient with a long-standing upper eyelid ptosis due to complete detachment of the levator aponeurosis from the upper tarsus attachments. She has bilateral frontalis muscle hyperactivity. Even this compensation has failed; she has to hold her upper eyelids with her fingers in a higher position to be able to see properly. The detached edge of the levator mechanism is still pulling the skin forming an unusually high supratarsal fold (*arrows*).

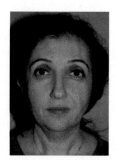

FIG 8 • A 49-year-old female with unusually high supratarsal fold distance. She almost has no preaponeurotic fat to fill the upper sulcus. Notice that the upper orbital rim is clearly visible throughout its course. The medial two-thirds of the brow is elevated to compensate for the upper lid ptosis.

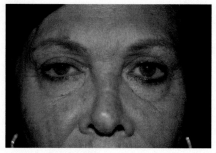 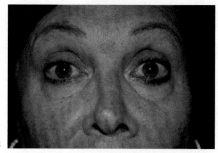

FIG 9 • A. A 60-year-old female presents with asymmetric upper eyelid levels and levator function. The supratarsal fold height is surprisingly symmetric due to the presence of excess upper eyelid skin. Brow ptosis masks the levator-upper tarsal border interface. **B.** When the patient is asked to elevate the brows, the deformity becomes visible. She has almost no upper eyelid fat, and the levator is detached, pulling the skin at a much higher level than normal. The normal level of the supratarsal folds is completely deceiving. Skin resection type of upper blepharoplasty will give her a sunken eye appearance.

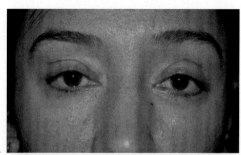

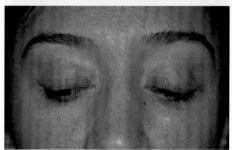

FIG 10 • **A,B.** A 39-year-old patient who had Fasanella-Servat procedure for the treatment of her ptosis. She also had resection of her upper eyelid medial fat pads through a stab incision. She still has compensatory frontalis muscle hyperactivity and residual ptosis. Notice the high skin attachment of the levator system, more on the left. Upper orbital sulcus appears relatively empty.

- The unilateral ptosis cases are more difficult to assess preoperatively (**FIG 11**). The ptotic upper eyelid should be elevated to a normal position with the finger, and the contralateral side should be watched carefully. If the normal upper eyelid level drops as a result of this maneuver, this is a sure sign of an occult ptosis. In this case, the surgical approach should involve both upper eyelids to achieve symmetry postoperatively.

IMAGING

- The assessment of the levator function is of utmost importance in surgical candidates. The measurement of the upper eyelid excursion between extreme upward and downward gaze gives the levator function, and a measurement above 10 mm guarantees successful outcomes with levator advancement technique.

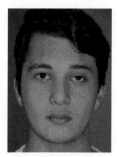

FIG 11 • A 17-year-old male patient presents with left upper eyelid ptosis. He has slight elevation of the left medial eyebrow.

DIFFERENTIAL DIAGNOSIS

- Congenital ptosis
- Muscle disease
- Fatty infiltration of the levator muscle

SURGICAL MANAGEMENT

Preoperative Planning

- The patient should not take any blood thinning agents for 3 weeks preoperatively. A bloodless field and loupe magnification are much needed for proper dissection and recognition of the pertinent anatomy.

Positioning

- The patient is placed on the surgical table in the supine position. A reverse Trendelenburg positioning of the patient is best for a bloodless surgical field.

Approach

- The supratarsal crease incision is used. It is not preferable to use the original crease of the patient because it might be displaced higher due to the pull of the levator muscle on the skin. I prefer to place my incision 8 mm from the upper eyelid lash border. This unfortunately coincides with the junction of the levator aponeurosis with the upper orbital septum and is a difficult area to delineate the anatomy. This requires surgical expertise and the use of loupe magnification.

■ Levator Advancement Technique for the Treatment of Upper Eyelid Ptosis

- The patient is a 17-year-old who presents with left upper eyelid ptosis and slight left eyebrow asymmetry. He has quite equal skin folds on both sides and this

ensures a good outcome. He has asymmetric levator function, 14 mm on the right and 11 mm on the left (**TECH FIG 1A,B**). A surgical simulation is performed by elevating the ptotic lid to a higher level with the index finger while watching the normal side to detect a positional change. In his case, the upper lid level drops on the normal side; hence, the surgery is performed on both sides (**TECH FIG 1C**).

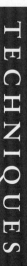

TECHNIQUES

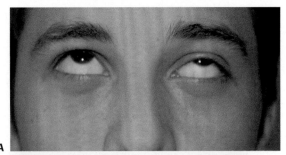
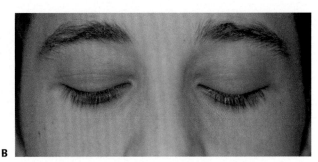
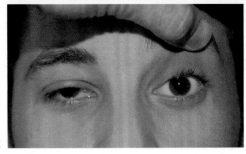

TECH FIG 1 • A,B. The patient has asymmetric levator function, 14 mm on the right and 11 mm on the left. **C.** Hering law in effect: if the left upper eyelid is pulled to a higher level to simulate surgery, the right lid drops. This shows the occult ptosis of the contralateral side. In this case, a bilateral approach is mandatory.

■ Incision and Dissection

- The upper eyelid incision is injected with local anesthetic and adrenaline solution, and 7 to 10 minutes are allowed to pass before skin incision. The surgical incision is placed at 8 mm from the eyelash margin in the middle and both ends at 5 mm. Laterally, the lateral canthus is the outer limit, and medially, the limit is the punctum (**TECH FIG 2A**).
- The upper eyelid incision is performed very superficially, and then the dermis is cut with the cautery to prevent bleeding. The dissection continues with the muscle layer. There is uneven thickness of the orbicularis muscle in the upper eyelid due to the convexity of the eye globe; the muscle is thicker laterally and medially. It is advisable to advance along the medial incision first, because there is a more significant adipose layer in between the muscle and the upper orbital septum in this area. Once the dissection reaches this layer, it is easier to extend toward the middle

and then laterally, staying on top of the orbital septum (**TECH FIG 2B**). Under loupe magnification, the upper flap is dissected toward the upper orbital rim for another 10 mm, staying immediately adjacent to the muscle layer (**TECH FIG 2C**). This facilitates the closure at the end of the surgery.

- The upper orbital septum is punctured, and 1 cc of saline is injected staying close to the undersurface of the septum (**TECH FIG 2D**). This type of hydrodissection facilitates the separation of the septum from the levator aponeurosis. In most of the ptosis cases, there is not much of a tissue space in between these layers, and this increases the risk for inadvertent levator system surgical damage. If the patient has well-developed preaponeurotic fat pads, these lie immediately under the septum (**TECH FIG 2E**). There are fibrous connections in between the levator system and the fat pads; they are released and the fat pad is retracted to visualize the levator muscle (**TECH FIG 2F**).

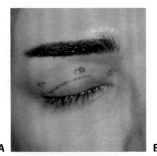
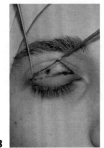
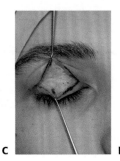
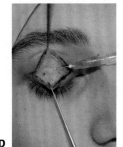
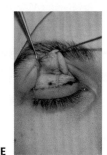
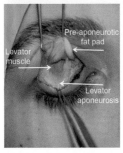

TECH FIG 2 • A. The surgical incision is planned 8 mm from the lash margin, and the corners have 5 mm distance to maintain the natural curve of the supratarsal crease. **B,C.** The upper eyelid skin and muscle are incised, and the upper edge of the flap is elevated off of the orbital septum. **D,E.** The injection of saline into the upper orbital space helps with the separation of the levator system from the septum. The elevation of the upper orbital fat pad helps to visualize the levator muscle. **F.** The levator muscle and the aponeurosis are clearly visible immediately under the preaponeurotic fat pad.

TECHNIQUES

■ Suturing

- There is a strong fibrous tissue layer along the anterior surface of the upper tarsal plate immediately deep to the orbicularis muscle layer. A 6-0 nylon suture is passed through this strong layer without penetrating the cartilaginous tarsal plate. This prevents the unnecessary manipulation of the upper eyelid tarsal plate (**TECH FIG 3A**).
- The second suture is then passed through the aponeurosis close to the distal edge of the levator muscle (**TECH FIG 3B**). The decision-making process for the amount of aponeurosis shortening depends on the severity of the ptosis and experience. The suture is then tied, which will effectively pull the levator muscle closer to the upper tarsal edge (**TECH FIG 3C**).

- The aponeurosis shortening sutures are placed on both eyes, and the patient is asked to open the eyes and look forward (**TECH FIG 3D**). There should be perfect symmetry of the upper eyelid levels. If not, the sutures are removed and arranged accordingly. When equal upper eyelid levels are maintained, two more additional sutures are placed on both sides of the midline suture to reinforce the attachment of the system to the anterior tarsal plate.
- The septum is closed with 6-0 poliglecaprone sutures, the upper flap is pulled down, and the skin excess is measured. The orbicularis muscle is never excised as the muscle fibers are more condensed close to the incision. The skin is injected with a local anesthetic solution and de-epithelialized with a surgical blade. Then the muscle is folded on itself and the skin is closed with a 6-0 nylon continuous suture.

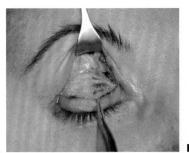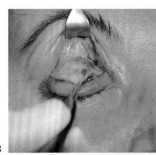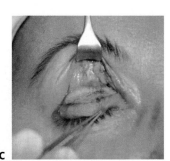

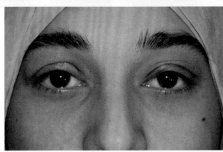

TECH FIG 3 • A. The 6-0 nylon suture is passed through the strong fibrous tissues of the anterior surface of the upper tarsal plate. The suture is then grasped and pulled up to see if it will hold the repair. **B.** The suture is then passed through the levator aponeurosis at a level closer to the muscle. The decision process for the placement of this suture is obtained with practice and time. **C.** The suture is then tied to pull the muscle closer to the upper tarsal border, hence the name levator advancement repair. **D.** After the levator is advanced on both sides, the patient is asked to open the eyes to check for symmetry. If this is not achieved, the levator system suture is removed, and a new level is obtained to provide equal upper eyelid levels.

PEARLS AND **PITFALLS**

Hemostasis	■ Instruct patient to stay away from blood thinning agents for at least 2 weeks. ■ Use freshly prepared local anesthetic and adrenaline solution. ■ Elevate the head of the bed. ■ Dissect with a Colorado tip cautery and obtain meticulous hemostasis.
Orbital septum incision	■ Inject saline for hydrodissection to prevent injury to the levator.
Levator muscle	■ The muscle is very fragile, and once it bleeds, its function is temporarily lost—no touch technique is mandatory.
Symmetry	■ The patient is asked to open the eyes and look up and down to check for function after placement of the aponeurosis shortening sutures.

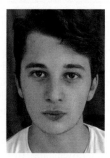

FIG 12 • The patient is seen 6 months after surgery with symmetric upper eyelid levels. There is better match of the left eyebrow position.

POSTOPERATIVE CARE

- Apply ice for 5 days.
- Elevate the head of the bed.
- Suture removal in 3 to 5 days

- Ophthalmic antibiotic ointment application for the first 3 days
- If the patient has compensatory frontalis muscle hyperactivity, he/she should be informed that it would take up to 3 to 6 months for the muscle to relax. In the early postoperative period, frontalis muscle activity might cause asymmetry and overelevation.
- The patient should understand that there is a period of 1 to 3 months of refractory changes in the postoperative phase.

OUTCOMES

- See **FIG 12**.
- The most common complication is a slight asymmetry in the postoperative period. This possibly is due to suture displacement in the healing phase. It is more frequent in asymmetric ptosis cases, and a proper consent should be obtained prior to initial surgery (**FIG 13**).

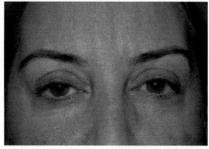
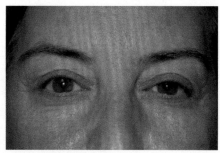

FIG 13 • **A.** A 37-year-old female presenting with right upper eyelid ptosis and an occult ptosis on the left side. She had levator advancement procedure on both sides with medial fat pad excision and grafting of the middle upper sulcus and 15-mm skin-only resection preserving the orbicularis muscle mass. **B.** The patient has asymmetric levels of the upper eyelids 4 months later. There is inadequate correction of her occult ptosis on the left side, even though the eyelid levels looked perfectly symmetric on the operative table at the end of the procedure.

REFERENCES

1. Carraway JH, Vincent MP. Levator advancement technique for upper eyelid ptosis. *Plast Reconstr Surg.* 1986;77(3):394-403.
2. Lambros V. Observations on periorbital and midface aging. *Plast Reconstr Surg.* 2007;120(5):1367-1376.
3. Faigen S. The role of the orbicularis oculi muscle ant the eyelid crease in optimizing results in aesthetic upper blepharoplasty: a new look at the surgical treatment of mild upper eyelid fissure and fold asymmetries. *Plast Reconstr Surg.* 2010;125(2):653-666.

Asian Blepharoplasty ("Double Eyelid" Surgery)

Clyde H. Ishii

DEFINITION

- Asian blepharoplasty or "double eyelid" surgery is a procedure to create a supratarsal fold.
- The fusion level of the orbital septum–levator aponeurosis and dermal insertions result in naturally occurring supratarsal folds.
- The incision height, amount of remaining upper eyelid skin, height of fixation, and levator function affect pretarsal exposure or "show."
- The shape of the desired fold varies according to patient preference.

ANATOMY

- Tissue connections between the levator aponeurosis and pretarsal skin result in the formation of the supratarsal fold[1,2] (**FIG 1**).
- Caucasians and Asians with naturally occurring supratarsal folds have a relatively higher fusion level of the orbital septum and levator aponeurosis.[3] In contrast, these structures fuse at a lower level in Asians with low or absent folds[4] (**FIG 2**).

PATIENT HISTORY AND PHYSICAL FINDINGS

- Ethnic differences must be considered when performing Asian blepharoplasty. Asian blepharoplasty is not simply Caucasian blepharoplasty applied to Asians. Asians undergoing this procedure want to enhance their appearance while maintaining their ethnicity. Most Asians do not want to end up with deep-set eyelids and tall supratarsal folds as seen in Caucasians.
- Physical examination:
  - The upper eyelid is examined for asymmetry, ptosis, abundance of skin/fat, and scarring or previous incision sites. The presence of brow ptosis should also be noted because this will affect the final appearance.
  - The chosen height of the supratarsal fold is key to the final result and must be discussed in detail with the patient. Patients are interested in the final amount of pretarsal exposure or "show." Most Asians prefer to end up with a pretarsal exposure of 3 mm or slightly less. Older patients and males tend to prefer a smaller amount of pretarsal exposure. Pressing a lacrimal probe or bent paper clip against the eyelid may simulate the desired pretarsal exposure (**FIG 3**).
  - The shape of the desired fold is also very important and must be discussed with the patient.
    - Medially, the fold may taper toward the medial canthus resulting in an "inside" fold[5] (**FIG 4**).
    - Folds that run outside the epicanthus ("outside" fold) will result in more of a Western appearance[5] (**FIG 4**). Some Asians prefer such an "outside" fold because it gives the illusion of a narrower intercanthal distance.
    - Most Asians prefer that the central third of the fold runs parallel to the lid margin.

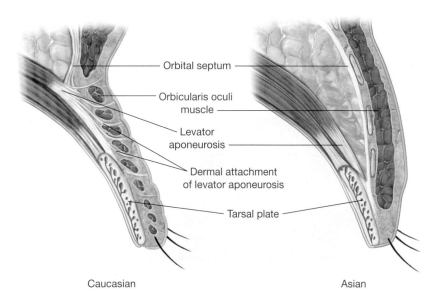

Orbital septum

Orbicularis oculi muscle

Levator aponeurosis

Dermal attachment of levator aponeurosis

Tarsal plate

FIG 1 • Dermal attachments from the levator aponeurosis result in the formation of the supratarsal fold.

Caucasian

Asian

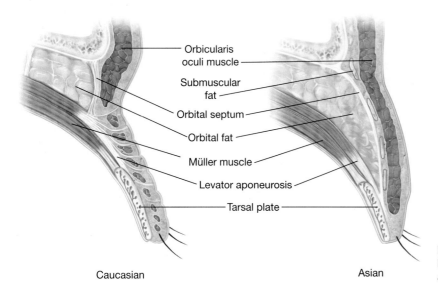

Caucasian

Asian

FIG 2 • Asians with short or absent folds have a lower fusion level of the orbital septum and levator aponeurosis.

- Orbicularis oculi muscle
- Submuscular fat
- Orbital septum
- Orbital fat
- Müller muscle
- Levator aponeurosis
- Tarsal plate

- Laterally, the fold may run parallel to the lid margin or have a slight lateral flare. This lateral flare produces an uplifted appearance and tends to mitigate the natural bunching of skin in this area that occurs with aging.

SURGICAL MANAGEMENT

- Surgical techniques to create a supratarsal fold include nonincisional methods (sutures alone), partial incisional methods (one or more small incisions combined with sutures), and incisional methods.
- Nonincisional methods are mainly used for young patients who do not need excision of skin or fat. Although these methods are associated with less postoperative edema than partial incision or incisional methods, the fixation is not as durable and loss of the fold is well-documented.
- Partial incisional methods allow for excision of excess fat and better fixation than nonincisional methods but any excess skin cannot be addressed.
- My preferred technique is the incisional method because it allows the surgeon to address redundancy of skin/fat and correct any accompanying blepharoptosis while providing secure fixation. These incisions heal well, and unsightly scars are rare. In my experience, the advantages of this technique far outweigh any disadvantages.

Preoperative Planning

- The desired height and shape of the fold are once again discussed with the patient.
- Marking of the eyelid is performed with the patient in the supine or semirecumbent position. Needed materials include vernier caliper, toothed forceps, and marking pen (**FIG 5**). An alcohol swab is used to clean the eyelid of makeup or oil film.
- The caliper is set to the desired fold height, and ink is applied to the distal tip of the caliper. With the eyelids closed, the surgeon gently lifts the superior lid/brow skin until slight eversion of the upper lid lashes is noted. The proximal tip of the caliper is placed at the lid margin and a marking is laid down in line with the midpupil. A similar marking is made laterally if a slight lateral flare of the fold shape is desired.

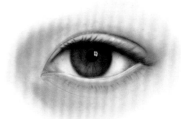

"Inside" fold

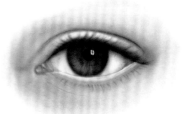

"Outside" fold

FIG 4 • Medially, the fold may taper toward the medial canthus ("inside" fold) or run outside the epicanthus ("outside" fold).

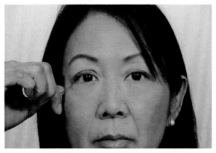

FIG 3 • Simulation of a supratarsal fold using a lacrimal probe or bent paper clip.

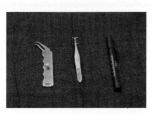

FIG 5 • Vernier caliper, toothed forceps, and marking pen.

If an "inside" fold is desired, the markings can taper toward the medial canthus. For an "outside" fold, the medial markings run several millimeters above the epicanthus.

■ Markings for skin excision depend on the amount of skin excess in a given patient. Younger patients usually need only 0 to 2 mm skin excision. In older patients, the amount of skin excess is determined by gently grasping the eyelid skin with toothed forceps. One tip of the forceps is placed on the fold height marking above while gathering the excess skin with the other tip. Mild eversion of the lid lashes is used as an end point. A third to half of the measured skin excess is marked centrally, and the markings taper medially and laterally to complete the elliptical marking. One should err on the more conservative side of skin excision in patients who desire a more subtle pretarsal exposure.

Positioning

■ The patient is positioned supine on the operating table.

Anesthesia

■ The procedure is performed under local anesthesia with mild sedation.
■ The sedation must be mild so patients can open/close their eyelids on command after the fixation sutures are placed. This allows the surgeon to check for symmetry regarding fold height and shape.

Approach

■ An incisional approach is used because of its versatility while providing very secure fixation.

■ With the eyelid under stretch, the elliptical skin incisions are made and a strip of skin is excised. A strip of orbicularis is also removed along with any excess submuscular fat. The fusion of the orbital septum and levator aponeurosis is thus exposed as it approaches the tarsal plate (**TECH FIG 1**). The orbital septum may be entered to address any excess retroseptal fat. Care should be taken to leave some fat behind to avoid unnatural accessory folds from forming above the fixation line.

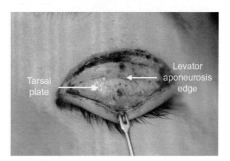

TECH FIG 1 • Exposure of fusion involving orbital the septum and levator aponeurosis.

■ Skin-Aponeurosis Fixation Technique

■ Three or four 7-0 nylon sutures are placed to secure the levator aponeurosis to the muscle-dermis of the pretarsal skin edge (**TECH FIG 2**).

■ The sutures may be either of the buried internal variety or external in nature.
■ I prefer buried internal sutures because I like to remove all external sutures on postoperative days 4 to 5.

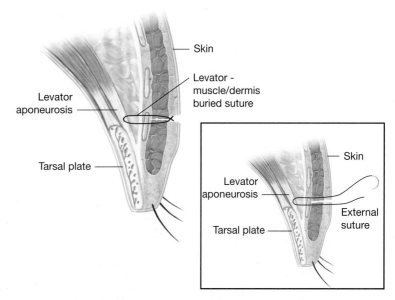

TECH FIG 2 • Skin fixation to the levator aponeurosis.

T E C H N I Q U E S

■ Skin-Tarsus Fixation Technique

- The caliper is used to place markings on the tarsus in the mid pupil line and laterally according to the patient's desired fold height. Medially, the markings parallel the pretarsal skin edge.
- 7-0 nylon sutures are placed to secure the markings on the tarsus to the muscle-dermis of the pretarsal skin edge (**TECH FIG 3**).

- At the medial and lateral extremes where the tarsus tapers narrowly, the sutures fix the aponeurosis to the muscle-dermis of the skin edge. As noted above, the sutures in this technique may be of the buried internal variety or external in nature.
- The skin-tarsus fixation technique results in a more static and well-defined fold when compared to the skin-aponeurosis fixation technique described above.
- **Closure:** Skin closure is performed using a 7-0 nylon running suture for both techniques.

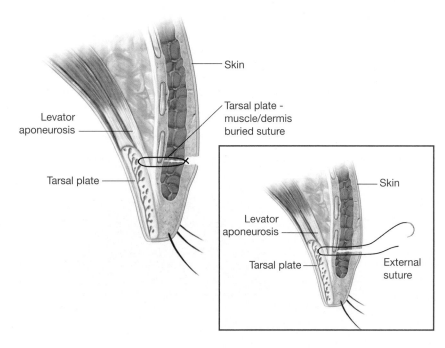

TECH FIG 3 • Skin fixation to the tarsal plate.

PEARLS AND PITFALLS

Planning	■ Most Asians prefer only a modest amount of pretarsal exposure (3 mm or less) compared to their Western counterparts. ■ Creating an "outside" fold or eyelids with significant pretarsal exposure will tend to Westernize the eye, and many patients will find this distressing. ■ The desired fold height, shape, and pretarsal exposure should be carefully discussed with the patient preoperatively. ■ Reviewing preoperative and postoperative images of other patients or models may be helpful.
Technique	■ The leading edge of the levator aponeurosis must be carefully identified when using the skin-aponeurosis fixation technique. Failure to identify and secure the proper anatomic structures will lead to incomplete/lack of folds.
Postoperative care	■ Patients desiring a taller supratarsal fold with more pretarsal exposure will show more pretarsal edema postoperatively, and this will persist for several months. Accordingly, patients should be informed of this preoperatively.

POSTOPERATIVE CARE

- Apply cold compresses during the first 24 hours.
- Cleanse the suture line with water and apply a light coat of antibiotic ointment two to three times a day.
- Avoid use of cosmetics to the upper eyelid for 10 days.
- Avoid bending, straining, or strenuous activities for 1 week.

OUTCOMES

- A highly satisfactory outcome is likely if the patient's desired final appearance is properly understood and the procedure is performed with the above guidelines in mind.
- Pre-existing asymmetry involving a patient's brow or lid level may affect the final result. Such asymmetry must be discussed with the patient prior to surgery.

COMPLICATIONS

- Bleeding/hematoma
- Excessive swelling
- Asymmetry in fold height/shape
- Dehiscence
- Infection
- Incomplete/loss of folds
- Multiple folds
- Milia
- Suture granuloma
- Hypertrophic scarring

REFERENCES

1. Sayoc BT. Anatomic considerations in the plastic construction of a palpebral fold in the full upper eyelid. *Am J Ophthalmol.* 1967;63(1): 155-158.
2. Cheng J, Xu FZ. Anatomic microstructure of the upper eyelid in the oriental double eyelid. *Plast Reconstr Surg.* 2001;107:1665-1668.
3. Yoon KC, Park S. Systemic approach and selective tissue removal in blepharoplasty for young Asians. *Plast Reconstr Surg.* 1998;102(2): 502-508.
4. Siegel R. Surgical anatomy of the upper eyelid fascia. *Ann Plast Surg.* 1984;13(4):263-273.
5. Zubiri JS. Correction of the oriental eyelid. *Clin Plast Surg.* 1981;8(4): 725-737.

31

CHAPTER

Section IX: Lower Blepharoplasty
Transconjunctival Approach to Resection and/or Repositioning of Lower Eyelid Herniated Orbital Fat

Allen Putterman

DEFINITION

- This procedure is undertaken to treat baggy lower eyelids and inferior orbital rim hollowing.

ANATOMY

- Pertinent anatomic structures are the lower eyelid conjunctiva, Müller muscle, capsulopalpebral fascia, orbital fat, and orbital septum (**FIG 1**).
- There are three distinct lower eyelid orbital fat pads (nasally, centrally, and temporally).
  - The nasal and central fat pads are divided by the inferior oblique muscle, and the central and temporal fat pads are separated by the temporozygomatic ligament.
  - There may be a second temporal fat pad.[1]

PATIENT HISTORY AND PHYSICAL FINDINGS

- Patients note fullness and bagginess of their lower eyelids. Some patients also notice a hollowing appearance in the inferior orbital rim area.

- This technique is also especially advantageous for:
  - Younger patients with large amounts of herniated orbital fat
  - Patients who have had previous blepharoplasties and for whom an external approach might lead to eyelid retraction or ectropion
  - Fat repositioning is advocated for patients with inferior orbital rim hollowness.

SURGICAL MANAGEMENT

- The transconjunctival approach to removal of herniated orbital fat is the preferred method of treatment in patients who have only herniated orbital fat with minimal or no evidence of dermatochalasis (excess skin) and no hypertrophic orbicularis oculi muscle.

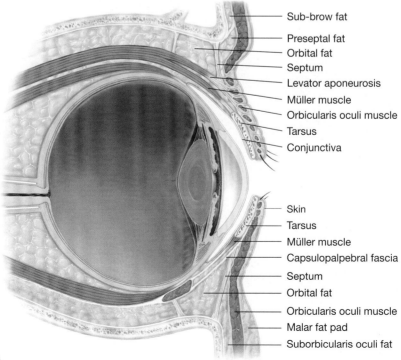

Sub-brow fat
Preseptal fat
Orbital fat
Septum
Levator aponeurosis
Müller muscle
Orbicularis oculi muscle
Tarsus
Conjunctiva

Skin
Tarsus
Müller muscle
Capsulopalpebral fascia
Septum
Orbital fat
Orbicularis oculi muscle
Malar fat pad
Suborbicularis oculi fat

A

FIG 1 • Eyelid anatomy.

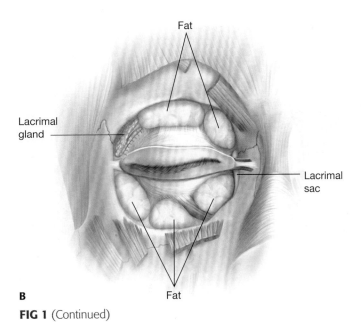

B

FIG 1 (Continued)

T E C H N I Q U E S

■ Anesthesia and Eye Preparation

- Two percent lidocaine (Xylocaine) with 1:100 000 epinephrine is injected subcutaneously at the center of the lower eyelid just beneath the lashes.
- An additional anesthetic agent is injected into each fat pad.
  - To inject the anesthetic into the nasal, central, or temporal fat pad, the surgeon inserts a 25-gauge, 0.8-cm needle just above the inferior orbital rim and directs it downward slightly until it penetrates its entire length (0.8 cm).
  - The barrel of the syringe is withdrawn to make sure that no blood vessel has been entered and approximately 0.5 mL of the agent is injected into each of the three fat pads.
- Topical tetracaine is instilled over the eye, and a scleral lens is placed over the eye to protect it.
- A 4-0 black silk traction suture is placed through the skin, orbicularis muscle, and superficial fascia at the center of the eyelid. The surgeon pulls the eyelid downward with a traction suture as the assistant everts the lower eyelid over a small Desmarres retractor to expose the inferior palpebral conjunctiva.
- Additional anesthetic is injected subconjunctivally over the inferior palpebral conjunctiva across the eyelid.

■ Isolating the Eyelid Retractors

- A Colorado needle is used to cut the conjunctiva from the medial to temporal end of the eyelid halfway between the inferior palpebral fornix and the inferior tarsal border (**TECH FIG 1A**).
- The surgeon grasps the inferior edge of the severed palpebral conjunctiva, while the assistants grasps the adjacent, more superior edge with forceps, and the assistant pulls the Desmarres retractors downward (**TECH FIG 1B**).
  - The two forceps are pulled apart.
  - Further dissection with the Colorado needle is carried out through the Müller muscle, and capsulopalpebral fascia until fat is seen.
- A 4-0 black silk double-armed suture is passed through the inferior edge of the conjunctiva, the Müller muscle, and the capsulopalpebral fascia, and the suture arms are pulled upward and clamped to the drape (**TECH FIG 1C**).

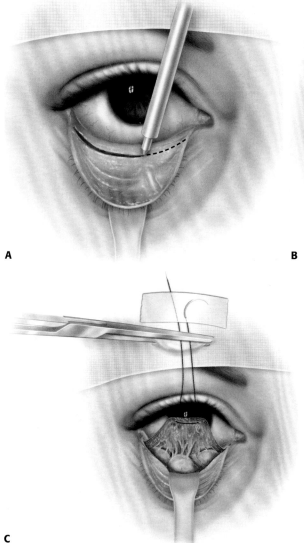

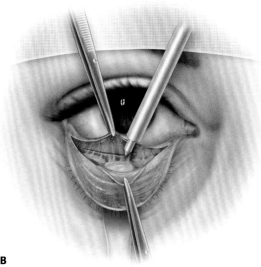

TECH FIG 1 • A. A Colorado needle is applied to the inferior palpebral conjunctiva halfway between the fornix and the inferior tarsal border and is used to sever the conjunctiva from medial to temporal end of the eyelid. **B.** With forceps, the surgeon and surgeon's assistant grasp the inferior and superior edges, respectively, of the severed palpebral conjunctiva to facilitate dissection of the Müller muscle and capsulopalpebral fascia with the Colorado needle. **C.** A 4-0 double-armed black silk suture is placed through the inferior edge of the conjunctiva, Müller muscle, and capsulopalpebral fascia and is pulled upward and clamped and taped to the drapes.

■ Excision of Orbital Fat

- A small Desmarres retractor is placed over the lower eyelid and is pulled downward and outward to expose the orbital fat.
- With the use of a disposable cautery and Westcott scissors, blunt dissection is carried out to isolate the three orbital fat pads.
- The temporal herniated orbital fat is isolated, and the fat that prolapses with gentle pressure on the eye is clamped with a hemostat and cut along the hemostat blade with a no. 15 Bard-Parker blade (**TECH FIG 2A**).
- Cotton-tip applicators are placed underneath the hemostat as a Bovie cautery is applied over the fat stump.

- The surgeon grasps the fat with forceps before it is allowed to slide back into the orbit to make sure that there is no residual bleeding that might cause a retrobulbar hemorrhage.[2]
- After the first temporal fat pad is removed, the surgeon applies additional pressure to the eye to determine whether there is a second temporal fat pad:[1]
- If a second temporal fat pad is found, it is also removed. The central and nasal fat pads are then removed in a similar manner.
- The retractor suture is removed, and then the conjunctiva is reapproximated with three 6-0 plain catgut buried sutures (**TECH FIG 2B**).

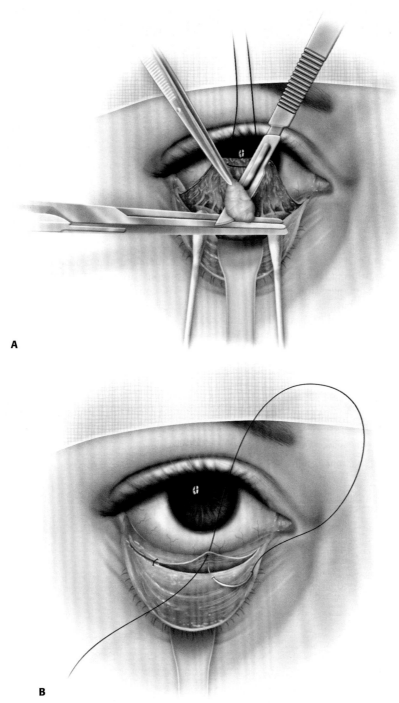

A

B

TECH FIG 2 • A. The surgeon removes the temporal, central, and nasal fat orbital fat pads by cutting along the hemostat blade with a no. 15 Bard-Parker blade and then applying a Bovie cautery to the fat stump. **B.** The conjunctiva is reapproximated with three 6-0 plain catgut buried sutures.

■ Orbital Fat Repositioning

- If there is both herniated orbital fat and inferior orbital rim hollowing, fat repositioning is performed.
- After the isolation of the orbital fat pads, an incision is made over the nasal inferior orbital rim, and periosteum is dissected for approximately 1 cm inferior to the orbital rim from the orbital bone (**TECH FIG 3A**).

- A 4-0 Prolene double-armed suture is threaded through the distal end of the nasal orbital fat pad, and then each arm of the suture passes subperiosteally 1 cm beneath the inferior orbital rim and exits through the skin (**TECH FIG 3B**).
  - The central fat pad at times will also be repositioned in a similar manner.

TECHNIQUES

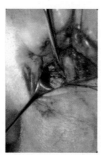 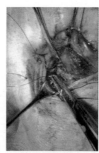 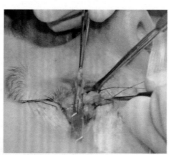 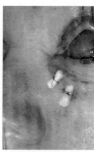

A   B   C   D

TECH FIG 3 • **A.** Orbital fat repositioning. Periosteum is dissected from orbital bone over the nasal half of the lower eyelid for approximately 1 cm. **B.** A 4-0 Prolene double-armed suture is threaded through the nasal lower eyelid distal fat stump. Each arm of the suture is passed sub-periosteally approximately 1 cm beneath the inferior orbital rim and exits through skin inferior to the hollowed areas. **C.** If there is excessive lower eyelid fat, the nasal and or central fat pads are divided into pedicles and parts of the fat pads are excised and parts repositioned. **D.** The 4-0 Prolene sutures are tied over cotton pledgets to allow the nasal and central fat to be repositioned into the nasal inferior orbital rim hollowed areas.

- The arms of the suture are tied over cotton pledgets to allow the nasal and central fat pads to be repositioned into the inferior orbital rim hollowed area and to fill this area as well as to decrease the bagginess of the lower lid.
- At times, if there is too much nasal or central fad, pedicles are used to divide the nasal and/or central fat, parts

of the nasal and central fat pads are excised, and parts are repositioned (**TECH FIG 3C**).[3]
- The cotton pledgets and 4-0 Prolene sutures are removed approximately 1 week postoperatively (**TECH FIG 3D**).

PEARLS AND PITFALLS

Inferior oblique muscle	■ Identify inferior oblique muscle to avoid injury with secondary diplopia.
Temporal fat	■ Check for the second or deeper temporal fat pad after initial temporal fat pad is removed to avoid residual temporal lower lid postoperative fullness.[1]
Fat transposition	■ Perform fat pedicles with fat repositioning if there is a large amount of fat to avoid inferior orbital rim overfill and bulging.[3]
Selective fat removal	■ Only remove the fat that flows forward when gentle pressure is applied to the eye through the eyelids to avoid overcorrection with secondary inferior orbital rim hollowing.
Excess swelling	■ Apply pressure to closed eyelids over areas of postoperative conjunctival chalasis to speed resolution of conjunctival chalasis.[4] ■ If there is a retrobulbar hemorrhage, remove the conjunctival sutures and do a lateral canthotomy.[2]

POSTOPERATIVE CARE

- No dressings are used after surgery.
- The patient is instructed to apply ice cold compresses on the eyelids, and pads (4 × 4 in.) soaked in a bucket of saline and ice are applied with slight general pressure to the eyelids:
  - When the pads become warm, they are dipped again into the saline and ice and reapplied.
  - This process is repeated for 24 hours but is not necessary during sleep.
  - The application should be fairly constant, especially for the first postoperative hours. After that, the compresses are applied for about 15 minutes with a 15-minute rest period in between until bedtime. The applications are resumed on awakening.
- To reduce edema postoperatively, the patient lies in a bed with the head approximately 45 degrees higher than the rest of the body:

- Nurses should check for bleeding associated with proptosis, pain, or loss of vision every 15 minutes for the first 2 to 3 hours postoperatively or until the patient leaves the surgical facility.
- Every hour thereafter until bedtime, the family or patient should monitor the patient's ability to count fingers and should check the residual proptosis and pain.
- If the patient cannot count fingers or has marked proptosis or pain, the family should take him or her to the emergency room.
- If loss of vision occurs secondary to retrobulbar hemorrhage, it could be treated by opening the incision involved and doing a lateral canthotomy.[2]
- Neomycin ointment is applied to the eyes twice a day for the first 2 weeks.

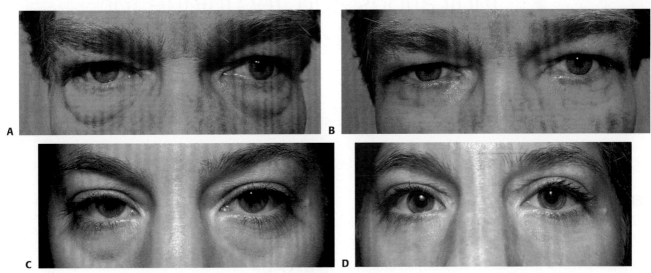

FIG 2 • **A.** A patient with lower eyelid herniated orbital fat preoperatively. **B.** Postoperative appearance after removal of herniated fat with a transconjunctival approach. **C.** A patient with lower eyelid herniated orbital fat and inferior orbital rim hollowing areas. **D.** Postoperative photograph showing resolution of the baggy lower lids and filling in of the inferior orbital rim hollowed areas.

OUTCOMES

- I have performed the transconjunctival approach in more than 1000 patients (**FIG 2A–D**).
- The procedure has the advantages of causing less eyelid retraction and ectropion than with the skin flap or skin muscle flap approaches because the external lamellae are not manipulated.
    - I believe there is less ecchymosis because the orbicularis muscle and skin are not severed.
- There tends to be more conjunctival chemosis immediately postoperatively with this procedure than with the external technique. If it occurs, it is treated with pressure applied over the closed eyelids.[4]
- With the fat repositioning, there is always the concern of overfill of the inferior orbital rim hollowed areas. I have performed fat repositioning for the last 25 years and so far have not had to repeat the procedure or to remove overfill of herniated orbital fat. Titrating the amount of fat reposition, I believe, has been the secret to that success.[3]

- I have had several patients who initially postoperatively had diplopia, but this has resolved in all patients, and I have not had any permanent diplopia from fat repositioning.

COMPLICATIONS

- Several patients in whom I have performed a transconjunctival approach had postoperative residual dermatochalasis, which needed to be removed through an external approach.
    - Better patient selection or combined initial procedure with a skin flap excision or orbicularis muscle plication could have presented this problem.

REFERENCES

1. Putterman AM. The mysterious second temporal fat pad. *Ophthalmic Plast Reconstr Surg.* 1985;1:83-86.
2. Putterman AM. Temporary blindness after cosmetic blepharoplasty. *Am J Ophthalmol.* 1975;80:1081-1083.
3. Aakalu VK, Putterman AM. Fat repositioning in lower lid blepharoplasty: the role of titrated excision. *Ophthal Plast Reconstr Surg.* 2011;27:462.
4. Putterman AM. Treatment of conjunctival prolapse. *Arch Ophthalmol.* 1995;113:553-554.

32

CHAPTER

Indications and Technique for Skin Pinch Skin Excision in the Lower Eyelids

Charles H. Thorne and Sammy Sinno

DEFINITION

- *Skin pinch skin excision* is a technique in which excess lower eyelid skin is simply grasped and excised without performing any subcutaneous dissection.
- *Dermatochalasis* is the condition of excess and loose eyelid skin. It is important to distinguish this condition from blepharochalasis.
- *Blepharochalasis* is a syndrome of recurrent eyelid edema that causes thinning and fine wrinkling of eyelid skin.

ANATOMY

- The skin of the eyelid is the thinnest of the body at less than 1 mm and has a high concentration of sebaceous glands.

PATIENT HISTORY AND PHYSICAL FINDINGS

- All patient undergoing eyelid surgery should have a detailed ophthalmologic history. History of previous periorbital surgery, visual disturbances, and relevant medications are noted.
- Patients who are candidates for skin pinch lower eyelid blepharoplasty have redundant and lax skin and often complain of a "tired" look. The stimulated effect of surgery can be reproduced preoperatively by providing gentle lateral traction on the lower eyelids.

- Patients who undergo this procedure may undergo additional procedures to correct other periorbital deformities, ie, transconjunctival lower eyelid fat removal for "puffy eyelids."

IMAGING

- No imaging is needed for this procedure.

SURGICAL MANAGEMENT

- The procedure is relatively simple and straightforward if carefully planned.

Preoperative Planning

- Skin pinch lower blepharoplasty can be performed under general anesthesia or local anesthesia. If local infiltration is used, the surgeon must be aware that skin excision may be less precise because the field has been distorted.

Positioning

- The patient is positioned supine. Corneal protectors can be used but are associated with increased risk of corneal abrasion.

Approach

- The removal is performed just under the ciliary margin.

TECHNIQUE

■ Excess Eyelid Skin Removal

- Using two Adson-Brown forceps, the skin of the lower eyelid near the ciliary margin is grasped and moved cephalically.
- The skin is then tented up sequentially from lateral to medial and crushed with a fine hemostat for hemostasis

and to precisely outline the amount of skin to be removed (**TECH FIG 1A–C**).
- Using a Stevens scissors, the tented skin only is excised. The skin is trimmed from medial to most commonly just lateral to the lateral canthus (**TECH FIG 2A–C**).
- Closure is performed using a running 6-0 silk suture (**TECH FIG 3A,B**).

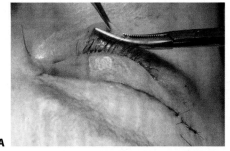

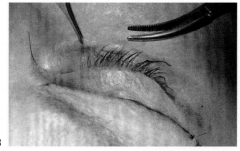

A   **B**

TECH FIG 1 • A–C. A hemostat is used to precisely and sequentially outline the planned skin resection.

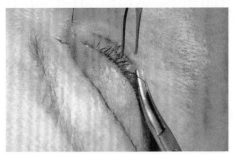

TECH FIG 1 (Continued)

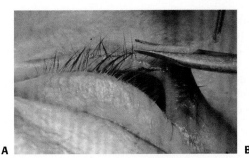 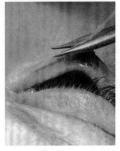 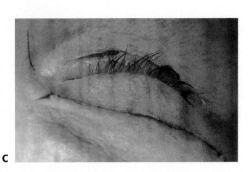

TECH FIG 2 • A–C. The skin is excised using Steven scissors.

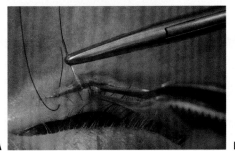 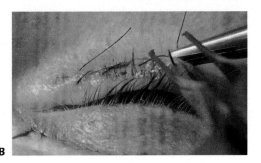

TECH FIG 3 • A,B. Closure with 6-0 silk suture.

PEARLS AND PITFALLS

Preoperative counseling	■ Patients must be counseled that all lower eyelid laxity cannot be removed to avoid lower eyelid malposition. ■ This procedure should be avoided with patients who exhibit lower eyelid malposition and/or poor lower eyelid tone.
Local anesthesia	■ Injected volume can reduce precision of the procedure.
Lateral extension of excision	■ If excision is not carried out lateral to the lateral canthus, bunching and incomplete correction can result.

POSTOPERATIVE CARE

- Patients are instructed to apply cold compresses to the eyes continuously for 12 hours after surgery.
- Sutures are removed at 3 days.
- Alcohol should be avoided for 2 to 3 days and heavy exercise avoided for 2 weeks.
- Patients are encouraged to sleep on their backs.

OUTCOMES

- Excellent contour is restored to the lower periorbita following excess skin excision.

- This technique does not require any dissection, so complications such as excess bruising, swelling, and eyelid malposition are nonexistent.

COMPLICATIONS

- If too much skin is excised, there is a possibility for excess tension on the incision at closure. Typically, delayed healing will occur spontaneously.

33 CHAPTER

Indications and Technique for Transconjunctival Fat Removal and Redraping in the Lower Eyelids

Francisco G. Bravo

DEFINITION

- Patients with good skin quality who present with prominent lower eyelid bags and evident nasojugal and palpebromalar grooves may benefit from transconjunctival fat removal and redraping of excess fat over the inferior orbital rim.[1-4]
- This procedure avoids the need for external incisions, which may be visible in younger patients and may be associated with a higher incidence of complications such as lower lid retraction, scleral show, and prolonged swelling.
- The need for routine use of canthal support techniques is also generally avoided through this approach.
- A recessed lower orbital rim and an evident tear trough deformity may be augmented and attenuated, respectively, with the patient's own prominent lower eyelid bags without the need for fat grafting or synthetic filler injections.

ANATOMY

- The lower eyelid consists of an anterior, middle, and posterior lamella[5] (**FIG 1A**).
- Skin and the *orbicularis oculi* muscle form the anterior lamella.
- The orbital septum, orbital fat, and suborbicularis adipose tissue form the middle lamella.
- The tarsal plate, lower eyelid retractors (capsulopalpebral head and fascia), and the conjunctiva form the posterior lamella.
- The *orbicularis oculi* muscle is subdivided into the pretarsal, preseptal, and orbital components.

- There are three postseptal fat compartments in the lower eyelid (**FIG 1B**).
- Nasal and central fat pads are separated by the inferior oblique muscle.
- Central and lateral fat pads are separated by the arcuate expansion of the Lockwood ligament (**FIG 1C**).
- The *orbicularis* retaining ligament or orbitomalar ligament attaches the palpebral *orbicularis oculi* muscle to the underlying maxilla (**FIG 2A**).
- The tear trough or nasojugal groove and the lid-cheek junction or palpebromalar groove extend below the orbital rim and are explained by anatomical features in the subcutaneous plane[6] (**FIG 2B**).

PATIENT HISTORY AND PHYSICAL FINDINGS

- The preoperative evaluation for patients seeking lower eyelid surgery includes a detailed assessment of the patient's medical history and a thorough physical examination.[7]
- Medical history
  - Special attention should be paid to risk factors that may predispose to postoperative complications.
  - Thyroid pathology, diabetes, hypertension, heart disease, coagulopathy, and any previous periorbital surgery or trauma should be documented.
  - Vision disorders such as impaired visual acuity or the need to use corrective glasses or contact lenses should be noted before surgery.
  - The use of medications such as aspirin and other nonsteroidal anti-inflammatory drugs, anticoagulants, and

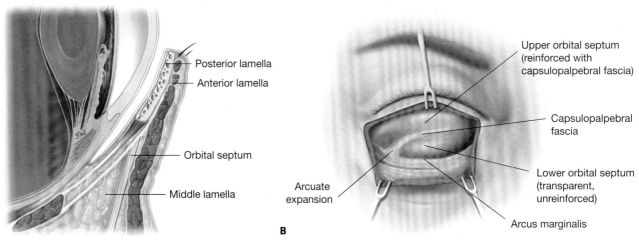

A   **B**

FIG 1 • A. The lower eyelid consists of an anterior, middle, and posterior lamella. **B.** There are three postseptal fat compartments in the lower eyelid.

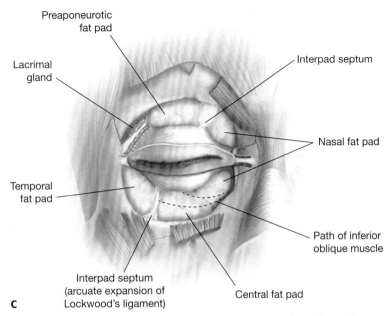

Preaponeurotic fat pad

Lacrimal gland

Interpad septum

Nasal fat pad

Temporal fat pad

Path of inferior oblique muscle

Interpad septum (arcuate expansion of Lockwood's ligament)

Central fat pad

C

FIG 1 (Continued) • **C.** Central and lateral fat pads are separated by the arcuate expansion of the Lockwood ligament.

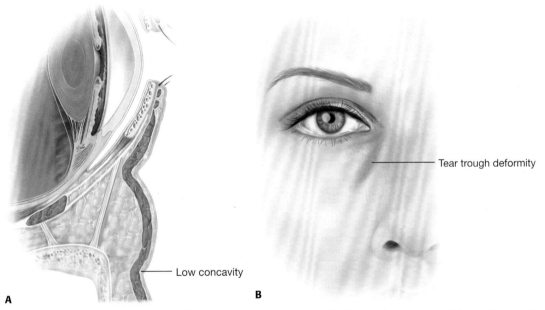

Low concavity

Tear trough deformity

A

B

FIG 2 • **A.** The *orbicularis* retaining ligament or orbitomalar ligament attaches the palpebral *orbicularis oculi* muscle to the underlying maxilla. **B.** The tear trough or nasojugal groove and the lid-cheek junction or palpebromalar groove extend below the orbital rim and are explained by anatomical features in the subcutaneous plane.

certain vitamins and herbal supplements such as vitamin E and ginkgo should be recorded and suspended 2 weeks prior to surgery.
- Smoking history should also be documented and interrupted preferably for 4 weeks prior and 2 weeks after surgery.
- A history suggestive of dry eye syndrome should be clarified, and if present, the decision to proceed should be discussed carefully with the patient.

- Physical examination
  - Evaluation should be performed with three goals in mind:
    - To document preoperative eye function
    - To identify anatomical features that may predispose patients to developing postoperative complications
    - To identify the specific anatomical features that are causing the patient's concern in order to customize the procedure

- Functional evaluation should include an examination and documentation of visual acuity, extraocular muscular movements, Bell phenomenon, pupillary response, and adequate tear production through a Schirmer or tear break-apart time test.[7]
- Anatomic features that may predispose to postoperative complications such as lower eyelid retraction, ectropion, or malposition[8] include the following:
  - A negative vector caused by a prominent eye or a retruded maxilla, which may be measured by a Hertel exophthalmometer
  - Tarsoligamentous or horizontal lid margin laxity with a measurable lag in the snapback test and a greater than 6-mm distraction test
  - A negative canthal tilt in which the lateral canthus lies at a lower position in relationship to the medial canthus
  - Scleral show in which the lid margin rests below the corneoscleral limbus
- Specific anatomic features[9,10] that need to be identified as possible causes of the morphological concerns the patient might wish to address are as follows:
  - Orbital fat herniation or prolapse due to fat pad hypertrophy or to excessive laxity of the orbital septum and orbicularis oculi muscle
  - Tear trough deformity and a deep lid-cheek junction
  - Dark circles due to skin pigmentation or prominent intramuscular vasculature in patients with thin, translucent skin and subcutaneous fat atrophy
  - Dermatochalasis or skin excess and rhytides
  - Orbicularis prominence or hypertrophy
  - Malar bags and festoons

IMAGING

- The use of high-quality preoperative photography is a key element to plan and carry out eyelid surgery, as well as to document and serve as reference for clinical examination.
- Standardization in patient positioning, lighting, lens focal length, and background is crucial to avoid misinterpretation and distortion of the patient's anatomic features.[11]
- The photographic series should include frontal, oblique, and profile views (**FIG 3**), as well as frontal views while smiling, rising the eyebrows, frowning, gazing upward, closing the eyes, and also with slight posterior and anterior head tilts while looking into the lens.
- High-quality video capture should also be considered to appropriately document ocular and eyelid function preoperatively.

- Digital imaging software may be an important adjunct to precisely evaluate eyelid morphology and to detect asymmetries, which are common in the lower eyelid.[12]

NONOPERATIVE MANAGEMENT

- With the popularity and appeal of noninvasive procedures among cosmetic surgery patients, a thorough and earnest discussion should be maintained regarding the advantages and disadvantages of such techniques versus surgical options by attending to the patient's particular anatomic features and concerns.
- Botulinum toxin may be employed to reduce skin wrinkles and expression lines along the lateral portion of the lower eyelid, as well as to soften *orbicularis* hypertrophy or protrusion.
- Skin resurfacing techniques with either lasers or chemical peels such as trichloroacetic acid or phenol/croton oil may be performed to improve skin quality and dermatochalasis.
- The use of fillers such as hyaluronic acid, collagen, or the patient's own fat may be infiltrated around the lower eyelid to correct an evident tear trough or deep lid-cheek junction or to augment the inferior orbital rim and malar area to provide better support and contour in a negative vector patient.
- The use of nonsurgical procedures should not be discarded even if surgery is indicated as they may be valuable adjuncts to improve and enhance the results after lower blepharoplasty.

SURGICAL MANAGEMENT

- The decision to proceed with surgery depends on the specific anatomic concerns of the patient as well as on the degree and duration of the result sought.[13]
- Indications for surgery include herniated and prolapsed bags appearing together with an evident tear trough deformity or deep lid-cheek junction.
- Patients with poor skin quality or noticeable dermatochalasis are not good candidates for transconjunctival fat removal and redraping in the lower eyelid. They must be informed that this procedure alone will not improve and may even worsen this specific condition.
- Risks to the patient include hematoma, infection, and scarring
- Determining the correct amount of fat to resect directly impacts the result of the procedure. Excessive resection may result in insufficient tear trough correction, whereas inadequate resection may leave a bulge that could require revision.[14]

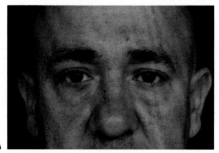
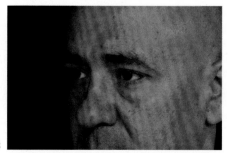

FIG 3 • **A.** Preoperative frontal. **B.** Preoperative three-quarters views of a male patient with protruding eyelid bags and marked nasojugal and palpebromalar grooves.

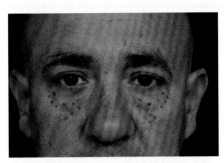

FIG 4 • Preoperative markings.

Preoperative Planning

- The complete eyelid photographic series of the patient should be carefully reviewed before surgery and should be available in the operating room.
- Markings on the patient should be performed in the upright position. The tear trough and lid-cheek junction should be outlined, as well as the areas of maximal protrusion of the fat pads (**FIG 4**).
- The patient should be inquired as to whether having taken aspirin in the days prior to surgery and the procedure suspended if aspirin is still taken.
- The surgeon must be familiar with techniques for canthal support and tarsorrhaphy should they be necessary at the end of the procedure.

Positioning

- The patient is positioned supine on the operating table.
- Prepping is performed with a low concentration chlorhexidine solution without alcohol, avoiding penetration into the eyes.
- Intravenous sedation is started and corneal protectors are placed.
- Oxygen is administered through a nasal catheter at a low flow and concentration. Instructions should be given to the anesthetist to momentarily interrupt flow when using electrocautery to avoid accidental fires in the operating room.
- The conjunctiva, lower eyelid, and tear trough are infiltrated with a 1% lidocaine with 1:100,000 epinephrine solution.

Approach

- Approach to the lower eyelid bags and tear trough is achieved preseptally through a transconjunctival incision made midway between the tarsal plate and fornix.
- Alternatively, the transconjunctival incision may be shortened and the lateral bag may be approached through an upper blepharoplasty incision if performed concomitantly.[15]
- Dissection over the orbital rim to create a pocket for the fat pads to be transposed may be performed in a supra- or subperiosteal plane.

■ Exposure

- A 5/0 silk traction suture with a noncutting needle is placed through the lower eyelid to expose the conjunctiva.
- An incision with needle-tip electrocautery is performed just above the fornix through the conjunctiva (**TECH FIG 1A**).
- A traction suture is placed through the posterior conjunctival flap and held with a mosquito clamp over the

corneal protector (**TECH FIG 1B**). The incision through the conjunctiva is then completed (**TECH FIG 1C**).
- Vertical dissection with Stevens scissors divides the capsulopalpebral fascia, and an insulated Desmarres retractor is used to elevate caudally the palpebral edge of the divided conjunctiva (**TECH FIG 1D**).

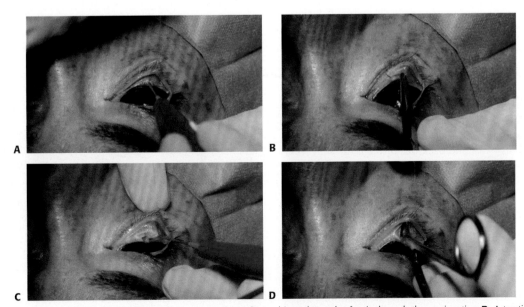

TECH FIG 1 • **A.** An incision with needle-tip electrocautery is performed just above the fornix through the conjunctiva. **B.** A traction suture is placed through the posterior conjunctival flap and held with a mosquito clamp over the corneal protector. **C.** The incision through the conjunctiva is then completed. **D.** Vertical dissection with Stevens scissors divides the capsulopalpebral fascia, and an insulated Desmarres retractor is used to elevate caudally the palpebral edge of divided conjunctiva.

TECHNIQUES

Fat Pad Resection

- The orbital septum is visualized and the fat compartments identified with the help of sterile cotton tips (**TECH FIG 2A**).
- The septum is incised and gentle, continuous pressure is applied to the globe to allow the fat to herniate.
- Fat is conservatively excised with electrocautery according to the preoperative plan from the medial, central, and lateral fat compartments (**TECH FIG 2B**).
- The *arcus marginalis* is released and a 7- to 15-mm subperiosteal dissection over the inferior orbital rim is performed and extended laterally by releasing the *orbicularis* retaining ligament with cautery and a periosteal elevator[3] (**TECH FIG 2C**).
- Alternatively, the dissection can be carried out in the suborbicularis plane supraperiostally, although more bleeding may be encountered.
- Fat transposition is performed with the aid of two to three percutaneous sutures by securing the medial and central fat pads over the inferior orbital rim to ablating the tear trough deformity and blending the lid-cheek junction[14] (**TECH FIG 2D**).
- Transposition of the lateral fat pad is seldom indicated although it may be performed after releasing the lateral orbital thickening.

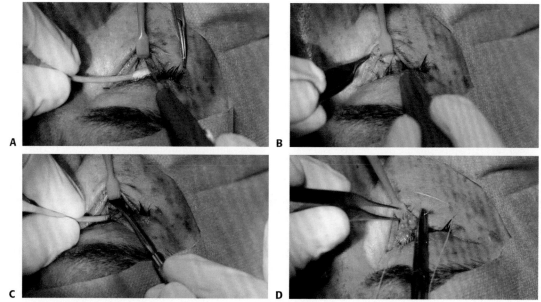

TECH FIG 2 • A. The orbital septum is visualized and the fat compartments identified with the help of sterile cotton tips. **B.** Fat is conservatively excised with electrocautery according to the preoperative plan from the medial, central, and lateral fat compartments. **C.** The *arcus marginalis* is released and a 7- to 15-mm subperiosteal dissection over the inferior orbital rim is performed and extended laterally by releasing the *orbicularis* retaining ligament with cautery and a periosteal elevator. **D.** Fat transposition is performed with the aid of two to three percutaneous sutures securing the medial and central fat pads over the inferior orbital rim ablating the tear trough deformity and blending the lid-cheek junction.

Completion

- A 4/0 fast resorbing suture on a noncutting needle is passed percutaneously deep to the *orbicularis*, through the fat pads twice and back out through the skin (**TECH FIG 3A**).
- The sutures are secured over a Xeroform or cotton bolster or simply held in place using Steri-Strips[2] (**TECH FIG 3B–D**).
- Hemostasis is revised and the wound is thoroughly cleansed with saline. The traction suture and corneal protector are removed. It is not necessary to suture the conjunctiva.
- Secondary procedures such as a lower eyelid skin excision/resurfacing or canthopexy may be performed at this stage.

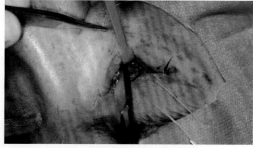

TECH FIG 3 • A. A 4/0 fast resorbing suture on a noncutting needle is passed percutaneously deep to the *orbicularis*, through the fat pads twice and back out through the skin.

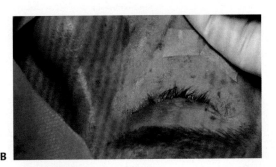

TECH FIG 3 (Continued) • **B.** The sutures are secured over a Xeroform or cotton bolster or simply held in place using Steri-Strips. **C,D.** Illustration showing the lower eyelid fat pads before being secured over the inferior orbital rim through percutaneous sutures.

Orbital fat

Tear trough

Arcus

C SOOF fat

D

PEARLS AND PITFALLS

Patient evaluation	■ Failure to identify adequate candidates for the procedure will inevitably lead to suboptimal results. ■ A tear trough deformity caused by a sagging *orbicularis* muscle or excessive skin will not be corrected by transconjunctival fat pad redraping alone.
Hemostasis	■ Bleeding should be avoided from beginning to end of the procedure through adequate infiltration and use of needle-tip cautery for dissection and fat excision.
Exposure	■ Inadequate exposure of the surgical field should be avoided. The length of the transconjunctival incision should be long enough to ensure correct visualization. ■ Alternatively, the lateral fat pad may be approached through the upper eyelid incision if an upper blepharoplasty is planned concomitantly.
Fat resection	■ Fat pad resection should be performed cautiously on the medial and central compartments to avoid ending up with too little fat to transpose. ■ Excision of the lateral fat pad is often more ample because correction of a deep lid-cheek junction laterally is usually insufficient through transposition alone.
Orbital rim dissection	■ Dissection over the inferior orbital rim should be generous to accommodate for the transposed fat pads and allow them to adequately redrape caudally. Care should be taken to avoid injury to the inferior orbital nerve.
Percutaneous sutures	■ Placement of the percutaneous sutures should be performed far enough caudally to provide sufficient tension to the transposed fat pads to avoid their retraction back to their original position. ■ A de la Plaza retractor or a small Langenbeck-type retractor may be employed instead of a Desmarres to aid in the placement of the sutures. ■ A blunt tip needle should be employed and passed twice through the fat pads to avoid cheese wiring of the sutures. ■ Caution should be taken not to tie the sutures excessively tight over the bolsters to avoid dents or injury to the skin over the inferior orbital rim due to postoperative facial swelling. ■ Alternatively, Steri-Strips may be employed to hold the sutures in place.

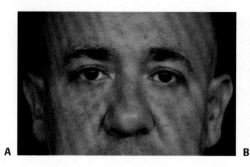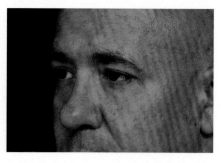

FIG 5 • **A.** Postoperative frontal. **B.** Postoperative three-quarters views of the patient.

POSTOPERATIVE CARE

- The bolsters or Steri-strips are removed after 6 days.
- Patients are instructed to apply cold packs and slight compression for 48 hours.
- Artificial tear drops are prescribed as well as oral antibiotics and pain medication.
- Patients should be carefully followed the evening and day after surgery. Any suspicion of retrobulbar hematoma such as excessive pain, pressure, or nausea and vomiting should be managed urgently through canthotomy with cantholysis and hematoma drainage.
- Patients should start early with massage if lower lid retraction or hardness appears.
- Patients are advised to sleep for 5 days with their head elevated and to avoid activity, medication, or food, which may increase blood pressure or swelling.

OUTCOMES

- Patients with protruding fat pads and an evident tear trough deformity should expect good outcomes when no skin excess is present preoperatively (**FIGS 5–7**).
- Hidalgo performed transconjunctival fat transposition in 61% of 248 consecutive lower blepharoplasties in which an integrated approach was employed. Only 2.4% required revision to remove excess fat or skin.[14]
- Goldberg reviewed the results of 24 consecutive patients who underwent subperiosteal transconjunctival fat repositioning and noted hardening of the transposed fat that resolved by 6 months. Four patients required revision for undercorrection of the tear trough deformity.[3]
- A recurrence of the initial deformity may appear if fixation of the extruded fat pads over the inferior orbital rim is insufficient or if excess fat was not adequately removed.

COMPLICATIONS

- Apart from prolonging postoperative downtime, a hematoma may constitute a true surgical emergency if the bleeding accumulates in the retrobulbar space, which may lead to optic nerve compression and blindness.[16]
- Although an infrequent complication, an infection should be treated promptly with topical or systemic antibiotics if necessary.
- Patients should be informed of the possibility of lid margin malposition or retraction despite avoiding an external incision. Excessive or inadequate scarring in the middle or posterior lamella may be responsible for this complication.

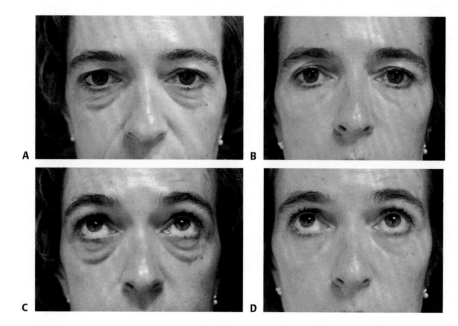

FIG 6 • Female patient with protruding eyelid bags and marked nasojugal and palpebromalar grooves. **A.** Preoperative frontal view. **B.** Postoperative frontal view. **C.** Preoperative view in upward gaze. **D.** Postoperative view in upward gaze.

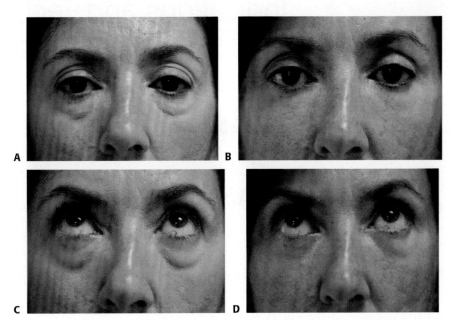

FIG 7 • Female patient with protruding eyelid bags and marked nasojugal and palpebromalar grooves. **A.** Preoperative frontal view. **B.** Postoperative frontal view. **C.** Preoperative view in upward gaze. **D.** Postoperative view in upward gaze.

Surgical revision may be required to correct it, although early management with vertical massage and taping may be sufficient to avoid surgery.

- Prolonged edema may be seen more frequently when fat transposition is performed, due to the more extensive infraorbital dissection required, which produces more disruption of lymphatic channels draining the orbit.
- Patients may also experience various degrees of hardening and fibrosis around the infraorbital rim where the fat is transposed, especially in the first 3 months.[3]
- Inclusion cysts or granulomas may occur after a transconjunctival approach, especially if a long incision was employed and topical ointment was prescribed postoperatively.
- Chemosis is less common through the transconjunctival approach but may occur more frequently if canthal support techniques were added to the procedure.

REFERENCES

1. Barton FE, Ha R, Awada M. Fat extrusion and septal reset in patients with the tear trough triad: a critical appraisal. *Plast Reconstr Surg.* 2004;113(7):2115-2121.
2. Davison SP, Irio M, Oh C. Transconjunctival lower lid blepharoplasty with and without fat repositioning. *Clin Plast Surg.* 2015;42(1):51-56.
3. Goldberg RA. Transconjunctival orbital fat repositioning: transposition of orbital fat pedicles into a subperiosteal pocket. *Plast Reconstr Surg.* 2000;105(2):743-748.
4. Hamra ST. The role of the septal reset in creating a youthful eyelid-cheek complex in facial rejuvenation. *Plast Reconstr Surg.* 2004;113(7):2124-2141.
5. Kakizaki H, Malhotra R, Madge SN, Selva D. Lower eyelid anatomy: an update. *Ann Plast Surg.* 2009;63(3):344-351.
6. Haddock NT, Saadeh PB, Boutros S, Thorne CH. The tear trough and lid/cheek junction: anatomy and implications for surgical correction. *Plast Reconstr Surg.* 2009;123(4):1332-1340.
7. Jindal K, Sarcia M, Codner MA. Functional considerations in aesthetic eyelid surgery. *Plast Reconstr Surg.* 2014;134(6):1154-1170.
8. Tepper OM, Steinbrech D, Howell MH, et al. A retrospective review of patients undergoing lateral canthoplasty techniques to manage existing or potential lower eyelid malposition: identification of seven key preoperative findings. *Plast Reconstr Surg.* 2015;136(1):40-49.
9. Friedmann DP, Goldman MP. Dark circles: etiology and management options. *Clin Plast Surg.* 2015;42(1):33-50.
10. Goldberg RA, McCann JD, Fiaschetti D, Simon GJB. What causes eyelid bags? Analysis of 114 consecutive patients. *Plast Reconstr Surg.* 2005;115(5):1395-1402.
11. Archibald DJ, Carlson ML, Friedman O. Pitfalls of nonstandardized photography. *Facial Plast Surg Clin North Am.* 2010;18(2):253-266.
12. Bravo FG, Kufeke M & Pascual D. Incidence of lower eyelid asymmetry: an anthropometric analysis of 204 patients. *Aesthet Surg J.* 2013;33(6):783-788.
13. Bravo FG. The aesthetic-health pyramid: a tool for patient education. *Plast Reconstr Surg.* 2010;126(2):112e-113e.
14. Hidalgo DA. An integrated approach to lower blepharoplasty. *Plast Reconstr Surg.* 2011;127(1):386-395.
15. Jelks GW, Jelks EB. The influence of orbital and eyelid anatomy on the palpebral aperture. *Clin Plast Surg.* 1991;18(1):183.
16. Mejia JD, Egro FM, Ergo FM, Nahai F. Visual loss after blepharoplasty: incidence, management, and preventive measures. *Aesthet Surg J.* 2011;31(1):21-29.

34
CHAPTER

Indications and Technique for Lower Blepharoplasty via Subciliary Incision

Francisco G. Bravo

DEFINITION

- Patients concerned with the aesthetic appearance of their lower eyelids may be managed surgically through a direct external approach bellow the lid margin.
- Patients with poor skin quality or dermatochalasis associated with prominent bags and orbicularis laxity are good candidates for this approach.
- Canthal support techniques as well as orbicularis suspension maneuvers are usually required and are frequently performed routinely to avoid postoperative lid malposition.

ANATOMY

- The lower eyelid consists of an anterior, middle, and posterior lamella[1] (**FIG 1A**).
- The skin and the orbicularis oculi muscle form the anterior lamella.
- The orbital septum, orbital fat, and suborbicularis adipose tissue form the middle lamella.
- The tarsal plate, lower eyelid retractors (capsulopalpebral head and fascia), and the conjunctiva form the posterior lamella.
- The orbicularis oculi muscle is subdivided into the pretarsal, preseptal, and orbital components.
- There are three postseptal fat compartments in the lower eyelid (**FIG 1B**).
- Nasal and central fat pads are separated by the inferior oblique muscle.
- Central and lateral fat pads are separated by the arcuate expansion of the Lockwood ligament (**FIG 1C**).
- The orbicularis retaining ligament or orbitomalar ligament attaches the palpebral orbicularis oculi muscle to the underlying maxilla (**FIG 2A**).
- The tear trough or nasojugal groove and the lid-cheek junction or palpebromalar groove extend below the orbital rim and are explained by anatomical features in the subcutaneous plane[2] (**FIG 2B**).

PATIENT HISTORY AND PHYSICAL FINDINGS

- The preoperative evaluation for patients seeking lower eyelid surgery includes a detailed assessment of the patient's medical history and a thorough physical examination.[3]
- Medical history
  - Special attention should be paid to risk factors that may predispose to postoperative complications.

- Thyroid pathology, diabetes, hypertension, heart disease, coagulopathy, and any previous periorbital surgery or trauma should be documented.
- Vision disorders such as impaired visual acuity or the need to use corrective glasses or contact lenses should be noted before surgery.
- The use of medications such as aspirin and other non-steroidal anti-inflammatory drugs, anticoagulants, and certain vitamins and herbal supplements such as vitamin E and ginkgo should be recorded and suspended 2 weeks prior to surgery.
- Smoking history should also be documented and interrupted preferably for 4 weeks prior and 2 weeks after surgery.
- A history suggestive of dry eye syndrome should be clarified, and if present, the decision to proceed should be discussed carefully with the patient.
- Physical examination
- Evaluation should be performed with three goals in mind:
  - Document preoperative eye function
  - Identify anatomic features that may predispose patients to developing postoperative complications.
  - Identify the specific anatomical features that are causing the patient's concern in order to customize the procedure.
- Functional evaluation should include an examination and documentation of visual acuity, extraocular muscular movements, Bell phenomenon, pupillary response, and adequate tear production through a Schirmer or tear break-apart time test.[3]
- Anatomic features that may predispose to postoperative complications such as lower eyelid retraction, ectropion, or malposition include the following:
  - A negative vector caused by a prominent eye or a retruded maxilla, which may be measured by a Hertel exophthalmometer.
  - Tarsoligamentous or horizontal lid margin laxity with a measurable lag in the snap-back test and a greater than 6 mm distraction test.
  - A negative canthal tilt in which the lateral canthus lies at a lower position in relationship to the medial canthus.
  - Scleral show in which the lid margin rests below the corneoscleral limbus.
- Specific anatomic features that need to be identified as possible causes of the morphological concerns the patient might wish to address include[4,5]

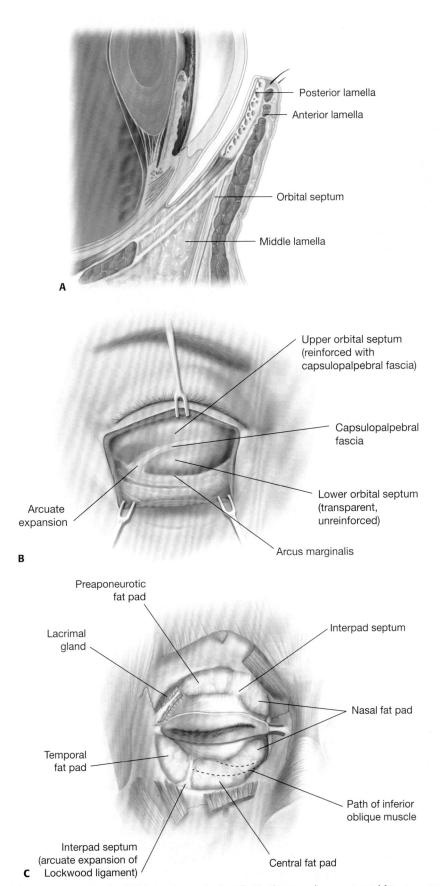

FIG 1 • **A.** The lower eyelid consists of an anterior, middle, and posterior lamella. **B.** There are three postseptal fat compartments in the lower eyelid. **C.** Central and lateral fat pads are separated by the arcuate expansion of the Lockwood ligament.

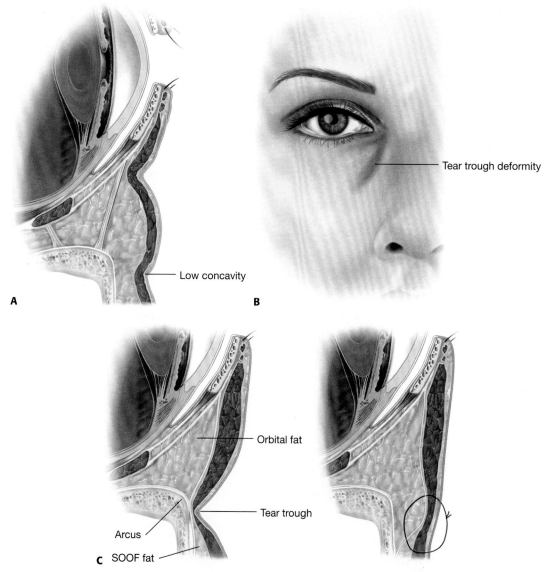

FIG 2 • A. The orbicularis retaining ligament or orbitomalar ligament attaches the palpebral orbicularis oculi muscle to the underlying maxilla. **B,C.** The tear trough or nasojugal groove and the lid-cheek junction or palpebromalar groove extend below the orbital rim and are explained by anatomical features in the subcutaneous plane.

- Orbital fat herniation or prolapse due to fat pad hypertrophy or caused by excessive laxity of the orbital septum and orbicularis oculi muscle
- Tear trough deformity and a deep lid-cheek junction
- Dark circles due to skin pigmentation or prominent intramuscular vasculature in patients with thin, translucent skin and subcutaneous fat atrophy
- Dermatochalasis or skin excess and rhytides
- Orbicularis prominence or hypertrophy
- Malar bags and festoons

IMAGING

- The use of high-quality preoperative photography is a key element to plan and carry out eyelid surgery, as well as to document and serve as reference for clinical examination.

- Standardization in patient positioning, lighting, lens focal length, and background is crucial to avoid misinterpretation and distortion of the patient's anatomic features.[6]
- The photographic series should include frontal, oblique, and profile views, as well as frontal views while smiling, rising the eyebrows, frowning, gazing upward, and closing the eyes, and also with slight posterior and anterior head tilts while looking into the lens.
- High-quality video capture should also be considered to appropriately document ocular and eyelid function preoperatively.
- Digital imaging software may be an important adjunct to precisely evaluate eyelid morphology and to detect asymmetries, which are common in the lower eyelid.[7]

NONOPERATIVE MANAGEMENT

- With the popularity and appeal of noninvasive procedures among cosmetic surgery patients, a thorough and earnest discussion should be maintained regarding the advantages and disadvantages of such techniques vs surgical options attending to the patient's particular anatomic features and concerns.
- Botulinum toxin may be employed to reduce skin wrinkles and expression lines along the lateral portion of the lower eyelid, as well as to soften orbicularis hypertrophy or protrusion.
- Skin resurfacing techniques with either lasers or chemical peels such as trichloroacetic acid or phenol-croton oil may be performed to improve skin quality and dermatochalasis.
- The use of fillers such as hyaluronic acid, collagen, or the patient's own fat may be infiltrated around the lower eyelid to correct an evident tear trough or deep lid-cheek junction or to augment the inferior orbital rim and malar area to provide better support and contour in a negative vector patient.
- The use of nonsurgical procedures should not be discarded even if surgery is indicated as they may be valuable adjuncts to improve and enhance the results after lower blepharoplasty.

SURGICAL MANAGEMENT

- The decision to proceed with surgery depends on the specific anatomic concerns of the patient as well as on the degree and duration of the result sought.[8]
- Indications for surgery include herniated and prolapsed bags, an evident tear trough deformity or deep lid-cheek junction and orbicularis muscle laxity or excess skin.
- Patients with good skin quality might be better candidates for a transconjunctival approach.
- Risks to the patient include hematoma, infection, and lower eyelid retraction or malposition.
- The main steps include access to the eyelid bags through a subciliary incision, release of the arcus marginalis and orbitomalar ligament, removal of lower eyelid fat, lateral canthopexy, and resuspension or tightening of the orbicularis muscle.
- The skin should be excised conservatively in most cases, and canthal support techniques should be employed routinely to decrease the incidence of lower lid retraction or scleral show.

Preoperative Planning

- The complete eyelid photographic series of the patient should be carefully reviewed before surgery and should be available in the operating room.
- Markings on the patient should be performed in the upright position. The tear trough and lid-cheek junction should be outlined, as well as the areas of maximal protrusion of the fat pads.

- The patient should be inquired as to whether having taken aspirin in the days prior to surgery and the procedure suspended if a positive response was given.
- The surgeon must be familiar with techniques for canthal support and tarsorrhaphy as they are often necessary at the end of the procedure.

Positioning

- The patient is positioned supine on the operating table.
- Prepping is performed with a low concentration chlorhexidine solution without alcohol, avoiding penetration into the eyes.
- Intravenous sedation is started, and corneal protectors are placed.
- Oxygen is administered through a nasal catheter at a low flow and concentration. Instructions should be given to the anesthetist to momentarily interrupt flow when using electrocautery to avoid accidental fires in the operating room.
- The lower eyelid and inferior orbital rim are infiltrated with a 1% lidocaine with 1:100 000 epinephrine solution.

Approach

- Skin-muscle flap approach with orbicularis oculi resuspension:
  - Exposure to the lower eyelid bags and orbital septum is achieved through the subciliary incision, dividing the muscle in a stair-step fashion to preserve the pretarsal segment.
  - Undermining of the skin-muscle flap is performed to achieve adequate exposure of the orbital septum and inferior orbital rim for fat reduction.
  - A strong resuspension of the orbicularis to the periosteum is required after skin excision, so as to avoid lid malposition or retraction postoperatively.
- Skin-only flap approach with reverse orbicularis oculi tightening (ROOT):
  - Exposure of the pretarsal and preseptal segments of the orbicularis is achieved through the subciliary incision by undermining a skin-only flap extending to the infraorbital rim.
  - The orbital septum and fat pads are exposed through an incision in the caudal aspect of the preseptal orbicularis taking care to avoid the medial portion that provides innervation through buccal branches to the pretarsal segment.
  - After fat reduction is performed, tightening of the lax orbicularis muscle is performed in a reverse fashion by excising a segment of the muscle caudally and repairing the orbicularis without tension.
  - Skin excision and muscle tightening are performed independently through this approach, which may be useful in patients with evident muscular laxity and excess skin.

T E C H N I Q U E S

■ Skin-Muscle Flap Approach With Orbicularis Oculi Resuspension

- The skin is incised 5 mm from the canthal angle with a slight downward slant to run parallel or within and existing crow's foot.
- Straight scissors are employed to undermine the skin from the pretarsal muscle through careful spreading, pointing the tips of the scissors to the medial canthus (**TECH FIG 1A**).
- A 5-0 silk traction suture with a noncutting needle is placed through the lower eyelid, and the lid margin is retracted upward covering the eye (**TECH FIG 1B**).
  - The subciliary incision is performed through skin only with straight scissors, 2 to 3 mm below the lid margin.
- The muscle is divided in a stair-step fashion[9] 2 to 3 mm below the skin incision to preserve at least 5 mm of pretarsal orbicularis muscle (**TECH FIG 1C**).
- The skin-muscle flap is elevated inferiorly in a preseptal plane to the inferior orbital rim.
- The orbital septum is visualized and the fat compartments identified with the help of sterile cotton tips.
- The septum is incised and gentle, continuous pressure is applied to the globe to allow the fat to herniate.

- Fat is conservatively excised with electrocautery according to the preoperative plan (**TECH FIG 1D**).
- The arcus marginalis is released, and dissection over the inferior orbital rim is performed and extended laterally by releasing the orbicularis retaining ligament with cautery and a periosteal elevator.
  - Alternatively, the dissection can be carried out in the suborbicularis plane supraperiosteally, although more bleeding may be encountered.
- Excess fat may be transposed or grafted over the inferior orbital rim to blend the lid-cheek junction or improve a tear trough deformity.
- Canthopexy is performed to correct lid laxity and prevent scleral show postoperatively. Care is taken to maintain the lid margin against the globe at the lateral canthus and to remove the corneal protector before tightening the canthopexy suture[9] (**TECH FIG 1E–G**).
- Hemostasis is revised, and the wound is thoroughly cleansed with saline.
- The skin-muscle flap is redraped in a superior lateral vector, and excess skin and muscle are excised conservatively (**TECH FIG 1H,I**).
  - Remaining excess muscle is excised with cautery.

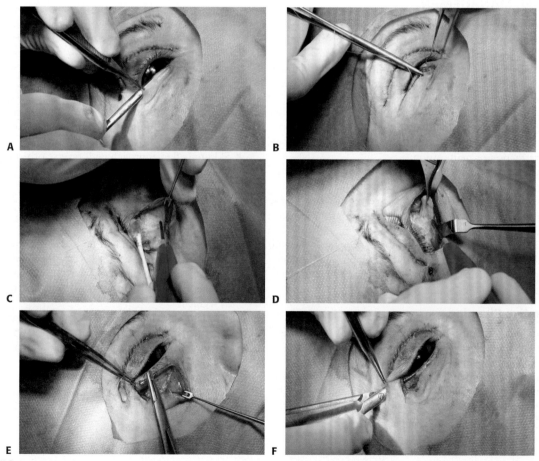

TECH FIG 1 • **A.** After the skin is incised, straight scissors are used to undermine the skin from the pretarsal muscle. **B.** A 5-0 Silk traction suture with a noncutting needle is placed through the lower eyelid, and the lid margin is retracted upward covering the eye. **C.** The muscle is divided in a stair-step fashion[9] 2 to 3 mm below the skin incision to preserve at least 5 mm of pretarsal orbicularis muscle. **D.** Fat is conservatively excised with electrocautery according to the preoperative plan from the lateral, central (shown), and medial fat compartments. **E.** A 4-0 white Ethibond or Mersilene suture is placed on the tarsal plate and lateral retinaculum. **F.** Right angle scissors are employed to connect the lateral orbital rim to the inferior incision.

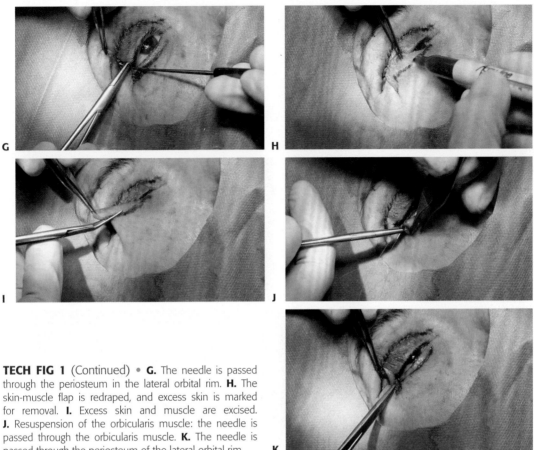

TECH FIG 1 (Continued) • **G.** The needle is passed through the periosteum in the lateral orbital rim. **H.** The skin-muscle flap is redraped, and excess skin is marked for removal. **I.** Excess skin and muscle are excised. **J.** Resuspension of the orbicularis muscle: the needle is passed through the orbicularis muscle. **K.** The needle is passed through the periosteum of the lateral orbital rim.

- Resuspension of the orbicularis muscle is performed with direct periosteal fixation of the muscle to the lateral orbital rim using a 4-0 resorbable suture (**TECH FIG 1J,K**).
- A 6-0 fast resorbing or a 7-0 Prolene suture is employed to close the subciliary incision.
- The initial traction suture may be employed as a temporary Frost suture in patients who might be prone to lower lid retraction or scleral show and left in place for 24 to 72 hours.
- A temporary lateral tarsorrhaphy using a 5-0 Prolene suture is performed in patients who develop chemosis intraoperatively or in those that required more extensive canthal support and left in place for 3 days.

■ Skin-Only Flap Approach With Reverse Orbicularis Oculi Tightening (ROOT)

- A 5-0 silk traction suture with a noncutting needle is placed through the lower eyelid, and the lid margin is retracted upward to cover the eye.
- The skin is incised 5 mm from the canthal angle with a slight downward slant to run parallel or within and existing crow's foot and continued medially toward the medial canthus 2 to 3 mm below the lid margin (**TECH FIG 2A**).
- A skin-only flap is elevated to the level of the orbital rim exposing the pretarsal and preseptal portions of the orbicularis muscle. Countertraction with sterile cotton tips and transillumination are helpful in this dissection (**TECH FIG 2B**).
- Orbicularis muscle laxity is assessed, and a small strip of muscle is marked for removal near the inferior orbital rim.

- The muscle is incised along the markings, and a small strip of orbicularis is elevated as a flap from lateral to medial (**TECH FIG 2C**).
  - Care is taken to avoid extending the incision too far medially in order to preserve buccal branches that provide innervation to the pretarsal orbicularis.
- Through the resulting gap in the muscle, the orbicularis is undermined in a preseptal plane cranially to expose the fat compartments and caudally to access the inferior orbital rim.
- The orbital septum is visualized, and the fat compartments are identified with the help of sterile cotton tips.
- The septum is incised, and gentle, continuous pressure is applied to the globe to allow the fat to herniate.
- Fat is conservatively excised with electrocautery according to the preoperative plan from the medial, central, and lateral fat compartments (**TECH FIG 2D**).

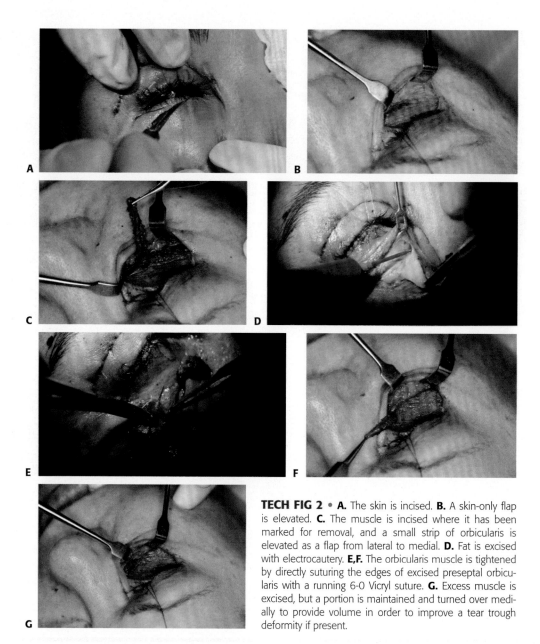

TECH FIG 2 • **A.** The skin is incised. **B.** A skin-only flap is elevated. **C.** The muscle is incised where it has been marked for removal, and a small strip of orbicularis is elevated as a flap from lateral to medial. **D.** Fat is excised with electrocautery. **E,F.** The orbicularis muscle is tightened by directly suturing the edges of excised preseptal orbicularis with a running 6-0 Vicryl suture. **G.** Excess muscle is excised, but a portion is maintained and turned over medially to provide volume in order to improve a tear trough deformity if present.

- The arcus marginalis is released, and dissection over the inferior orbital rim is performed and extended laterally by releasing the orbicularis retaining ligament with cautery and a periosteal elevator.
- Alternatively, the dissection may be carried out in the suborbicularis plane supraperiostally, although more bleeding may be encountered.
- Excess fat may be transposed or grafted over the inferior orbital rim to blend the lid-cheek junction or improve a tear trough deformity.
- Canthopexy is performed to correct lid laxity and prevent scleral show postoperatively. A white Ethibond or Mersilene suture is employed to fix the tarsal plate and lateral retinaculum to the periosteum in the lateral orbital rim. Care is taken to maintain the lid margin against the globe at the lateral canthus and to remove the corneal protector before tightening the canthopexy suture.

- Hemostasis is achieved, and the wound is thoroughly cleansed with saline.
- The orbicularis muscle is tightened by directly suturing the edges of excised preseptal orbicularis with a running 6-0 Vicryl suture. Excess muscle is excised, and a portion is maintained and turned over medially to provide volume to improve a tear trough deformity if present (**TECH FIG 2E–G**).
- The skin-only flap is redraped in a superior lateral vector, and excess skin is excised conservatively.
- A 6-0 fast resorbing or a 7-0 Prolene suture is employed to close the subciliary incision.
- The initial traction suture may be employed as a temporary Frost suture in patients who may be prone to lower lid retraction or scleral show.
- A temporary lateral tarsorrhaphy using a 5-0 Prolene suture is performed in patients who develop chemosis intraoperatively or in those who required more extensive canthal support. The suture is left in place for 3 days.

PEARLS AND PITFALLS

Patient evaluation	▪ Failure to identify adequate candidates for the procedure will inevitably lead to suboptimal results. ▪ Patients with good skin quality and minimal orbicularis laxity may benefit more from a transconjunctival approach.
Hemostasis	▪ Bleeding should be avoided from the beginning to the end of the procedure through adequate infiltration and use of needle-tip cautery for dissection and fat excision.
Canthopexy	▪ Although the standard position of the lateral canthopexy suture is at the lower level of the pupil, patients with prominent eyes or negative vectors require a higher fixation at the upper level of the pupil, whereas patients with deep set eyes will require positioning at a lower level. ▪ Patients with asymmetric lower eyelids, as is often the case, will also require a higher fixation on the side in which the lateral canthus is initially lower. ▪ Special attention must be paid to maintaining the lid margin against the globe when tightening the canthopexy suture. The anchoring point in the periosteum should be well inside the lateral orbit at the depth of Whitnall tubercle.
Orbicularis muscle incision	▪ Care must be taken to leave a segment of at least 5 mm of pretarsal orbicularis when incising the muscle through the subciliary skin-muscle approach. ▪ The incision should not extend excessively past the medial corneal limbus to avoid injury to the buccal nerve branches that are responsible for pretarsal orbicularis innervation.
Orbicularis muscle tightening	▪ A strong canthal support and a secure orbicularis resuspension to periosteum are imperative to avoid lower lid malposition and retraction when the skin-muscle flap approach is employed. ▪ Muscle resection must be conservative and not extended medially when performing a reverse orbicularis oculi tightening procedure through a skin-only flap.
Skin excision	▪ The skin should be removed very conservatively. ▪ A slight upward pull should be applied on the lid margin until it lies above the inferior corneal limbus before assessing the skin that should be excised.
Postoperative care	▪ Frost and tarsorrhaphy sutures must be employed readily in patients morphologically prone to develop postoperative lid malposition or retraction. ▪ Slight compression with a loose elastic head band applied over the eyes may prove useful to control swelling during the initial postoperative period. Adequate padding over the eyelids and midface is essential.

POSTOPERATIVE CARE

▪ Patients are instructed to apply cold packs and slight compression for 48 hours.
▪ Artificial tear drops are prescribed as well as oral antibiotics and pain medication.
▪ Patients are advised to sleep for 5 days with their head elevated and to avoid activity, medication, or food that may increase blood pressure or swelling.
▪ Sutures are removed at the 6th postoperative day.

OUTCOMES

▪ Patients with protruding fat pads and an evident tear trough deformity, who also have excess skin in the lower eyelid and a lax orbicularis muscle, should expect good outcomes (**FIG 3A–D**).
▪ Although excellent results may be obtained, patients should be well informed of the risks associated with the procedure that may require surgical revision as well as of the prolonged swelling that may occur.
▪ Codner reviewed the results of 264 patients who underwent transcutaneous lower lid blepharoplasty.[9]
  ▪ Chemosis was the most common complication occurring in over 12% of the patients.
  ▪ Blepharitis developed in 10 patients (3.8%) and required antimicrobial eye ointment in combination with steroids.
  ▪ Temporary lid malposition was encountered in 16 patients (6.1%) and resolved completely with conservative lid massage.

▪ Lower lid retraction requiring surgical correction occurred seven patients (2.7%), whereas frank bilateral ectropion with symptoms of corneal exposure occurred in two patients (0.8%) who also required revision of the lateral canthoplasty.
▪ Another 11.7% of the patients required revision for minor complications such as cysts or granulomas developing from the incision line, inadequate scars, canthal suture palpability, or inflammation and canthal webbing.

COMPLICATIONS

▪ Apart from prolonging postoperative downtime, a hematoma may constitute a true surgical emergency if the bleeding accumulates in the retrobulbar space, which may lead to optic nerve compression and blindness.
▪ Although an infrequent complication, an infection should be treated promptly with topical or systemic antibiotics if necessary.
▪ Patients should be informed of the possibility of lid margin malposition. Surgical revision may be required to correct this complication, although early management with vertical massage and taping may be sufficient to avoid surgery.[10]
▪ Prolonged edema may be seen more frequently when the transcutaneous approach is performed, due to the more extensive dissection required that produces more disruption of lymphatic channels draining the orbit.

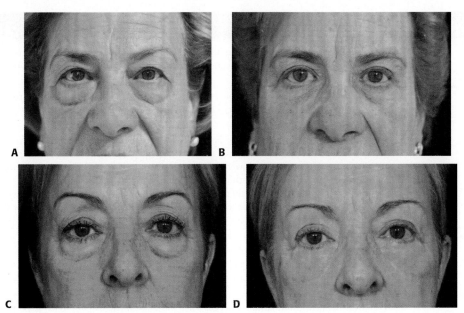

FIG 3 • A. Patient shown preoperatively and postoperatively **(B)** after lower blepharoplasty through a subciliary incision with a skin-muscle flap and orbicularis resuspension. **C.** Patient shown preoperatively and postoperatively **(D)** after lower blepharoplasty through a subciliary incision with a skin-only flap and reverse orbicularis oculi tightening (ROOT).

- Patients may also experience various degrees of hardening and fibrosis around the infraorbital rim if fat was transposed or grafted, which normally resolves by 3 months.
- Chemosis may occur frequently when canthal support techniques are used, due to postoperative edema with poor lymphatic drainage. Treatment includes prescription of mild topical steroid eye drops or short-term eye patching. A temporal lateral tarsorrhaphy may prevent corneal exposure and avoid chemosis in selected patients. Conjunctival incision and drainage may be required in recalcitrant cases.[9]

REFERENCES

1. Kakizaki H, Malhotra R, Madge SN, Selva D. Lower eyelid anatomy: an update. *Ann Plast Surg.* 2009;63(3):344-351.
2. Haddock NT, Saadeh PB, Boutros S, Thorne CH. The tear trough and lid/cheek junction: anatomy and implications for surgical correction. *Plast Reconstr Surg.* 2009;123(4):1332-1340.
3. Jindal K, Sarcia M, Codner MA. Functional considerations in aesthetic eyelid surgery. *Plast Reconstr Surg.* 2014;134(6):1154-1170.
4. Friedmann DP, Goldman MP. Dark circles: etiology and management options. *Clin Plast Surg.* 2015;42(1):33-50.
5. Goldberg RA, McCann JD, Fiaschetti D, Simon GJB. What causes eyelid bags? Analysis of 114 consecutive patients. *Plast Reconstr Surg.* 2005;115(5):1395-1402.
6. Archibald DJ, Carlson ML, Friedman O. Pitfalls of nonstandardized photography. *Facial Plast Surg Clin North Am.* 2010;18(2):253-266.
7. Bravo FG, Kufeke M, Pascual D. Incidence of lower eyelid asymmetry: an anthropometric analysis of 204 patients. *Aesthet Surg J.* 2013;33(6):783-788.
8. Bravo FG. The aesthetic-health pyramid: a tool for patient education. *Plast Reconstr Surg.* 2010;126(2):112e-113e.
9. Codner MA, Wolfli JN, Anzarut A. Primary transcutaneous lower blepharoplasty with routine lateral canthal support: a comprehensive 10-year review. *Plast Reconstr Surg.* 2008;121(1):241-250.
10. Pepper JP, Baker SR. Transcutaneous lower blepharoplasty with fat transposition. *Clin Plast Surg.* 2015;42(1):57-62.

Lateral Canthal Manipulation With Canthopexy or Canthoplasty

35

CHAPTER

George N. Kamel, Glenn W. Jelks, and Oren M. Tepper

DEFINITION

- The lateral canthus or lateral retinaculum is a continuation of the preseptal and pretarsal orbicularis muscle and receives contributions from the following anatomic structures: the lateral horn of the levator aponeurosis, the lateral extension of the preseptal and pretarsal orbicularis oculi muscle (lateral canthal tendon), the Lockwood ligament, and the check ligament of the lateral rectus muscle.
- The inferior retinaculum refers to the lower eyelid's contribution to the lateral retinaculum.
- Lateral canthopexy refers to repositioning of the lateral canthus without disinsertion from the orbital tubercle, whereas in a lateral canthoplasty, the lateral canthus is disinserted and repositioned.

ANATOMY

- A thorough understanding of the periorbital anatomy is necessary to achieve optimal aesthetic surgical results while avoiding potential complications.
- The eyelids and surrounding structures can be divided into five anatomical zones (**FIG 1**).[1,2] Zone I and zone II represent the upper and lower eyelid, respectively. Zone III represents the medial canthus and lacrimal drainage system. Zone IV includes the lateral canthal region and lateral retinaculum. Zone V represents the surrounding periorbital structures and includes the forehead, brow, glabellar, temple, malar, and nasal regions.
- Lower eyelid procedures including lower eyelid blepharoplasty and lateral canthopexy or canthoplasty focus on zones II and IV. The lower eyelid or zone II can be thought of as a trilamellar structure that consists of an anterior, middle, and posterior lamella. The anterior lamella consists of skin and orbicularis oculi muscle that is further divided into

pretarsal, preseptal, and orbital components. The pretarsal and preseptal components are often referred to as palpebral portions. The middle lamella includes the tarsus, orbital septum, and retroseptal fat, while the posterior lamella denotes the capsulopalpebral fascia and conjunctiva.
- The tarsal plate of the lower eyelid on average measures 25 mm wide, 4 mm in height, and 1 mm in thickness and provides structural integrity to the eyelid.
- The lateral canthus or lateral retinaculum (zone IV) is a three-dimensional fibrous structure that connects the upper and lower tarsal plates to the Whitnall tubercle, located 8 mm posterior to the lateral orbital rim (**FIG 2**). These structures converge at the lateral canthal angle, typically approximately 1.5 to 2.0 mm above the medial canthal angle. This aesthetically pleasing and favorable relationship of the lateral canthus above the medial canthus is often referred to as a positive canthal tilt. When the lateral canthus is at the level of or below the medial canthus, this is referred to as neutral or negative canthal tilt, respectively. It is the lower eyelid portion of the lateral retinaculum or the "inferior retinaculum" that is the focus of the lateral canthopexy or canthoplasty techniques that will be described in this chapter.

PATHOGENESIS

- Despite distinct ethnic and cultural differences, the youthful eye resembles an almond shape, which has a long and narrow palpebral fissure and an upward inclination of approximately four degrees laterally. In patients with loss of lateral canthal support, the lateral palpebral fissure takes on a more rounded appearance with concomitant laxity of the lower eyelid margin. The pathophysiology of lateral canthal disorders is attributed to the loss of canthal support from gravitational, mechanical, or involutional factors.

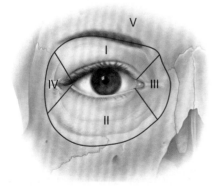

FIG 1 • The five zones of the periorbital region.

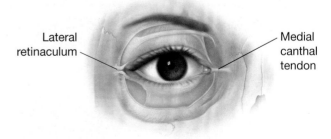

FIG 2 • Supporting structures of the upper and lower eyelid. Note the lateral retinaculum receives contributions from both the upper and lower eyelids.

7 Step Preoperative Checklist			
1. Vector analysis	☐ Positive	☐ Neutral	☐ Negative
2. Snap distraction	☐ Brisk	☐ Delayed	
3. Scleral show	☐ <4 mm	☐ >4 mm	
4. Canthal tilt	☐ Positive	☐ Neutral	☐ Negative
5. Lateral canthal-orbital rim distance	☐ <1 cm	☐ >1 cm	
6. Midface position	☐ Normal	☐ Descended	
7. Vertical restriction	☐ Absent	☐ Present	

FIG 3 • Key seven-step preoperative checklist.

- A subset of patients are at increased risk for lower eyelid malposition resulting from lower blepharoplasty. In such patients, lateral canthal tightening may be indicated to help prevent these sequelae.

PATIENT HISTORY AND PHYSICAL FINDINGS

- The preoperative assessment begins with a detailed medical history with emphasis on risk factors that may lead to postoperative complications. A past medical history of hypertension, diabetes, thyroid disease, bleeding diathesis, glaucoma, dry eyes, trauma, and periorbital and facial operations, including refractive surgery, is of particular significance and should be documented. Furthermore, the use of medications that include nonsteroidal anti-inflammatory, anticoagulants, and aspirin should be recorded and held for a minimum of 2 weeks prior to surgery.
- The physical exam should be performed with the patient sitting in an upright, relaxed position and should begin with an assessment of visual acuity, pupillary reflexes, extraocular muscle movement, and an intact Bell phenomenon.[3] A focused lower eyelid exam should document the presence of malar bags, fat herniation, dermatochalasis, tear trough deformities, and skin pigmentation. In addition, the senior authors have previously identified seven key features that should be assessed in patients undergoing lower eyelid procedures and include the following: canthal tilt, vector analysis, scleral show, tarsoligamentous integrity, lateral canthal-orbital rim distance, midface position, and vertical restriction.[2] This standard preoperative checklist is provided in **FIG 3**.
- Canthal tilt assesses the relationship of the medial and lateral canthus (**FIG 4**). The average position of the lateral canthus is approximately 1.5 to 2 mm cephalad to the medial canthus thus resulting in a positive tilt. Canthal tilt can be described as positive, negative, or neutral.
- Vector analysis describes the relationship of the anterior cornea of the globe to the malar eminence and can be neutral, positive, or negative. A positive vector is defined by a posterior relationship of the anterior cornea to the malar eminence, whereas in a negative vector, the anterior cornea projects in front of the malar eminence. It is negative vector anatomy that is associated with prominent fat pads, midface descent, and greater risk of lower eyelid malposition post blepharoplasty.
- Scleral show defines the relationship between the lower eyelid margin and the inferior limbus of the cornea, which is normally present at the same level precluding visualization of the sclera. Scleral show below the level of the inferior limbus suggests tarsoligamentous laxity.
- Tarsoligamentous integrity defines the tone of the lower eyelid and is examined with a snapback test and lid distraction test. The snapback test is performed by having the patient in primary gaze without blinking, displacing the lower eyelid inferiorly, and measuring the time required for the lower eyelid to return to its normal position. Measurements greater than 1 second are considered abnormal and can be associated with loss of orbicularis oculi muscle tone. The lid distraction test involves anterior traction on the lower eyelid away from the globe and measuring the distance between the globe and lower eyelid. Measurements less than 4 mm are considered normal, whereas distraction greater than 8 mm indicates tarsoligamentous laxity and the possible need for horizontal lower eyelid shortening.
- Lateral canthal-orbital rim distance (LC-OR) is a clinically valuable measurement and can be categorized as either

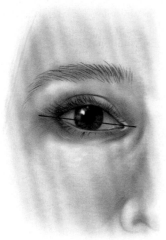
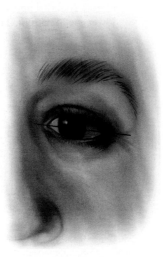

Positive tilt   Negative tilt

FIG 4 • Canthal tilt: The canthal tilt defines the relationship between the medial and lateral canthus.

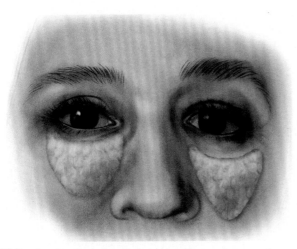

FIG 5 • A comparison of normal malar position as shown on the reader's right to descent.

being greater than or less than 1 cm. This measurement becomes important when determining which procedure to use for patients requiring correction of significant lower eyelid malposition.

- Midface position is an important consideration of the lower eyelid-cheek junction. Patients with midface descent may benefit from a cheek suspension to support the lower eyelid and relieve tension on the lateral canthus (**FIG 5**).
- This 7-step analysis helps to determine the proper procedures for the patient undergoing primary blepharoplasty or correcting pre-existing lower eyelid malposition. As shown (see **FIG 3**), patients with anatomic features on the left side have favorable conditions as compared to those with findings that line up on the right side.
- During the preoperative exam, one must assess for vertical restriction, which is measured by elevating the lower eyelid and ensuring that the eyelid margin reaches a level above the pupil. In cases of vertical restriction, one must decipher the origin as resulting from the anterior, middle, or posterior lamella. When restriction is present, additional corrective procedures may include release of cicatrix, placement of spacer graft, cheek suspension, or Mitek anchor fixation.

IMAGING

- Radiographic imaging is generally not indicated in the preoperative workup in patients undergoing procedures that include lower eyelid rejuvenation with lateral canthopexy or canthoplasty.

SURGICAL MANAGEMENT

- The inferior retinacular canthopexy was designed to improve eyelid aesthetics and prevent lower eyelid malposition in patients undergoing a primary blepharoplasty without separating the lower eyelid from the lateral palpebral commissure. Furthermore, its utility can be seen in correcting lower eyelid malposition in patients with a negative vector relationship. The lateral tension and pull achieved from the inferior retinacular canthopexy may provide significant improvement to lower eyelid aesthetics by smoothing the lower eyelid skin and diminishing or obviating the need for lower eyelid skin resection. Patients with more severe laxity or retraction may require canthoplasty in place of canthopexy.

Preoperative Planning

- The 7-step checklist previously described can aid the surgeon in stratifying patients into an appropriate surgical treatment plan.

Positioning

- Lower eyelid blepharoplasty with or without canthal manipulation is performed with the surgeon standing at the head of the patient looking toward the feet. Loupe magnification as well as a focused headlight is recommended to aid with visualization of key structures.

Approach

- Numerous surgical techniques have been described to address lateral canthal position and to correct lower eyelid malposition. These include dermal orbicular pennant lateral canthoplasty, tarsal strip lateral canthoplasty cheek suspension with Mitek anchor fixation, and bride of bone canthopexy.[1,4] The specifics of these is beyond the scope of this chapter; we will focus on inferior retinacular lateral canthopexy and canthoplasty techniques.

■ Inferior Retinacular Lateral Canthopexy/Canthoplasty

- The inferior retinacular lateral canthopexy/canthoplasty can be performed through a horizontal canthal incision or an upper lateral eyelid incision.[5]
- The advantage of an upper eyelid incision is that this incision is already being applied to patients undergoing concomitant upper blepharoplasty.
- The inferior edge of the lateral upper eyelid incision is grasped, and a submuscular dissection is performed in a supraperiosteal plane heading in an inferomedial direction.
- The skin and muscle flap is then elevated 2 cm around the lateral canthus and lower eyelid using a combination

of blunt scissor dissection and fine-point electrosurgical dissection.

- An insulated Desmarres retractor is used to retract the skin and muscle flap and help expose the lateral retinaculum, which is located just superior to the lower eyelid lateral fat.
- One additional advantage of this approach is that lower eyelid fat can also be removed at this stage, which creates an open space (Jelks cave) and allows visualization of the lateral retinaculum as it inserts on Whitnall tubercle (**TECH FIG 1A**).
- In a canthopexy, forceps are then used to grasp the inferior retinaculum (**TECH FIG 1B**), and U-stitch is placed through with two passes of permanent or semipermanent suture (Mersilene 4-0, Polydek Silky II-ME2).

T E C H N I Q U E S

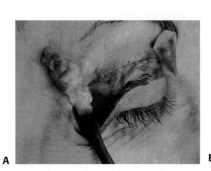
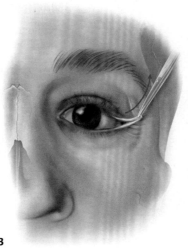

TECH FIG 1 • **A.** The inferior retinacular lateral canthopexy is performed through the lateral aspect of an upper eyelid blepharoplasty incision. **B.** The inferior retinaculum is grasped with forceps and fixated to the inner periosteum of lateral orbital rim.

- In a canthoplasty, the inferior retinaculum is divided from its insertion so that repositioning is possible.
- The lower eyelid is then everted to confirm that the suture has not violated the conjunctiva.
- In a canthoplasty, the inferior retinaculum is cut, thereby detaching the lower lid from the lateral orbital wall, before the suspension suture is placed.
- Fixation of the suture is then performed to the inner periosteum at the lateral orbital rim at the level of the superior aspect of the pupil in primary gaze. Placement of this stitch should be performed with great care, as this

sets the new height of the lateral canthal tendon. Of note, corneal shields may limit one's ability to assess the level of the pupil. In the orbit, this represents the portion of the lateral orbital rim that starts to take an inward curve.
- The wound is closed as a single layer.
- The same principles and surgical technique apply when using a horizontal canthal incision. If an upper blepharoplasty incision is not being used, one may also perform a transcanthal canthopexy. In this case, the lateral retinaculum is approached directly and grasped from below, but similar principles apply.

PEARLS AND PITFALLS

Indications	▪ Inferior retinacular lateral canthopexy was developed to help prevent lower eyelid malposition in primary blepharoplasty patients.
	▪ A canthoplasty can be used for correction of secondary lower eyelid malposition associated with a negative vector.
	▪ Lateral canthal tightening can address redundant lower eyelid skin, thus diminishing or obviating the need for more skin excision.
Advantage	▪ Inferior retinacular lateral canthopexy does not separate the lower eyelid from the lateral palpebral commissure.
Approach	▪ The lower eyelid should appear overcorrected and cover approximately 1–2 mm of the inferior limbus as it settles into position in 2 to 6 weeks.

POSTOPERATIVE CARE

- Minimal activity for 24 hours and head of bed elevation to at least 45 degrees should be maintained.
- Cool compresses may be applied for the first 24 hours.
- Ophthalmic antibiotic ointment is used two to three times per day for the eyelid suture lines. Steroid ophthalmic solutions are prescribed for 3 to 5 days.
- Tear supplements may be used for the 1st week, but are usually not necessary.
- Patients should sleep at 30 to 45 degrees elevation for 2 to 3 weeks.

- Patients may resume preoperative physical activity by 3 to 4 weeks postoperatively.
- Patients follow up 5 days postoperatively for suture removal and are followed 4 weeks, 3 months, 6 months, 9 months, and 1 year postoperatively.
- Photographs are taken at 1-year follow-up.

OUTCOMES

- See **FIG 6**.

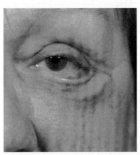 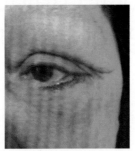

FIG 6 • **A.** A preoperative photograph of a patient with lower eyelid malposition. **B.** The inferior retinacular lateral canthopexy allows for proper lower eyelid positioning as well as improving canthal tilt.

COMPLICATIONS

- Postoperative complications from proper lateral canthal support are uncommon but may include the following:
  - Bleeding
  - Infection
  - Lower lid malposition
  - Scar formation
  - Chemosis

ACKNOWLEDGMENTS

We thank Steve Sultan and Elizabeth Jelks for their assistance in the preparation of this chapter.

REFERENCES

1. Jelks GW, Elizabeth BJ. "Lateral canthal suspension techniques". *Aesthet Plast Surg.* 2009:329.
2. Tepper O, Steinbrech D, Howell MH, et al. A retrospective review of patients undergoing lateral canthal techniques to manage existing or potential lower eyelid malposition: identification of seven key preoperative findings. *Plast Reconstr Surg.* 2015;136(1):40-49.
3. Jindal K, Sarcia M, Codner MA. Functional considerations in aesthetic eyelid surgery. *Plast Reconstr Surg.* 2014;134(6):1154-1170.
4. Yaremchuk MJ, Chen YC. Bridge of bone canthopexy. *Aesthet Surg J.* 2009;29:323-329.
5. Jelks GW, Glat PM, Jelks EB, Longaker MT. The inferior retinacular lateral canthoplasty: a new technique. *Plast Reconstr Surg.* 1997;100(5):1262-1270.

36
CHAPTER

Indications and Techniques for Fat Grafting for Periorbital Rejuvenation

Oren M. Tepper, Jillian Schreiber, Elizabeth B. Jelks, and Glenn W. Jelks

DEFINITION

- The periorbital region is an essential component of a youthful appearing face. Aesthetic rejuvenation of the eyelids is a frequently requested and challenging procedure offered by most plastic surgery practices. Although soft tissue descent and cutaneous changes have long been recognized as a sign of periorbital aging, volume loss or deflation has more recently been appreciated as an important contributing factor as well.[1,2]
- Traditional blepharoplasty is subtractive in nature. Conventional approaches to upper and lower blepharoplasty include excision of excess skin and fat, with potential risk of creating a hollowed or "operated" appearance.[2–4] In light of the importance of periorbital fat to provide support and contour in the youthful eyelid, there has been a shift in blepharoplasty techniques away from excision alone toward preservation and restoration of periorbital volume.[2,5–7] The goals of this chapter are to provide an updated approach to fat grafting in the periorbital region as a primary means of achieving upper and lower eyelid rejuvenation and/or correction of secondary deformities.
- Autologous fat grafting has gained widespread popularity as an effective means of volume augmentation for various facial procedures due to its ease of harvest, longevity, rapid execution, and relative safety.[8–10] Autologous fat grafting is used to address changes due to aging in the upper and lower eyelid, the brow, and the eyelid-cheek junction.[1]

Upper Eyelid

- Atrophy of fat and skin in the upper eyelid and surrounding regions can result in skeletonization of the bony orbit, protuberance of remaining periorbital fat, poor soft tissue support, and eyebrow descent.
- In general, fat grafting of the upper eyelid is most commonly performed for correction of a hollowed appearance to the upper eyelid sulcus. This may be the result from aging or secondary to over-resection of retroseptal fat during an upper blepharoplasty procedure.

Lower Eyelid

- A prominent nasojugal groove, often described as the "tear trough," is a common finding in patients seeking periorbital rejuvenation. The anatomical junction of the lower eyelid and cheek (palpebral malar interface) extends from the medial canthus inferolaterally above cheek tissue to form a depression (nasojugal groove). This is distinct from colloquial terms such as "dark circles" and "puffiness" of the lower eyelid that are commonly used interchangeably.

- Fat grafting to the eyelid-cheek junction, with or without skin and fat excision, is an effective means to treat a tear trough deformity and camouflage the prominence of fat in the lower eyelid compartments.

ANATOMY

- The periorbital region is composed of the bony orbital rim, orbicularis oculi muscle, orbital fat compartments, and the upper and lower eyelids. The upper and lower eyelids are layered structures composed of an anterior and posterior lamella divided by the orbital septum (**FIG 1**).
- The thin eyelid skin and orbicularis oculi muscle constitute the anterior lamella of the upper and lower eyelids. The orbicularis oculi muscle is divided into pretarsal, preseptal, and orbital components. The pretarsal and preseptal portions make up the palpebral segment and provide involuntary blink, whereas the orbital portion provides voluntary eyelid closing.
- The posterior lamella is composed of different but analogous structures between the upper and lower eyelids. The upper eyelid posterior lamella includes the palpebral conjunctiva and tarsal plate. Above the tarsal plate, it is composed of the palpebral conjunctiva and Müller muscle. The posterior lamella of the lower eyelid is similarly made up of the palpebral conjunctiva and tarsal plate and inferior to the tarsal plate the conjunctiva and capsulopalpebral fascia and inferior tarsal muscle.

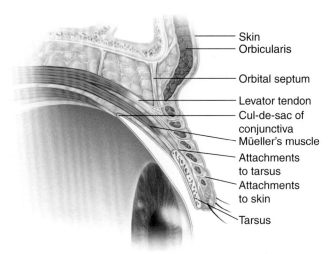

Skin
Orbicularis

Orbital septum

Levator tendon
Cul-de-sac of conjunctiva
Müeller's muscle
Attachments to tarsus
Attachments to skin

Tarsus

FIG 1 • Upper eyelid anatomy. Sagittal section through the upper eyelid demonstrating the anterior and posterior lamella and the relationship with the orbital septum.

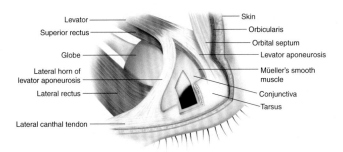

FIG 2 • Upper eyelid anatomy highlighting the relationship between the levator muscle, the tarsus, and lateral canthal tendon.

- The upper eyelid retractors are the levator palpebrae superioris innervated by the oculomotor nerve and the sympathetically innervated Müller muscle (**FIG 2**). The lower eyelid retractors include the capsulopalpebral fascia and inferior tarsal muscle.

- The prominent tear trough is often addressed in periorbital rejuvenation. Factors that contribute to a prominent palpebral malar interface include alterations in the quality and elasticity of the overlying skin, subcutaneous tissue, orbicularis oculi muscle, orbital septum, capsulopalpebral fascia, and retroseptal orbital fat.[2] The anatomical position of the arcus marginalis on the zygomatic and maxillary bones determines the location of the palpebral malar interface[2,3] (**FIG 4**).

- The arcus marginalis is defined by the bony origin of the orbital septum, orbital periosteum, and the maxillary periosteum. The origins of the preseptal and orbital orbicularis oculi muscle, the orbital retaining ligaments, malar septum, prezygomatic space, and arcuate bands are related to the arcus marginalis.

- The upper eyelid fat is composed of the medial and lateral fat compartments. In the lower eyelid, three distinct fat compartments of retroseptal fat exist: lateral, central, and nasal. The nasal and central compartments are divided by the inferior oblique muscle tendon. The medial (nasal)

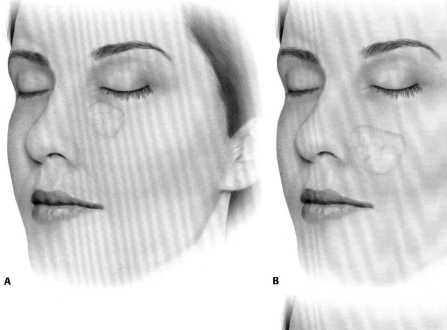

A

B

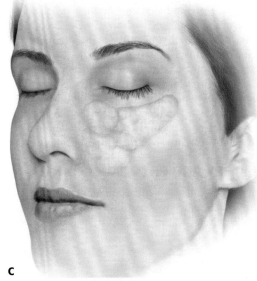

FIG 3 • Periorbital fat compartments of the lower eyelid and cheek. **A.** The medial suborbicularis oculi fat compartment (MSOOF). **B.** The deep medial cheek fat compartment. **C.** Addition of the MSOOF, DMC, and the lateral suborbicularis oculi fat compartment (LSOOF).

C

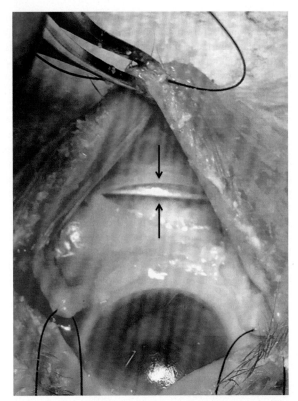

FIG 4 • The arcus marginalis is shown on cadaveric dissection. It is the bony origin of the orbital septum, orbital periosteum, and the maxillary periosteum.

compartment is derived from the white orbital fat and the lateral (central) fat compartment from the less dense, yellow preaponeurotic fat.[1]

- Emerging research demonstrates facial fat is divided into discrete fat compartments.[11–13] However, the exact anatomy of the periorbital fat compartments somewhat varies within the literature. Recent cadaveric studies by Rohrich et al. describe two suborbicularis fat compartments: the medial suborbicularis oculi compartment extending from the medial limbus to the lateral canthus along the infraorbital rim and the lateral orbicularis oculi compartment from the lateral canthus to the temporal fat pad.[11] Regardless of the exact nomenclature and anatomic boundaries of these compartments, eyelid aesthetics needs to go well beyond the traditional retroseptal compartments and consider the periorbital fat compartments as well (**FIG 3**).

- The temporal hallows are an underappreciated yet important region when approaching the aged face. Temporal wasting leads to an "hourglass" appearance to the upper face that can be corrected with autologous fat grafting. A smooth transition may be achieved between the forehead and malar region when volume is replaced in the temporal hallow.

PATIENT HISTORY AND PHYSICAL FINDINGS

- A thorough history and physical examination is vital to effectively approach rejuvenation of the periorbital region. This includes a general history and physical examination,

as well as a complete ophthalmologic examination. Anticoagulant and antiplatelet medications should be documented and stopped prior to surgery to avoid complications due to bleeding. Assessment of all periorbital and adjacent structures, including malar, temporal, and glabellar regions, are vital to achieving a harmonious and balanced result.

- The periorbital region is evaluated in detail. Upper and lower eyelid skin quality, excess skin, and pseudoherniation of orbital fat are documented.

- A functional examination of the orbital region is performed. Lateral canthal descent, lid laxity, scleral show, and ectropion are all evaluated. Symmetry is appreciated.
  - The vector between the globe and malar region is characterized as positive or negative. This relationship aids the surgeon in assessing malar descent and selecting patients who would benefit from malar augmentation to provide support to the lower lid as well as restore a positive vector. When assessing patients for correction of lower eyelid aging, it is essential to consider not only the lower eyelid but also the cheek and the interface of the two. Midfacial volume loss and descent lead to loss of anterior projection and contour and decreased support to the lower eyelid.
  - The seven-step preoperative checklist, developed by the senior authors of this chapter, is used for preoperative planning for blepharoplasty patients.[14] This examination included seven key findings: vector analysis, snap, distraction, scleral show, canthal tilt, lateral canthal-orbital rim distance, midface position, and vertical restriction. This standardized physical examination characterizes the severity of hollowing, skin quality, and descent of the periorbital region to guide treatment (**FIG 5**).
  - Periorbital aging is a combination of volume loss, soft tissue descent, and cutaneous changes.[1,2] Brow descent with atrophy of superior orbital fat and hollowing lead to a tired, aged appearance. The extent of these changes needs to be considered when evaluating patients.

NONOPERATIVE MANAGEMENT

- Hyaluronic acid fillers are an effective temporary alterative to autologous fat grafting for periorbital rejuvenation. This approach is a nonpermanent option for patients who wish to achieve added volume of the periorbital region and wish to avoid surgical intervention. The best candidates for hyaluronic acid injection are those with good skin tone and minimal skin laxity with minimal to moderate volume loss in the periorbital region.[15] These characteristics help minimize the injection volume required and risk of palpable or visible deformities that are associate with fillers in this region.

SURGICAL MANAGEMENT

Positioning

- The patient is positioned supine.

7-step Lower Eyelid Checklist

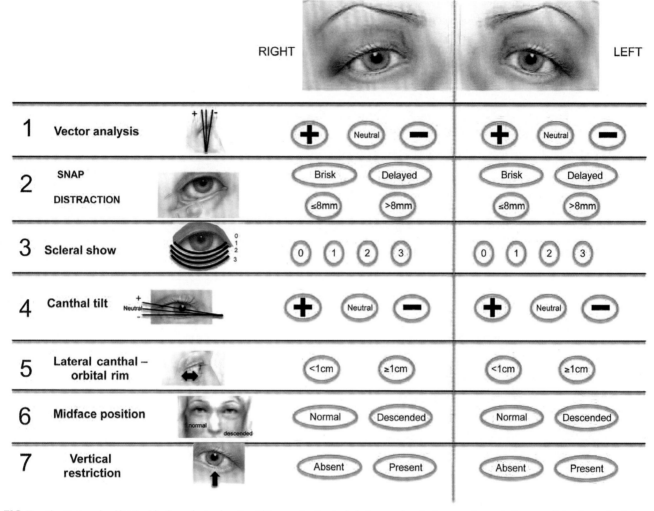

	RIGHT			LEFT		
1 Vector analysis	+ -	**+** Neutral **-**			**+** Neutral **-**	
2 SNAP DISTRACTION		Brisk Delayed ≤8mm >8mm			Brisk Delayed ≤8mm >8mm	
3 Scleral show	0 1 2 3	0 1 2 3			0 1 2 3	
4 Canthal tilt	+ Neutral -	**+** Neutral **-**			**+** Neutral **-**	
5 Lateral canthal – orbital rim		<1cm ≥1cm			<1cm ≥1cm	
6 Midface position	normal descended	Normal Descended			Normal Descended	
7 Vertical restriction		Absent Present			Absent Present	

FIG 5 • The 7-step checklist for blepharoplasty planning. This examination included seven key findings: vector analysis, snap, distraction, scleral show, canthal tilt, lateral canthal-orbital rim distance, midface position, and vertical restriction.

■ Fat Harvest and Injection Technique

- Autologous fat is most commonly harvested from the anterior abdomen or the medial or lateral thigh or anterior abdomen. The patient is positioned supine, and these locations are easily accessed for fat harvest.
- Autologous fat may be processed according to surgeon preference. The authors of this paper prefer harvesting with 10-cc syringes under negative suction, allowing for gravitational sedimentation. Fat is then transferred to 1-cc syringes for injection with 0.9-mm blunt cannulas. Fat is deposited deep at the level superficial to the periosteum. Fat may be injected in multiple passes of small aliquots into the individual compartments.[1]

■ Eye Brow and Temporal Region

- Fat grafting of the eyebrow and temporal is routinely performed in our practice to achieve facial rejuvenation.
- The upper brow and temporal region may be accessed approximately 15 to 20 mm above the central brow. For treatment of the eyebrow region, fat is injected deep in the supraperiosteal plane into the central and lateral brow. This not only provides volume but also has a "lifting" effect on the brow. Typical volumes are approximately 1 to 3 mL in this region, depending on the overall aesthetic goals.
- Lipostructural fat grafting to the temporal region can also be achieved through this port site or accesses via a separate point along the lateral forehead hairline. The layer of injection is targeted between the superficial and deep temporal fascia to minimize risk of visible deformity while still achieving an added volume effect on the surface.

TECHNIQUES

T
E
C
H
N
I
Q
U
E
S

■ Upper Eyelid

■ Fat grafting in the upper eyelid corrects hollowing due to aging, however more commonly treats secondary deformity due to over-resection during prior blepharoplasty.

■ The upper eyelid fat compartments are accessed by a port site located 10 to 15 mm lateral to the lateral canthus.[1] Fat is injected into the preseptal space, directly beneath the orbicularis muscle, as to avoid obvious irregularities of superficial injection beneath the thin eyelid skin. This injection is placed at the edge of the orbital rim.

■ Lower Eyelid/Malar Fat Grafting

■ Fat grafting to the malar compartments is performed using a technique modified from Surek et al.[16] The deep medial cheek compartment is accessed via the "nasolabial insertion port" located 1.5 to 2 cm inferolateral to the ipsilateral alar base within the nasolabial fold and the lateral cheek compartment via the "lateral cheek insertion port" located 1.5 to 2 cm inferolaterally to the lateral canthus, as described (**TECH FIG 1**).

■ An alternative approach practiced by the authors of this paper is the use of a single port (nasolabial insertion port) to access the malar and lower eyelid fat compartments. Adding volume of the deep medial cheek provides anterior projection to the midface as well as effacement of the nasojugal groove. Via the nasolabial port, a blunt cannula is used to inject 1 to 2 cc of autologous fat. The lateral cheek compartment is accessed, and a 1 to 2 cc of autologous fat is injected.

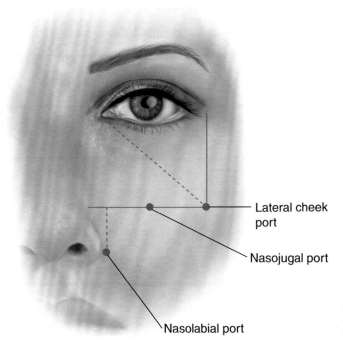

Lateral cheek port

Nasojugal port

Nasolabial port

TECH FIG 1 • Malar fat grafting port sites for injection. The nasolabial, nasojugal, and lateral cheek port sites are shown. Alternatively, all three cheek compartments may be accessed via a single port (lateral cheek port site).

■ Arcus Marginalis Release

■ Arcus marginalis release in conjunction with fat grafting may be an effective means of treating a severe tear trough deformity. This is performed with a horizontal incision 8 mm from the posterior lower eyelid margin through the conjunctiva and capsulopalpebral fascia to access the retroseptal space (**TECH FIG 2A**).

■ Retroseptal fat is retracted to visualize the arcus marginalis, which is sharply released from the medial canthus along the infraorbital rim to the level of the mid-pupil.[17] The origin of the preseptal and orbital orbicularis oculi muscle is also released with this maneuver (**TECH FIG 2B**).

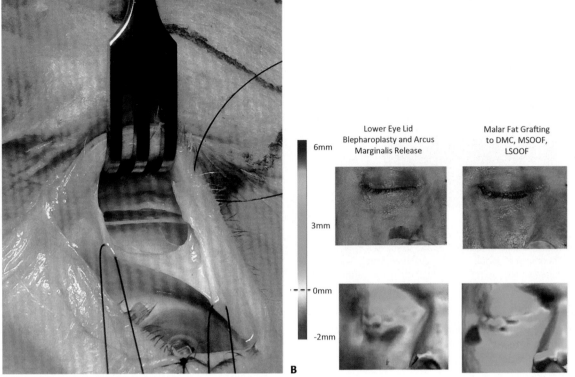

TECH FIG 2 • A. Arcus marginalis on cadaveric specimen is shown after release from the medial canthus along the infraorbital rim to the level of the mid-pupil. **B.** Color map analysis of clinical patient following lower blepharoplasty with fat excision followed by arcus marginalis release. Color spectrum shows change in surface projection as compared to the baseline surface. Color spectrum ranges from no change (*green*) to most significant volume loss (*red*) and volume gain (*blue*). Note volume loss during fat excision (*red*) and a volume gain following arcus marginalis release (less red medially) and maximum volume following malar fat grafting (*blue*).

PEARLS AND PITFALLS

Indications	■ Periorbital volume loss contributes to aging in the upper face. 　■ Brow descent, upper eyelid hollowing, temporal hollowing, malar descent, and a prominent nasojugal groove (or "tear trough deformity") may be addressed by way of autologous fat grafting to various facial fat compartments.
Advantage	■ Volume addition of the periorbital restores youthful contour and may provide support to the lower eyelid and brow. ■ Hyaluronic acid fillers are an effective yet temporary option for patients to be reserved for patients with good skin quality and minimal to moderate volume loss. ■ Patients with moderate to severe periorbital atrophy and descent of the upper and midface benefit for autologous fat grafting. ■ Arcus marginalis release in conjunction with fat grafting may be an effective means of treating a severe tear trough deformity. ■ A single port (nasolabial insertion port) may be used to access the malar and lower eyelid fat compartments.
Pitfalls	■ A thorough history and physical examination, including ophthalmologic examination, are vital to successful patient selection and outcomes in periorbital rejuvenation. ■ Anatomical knowledge of facial fat compartments permits precise placement of fat and reproducible results.

POSTOPERATIVE CARE

■ Patients should maintain head of bed elevation of at least 45 degrees for the first 24 hours postoperatively.
■ Cool compresses may be applied for comfort.
■ Patients may resume preoperative physical activity by 3 to 4 weeks postoperatively.

■ Postoperative photographs are taken at 3 and 6 months and at 1 year follow-up.

OUTCOMES

■ See **FIGS 6** and **7.**

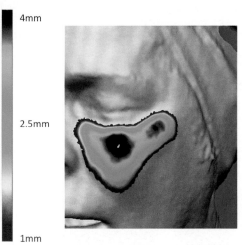

Deep Medial
Cheek 1cc,
MSOOF 1cc,
LSOOF 2cc

4mm

2.5mm

1mm

FIG 6 • 3D color map of clinical patient following malar augmentation to the deep medial cheek, medial SOOF, and lateral SOOF. Note the characteristic "boomerang" shape with the gradient of projection from the boundary in *red* (1 mm) to maximal projection in *blue* (4 mm).[18]

COMPLICATIONS

- Complications from autologous fat grafting to the periorbital region are rare but may be significant.
- Contour irregularities, particularly in areas of thin eyelid skin, may arise.
- Complications during fat harvest include pain, ecchymosis, and perforation of the abdominal wall and intra-abdominal viscera.

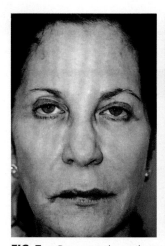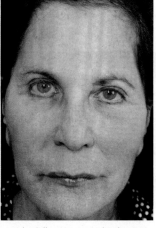

FIG 7 • Representative patient example following periorbital rejuvenation. This patient underwent autologous fat grafting to the MSOOF, LSOOF, DMC, and temporal hollows.

- Periocular complications following hyaluronic acid filler injections are exceedingly rare and due to retrograde displacement of product into the central retinal artery. Ptosis, ophthalmoplegia, enophthalmos, and blindness have been reported.[19]

REFERENCES

1. Massry GG, Azizzadeh B. Periorbital fat grafting. *Facial Plast Surg.* 2013;29(1):46-57.
2. Hamra ST. Arcus marginalis release and orbital fat preservation in midface rejuvenation. *Plast Reconstr Surg.* 1995;96(2):354-362.
3. Goldberg RA. Transconjunctival orbital fat repositioning: transposition of orbital fat pedicles into a subperiosteal pocket. *Plast Reconstr Surg.* 2000;105(2):743-748.
4. Carraway JH. Volume correction for nasojugal groove with blepharoplasty. *Aesthet Surg J.* 2010;30(1):101-109.
5. Hester TR Jr, Ashinoff RL, McCord CD. Managing postseptal fat in periorbital rejuvenation: anatomic intraorbital replacement using passive septal tightening. *Aesthet Surg J.* 2006;26(6):717-724.
6. Lambros V. Observations on periorbital and midface aging. *Plast Reconstr Surg.* 2007;120(5):1367-1376.
7. Lambros VS. Hyaluronic acid injections for correction of the tear trough deformity. *Plast Reconstr Surg.* 2007;120(6 suppl):74S-80S.
8. Coleman SR. Structural fat grafting. *Aesthet Surg J.* 1998;18(5):386-388.
9. Coleman SR. Facial augmentation with structural fat grafting. *Clin Plast Surg.* 2006;33(4):567-577.
10. Coleman SR. Structural fat grafting: more than a permanent filler. *Plast Reconstr Surg.* 2006;118(3 suppl):108S-120S.
11. Rohrich RJ, Arbique GM, Wong C, et al. The anatomy of suborbicularis fat: implications for periorbital rejuvenation. *Plast Reconstr Surg.* 2009;124(3):946-951.
12. Rohrich RJ, Pessa JE. The retaining system of the face: histologic evaluation of the septal boundaries of the subcutaneous fat compartments. *Plast Reconstr Surg.* 2008;121(5):1804-1809.
13. Stern CS, Schreiber JE, Surek CC, et al. Three-dimensional topographic surface changes in response to compartmental volumization of the medial cheek: defining a malar augmentation zone. *Plast Reconstr Surg.* 2016;137(5):1401-1408.
14. Tepper OM, Steinbrech D, Howell MH, et al. A retrospective review of patients undergoing lateral canthoplasty techniques to manage existing or potential lower eyelid malposition: identification of seven key preoperative findings. *Plast Reconstr Surg.* 2015;136(1):40-49.
15. Hirmand H. Correction of the tear trough deformity with hyaluronic acid. 2009.
16. Surek C, Beut J, Stephens R, et al. Volumizing viaducts of the midface: defining the beut techniques. *Aesthet Surg J.* 2015;35(2):121-134.
17. Wong CH, Mendelson B. Facial soft-tissue spaces and retaining ligaments of the midcheek: defining the premaxillary space. *Plast Reconstr Surg.* 2013;132(1):49-56.
18. Schreiber JE, Terner J, Stern CS, et al. The "Boomerang Lift": a 3-step compartment based approach to the youthful cheek. *Plast Reconstr Surg.* 2018;141(4):910-913.
19. Myung Y, Yim S, Jeong JH, et al. The classification and prognosis of periocular complications related to blindness following cosmetic filler injection. *Plast Reconstr Surg.* 2017;140(1):61-64.

Indications and Techniques for Upper and Lower Blepharoplasty With Microfat Injections

Nuri A. Celik

DEFINITION

Upper Blepharoplasty

- Upper blepharoplasty is considered an easy operation; however, depending on your level of expertise and ability to systematically analyze the inherent problems, it might be considered one of the most complex operations of aesthetic surgery practice.
- The complex component is the patient evaluation. There is more to a periorbital rejuvenation than just excision of fat, muscle, and skin. We should be able to answer the question: what makes an eye beautiful?
- The upper blepharoplasty evaluation should always involve the brow level and shape considerations. Although a high and arched eyebrow is a common feature in female beauty, transverse and low eyebrows are a masculine characteristic in the majority of the male models.
- One should always keep in mind that the facial skeleton also plays a major role in the perception of beauty.
- A convex area beneath the middle and lateral brow:
  - A surgeon should always examine the lateral brow mobility before performing an upper blepharoplasty. There are conflicting reports about the brow positional changes following an upper blepharoplasty.[1,2] The author has two main criteria for this assessment.

- The lateral brow response to a downward pull. This is a sure sign that the skin resection at the end of the upper blepharoplasty procedure will easily displace the lateral brow tissues to a lower position.
- Any skin excess lateral to the lateral canthus. This is an indication for a brow lift by the author who never extends the upper blepharoplasty incision beyond the lateral orbital rim, because in thick skin individuals, scars lateral to the rim are visible.
- The fullness beneath the lateral brow area is a beauty feature in women[3] and can also be a positive factor of masculinity in a low running male eyebrow. The fullness in this area is related to the fullness over the lateral orbital rim, and this can be surgically achieved with fat injection into the area (**FIG 1**) and also dermofat grafting (**FIG 2**).
- A short supratarsal distance is a significant feature of youth. It is directly associated with the periorbital soft tissue volume and an indicator of the upper sulcus fat content and the levator function.
  - The skeletonized upper sulcus becomes prominent in the elderly (**FIG 3**), and the majority of these patients have an increased supratarsal distance. This shows the necessity of the addition of the intraseptal fat management and the levator procedures in our upper blepharoplasty practices.

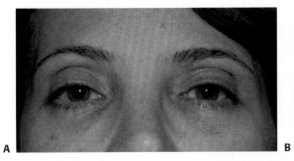
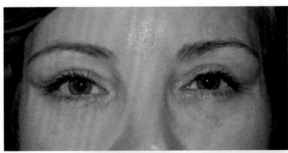
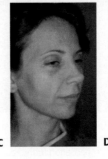
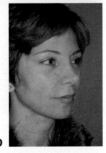

FIG 1 • **A,B.** A 45-year-old female who underwent upper blepharoplasty and lateral brow lift with fat injection. The levator advancement technique was used to correct the ptosis. **C,D.** The 2-year postoperative brow contour is achieved with the help of lateral subperiosteal brow lift and fat injection of lateral infrabrow area.

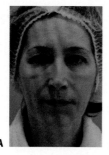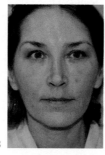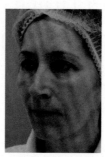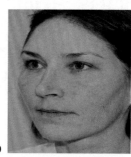

FIG 2 • A,B. A 42-year-old female patient before-after pictures. Upper eyelid ptosis corrected with levator advancement. Notice the raised lateral brow and the fullness of the infrabrow area. **C,D.** She had lateral brow lift through the upper blepharoplasty incision and dermofat grafting of the upper lateral orbital rim and the upper sulcus. The periorbital contours were obtained with 42-cc fat injection.

- The almond shape of the eye aperture:
  - In young individuals, the medial portion of the eye aperture has a higher measurement vertically than the lateral half.
  - The better support offered by the lateral canthus during early decades of life provides a higher lateral lower eyelid topography. This decreases the angle of convergence at the lateral corner of the eye and narrows the aperture in the lateral half.
  - The aging changes of the inferolateral orbital rim bone and dimension are mainly responsible for the sagging of the lateral part of the lower eyelid resulting in the change in shape of the eye to oval.[4,5]
- An upper eyelid covering 1 to 2 mm of the limbus:
  - This is maintained with intact levator function and proper attachment of the aponeurosis on the anterior surface of the upper tarsus.
  - The upper eyelid level should be evaluated in conjunction with the frontalis muscle activity because the frequent transverse horizontal wrinkles of the elderly show involvement of this muscle as a compensation for the failure of the levator system.
- Lateral and medial canthal position and stability:
  - The effect of the lateral canthal placement and resistance on the position of the lower eyelid is well documented in the literature.
  - The lateral canthal laxity is not age specific; it might be present in the young (**FIG 4A**), and surprisingly, the lateral canthus might have good stability in the elderly (**FIG 4B**).
  - The medial canthal position and symmetry are also significant factors in the lower eyelid stability because the lower tarsus is attached to both canthi.

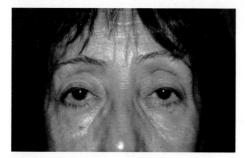

FIG 3 • A 64-year-old female presenting with the typical superior sulcus fat deficiency, ptosis of the upper eyelids, and asymmetrically elevated eyebrows due to frontalis muscle compensation further accentuating the upper eyelid deformity.

- Slight asymmetries of the medial canthal origin will alter the hammock-type support of the lower eyelid, interfering with the postoperative results.
- The occasional patient who has slight displacement of the medial canthal attachment should be informed preoperatively that the possibility of obtaining perfectly symmetric lower eyelids is compromised (**FIG 5**).
- Medial and lateral canthal laxity is responsible for the majority of postoperative complications and should be taken into account to achieve good results with lower eyelid surgery.
- Nasojugal fold:
  - It is important to obtain a smooth pass from the lower eyelid to the cheek to decrease the shadows that increase with age.
  - The transformation of the orbital cavity with the aging process decreases the support to the lower lateral orbital rim and the lateral canthus with increased fat herniation and degree of negative factor.[6]

Lower Blepharoplasty

- Lower blepharoplasty is a challenging operation because there are many factors that affect the outcome of surgery. The most important factors are medial and lateral canthal stability, presence of negative vector of the lower orbital rim, and orbital prominence or a shallow orbit.
- The need for a concomitant lateral canthal procedure during lower blepharoplasty procedure is not debatable in the author's opinion.[7] It is the author's experience that patients with a medial canthal attachment at or below the level of the inferior limbus are at increased risk for lower eyelid retraction, no matter what type of maneuver is used for the lateral canthal support.[8]

Fat Injection

- As mentioned before, the telltale sign of periorbital aging is skeletonization; decreased subcutaneous fat fails to camouflage the upper and lower orbital rim bony contours.
- With the concomitant brow lift procedures, the relatively thin eyelid skin is pulled superiorly, leaving a depression over the superolateral orbital bony rim.
- This area needs augmentation in conjunction with the subbrow area, and the relative prominence of this fill creates a need for temporal hollow, glabellar, and frontal regions and, in select cases, zygomatic arch and midface to be augmented with fat injections.[9]

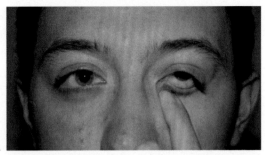 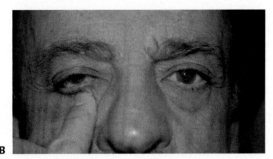

FIG 4 • A. A surprisingly slack lower eyelid in a 24-year-old male patient. Notice the curved contour of the lower eyelid and excessive scleral show for his age. **B.** A 67-year-old male with good lateral canthal support.

ANATOMY

- The upper eyelid is a complex structure that consists of multiple tissue layers that seem to adhere to each other around the upper anterior tarsal surface.
- When the skin and muscle layers are incised and a skin muscle flap is elevated as a superiorly based flap, one notices a thin layer of adipose tissue on top of the upper orbital septum that is more defined medially and somewhat less laterally.
- The increased convexity of the globe is possibly responsible for this uneven distribution of the fat layer. The underlying septum should always be incised laterally and higher than the upper tarsal border in order not to injure the levator mechanism inadvertently.
- There usually is a preaponeurotic fat pad present, if not previously excised or developmentally absent.
- Under the fat pad, toward the upper orbital rim, one can find the vertically oriented fibers of the levator muscle. The surgeon should always keep in mind that, immediately below the levator aponeurosis, there is the vertically oriented arterial loop of the supratarsal arch that might resemble the fibers of the levator muscle.

- The lower eyelid has similar tissue layers converging and attaching to the lower end of the lower tarsus, mainly the septum under the muscle and, in deeper layers, the lower lid retractors and the conjunctiva.
- The lower half of the orbital septum is almost always attenuated and the lower eyelid fat pads are herniated in individuals with protruding fat pockets.
- One important surgical landmark is the periosteal attachment of the orbicularis oculi muscle that extends around 1 cm along the medial part of the lower orbital rim.[9]
- The middle and lateral portions of the surface of the bony rim periosteum are covered by the SOOF to a variable degree in every individual. This creates two separate surgical dissection layers: around the midportion of the lower orbital rim, the medial part elevation should always be subperiosteal, whereas the more lateral portions allow a supraperiosteal dissection.

PATHOGENESIS

- Many complex mechanisms are involved in the aging process with various contributions from different tissue layers presenting as the individual aging patterns seen in different races and skin types.

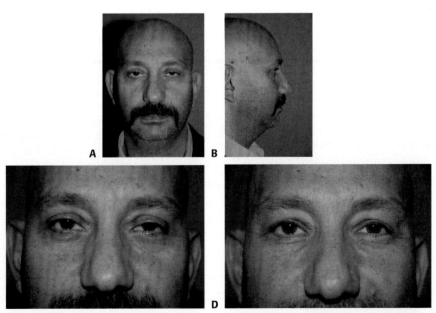

FIG 5 • A,B. A 44-year-old male seeking correction for his asymmetric ptosis, scleral show, and premature facial aging. Notice the low insertion of the medial canthi in relation to the lower limbus. This puts the patient in a "surgical risk" category. **C,D.** The patient was informed of the asymmetry of his medial canthal insertion and possibility of lower eyelid level and shape mismatch. The postoperative level of the right lower eyelid is slightly lower than the left due to lower insertion of the medial canthus on that side.

- Camirand's paper[10] deals with mainly the soft tissue changes, whereas recent investigations[4-6] point to concomitant bony topographical alterations.
- With time, the ligaments attenuate and the subcutaneous thinning ensues, whereas the compensatory powerful muscle contractions create furrows and lines.

PATIENT HISTORY AND PHYSICAL FINDINGS

- The variable pattern of the individual aging process makes it impossible to specifically organize the deformities that the patients present with.
  - There are patients who present mainly with tissue loss as well as the ones who complain of increased fat pockets around the eyes (**FIG 6**).
  - Although the thin-skinned patients mainly complain of wrinkles, the thick-skinned individuals would like more of a "lift" because of the higher incidence of sagging of the periorbital tissues.
- It is advisable to obtain pictures of patients from their early decades of life. This gives the surgeon the ability to assess the aging changes and the pattern and shed light to a sound surgical planning.

DIFFERENTIAL DIAGNOSIS

- Myasthenia gravis
- Thyroid disease

NONOPERATIVE MANAGEMENT

- There are many different treatment options for this area, including lasers, ultrasonic devices, peels, and fillers.

SURGICAL MANAGEMENT

Preoperative Planning

- Consider
  - Skin thickness
  - Brow ptosis: horizontal frontal wrinkles

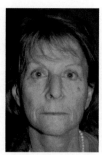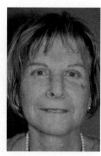

FIG 6 • **A,B.** A 72-year-old female before and after face-lift with upper and lower blepharoplasty 7 years ago. She was treated with 200-cc single-stage periorbital and perioral fat grafting and upper lip shortening of 7 mm.

- Upper eyelid ptosis
- Loss of upper eyelid curve
- Asymmetric or high supratarsal fold
- Upper eyelid fat and skin
- Lateral canthal ligament laxity
- Medial canthal ligament laxity
- Medial canthal ligament insertion variations
- Any asymmetry
- Lower eyelid fat pads, pretarsal muscle activity, and tone
- Nasojugal fold

Positioning

- Patient is operated supine and in a reverse Trendelenburg position.

Approach

- The upper blepharoplasty incision follows the natural curve of the supratarsal crease and is situated at 8 mm from the eyelash border in the middle, closing to a 5-mm distance at both corners. The lateral extension should not go beyond the lateral orbital rim.
- The lower blepharoplasty incision is a subciliary incision and does not cross the level of the lateral corner of the eye.

■ Upper Blepharoplasty

Preparation

- The surgery starts with the upper blepharoplasty markings (**TECH FIG 1**) and the injection of a freshly prepared local anesthetic and adrenalin mixture.

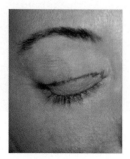

TECH FIG 1 • Upper blepharoplasty marking.

Incision

- It is important to wait for at least 7 minutes for vasoconstriction, and then a superficial skin incision is performed with the surgical blade (**TECH FIG 2A**). A Colorado tip cautery is used to incise the dermis and the muscle to prevent bleeding.

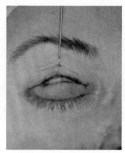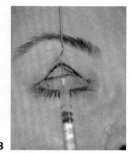

TECH FIG 2 • **A.** Dermal incision performed with Colorado tip cautery to prevent bleeding. **B.** Injection of local anesthetic into the muscle.

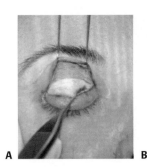
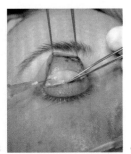
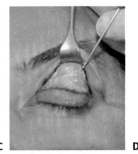
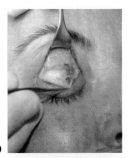
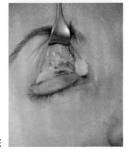

TECH FIG 3 • A. Orbicularis oculi muscle preseptal portion elevated off of the upper orbital septum. **B.** Injection of saline into the preaponeurotic cavity. **C.** Upper orbital septum opened medially to reveal preaponeurotic fat pad. **D.** Upper orbital septum opened at its full width. **E.** Medial fat pad resected.

- After incision of the full thickness of the muscle, the local anesthetic is injected into the superior flap superficially (**TECH FIG 2B**).

Dissection

- Then, the dissection continues immediately adjacent to the undersurface of the orbicularis muscle layer on top of the upper orbital septum (**TECH FIG 3A**).
- With time, one recognizes a very thin layer of fatty tissue on top of the septum, more pronounced medially and laterally. It is advisable to use loupe magnification and start the submuscular dissection either medially or laterally to be able to distinguish the tissue layers.
- The elevation of the muscle flap also allows easy access to the plane of the corrugator for resection and the brow region for brow fixation.
- The upper orbital septum and levator aponeurosis layers lie almost adjacent to each other in the area of our

incisions, so it is advisable to inject 1 cc of saline into the subseptal space for hydrodissection (**TECH FIG 3B**).
- This facilitates the separation of the layers, and a laterally placed incision of the septum is then advanced to completely open the preaponeurotic space. The fat pads lie in this layer (**TECH FIG 3C**).
- The preaponeurotic fat pad is gently dissected free from the underlying levator muscle (**TECH FIG 3D**), and if necessary, levator procedure is performed.
- The medial fat pad, almost always excessive, is dissected and excised (**TECH FIG 3E**).
- There is no need for preaponeurotic fat pad resection except in very rare cases. Instead, the upper sulcus needs to be augmented in the majority of the aging patients.

Suturing

- The resected medial fat pad is used to graft the middle upper sulcus, and for a better take, the fat graft is placed under the existing fat pad (**TECH FIG 4A–C**).

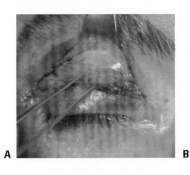
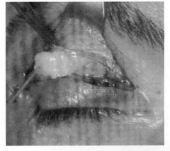
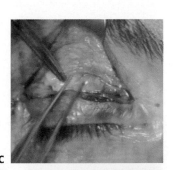
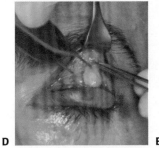
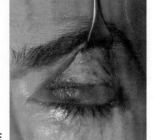

TECH FIG 4 • A. Upper orbital septum opened. **B.** Resected medial fat pad brought on site. **C.** The medial fat pad is grafted to the upper middle sulcus to treat the superior sulcus fat deficiency. **D.** Intraseptal fat graft in place. **E.** Septum is closed over the graft.

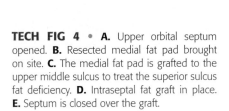

- The upper edge of the septum is then found and pulled down with a forceps to cover over the upper orbital fat pad, and the fullness and convexity are checked to obtain a smooth pass from the brow to the upper eyelid (**TECH FIG 4D**).
- The upper orbital septum is then sutured with a 6-0 poliglecaprone suture (**TECH FIG 4E**).

Closure

- The skin muscle flap is pulled down and skin excess is marked.
- The muscle fibers of the orbicularis muscle of the upper eyelid are more condensed around the supratarsal area (**TECH FIG 5**), and unfortunately, this is the region where we resect the skin and muscle at the end of our blepharoplasty procedures.
  - This may interfere with proper eye closure in the early postoperative period. This is the reason why the author

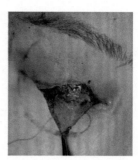

TECH FIG 5 • The skin is de-epithelialized and the orbicularis muscle left intact. The orbicularis oculi fibers are more condensed in the area of resection in conventional blepharoplasty.

prefers to de-epithelialize the skin and leave the muscle intact to turn in during closure, also helping with the upper orbital sulcus fullness.
- The closure of the skin is done with 6-0 nylon sutures.

■ Lower Blepharoplasty

Preparation

- The upper and lower eyelids are sutured together at the start of the lower blepharoplasty procedure, and this suture is used for traction.
- Similar to the upper blepharoplasty technique described above, the injection of the local anesthetic and epinephrine solution is followed by the subciliary incision.

Incision

- The thin skin of the lower eyelid is then separated from the underlying orbicularis muscle fibers with the help of the Colorado needle tip cautery for 10 to 15 mm to facilitate muscle and skin excision at the time of the closure (**TECH FIG 6A**).

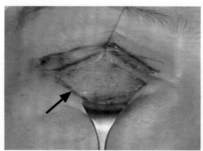

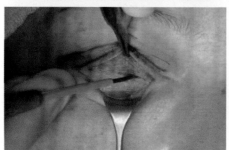

TECH FIG 6 • A. The skin is elevated off of the orbicularis fibers through a subciliary incision at the start of the lower blepharoplasty. **B.** The pretarsal portion of the orbicularis is protected, and the muscle is cut below the level of the lower rim of the tarsal plate.

- The lower pretarsal muscle is marked, and an incision is performed with the cautery to reach the preseptal space of the lower eyelid (**TECH FIG 6B**).

Dissection

- The dissection is continued to reach the lower orbital rim. The lower eyelid septum is most often attenuated in this region, so it is better to stay close to the fibers of the orbicularis muscle during the dissection.
- Once the surgeon reaches the lower orbital rim, the attention is focused on the most medial portion of the rim first.
- The insertion of the orbicularis muscle on the periosteum of the medial orbital rim forms the nasojugal fold (**TECH FIG 7**), and therefore, the dissection continues in a subperiosteal plane medially to reach the level of the nasal bone suture line, creating a pocket.

Suturing

- A fat flap is formed with the already herniated medial fat pad, and it is then advanced to this space to prevent the attachment of the muscle again.
- The fat flap is sutured to the periosteum medially with 5-0 nylon sutures. The suture should be strong enough to hold the fat flap in position to cover the medial lower orbital rim.

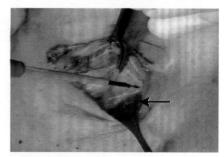

TECH FIG 7 • The dissection reveals the anatomy of the medial lower orbital rim. The *arrow* points the orbicularis muscle insertion on the periosteum.

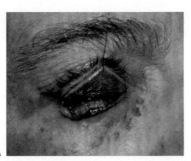 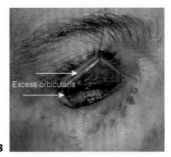 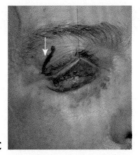

TECH FIG 8 • **A.** At the time of closure, the lower eyelid muscle layer is pulled up and the excess orbicularis is marked. **B.** The excess orbicularis muscle. **C.** The excess muscle is elevated as a laterally based Anderson flap, and the edges of the lower orbicularis muscle are sutured together.

- This effective fat transposition fills the nasojugal fold depression that is caused by the orbicularis attachments on the rim periosteum.[12]
- The lateral fat pad is almost always excessive and is excised.
- The lower eyelid is then pulled up with the help of the traction suture. The decision of skin and muscle excision should be done in this position to prevent complications.

Closure

- The muscle is pulled up gently and excess muscle is marked, if there is any (**TECH FIG 8A**).
- It is advisable not to resect the muscle (**TECH FIG 8B**) and, instead, prepare it as a laterally based Adamson flap (**TECH FIG 8C**) to suture to the lateral rim periosteum to act as an efficient canthopexy in individuals with a proper canthal tilt.
  - If the patient does not have a proper canthal tilt to start with preoperatively, then a transpositional type of canthal surgery should be undertaken.
- The cut edges of the muscle are then sutured with 6-0 inverted polydioxanon suture to prevent muscle retraction in the early postoperative period. With the help of this measure, it is possible to see early intact pretarsal muscle activity in the lower blepharoplasty patients (**TECH FIG 9**).
- There usually is no need for skin excision other than a marginal correction.
- The subciliary incision is then closed with 6-0 nylon sutures.

TECH FIG 9 • **A,B.** The patient force closes the eyes on the 5th postoperative day. Notice the upward movement of the lower eyelid. This is due to the early intact function of the lower eyelid orbicularis muscle, possibly due to the atraumatic technique and suturing of the muscle edges together to prevent avulsion.

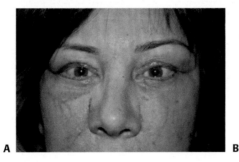 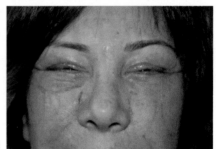

■ Periorbital Fat Injection

- Injecting fat in the periorbital area is a sculpting measure to help with the surgical fat preservation and reorganization principle observed during the upper and lower blepharoplasty.
  - Midfacial, frontal, glabellar, root of the nose, zygomatic, and brow fat injections are done at deeper tissue layers, over the periosteum.

- The temporal area injections are superficial in the subcutaneous plane.
- The microfat grafts pass through tuberculin syringes and are used to directly inject into the wrinkles (**TECH FIG 10**).
  - It is advisable to use an average of 45 to 60 cc of fat grafting in the periorbital area.

TECH FIG 10 • **A,B.** A 47-year-old female underwent a periorbital lift with upper and lower blepharoplasty with fat preservation and additional fat injection. **C,D.** The profile view of the patient. Notice the change in the periorbital and perioral profile as a result of the brow and midface lift, upper lip shortening, and 60 cc of facial fat grafting.

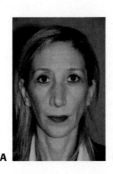 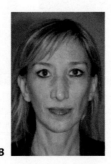 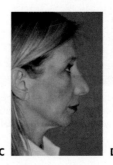 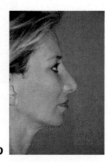

TECHNIQUES

PEARLS AND PITFALLS

Hemostasis	■ Hemostasis is the key to the success of the surgical dissection and tissue healing.
	■ Stop any coagulants 3 weeks before surgery.
	■ Postoperatively, use only opioids for pain.
Incisions	■ Never extend incisions beyond the level of the lateral canthus; estimate skin excess at the end of the procedure.
Technique	■ Use loupe magnification and Colorado tip cautery.
	■ Do not aim excision; plan to preserve fat and muscle.
	■ Assess lateral and medial canthal stability before surgery and plan necessary measures to increase lower eyelid support.
	■ Skin and muscle excision of the lower eyelid is performed with the lid pulled up.

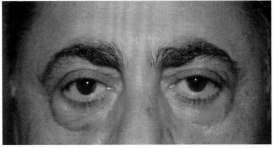 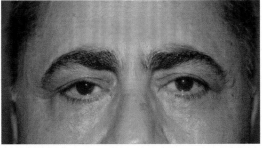

FIG 7 • A,B. A 62-year-old male presented with medial fat pad herniation of the ptotic upper eyelids, periorbital skeletonization, lower eyelid medial and lateral fat pad herniation, midfacial atrophy R greater than L, lower eyelid laxity, and rather low medial canthal attachment. He was treated with resection of only the medial fat pad of the upper eyelid and the lateral from the lower. The medial fat pad of the lower eyelid was maintained and advanced subperiosteally to efface the nasojugal fold. Periorbital and midfacial fat injection helped achieve better contours. Levator advancement procedure corrects his upper eyelid senile ptosis, and a tensor fascia lata suspension of the lower eyelid overcomes the possible complications.

POSTOPERATIVE CARE

■ The head of the bed is elevated.
■ No NSAID at any time, intra- or postoperatively.
■ Constant application of ice for 5 days over a wet sponge.
■ Suture removal 3 to 5 days.

OUTCOMES

■ The principles of fat and muscle preservation, judicious fat grafting help accomplish good results with upper and lower blepharoplasty surgery.
  ■ The surgeon's awareness before surgery about the inherent problems of the medial and lateral canthal position

and stability will help prevent the possible complications of lower eyelid surgery (**FIGS 7** and **8**).

COMPLICATIONS

■ The most common complication of the upper eyelid surgery is caused by excessive removal of the fat pads. This causes superior sulcus fat deficiency and increased supratarsal fold distance and is a telltale sign of poor surgical evaluation (see **FIG 8**).
■ The fibrosis associated with the poor technique when performing a lower blepharoplasty will increase the fibrous tissue (**FIG 9**) and exert a pull and cause shortening of the lower eyelid causing scleral show.

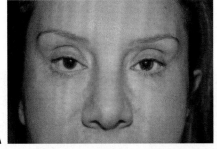 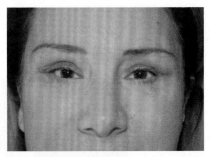

FIG 8 • A. A 44-year-old female S/P upper and lower blepharoplasty and brow lift and six consecutive revisions. Notice the fat deficiency of the upper eyelid sulcus. She also has sagging of the right lower eyelid. **B.** The patient 2 years after dermofat grafting of the upper eyelids, tensor fascia lata suspension reconstruction of the lower eyelid, and periorbital fat grafting. The right upper eyelid still needs more fatty tissue support.

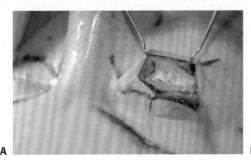
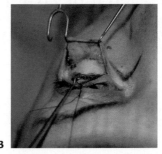

FIG 9 • A,B. The surgical dissection findings of a lower blepharoplasty complication. Notice the significant fibrous thickening of the orbital septum, shortening the lower eyelid.

REFERENCES

1. Nakra T, Modjtahedi S, Vrcek I, et al. The effect of upper eyelid blepharoplasty on eyelid and brow position. *Orbit.* 2016;35(6 suppl):324-327.
2. Hassanpour SE, Khajouei Kermani H, Brow ptosis after upper blepharoplasty: findings in 70 patients. *World J Plast Surg.* 2016;5(1 suppl):58-61.
3. Shaw RB Jr, Katzel EB, Koltz PF, et al. Aging of the facial skeleton: aesthetic implications and rejuvenation strategies. *Plast Reconstr Surg.* 2011;127(1 suppl):374-383. doi:10.1097/PRS.0b013e3181f95b2d.5).
4. Kahn DM, Shaw RB Jr. Aging of the bony orbit: a three-dimensional computed tomographic study. *Aesthet Surg J.* 2008;28(3 suppl):258-264.
5. Richard MJ, Morris C, Deen BF, et al. Analysis of the anatomic changes of the aging facial skeleton using computer-assisted tomography. *Ophthalmic Plast Reconstr Surg.* 2009;25(5 suppl):382-386.
6. DiFrancesco LM, Anjema CM, Codner MA, McCord CD. Evaluation of conventional subciliary incision used in blepharoplasty: preoperative and postoperative videography and electromyography findings. *Plast Reconstr Surg.* 2005;116(2 suppl):632-639.
7. Rohrich RJ, Arbique GM, Wong C, et al. The anatomy of suborbicularis fat: implications for periorbital rejuvenation. *Plast Reconstr Surg.* 2009;124(3 suppl):946-951.
8. Hwang K, Kim HJ, Kim H, et al. Origin of the lower orbicularis oculi muscle in relation to the nasojugal groove. *J Craniofac Surg.* 2015;26(4 suppl):1389-1393.
9. Camirand A, Doucet J, Harris J. Eyelid aging: the historical evolution of its management. *Aesthetic Plast Surg.* 2005;29(2 suppl) 65-73.
10. Carraway JH. Volume correction for nasojugal groove with blepharoplasty. *Aesthet Surg J.* 2010;30(1 suppl):101-109.

38 CHAPTER

Indications and Technique for Fat Grafting for Periorbital Rejuvenation

Dino Elyassnia and Timothy Marten

DEFINITION

- The hallmark of a youthful, attractive orbit is fullness. It has become clear that fat atrophy is a significant component of periorbital aging that results in volume loss and a hollow appearance around the eyes.
- Traditional blepharoplasty procedures have focused on treating skin laxity, fat herniation, canthal laxity, and levator dehiscence but have largely ignored fat atrophy. Often, blepharoplasty procedures aggressively remove fat from the eyelids, further compounding the problem of volume loss.
- Periorbital fat grafting represents a new paradigm in eyelid aesthetics that focuses on volumetric rejuvenation of the upper and lower eyelids. This approach produces a full, healthy appearance to the eyes that has not been possible with traditional blepharoplasty techniques.

ANATOMY

- In recent years, a great amount of work has been done to beautifully elucidate the detailed fat compartments of the face.[1]
- Although this work has been a great contribution to further understanding of facial anatomy, it plays a smaller role in technically carrying out periorbital fat grafting because the goal is not to inject fat in such a way that we aim to "refill" each deflated fat compartment.

PATIENT HISTORY AND PHYSICAL FINDINGS

- A focused history should include any ophthalmologic conditions, previous blepharoplasties, or other aesthetic treatments including filler use. As hyaluronic acid filler tends to last especially long in the upper and lower eyelids, knowledge of its use must be obtained so a decision can be made whether to dissolve the material prior to fat grafting.
- Physical exam of the eyelids should include looking for the presence of ptosis, dermatochalasis, lower lid fat herniation, canthal laxity, orbital vector, and degree of fat atrophy of the eyelids, midface, and cheek. If problems other than fat atrophy are present such as significant lower lid fat herniation or excess skin, traditional blepharoplasty techniques may need to be combined with fat grafting.
- A significant advantage of periorbital fat grafting over traditional lower lid blepharoplasty is that fat grafting is very safe in the setting of dry eye or the presence of canthal laxity, whereas these problems represent relative contraindications for lower blepharoplasty.
- Regarding fat harvest, thin patients should be examined at the time of their consultation because patients with limited

fat stores often present significant challenges. Extra time and effort will be required to obtain fat from them. Anesthesia and OR times must be calculated accordingly.
- Although the abdomen is often cited as the "best" and most convenient site for fat harvest, in our practice, the hip, waist, and outer thigh are the harvest sites of choice. The abdomen typically has thinner, less forgiving skin than the hip, waist, and outer thigh (especially in the face-lift age group) and is readily open to detailed inspection by the patient after the procedure. As such, it can be problematic as a sole donor site in many cases if more than a small amount of fat is needed. The hip, waist, and outer thigh taken together by contrast typically provide more volume and are less subject to surface irregularities, and fat harvest from these areas generally provides more overall improvement in the patient's silhouette.

IMAGING

- Typically, radiographs are not necessary for periorbital fat grafting.
- All patients should have standardized photographs taken preoperatively, and any markings made preoperatively on patients should be photographed as well.
- These photos should be used intraoperatively to help guide precise placement of fat injections.

NONOPERATIVE MANAGEMENT

- Fillers to the periorbital area are a viable alternative to fat grafting and have helped patients understand how volume loss contributes to the periorbital and facial aging process.
- Advantages of fillers are they have minimal downtime, they are easily adjustable, they can be reversed (if hyaluronic acid is used), and they last particularly long in the periorbital area compared to other regions of the face.
- Disadvantages are they require ongoing maintenance; they are time-consuming, painful, and expensive; and they can look unnatural requiring a high level of precision during injection.

SURGICAL MANAGEMENT

- Whether the result of illness, aging, or previous overzealous surgical treatment, filling the hollow upper orbit can produce a remarkable rejuvenation of the upper eyelid and eliminate an unnaturally hollow and elderly appearance sometimes referred to by patients as "nursing home" or "owl" eyes (**FIG 1**).
- Like the upper orbit, fat grafting the infraorbital area allows comprehensive correction of age-associated hollowness that lends the face an ill or haggard appearance, "shortens" the

FIG 1 • Correcting upper orbital hollowing. **A.** Patient with an unnaturally hollow upper eyelid appearance ("owl eyes") following blepharoplasty performed by an unknown surgeon. **B.** Same patient seen after fat injections to the upper orbit. A healthier, more youthful appearance can be seen (procedure performed by Timothy Marten, MD, FACS—Courtesy of Marten Clinic of Plastic Surgery).

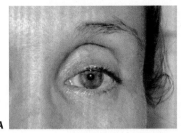
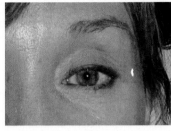

before   after

apparent length of the lower eyelid, and produces a youthful, attractive, and highly desirable smooth transition from the lower eyelid to the cheek. This effect is generally unobtainable by traditional lower eyelid surgery, fat transpositions, "septal resets," midface lifts, free fat grafts, and other like means (**FIG 2**).

■ Although the primary goal of fat harvest is to obtain the "best" tissue for the fat grafting procedure, fat harvesting should be thought of as an opportunity to improve the patient's figure. Thus, harvest must be undertaken in a thoughtful and artistic manner and generally in a bilateral and symmetrical fashion. Although any area can theoretically be used for a donor site, the hip, waist, and outer thigh are our primary choice for the reasons detailed above.

Preoperative Planning

■ Fat grafting cannot be performed casually, and deficient areas and key landmarks must be marked preoperatively with the patient in an upright position. Marking will require concentration and focus and is best carried out in an area that is free from distractions.

■ Creating a proposed plan on a full-page laser print of the patient's face is helpful in organizing the treatment plan and facilitates confirming with the patient the areas that will be treated.

■ If the patient wishes, marks can be made while she or he holds a hand mirror. Once markings are complete, a new series of photographs are taken and printed up for use during the procedure. These photographs typically provide the best information to the surgeon intraoperatively.

■ Regarding fat harvest, an estimate should be made as to the amount of fat that will be used and thus the amount that needs to be harvested. In estimating the amount that one needs to harvest, a helpful guideline is that after centrifugation, approximately 50% of what was harvested will be obtained as usable processed fat.

■ If one wishes to perform the fat grafting procedure predominantly with "stem cell"–rich fat (the bottom 2 cc of fat in the centrifuged 10-cc syringe consisting of high-density adipocytes), only 20% of what is harvested fat will be available for injection, and the total amount harvested will have to be adjusted accordingly.

■ As in the case of formal liposuction, the patient's torso must be marked preoperatively while she or he is standing if optimal contours are to be created and if irregularities are to be avoided at the harvest sites. Once markings are complete, marked areas should be photographed and the photos printed up for use during the harvesting part of the procedure.

Positioning

■ Fat is harvested after anesthesia is initiated but before prep and drape of the face. A complete prep of the torso is not necessary, and in all but the unusual case, a limited prep of the marked area is made and a sterile field is established.

■ If fat is to be harvested from the hip or lateral thigh, the patient is turned into a semilateral decubitus position; prep, drape and harvest is performed; and the patient then is turned to the opposite side where a similar procedure is performed.

■ This position can be used to simultaneously harvest fat from multiple sites including the hip, waist, flank, upper buttocks, outer and inner thigh, and knees (**FIG 3**). With practice, a

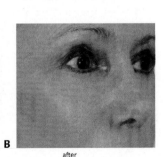

before   after

FIG 2 • Filling the hollow lower orbit with fat. **A.** Patient with an unnaturally hollow and elderly infraorbital appearance. The lower eyelid appears "long," and there is a distinct line of demarcation between the lower eyelid and the cheek. **B.** Same patient seen after face-lift and fat injections to the infraorbital area. There is a smooth transition from the lower eyelid to the cheek, and the patient has a healthier, youthful, and attractive appearance (note: the upper orbit, radix, cheek, and nasolabial crease have also been treated with fat injections, and the patient has undergone ptosis correction) (procedure performed by Timothy Marten, MD, FACS—Courtesy of Marten Clinic of Plastic Surgery).

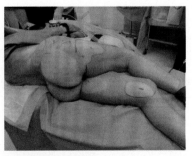

FIG 3 • Positioning patient for fat harvest. If the patient is carefully positioned in a semilateral decubitus position, fat can be simultaneously harvested from multiple sites including the hip waist, flank, inner knee, outer and inner thighs, buttocks, and inner knee. Obtaining fat from multiple sites is particularly important in thin patients with minimal fat stores or when multiple site fat grafting is being performed. Following harvest from one side, the patient is turned to the other where a similar harvest is performed.

well-organized OR team can complete this process expeditiously without undue delay of the procedure.

■ The patient is then returned to the supine position for fat grafting the periorbital area.

Approach

■ For upper orbit fat grafting, small stab incisions are made in the brow with a no. 11 blade scalpel or a 20-gauge needle. These incisions are so small that they will not require suturing upon completion of the procedure.

■ Injecting from two separate injection sites at the medial and lateral ends of the brow allows "crisscrossing" of cannula passes during graft placement parallel to the superior orbital rim.

■ This "crisscrossing" provides smoother fat infiltration and helps avert a "row of corn" effect that may result if injection is made from only one site.

■ Unlike the upper orbit, however, experience has shown that for the lower orbit, fat is best and most easily injected *perpendicular* to the infraorbital rim from stab incisions in the midcheek or perioral area. When this is done, lumps and irregularities are far less common. *Fat should not be injected parallel to the lid-cheek junction in the infraorbital area.*

■ Fat Harvest

■ Areas from which fat is to be harvested are infiltrated with a dilute 0.1% lidocaine with 1:1 000 000 epinephrine solution using a multiholed infiltration cannula (**TECH FIG 1**), and an adequate time is allowed for a proper anesthetic and hemostatic effect.

■ Approximately 1 cc of this solution is injected for every 3 cc of anticipated fat removal. It is not necessary or desirable to infiltrate in a "tumescent" fashion as overwetting the tissue will result in an overdilute harvest and more time spent in the harvesting process.

■ Local anesthetic should be injected even if general anesthesia is used to limit stimulation of the patient and the overall amount of general anesthetic needed.

■ Fat is harvested with a special harvesting cannula (see **TECH FIG 1**) ranging in size from 2.1 to 2.4 mm and 15 to 25 cm long attached to a 10-cc syringe using gently applied syringe suction to minimize vacuum barotrauma to the tissue.

■ Sharp hypodermic needles should not be used to harvest fat.

■ In general, and as mentioned previously, at least twice as much fat is harvested as is anticipated will be used to ensure an adequate amount of processed fat will be available for use on the face.

Processing Harvested Fat

■ Our preferred method of processing fat is centrifugation.

■ Before centrifugation is commenced, a sterile disposable plastic cap is placed on the end of the syringe to keep its contents inside it, and the syringe plunger is removed from the syringe barrel.

■ Capped syringe barrels containing unprocessed fat are then loaded into the centrifuge in a balanced fashion and spun for 1 to 3 minutes at 1000 RPM.

■ Many centrifuges available for this purpose have variable speed adjustments and rotors that can be sterilized so that the syringes the fat is in remain sterile and can be handled by the scrubbed surgical team. Other centrifuges have sterile tubes that fit into the rotor for this purpose (**TECH FIG 2**). The typical spin speeds of approximately 3500 RPM used by most single-speed desktop centrifuges sold for fat processing are said to not cause injury to fat or compromise its "take."

■ Once centrifuged, syringe barrels containing spun fat are removed, centrifuged fat will be seen to contain an upper oil (ruptured fat cells), central fat, and lower "water" (blood, lidocaine) components (**TECH FIG 3**).

■ The often blood-tinged "water" (local anesthetic) component is discarded by simply removing the syringe tip cap and allowing it to run out. The oil fraction is then poured off out of the top of the syringe. Telfa sponges can also be placed inside the syringe barrel to wick up the small amount of residual oil present after the majority of it has been poured off.

■ A laboratory "test tube"–type rack to hold and organize the syringes containing fat greatly facilitates fat processing activities (**TECH FIG 4**).

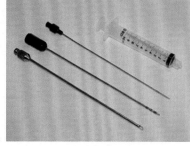 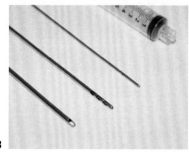

TECH FIG 1 • Fat harvesting instruments. **A.** Specially designed harvesting cannulas ranging in size from 2.1 to 2.4 mm are attached to 10-cc Luer-Lok syringes and are used to extract fat from donor sites using gentle syringe suction. Fat harvested with these cannulas easily passes through injection cannulas as small as 0.7 mm. Shown from top to down: (a) 10-cc Leur-Lok syringe, (b) 1.6-mm Coleman local anesthetic infiltration cannula, (c) 2.4-mm Tulip "Tri-Port" harvesting cannula, and (d) Coleman harvesting cannula. **B.** Close-up of instrument tips. Shown from top to down: (a) 10-cc Leur-Lok syringe, (b) Coleman infiltration cannula, (c) Tulip harvesting cannula, and (d) Coleman harvesting cannula.

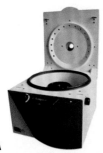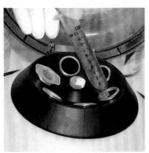

A   **B**

TECH FIG 2 • Centrifuging fat. Harvested fat is generally not uniform in character as extracted from donor sites as each syringe will contain a variable amount of fat, blood, local anesthetic, and ruptured fat cells ("oil"), and some type of processing is necessary to obtain uniform material for injection. Centrifugation allows separation of the "oil" and "water" fractions from the fat cells and concentrates high-density adipocytes ("stem cells"). **A.** Small portable countertop centrifuge (www.tulipmedical.com). **B.** Close-up view of centrifuge rotor being loaded with unprocessed fat in 10-cc syringes. Note that the syringe tip has been sealed with a disposable plastic cap. The removable and sterilizable metal sleeves shown to fit into rotor to keep syringe barrels containing fat sterile and allow them to be handled on the sterile field after spinning. Some centrifuges are designed to allow the entire rotor to be sterilized.

- After centrifugation and the separation and discarding of the resulting oil and water components have been accomplished, the resultant fat is transferred into 1-cc Luer-Lok syringes using a transfer coupler (**TECH FIG 5**). Proper infiltration of fat requires injection in very small amounts that cannot be reliably made with a 10-cc, 5-cc, or even 3-cc syringes.
- The bottom 2 cc of fat in the syringe containing the highest concentrations of high-density adipocytes (or adipose-derived regenerative cells [ADRC]) is segregated and is used preferentially in the procedure.

Upper Orbit Fat Grafting

- First, nerve blocks are performed with 0.25% bupivacaine with epinephrine 1:200 000 local anesthetic solution. It is typically not necessary to directly infiltrate areas to be treated with local anesthetic, if nerve blocks

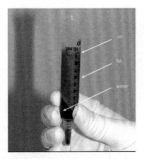

TECH FIG 3 • Centrifuged fat. Harvested fat seen after centrifugation. Three layers can be seen in the centrifuged material: an upper "oil" layer (ruptured fat cells), a middle layer of intact fat cells, and a bottom layer of blood and local anesthetic. Unlike straining of fat through a sieve, centrifugation may allow separation of the "oil" and "water" fractions from the fat cells with minimal loss of "stem cells," "growth factors," and "cellular messengers."

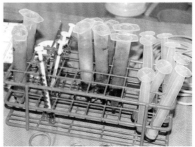

TECH FIG 4 • Syringe rack. A "test tube" rack to hold the syringes containing fat greatly facilitates fat processing activities. On the *left*, syringes containing unprocessed fat are present. In the *center*, syringes containing centrifuged fat can be seen. The rack also conveniently holds 1-cc syringes, syringe components, and other equipment used in the fat grafting procedure.

are properly performed and adequate sedation has been administered.

- Once nerve blocks have been administered, small stab incisions are made in the medial and lateral extent of the eyebrow.
- Infiltration is made in multiple passes injecting on both the in and out strokes. Approximately 0.05 cc or less should be injected per pass. This corresponds to 20 to 40 back and forth passes or more for each 1-cc syringe of processed fat.
- The goal is to inject the fat in a way that optimizes its chance of developing a blood supply and surviving, and the mental model should be one of scattering tiny particles of fat into the recipient site in multiple crisscrossing fine trails in such a way that each particle sits in its own compartment and has maximal surface contact with perfused tissue.
- Advancement and withdrawal of the injection cannula will typically be made slowly by the beginning injector, but as familiarity with the technique is acquired, the movements can and should be made faster. Ultimately, all other things being equal, faster movements are desirable in that if the injection cannula is constantly in motion, intravascular injection is less likely, and the likelihood that an accidental bolus injection into one area will be made is reduced.
- How the syringe is held is also important in avoiding overinjection and controlling the volume injected with each pass. If the syringe is held in the manner one would traditionally use to give an injection with the thumb on the end of the syringe plunger, it is easy to inject too much fat if tissue resistance changes or injection cannula resistance suddenly decreases. More control can generally be maintained, and overinjection more easily avoided, if the syringe is held with the end of the plunger in the palm of the hand (**TECH FIG 6**). Held in this manner, a slight closing of the hand results in a small amount of fat only being expressed from the cannula, and overinjection into any one area can more readily be avoided.
- To allow for the deposition of tiny aliquots of fat per pass, very fine cannulas must be used when fat grafting around the eyes. Currently, a 4-cm-long 0.7-mm (22-gauge) cannula is preferred. These newer fine cannulas have made injecting the upper orbit easier and more predictable

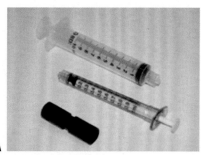
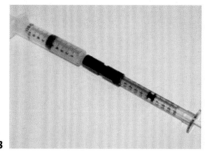

TECH FIG 5 • Transferring centrifuged fat to 1-cc syringes. Fat is transferred from 10-cc Luer-Lok syringes into 1-cc Luer-Lok syringes after centrifugation, and the oil and water fractions have been discarded using a transfer coupling. Proper injection in the very small quantities that are needed in the face cannot be made with larger syringes. **A.** 10-cc Luer-Lok syringe, 1-cc Luer-Lok syringe, and Luer to Luer transfer coupling. **B.** Transfer coupling in use.

than in the past as they can be advanced more smoothly and accurately through tissues.

- A common misconception in treating the hollow upper orbit is that fat is needed and should be grafted into the preseptal portion of the eyelid itself. The hollow upper eyelid is however more properly and practically restored by placing fat in a deep submuscular/preperiosteal position along the inferior margins of the supraorbital rim. The process is best conceptualized as one of *lowering the supraorbital rim* and filling the upper orbital area to push skin that has retracted up into the orbit down onto the preseptal eyelid to create a full and appropriately creased upper eyelid (**TECH FIG 7**).
- Once one accepts that improvement is obtained by grafting of the orbit, and not the eyelid itself, it becomes apparent that larger volumes than might otherwise be expected are required. In general, 2 to 3 cc of fat must be placed in each upper orbit to achieve the improvement typically sought.
- When grafting the upper orbit, it must always be remembered that when one is working in very close proximity to the eye, and although the injection cannulas are blunt tipped, they are easily capable of perforating the ocular globe.
- Fat grafting the upper orbit and "eyelid" is advanced in difficulty, and treatment of this area should be made only after experience has been gained treating more forgiving areas.

- Once that experience is obtained, fat grafting the upper orbit can be one of the most artistically rewarding uses of autologous fat and one that is likely to become a routine part of rejuvenating the upper eyelid in the future.

Lower Orbit Fat Grafting

- First, nerve blocks are performed as is done in the upper orbit.
- Unlike the upper orbit, for the lower orbit, fat is best and most easily injected *perpendicular* to the infraorbital rim through stab incisions placed in the midcheek or perioral area (**TECH FIG 8**). When this is done, lumps and irregularities are far less common.
- Like the upper orbit, fat grafting of the infraorbital area is typically performed with a 4-cm-long 0.7-mm (22-gauge) injection cannula with a focus on placing very small aliquots of fat per pass using the same basic injection technique described above.
- Also like the upper orbit, fat need not and should not be grafted in the pretarsal lower eyelid. Fat should be injected deep in a submuscular/preperiosteal plane, and the technical goal of the procedure should be thought of as raising up and anteriorly projecting the infraorbital rim rather that filling the lid itself.
- It is wise to avoid any subcutaneous injection in the infraorbital area due to the extremely thin skin present and the likelihood of creating visible lumps and irregularities. Thus, it is best to limit injections to a preperiosteal/suborbicularis oculi plane. The purported benefit

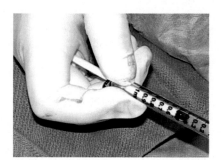

TECH FIG 6 • Method of holding syringe to control volume expressed during injection. If the syringe is held in the way one would traditionally use to give an injection, it is easy to inject too much fat if tissue or injection cannula resistance suddenly decreases. More control can be maintained, and overinjection better avoided, if the syringe is held with the end of the plunger in the palm of the hand. Held in this manner, a slight closing of the hand results in a small amount of fat only being expressed.

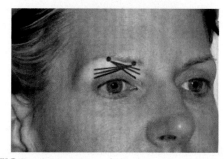

TECH FIG 7 • Incision sites and plan for injecting fat into the upper orbital ("upper eyelid") area. Fat grafting of the upper orbital area is typically performed with a 4-cm 0.7-mm (22-gauge) cannula, and fat is placed deep in a suborbicularis oculi/preperiosteal plane. Typically, 2 to 3 cc of fat is placed in each upper orbit. Level of difficulty: advanced.

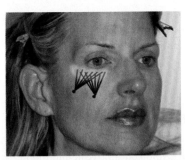

TECH FIG 8 • Incision sites and plan for injecting fat into the infra-orbital ("lower eyelid") area. Fat grafting of the infraorbital area is typically performed with a 4-cm 0.7-mm (22-gauge) cannula, and fat is placed deep in a suborbicularis oculi/preperiosteal plane. Typically, 2 to 3 cc of fat is placed on each side although occasionally more will be needed. Level of difficulty: advanced.

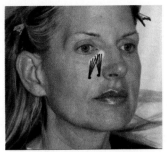

TECH FIG 9 • Incision sites and plan for injecting fat into the naso-jugal ("tear trough") areas. Fat grafting of the nasojugal "tear trough" area is typically performed with a 4-cm 0.7-mm (22-gauge) injection cannula, and fat is placed deep in a preperiosteal/suborbicularis oculi plane. Typically, 0.5 to 1.5 cc of fat is placed on each side depending on how far inferiorly and laterally the "tear trough" extends onto the cheek. Level of difficulty: advanced.

of superficial injections—improving skin texture and color—is too small an improvement in most cases for all but the expert injector to offset the all too likely occurrence that visible and difficult-to-correct irregularities will result.

- When injecting the lower orbit, the surgeon should place her or his index finger of the nondominant (noninjecting) hand firmly on the infraorbital rim to protect the ocular globe while injections are made.
- Volumes required to obtain corrections in the lower orbit are typically more than one might initially expect, and 2 to 3 cc per side is necessary to produce the desired effect in most cases.

"Tear Trough" Fat Grafting

- Where the infraorbital area ends and the "tear trough" and cheek areas begin is hard to precisely define, and in reality, the treatment of the infraorbital, cheek, and "tear trough" areas must be undertaken concurrently in most patients, and the treated areas will overlap each other to a certain extent.
- Treatment of the "tear tough" is most easily and best performed using incisions situated inferior to the medial orbit and placing fat predominantly perpendicularly as in the infraorbital areas (**TECH FIG 9**).
- A 4-cm-long 0.7-mm (22-gauge) cannula is typically used, and fat is placed deep in a preperiosteal/suborbicularis

oculi plane—especially superiorly and medially–where the skin is the thinnest. As experience is gained, and if care is taken, fat can be placed safely more superficially, especially in the lower more lateral part of the tear trough that is frequently seen to run down into and onto the cheek.

- Typically, 0.5 to 1.5 cc of fat is placed in the "tear trough" area, depending on how far inferiorly and laterally it extends onto the cheek (**TECH FIG 10**). Although ostensibly seeming simple to do, fat grafting the tear trough is advanced in difficulty.

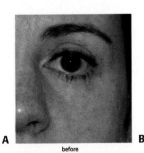
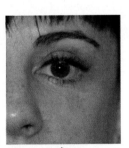

A   before   B   after

TECH FIG 10 • Filling the "tear trough" with Fat. **A.** Patient with hollow nasojugal groove ("tear trough") and an unnaturally hollow and elderly infra-orbital appearance. **B.** Same patient seen after fat injections. A healthier and youthful ocular appearance is noted (procedure performed by Timothy Marten, MD, FACS—Courtesy of Marten Clinic of Plastic Surgery).

PEARLS AND PITFALLS

Fat harvest	▪ The hip, waist, and outer thigh are the primary choice for fat harvest sites in our practice. ▪ They provide for abundant volume of fat, have less risk of surface irregularities, and produce the best improvement in the patient's silhouette.
Fat processing	▪ The bottom 2 cc of fat in the centrifuged 10-cc syringe consists of "stem cell"–rich fat. ▪ This fat should be isolated and used for more critical areas like the upper and lower orbits.
Instruments	▪ Special fine blunt cannulas are required to safely perform periorbital fat grafting. ▪ Sharp needle injection increases the risk of embolization and should be avoided.
Technique	▪ Fat should be placed in very tiny aliquots with each pass in a preperiosteal plane to produce optimal results and minimize complications.
Ocular injury	▪ For both the upper and lower orbit, the surgeon must always keep the nondominant index finger between the globe and the end of the cannula to protect the globe at all times.

POSTOPERATIVE CARE

- Regional fat grafting to the periorbital or more comprehensive facial fat grafting is performed on an outpatient basis. Patients having a combined face-lift with fat grafting are typically discharged to an aftercare specialist for the first night after surgery.
- Patients are asked to rest quietly and apply cool (but not ice or ice-cold) compresses to their face for 15 to 20 minutes of every hour that they are awake for the first 3 days after surgery.
- Patients are advised to take a soft diet that is easy to chew and digest for 2 weeks after surgery and are encouraged to avoid salty foods.
- When patients return to work or their social lives depends on how much fat is injected, their individual swelling response, their occupation, and need for secrecy. Patients are asked to set aside 2 to 3 weeks for recovery and 2 to 3 months prior to any major business presentation or important social function.
- Most of the change in facial contour seen at 4 to 6 months is likely to consist of living fat and represent a persistent improvement. Patients can be informed that most of what they see is what they get at that point because swelling has completely resolved.

OUTCOMES

- See before and after examples (**FIGS 4** to **6**).

COMPLICATIONS

- No major complications attributable to fat grafting, including infection, embolization, tissue infarction, or blindness, have been encountered in our clinic over the last 20 years.
- Embolization leading to tissue infarction or blindness has been reported and largely attributed to sharp needle injection.
- Other complications are largely minor aesthetic problems and include lumps, oil cysts, asymmetries, undercorrection, overcorrection, and donor-site irregularities.
- Though lumps or areas of overcorrection around the eyes have been exceedingly rare in our practice, they are best treated by opening the eyelid and removing the excess fat under direct vision.

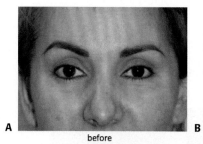
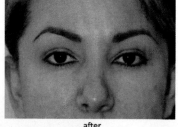

FIG 4 • Periorbital fat grafting case example. **A.** Patient with no previous surgery and hollow appearance around the eyes. **B.** Same patient seen after facial fat injections including the upper and lower orbit. A healthier, more youthful appearance can be seen (procedure performed by Timothy Marten, MD, FACS—Courtesy of Marten Clinic of Plastic Surgery).

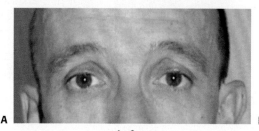
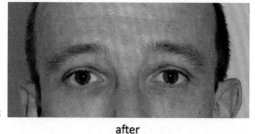

FIG 5 • Periorbital fat grafting case example. **A.** Patient with no previous surgery and hollow appearance around the eyes. **B.** Same patient seen after facial fat injections including to the upper and lower orbit. A healthier, more youthful appearance can be seen (procedure performed by Timothy Marten, MD, FACS—Courtesy of Marten Clinic of Plastic Surgery).

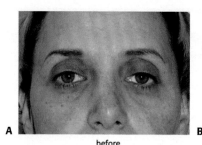
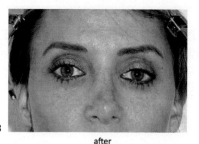

FIG 6 • Periorbital fat grafting case example. **A.** Patient with previous upper and lower blepharoplasty and hollow appearance around the eyes. **B.** Same patient seen after facial fat injections including to the upper and lower orbit along with face-lift and forehead lift. A healthier, more youthful appearance can be seen (procedure performed by Timothy Marten, MD, FACS—Courtesy of Marten Clinic of Plastic Surgery).

REFERENCE

1. Rohrich RJ, Pessa JE. The fat compartments of the face: anatomy and clinical implications for cosmetic surgery. *Plast Reconstr Surg.* 2007;119(7):2219-2227.

Indications and Techniques for Bridge of Bone Canthopexy

Dev Vibhakar, Erez Dayan, and Michael J. Yaremchuk

DEFINITION

- The positions of the lateral canthi are important functional and aesthetic facial landmarks. Their position is a fundamental determinant of the shape of the palpebral fissure.[1]
- The terminology of lateral canthal surgery may be confusing. A lateral canthopexy repositions the lateral canthal mechanism without violating the commissure. Canthoplasty procedures, by design, alter the shape of the palpebral fissure, because they disassemble and reassemble the lateral commissure while often shortening the lower lid margin.[2,3]
- Bridge of bone lateral canthopexy requires exposure of the lateral orbit and mobilization of the lateral canthus soft tissue mechanism. Its efficacy is based on the stable suture fixation point provided by drill holes placed relative to the zygomaticofrontal suture in the bone of the lateral orbit. It is our preferred technique for most surgical indications.

ANATOMY

- The lateral canthus is more correctly termed a lateral retinaculum. The retinaculum receives contributions from the lateral horn of the levator aponeurosis, the lateral extension of the preseptal and pretarsal orbicularis oculi muscle (lateral canthal tendon), the inferior suspensory ligament of the globe (Lockwood ligament), and the check ligament of the lateral rectus muscle. It has a broad attachment to the periosteum over the Whitnall tubercle (**FIG 1**).[4]
- Variations of the point of attachment or length of the retinaculum will alter eyelid shape, tension, and contour.[5]
- The lateral canthal angle is normally superior to the medial canthal angle, lying 4 ± 2 degrees or approximately 1.2 mm higher. This relationship is important for effective tear film distribution, and lacrimal drainage and for an aesthetically pleasing contour (**FIG 2**).[1]

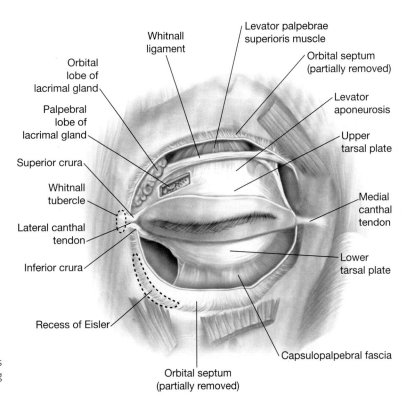

FIG 1 • Position of the medial and lateral canthal ligaments with respect to the bony orbit, tarsal plates, and underlying ligamentous structures

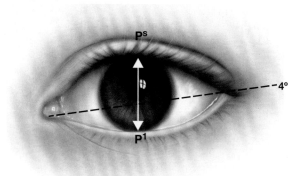

FIG 2 • Dimensions of the palpebral fissure measured in young Caucasian women. The mean height of the palpebral fissure measured from the upper lid (P^s) to lower lid (P^l) margin at the midpupil was 10.8 ± 1.2 mm ($n = 200$). The mean length of the eye fissure measured from medial commissure to lateral commissure was 30.7 ± 1.2 mm ($n = 200$). The mean inclination of the eye fissure was 4.1 ± 2.2 degrees.

PATHOGENESIS

- Medial and inferior canthal malposition changes the width and shape of the palpebral fissure as well as the position of lower eyelid resulting in the round eye deformity.[1]
- Inferior displacement of the lower eyelid may cause lagophthalmos leading to inadequate globe protection and exposure keratitis. Epiphora secondary to a displaced lower punctum and impaired tear drainage may also occur.
- The etiology of canthal malposition may be hereditary, senile, paralytic, traumatic, or iatrogenic.[4]
- Malposition of the lateral canthus most often occurs secondary to surgical access to the orbit and lower lid structures.[2,3]

PATIENT HISTORY AND PHYSICAL FINDINGS

- History and physical examination are the most important elements of preoperative assessment and planning for both reconstructive and cosmetic procedures. Standard preoperative photographs are taken and reviewed with the patient.
- History of recent eye surgery, dry eye, or visual acuity changes should be specifically elicited.
- Physical examination findings for lower eyelid malposition include canthal tilt, lid snapback test, lid distraction test, vector analysis, scleral show, and the presence of chemosis or keratoconjunctivitis. Other patient-directed examination includes visual acuity testing, Schirmer test for lacrimation, and slit-lamp evaluation.

IMAGING

- Whereas preoperative radiologic examination is uncommon for purely aesthetic surgery, computerized tomographic (CT) evaluation is almost routine for reconstructive procedures. CT scans provide the ability to view anatomic features in different planes and in three dimensions.

SURGICAL MANAGEMENT

Preoperative Planning

- Informed consent should include intrinsic risk of canthal malposition and potential for temporary postoperative chemosis.
- The patient's desired canthal position should be determined in aesthetic-focused procedures.
- This procedure may be performed under local or general anesthesia.

Positioning

- The patient is placed supine on the operating room table at a 90-degree perpendicular position relative to the anesthesiologist for maximal exposure.

TECHNIQUES

■ Preoperative Preparation

- Prior to antiseptic preparation and draping, a dilute solution of Marcaine and epinephrine (1:200 000) is infiltrated into the operative site for postoperative pain control and intraoperative hemostasis.
- Intravenous antibiotic prophylaxis is administered approximately 30 minutes preoperatively.

■ Operative Approach

- Bridge of bone lateral canthopexy requires access to the lateral orbital rim from the level of the Whitnall tubercle to the zygomaticofrontal suture. This can be accomplished through the lateral extent of an upper blepharoplasty incision. Most often, the lateral extent of both upper and lower blepharoplasty incisions is used (**TECH FIG 1**).
- The lower blepharoplasty incision provides superior visualization of the lateral canthal tissue.
- This anatomy may also be approached from the access provided by a bicoronal incision during exposure of traumatic fractures or aesthetic brow lift.

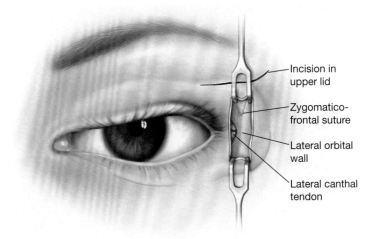

TECH FIG 1 • Through the lateral extent of the lower lid blepharoplasty incision, the lateral canthus is identified and released from the Whitnall tubercle by subperiosteal dissection.

- Incision in upper lid
- Zygomatico-frontal suture
- Lateral orbital wall
- Lateral canthal tendon

■ Figure-of-8 Suture Fixation of Lateral Canthus

- When only 1 or 2 mm of superior or lateral movement of the lateral canthus and adjacent lid margin are desired, one or both limbs of the lateral canthus may be purchased with a figure-of-8 suture without freeing of the lateral retinacular structures from the lateral orbit (**TECH FIG 2**). The amount of commissure movement will be limited by the length of the ligament, the point of suture purchase relative to the lateral commissure, and the position of the lateral orbit drill holes. This approach is most appropriate when there is minimal commissure malposition and no local scarring from previous lid surgery.
- When more significant movements of the lateral commissure and lid margin are desired, complete subperiosteal freeing of the lateral retinacular structures is required before figure-of-8 suture purchase of both limbs of the ligament.
- Through the lateral extent of the lower blepharoplasty incision, the lateral retinaculum is identified and dissected, and both limbs of the lateral canthus are purchased with a figure-of-8 nonabsorbable suture or 30- or 32-gauge titanium wire suture.

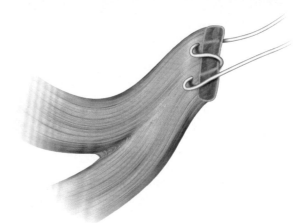

TECH FIG 2 • The lateral canthus is purchased by a figure-of-8 suture or 30-gauge titanium wire suture.

- If scarring from previous lower lid surgery restricts canthal movement, the lateral third of the middle lamellae is incised with needle-tip electrocautery to allow for sufficient mobility.

■ Drill Holes and Positioning of Lateral Canthus

- Through the upper access approach, the zygomaticofrontal suture is identified. This suture provides a landmark to allow symmetric placement of drill holes made in the lateral orbital rim.
- Using the zygomaticofrontal suture as a landmark, two drill holes are placed in the lateral orbital rim (**TECH FIG 3A**). The position of the lower drill hole is key, because it determines the maximum upward movement of the canthus. The upper drill hole is necessary to create the "bridge of bone"—a stable fixation point.
- The lateral canthal position and aperture shape are determined by the position of the drill holes, which should be 2 to 3 mm above the medial canthal plane to give the intercanthal axis a slight upward tilt. The drill holes should

also be placed in the internal orbit about 3 to 4 mm posterior to the anterior margin of the lateral orbital rim so the lateral lid will not be drawn away from the globe.
- To determine the ideal position of the drill holes, one can grasp the lateral canthus and tuck it against the lateral orbital rim until the desired canthal and lower lid position is obtained. The positions are marked and drill holes are made at that point. Most often, they are positioned just at, and 2 mm below, the zygomaticofrontal suture.
- The suture is then delivered in a subcutaneous plane from the lower to the upper incision (**TECH FIG 3B**).
- Each end of the suture is then passed from within the orbit through the drill holes to the lateral orbital rim. This is accomplished by bending a 28- or 30-gauge wire on itself and passing the bent end through the drill hole into the orbit (**TECH FIG 3C**).

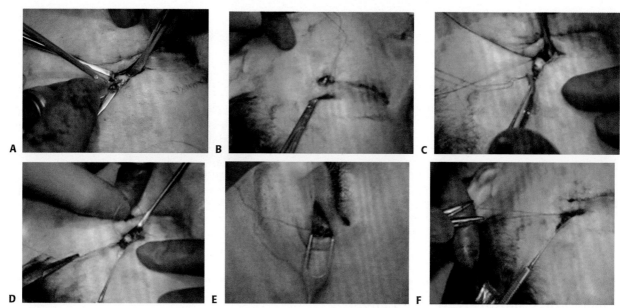

TECH FIG 3 • A. Using the zygomaticofrontal suture as a landmark, two drill holes are placed in the lateral orbital rim. **B.** Suture is then delivered in a subcutaneous plane from the lower to the upper incision. **C.** Each end of the suture is then passed from within the orbit through the drill holes to the lateral orbital rim. **D.** One end of the canthopexy stitch is placed into the "passing wire" loop to be pulled from inside the orbit through the drill hole to outside the orbit. **E.** The suture ends are then tied over the bridge of bone between the two holes. **F.** Tension on the sutures during their tying or tension on the wires during their twisting will determine canthal movement.

- One end of the canthopexy stitch is placed into the "passing wire" loop to be pulled from inside the orbit through the drill hole to outside the orbit (**TECH FIG 3D**).
- The suture ends are then tied over the bridge of bone between the two holes (**TECH FIG 3E**).
- Tension on the sutures during their tying or tension on the wires during their twisting will determine canthal

movement (**TECH FIG 3F**). The location of the lower drill hole dictates the limit of movement.
- Passage of the canthopexy sutures must occur from within the orbit to the outside. This allows tying the sutures over the bridge of bone (**TECH FIG 4A**) and allowing the lower lid to be applied to the globe (**TECH FIG 4B**).

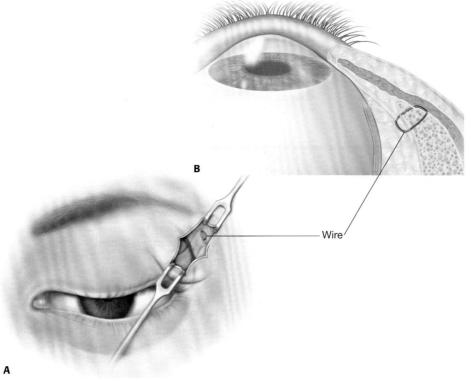

TECH FIG 4 • Passage of the canthopexy sutures must occur from within the orbit to the outside. This allows tying the sutures over the bridge of bone **(A)** and allowing the lower lid to be applied to the globe **(B)**.

- When wire fixation is used (most often for reconstructive cases), the wire ends are left approximately 5 mm long. This length of twisted wire has two advantages. First, it allows intraoperative (or postoperative) adjustment of the canthal position by simply twisting or untwisting the wires without repeating the suturing process. In addition, this length allows the ends to be placed into one of the drill holes or into the orbit. This maneuver avoids postoperative visibility or palpability of the wire ends.

■ Closure

- If local incisions are used for access, an ellipse of skin and muscle is removed from the lateral aspect of the upper lid to remove the lid redundancy caused by the upward movement of the canthus.
- The wounds are closed in layers.
- A temporary tarsorrhaphy stitch is often placed to avoid or minimize chemosis.

■ Postoperative Care

- Postoperatively, keep the patients head in a raised position to minimize edema and pain. Ice packs are applied to counteract swelling.
- Analgesia (narcotic and/or NSAIDs) as necessary for pain control.
- A single dose of IV antibiotics is given 30 to 60 minutes prior to incision. Oral antibiotics are continued no longer than 24 hours after surgery.
- Sutures are removed at 1 week after surgery.
- When extensive dissection is performed, postoperative chemosis is common. In addition to ophthalmic lubricants, a temporary tarsorrhaphy stitch is left in place for 5 to 7 days. The tarsorrhaphy is performed by placing a single 5-0 nylon suture through the upper and lower lid margins and adjacent skin approximately 2 to 3 mm lateral to the lateral limbus.

■ Outcomes

- Appropriate patient selection and sound surgical technique provide a vast majority of patients with satisfactory aesthetic outcomes (**FIGS 3** and **4**).
- When canthopexy is performed in heavily scarred tissues, wound contraction and contracture usually result in some loss of long-term canthal position. When bridge of bone canthopexy is performed in a nontraumatized field, canthal reposition is stable.

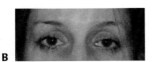

FIG 3 • A 27-year-old woman without any previous orbital surgery desired upward movement of her lateral canthus. **A.** Preoperative frontal view. **B.** Six-month postoperative view.

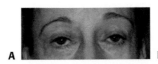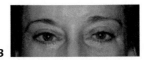

FIG 4 • **A.** Brow lift reversal was performed using a hairline incision in this patient who preoperatively had a high forehead. **B.** The patient also underwent infraorbital rim augmentation, subperiosteal midface lift, and bridge of bone lateral canthopexy as well as brow lift reversal.

■ Complications

- Complications are infrequent after bridge of bone canthopexy.
- Temporary chemosis is an anticipated short-term sequela. Some relapse may be anticipated when surgery is performed in heavily scarred fields.

REFERENCES

1. Yaremchuk MJ. Restoring palpebral fissure shape after previous lower blepharoplasty. *Plast Reconstr Surg.* 2003;111(1 suppl):441-450.
2. Fagien S. Lower-eyelid rejuvenation via transconjunctival blepharoplasty and lateral retinacular suspension: a simplified suture canthopexy and algorithm for treatment of the anterior lower eyelid lamella. *Oper Tech Plast Reconstr Surg.* 1998;5:121.
3. Fagien S. Algorithm for canthoplasty: the lateral retinacular suspension: a simplified suture canthopexy. *Plast Reconstr Surg.* 1999;103 (7 suppl):2042-2053.
4. Gioia VM, Linberg JV, McCormick SA. The anatomy of the lateral canthal tendon. *Arch Ophthalmol.* 1987;105(4 suppl):529-532.
5. Glat PM, Jelks GW, Jelks EB, et al. Evolution of the lateral canthoplasty: techniques and indications. *Plast Reconstr Surg.* 1997;100(6 suppl):1396-1405.

TECHNIQUES

40

CHAPTER

Indications and Techniques for Palatal Spacer Grafts

Dev Vibhakar, Erez Dayan, and Michael J. Yaremchuk

DEFINITION

- Retraction of the lower eyelid is a consequence of various surgical and medical conditions affecting the periorbital and midface region.
- Craniofacial trauma, tumors, facial paralysis, thyroid eye disease, and cosmetic blepharoplasty can alter the position of the normal lower eyelid.
- The clinical manifestation of this is inferior scleral show, lagophthalmos, and exposure keratitis. This can lead to dry eye syndrome, ocular discomfort, excessive tearing, photophobia, and blurred vision, as well as a cosmetically unappealing sad-eyed appearance.[1]
- Placement of a graft of palatal mucosa between the tarsal plate and lower lid retractors can elevate the lower lid margin.[2,3]

ANATOMY

- The normal lower eyelid lies at or just above the inferior corneal limbus.
- It is tethered medially and laterally by the canthal tendons.
- The lateral canthal angle is approximately 4.1 degrees or 1.2 mm higher than the medial canthal angle.
- It is considered a trilamellar structure—the anterior lamella (skin and orbicularis oculi muscle), the middle lamella (orbital septum), and the posterior lamella (lower eyelid retractors and conjunctiva (**FIG 1A**).

- The hard palate is composed of keratinized stratified squamous epithelium.
- There is no sex difference in mucosal thickness, and it increases with greater distance from the marginal gingiva, the mucosa being thinnest near the first molar.
- The bones of the hard palate are the palatine processes of the maxilla anteriorly and the horizontal plates of the palatine bones posteriorly.
- The greater palatine neurovascular bundles emerge bilaterally from the greater palatine foramina most commonly found medial to the upper second molar.
- They pass anteriorly along grooves in the palate to enter the incisive foramina (**FIG 1B**).

PATHOGENESIS

- Lower lid retraction can result from shortening of any of the lower eyelid lamella.
- This results in vertical contracture of the lower lid and is most commonly seen because of trauma or aggressive lower lid blepharoplasty.
- Patients with thyroid eye disease have a relative lower eyelid deficiency due to its inferior displacement caused by globe prominence.
- When lower lid malposition is caused by middle and posterior lamella inadequacy, grafts of palatal mucosa placed beneath the tarsal plate provide increase height and stiffness to support and elevate the lower lid margin (**FIG 2**).

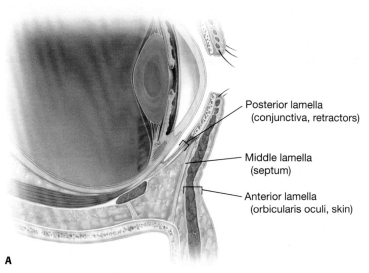

Posterior lamella
(conjunctiva, retractors)

Middle lamella
(septum)

Anterior lamella
(orbicularis oculi, skin)

A

FIG 1 • A. Lower eyelid anatomy demonstrating the anterior lamella (skin and orbicularis oculi muscle), the middle lamella (orbital septum), and the posterior lamella (lower eyelid retractors and conjunctiva).

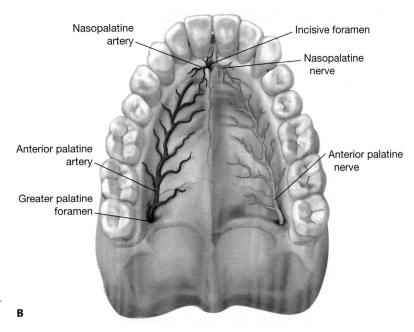

FIG 1 (Continued) • **B.** Relevant palatal neurovascular anatomy for donor-site harvest.

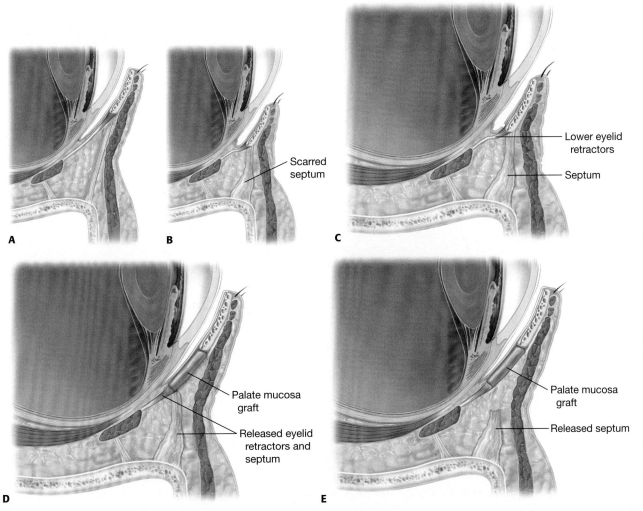

FIG 2 • **A,B.** Lower lid malposition secondary to vertical contracture of scarred septum. **C–E.** Hard palate mucosal graft used as a spacer between the lower tarsal plate and the recessed conjunctiva, lower eyelid retractors, and orbital septum.

PATIENT HISTORY AND PHYSICAL FINDINGS

- The underlying cause (previous surgery, metabolic disease, trauma, skeletal morphology) of lower eyelid retraction is determined.
- A thorough ophthalmologic examination is performed.
- Measuring the inferior scleral show assesses the degree of lower lid displacement.
- The status of the lower lid lamellae, skeletal morphology, and cheek prominence is assessed.
- Deficiencies of the middle and posterior lamellae are indications for the use of spacer grafts.

SURGICAL MANAGEMENT

Preoperative Planning

- Informed consent should include intrinsic risks and benefits of donor-site–related and lower lid complications. These include the possibility of infection, displacement, asymmetry, deformation, hematoma, seroma, motor/sensory nerve injury, donor-site discomfort, and palatal fistula.
- Prior to the induction of anesthesia, the amount of vertical height required to correct scleral show is measured medially and laterally with the patient in a sitting position.
- The authors' preference is to use general endotracheal or nasotracheal anesthesia. This allows optimal preparation of the donor site, operative site, and control of the airway.
- 0.12% chlorhexidine gluconate oral rinse is prescribed for daily use beginning 3 days preoperatively and including the day of surgery.

Positioning

- Intravenous cephalosporin or ciprofloxacin antibiotic prophylaxis is administered approximately 30 minutes preoperatively.
- Patients are placed supine on the operating room table at a 90-degree perpendicular position relative to the anesthesiologist to allow for maximal exposure.

T E C H N I Q U E S

■ Harvesting the Hard Palate Mucosa

- A side bite block is placed to facilitate exposure.
- A throat pack is placed.
- On average, a 25 × 10 mm graft is measured for harvesting. In cases of bilateral lid retraction, either one large central graft is taken and divided, or two separate grafts are taken from opposite sides of the palate.
- The junction of the hard and soft palate is identified laterally with forceps. The second molar is identified to assess the location of the greater palatine foramen.
- The graft is harvested in the canine-premolar region toward midline, where the palatal mucosa is thickest (**TECH FIG 1A**).

- The palate is then infiltrated with 1% lidocaine with epinephrine 1:100 000.
- A 15-blade scalpel is used to incise the mucosa and submucosa leaving the periosteum intact. A small layer of fat is harvested with the graft.
- Once the graft is harvested (**TECH FIG 1B**), bipolar cautery is used for selective hemostasis.
- The resulting defect is then covered with Surgicel (Johnson & Johnson, New Brunswick, NJ) that is secured in place with 4-0 chromic gut sutures.
- The graft is trimmed to remove all fatty tissue, mucosal glands, and submucosa from its undersurface (**TECH FIG 1C**).
- It is stored in saline-soaked gauze until ready for transfer to the eyelid.

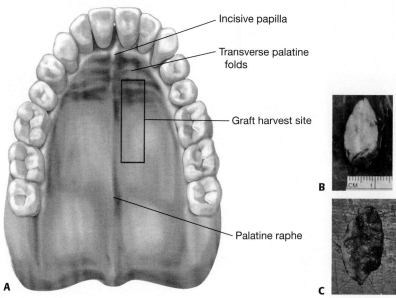

Incisive papilla

Transverse palatine folds

Graft harvest site

Palatine raphe

A

B

C

TECH FIG 1 • **A.** Graft harvest site. **B.** Average palatal graft is about 25 × 4 mm. **C.** Trimmed graft.

■ Lower Eyelid Surgery

- After markings are made (**TECH FIG 2A**), the lower lid is infiltrated with 1% lidocaine with epinephrine 1:100 000.
- Double skin hooks are used to expose the posterior lamella and identify the inferior border of the tarsal plate. A cotton-tipped applicator can facilitate palpating the transition.
- A 5-0 nylon suture is placed through the central portion of the lower fornix and retracted posteriorly over the eye to protect it and provide countertraction.
- A transconjunctival incision is made extending from below the punctum to the lateral canthus.
- Dissection is performed sharply to create a space between the inferior border of the tarsus and the superior edge of the recessed conjunctiva and lower lid retractors (**TECH FIG 2B**).
- The graft is placed within this space with the mucosal surface toward the globe (**TECH FIG 2C**).
- The inferior border of the graft is sutured to the recessed retractors and conjunctiva. The superior border of the graft is sutured to the inferior border of the tarsal plate.
- This is performed with double-armed 5-0 chromic sutures. The needles are passed full thickness through the lid, exiting the skin surface. Simple interrupted stitches are placed to ensure a flat transition and prevent any ridges.
- Each suture is then tied on the skin surface, ensuring that the knots are not secured tightly (**TECH FIG 2D**).
- A temporary tarsorrhaphy suture of 5-0 nylon is placed laterally if chemosis is a concern (**TECH FIG 2E**).

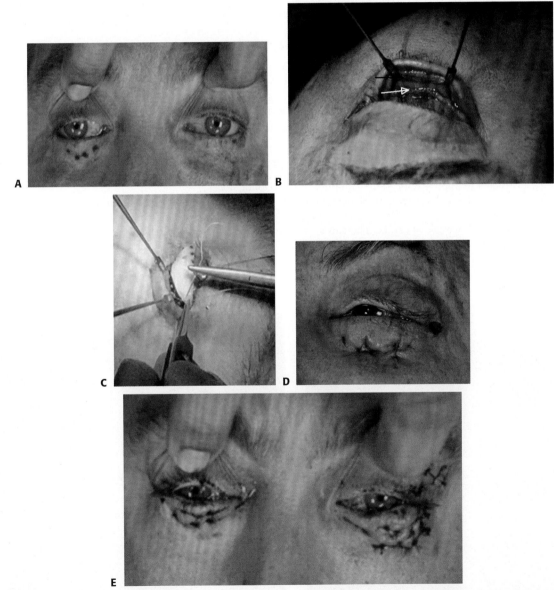

TECH FIG 2 • A. Patient markings. **B.** Transconjunctival exposure of the posterior lamella to identify the inferior border of the tarsal plate. **C.** Palatal graft is secured between the inferior border of the tarsus (*black arrow*) and the superior edge of the retracted conjunctiva (*white arrow*) and lower lid retractors with the mucosal surface toward the globe. **D.** The graft-securing sutures are tied on the skin surface. **E.** Immediate postoperative results.

PEARLS AND PITFALLS

Patient selection	▪ Many cases of lower lid retraction involve a multifactorial process requiring adjunct procedures such as a lateral canthopexy/canthoplasty, release of middle lamellar scarring, midface suspension, or infraorbital rim augmentation.
Surgical approach	▪ In the anterior palatal region, the neurovascular bundle runs toward the midline incisive canal and may be damaged if graft harvesting is not limited to the canine-premolar region.[2,3]
	▪ The donor site often oozes; it is important to not damage the periosteum or apply excessive electrocautery as this may cause necrosis of the underlying bone resulting in an oronasal fistula.
	▪ Donor site granulates and heals completely within 2 to 3 weeks.
	▪ The donor graft is typically trimmed medially. The majority of vertical height is required from the central lower limbus to the lateral canthus.
Donor-site selection	▪ Hard palate mucosa closely approximates lower lid tarsus in terms of contour, thickness, and stiffness.
	▪ It is abundant and easily obtained.
	▪ As an autograft, it is not at risk for rejection. It may undergo only minimal shrinkage following grafting for predictability in lid elevation.
	▪ It has a mucosal surface and is well tolerated when grafted into the lower lid.

POSTOPERATIVE CARE

▪ Oral antibiotics are prescribed for 7 days after surgery (cephalexin 500 mg q8h).

▪ Patients are asked to eat a soft diet for 7 days postoperatively.

▪ Frequent mouthwashes are advised as well as careful tooth brushing.

▪ Ocular lubricant ointment is applied every 12 hours.

▪ Patients are instructed to refrain from strenuous exercise for 2 to 3 weeks postoperatively.

▪ The patients are instructed to apply ice for 48 to 72 hours and sleep with head of bed elevated greater than 30 degrees or with three or four pillows.

▪ Follow up is at 1-, 2-, and 4-week intervals. Thereafter, long-term follow-up is at 6 months and 1 year.

▪ The external lower lid chromic sutures are trimmed at 1 week's time.

OUTCOMES

▪ Appropriate patient selection and sound surgical technique provides a vast majority of patients with satisfactory aesthetic outcomes (**FIG 3**).

▪ The improvement in scleral show and resolution of symptoms are noted once the swelling has resolved.

COMPLICATIONS

▪ Donor site

▪ Palatal fistula is typically self-limiting and allowed to granulate over time. A palatal splint or obturator can be made to provide symptomatic relief.

▪ Oral candidiasis will result in compromised healing. This resolves with oral antifungal treatment.

▪ Lower lid

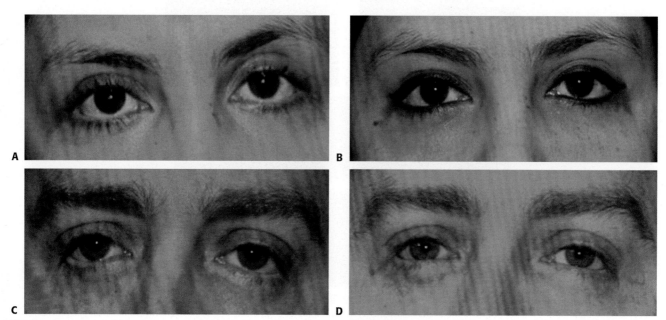

FIG 3 • A. A 45-year-old woman presented with lid descent after lower lid blepharoplasty with tarsal strip in negative vector patient. **B.** One year after infraorbital rim augmentation, subperiosteal midface lift, and palatal spacer graft. **C.** A 49-year-old man with lower lid descent after lower lid blepharoplasty and tarsal strip. **D.** Six months after subperiosteal midface lift and palatal graft placement.

- Corneal irritation can occur from hard palate suture grafts, but this is limited by placing the suture knots on the external skin surface.
- Ocular discharge is not uncommon in the initial postoperative period. The keratin layer of the hard palate graft continues to accumulate. Over time metaplasia to nonkeratinized mucosa occurs.

REFERENCES

1. Patel Munjal P, Shapiro Michael D, Spinelli Henry M. Combined hard palate spacer graft, midface suspension, and lateral canthoplasty for lower eyelid retraction: a tripartite approach. *Plast Reconstr Surg.* 2005;115(7):2105-2114.

2. Kersten RC, Kulwin DR, Levartovsky S, et al. Management of lower lid retraction with hard palate mucosa graft. *Arch Ophthalmol.* 1990;108:1339.

3. Wearne MJ, Sandy C, Rose GE, et al. Autogenous hard palate mucosa: the ideal lower eyelid spacer? *Br J Ophthalmol.* 2001;85:1183.

4. Mommaerts MY, DeRui G. Prevention of lid retraction after lower lid blepharoplasties: an overview. *J Craniomaxillofac Surg.* 2000; 28:189.

5. Patipa M. The evaluation and management of lower eyelid retraction following cosmetic surgery. *Plast Reconstr Surg.* 2000;106:438.

6. Patipa M. Complications of lower eyelid blepharoplasty. *Semin Ophthalmol.* 1996;11:183.

7. Spinelli HM, Jelks GW. Periocular reconstruction: a systematic approach. *Plast Reconstr Surg.* 1993;91:1017.

41
CHAPTER

Indication and Technique for Skin-Only Face- and Neck Lifting

James E. Zins and Gehaan D'Souza

DEFINITION

- Modern face and neck rejuvenation no longer focuses only on skin tightening but also may include fat contouring and volume restoration.
- Skin-only face-lift techniques avoid superficial musculoaponeurotic system (SMAS) manipulation. When combined with the release of major ligaments of the face, a skin-only face-lift may produce results equal to a more invasive technique.
- Knowledge of anatomical planes, three-dimensional relationship of the facial nerves, and location of the retaining ligaments is imperative.
- Procedures range from skin-only manipulation to alterations of the SMAS including minimal access cranial suspension (MACS) lift, lateral SMASectomy, extended SMAS, and the composite rhytidectomy.

ANATOMY

- Skin/fascial relationship
  - The facial soft tissue architecture can be described as being arranged in a series of concentric layers: skin, subcutaneous fat, superficial fascia, mimetic muscle, deep facial fascia (parotidomasseteric fascia), and the plane containing the facial nerve, parotid duct, and buccal fat pad.
  - Superficial fascial system invests mimetic muscles of facial expression, whereas deep fascial system covers and protects the facial nerve branches.[1]
- Ligaments and zones of adhesion
  - Retaining ligaments buttress the facial soft tissues against downward forces. These ligaments are in a constant location in relation to the facial nerve branches.[2,3]
  - Ligaments act as sentinels to the facial nerve branches.
    - True ligaments such as zygomatic and mandibular ligaments fixate the bone to the dermis and pass through SMAS.
    - False ligaments such as parotid and masseteric ligaments fixate fascial layers to superficial soft tissue.
  - Recent writings have emphasized the concept of adhesions rather than retaining ligaments. Adhesions such as the masseteric temporal and supraorbital ligaments are fibrous or fibrofatty attachments between superficial and deep tissue.
- Neck
  - Factors that provide a youthful and aesthetically pleasing neck include distinct mandibular border, subhyoid depression, thyroid bulge, a distinct border to the sternocleidomastoid muscle, and a cervicomental angle of 105 to 120 degrees.
- Facial nerve—five groups of branches are identified
  - Frontal (temporal) branches: Pitanguy delineated the course that extends from 0.5 cm below the tragus to 1.5 cm above the lateral eyebrow.[4] At the level of the zygomatic arch, the branches run 1.8 cm anterior to the helical crus, and 2 cm posterior to the lateral orbital rim deep to the SMAS and parotid masseteric fascia. Superior to the arch, the nerves travel in the innominate fascia—a fusion plane between superficial and deep fascia. One should remain superficial to the superficial layer of the deep temporal fascia or deep to the layer.[4]
  - Zygomatic and buccal branches: Interconnections between these branches account for natural recovery. The most commonly injured facial nerve is the buccal ramus.
  - Mandibular branches: The mandibular branch consists of a single nerve with few interconnections with other facial nerves that results in a risk of permanent injury. Posterior to the facial vessels, the mandibular rami travel within 1 cm cephalad to the mandibular border. Anterior to the facial vessels, the branches are always cranial to the border. The nerve travels deep to the parotid masseteric fascia and under the platysma by crossing superficial to the facial vessels.
  - Cervical branches: The nerve travels in close proximity to the gonial angle at the 1.74 mm inferior to the mandibular border.

PATHOGENESIS

- There is controversy between descent of soft tissue and volume loss in relation to facial aging. One camp suggests laxity of malar soft tissues as an etiology. The other side suggests that volume loss is the key factor leading toward facial aging.[1,5]
- Malar soft tissue migrates distal to the zygomatic cutaneous ligaments. This leads to soft tissue ptosis directly adjacent to the fixation of the nasolabial fold.
- Masseteric cutaneous ligaments support the cheek soft tissues that migrate downward inferior to the mandibular border to forming jowls.
- Jowling and loss of mandibular definition occurs by laxity of masseteric ligaments or deflation of the fat compartments of the face (submandibular).

NATURAL HISTORY

Upper third
- Aging is associated with
  - Eyebrow ptosis
  - Transverse forehead rhytides
  - Vertical glabellar lines
  - Hairline recession

Middle third
- Aging is associated with
  - Blepharochalasis

- Ptosis of malar soft tissue
- Laxity of lateral canthus and lid lead to rounding of palpebral fissure and ectropion
- Lower lid fat bulge
- Crow's feet
- Tear trough deformity
- Palpebromalar groove
- Malar mound

The lower third and neck
- Aging is associated with
  - Bulge superior to the nasolabial crease
  - Nasolabial crease deepening
  - Marionette lines
  - Exaggeration of the labiomental fold
  - Perioral wrinkles
  - Loss of the cervicomental angle secondary to skin ptosis, fat accumulation, and muscling banding
  - Platysmal bands

PATIENT HISTORY AND PHYSICAL FINDINGS

- Patients with medical comorbidities including cardiac and respiratory conditions should be excluded from surgery. Screening of bleeding complications should be undertaken.
- Antiplatelet medication must be ceased 2 weeks prior to surgery.
- Smoking must be stopped at least 4 weeks prior to operation.
- Patients with body dysmorphic disorder, unrealistic expectations, or psychiatric illness should also be excluded.
- Elderly patients (older than 65 years) are not at higher risk for complications compared to those younger than 65 years old when properly screened.

IMAGING

- No imaging is necessary prior to procedure.

NONOPERATIVE MANAGEMENT

- Nonsurgical interventions include botulinum toxin and soft tissue fillers. Skin resurfacing procedures include chemical peels, Ulthera, deoxycholic acid, and light amplification by stimulated emission of radiation (LASER) therapy such as fractionated CO_2 or erbium laser. Fat grafting is used for volume augmentation.

SURGICAL MANAGEMENT

- In the cheek a skin-only dissection can lead to good or excellent results when subcutaneous dissection is extensive by freeing the zygomatic cutaneous ligament, mandibular cutaneous ligament, and masseteric cutaneous ligament.
- Operative intervention for face-lift by elevating, advancing, and redraping of the skin.
- When aging affects the neck, one must proceed with fat removal and platysma tightening.

Preoperative Planning

- Soft tissue and skeletal cephalometrics may be helpful for assessment of facial aging. One should assess symmetry and proportions of regions of the face and identify differences between soft tissue and skeletal muscle pathology that cause facial aging.

- Assessment should begin with the head in straightforward gaze with the Frankfort horizontal parallel to the ground and the lips and eyebrows in a relaxed position.
  - When assessing the face, it can be divided into three horizontal thirds. The horizontal thirds are produced by lines drawn adjacent to the menton, nasal base, brows at the supraorbital notch level, and hairline.
  - The lower third can be divided into the upper third and the lower two-thirds by a line drawn through the oral commissures.
  - The lower third can be divided into halves by a horizontal line adjacent to the lowest pint of the lower lip vermilion.

Positioning

- The endotracheal tube is secured. Stainless steel dental wire (26 gauge) is used to affix the endotracheal tube to the first bicuspid.
- Face and hair are prepped entirely.
- Reinforced endotracheal tube is used and brought over the head rather than down toward the chin. The tube is attached to the anesthesia machine using a straight connector and extension tubing, which rests on a "Christmas tree" holder (Mainline Medical, Norcross, Georgia).
- Sterile stockinet is applied over the tubing and the "Christmas tree" connector.
- When eyelids and upper face access is required, the Christmas tree is removed from under the stockinet; the tube is directly placed onto the patient's draped torso and clipped to the drapes.

Approach

- Preauricular incision
  - Incision in the preauricular region has been shown to decrease scarring.
  - Incision should be carried out in a retrotragal or pretragal fashion (**FIG 1**).

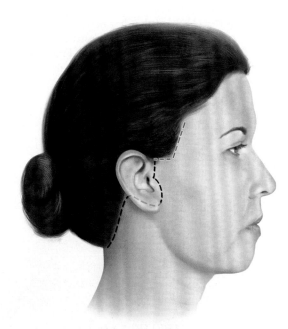

FIG 1 • The course of the preauricular and postauricular incision.

- Temporal incision
  - Temporal hairline incision is used when lateral canthus to temple distance is more than 5 cm.
  - When distance is less than 5 cm, temple scalp extension incision is made.
- Postauricular incision

- Incision in the postauricular sulcus and crosses the region of postauricular skin where the helix and postauricular hairline join
- This continues into the occipital scalp or follows the hairline.
- Submental incision
  - A 3 to 4 cm incision is centered over midline 5 mm caudal to the submental crease.[5]

■ Skin-Only Face and Neck Lifting

- Subcutaneous dissection (**TECH FIG 1**)
  - Local anesthetic
    - Infiltrate incision sites with 0.5% lidocaine with epinephrine (1:200 000). Regions of subcutaneous undermining are infiltrated with 0.5% lidocaine with epinephrine (1:200 000).
    - Inject each ipsilateral facial region prior to undermining to maintain tumescence and local block effect.
- Subcutaneous undermining
  - Skin flaps should be elevated under direct vision.
  - Preauricular dissection
    - Dissect anterior to the helix beginning in a superficial subcutaneous plane to avoid injury to the superficial temporal vessels. Care should be taken to avoid injury to tragal cartilage. In the area of the cheek, dissection should preserve fat on skin flap to provide for a robust flap. This plane should be consistent in the area of the upper neck and inferior mandibular border.
    - Dissect anteriorly to incise platysma-cutaneous ligaments and mandibular cutaneous ligaments when indicated.
  - Postauricular dissection
    - Elevate skin superficial to the sternocleidomastoid taking care to preserve fascia protecting the great auricular nerve (GAN).
    - Note: GAN location has been described (GAN fall within a 30-degree angle constructed using the vertical limb perpendicular to the Frankfort horizontal and a second limb drawn posteriorly from the midlobule).
  - Temporal region
    - Dissect in a plane superficial to the superficial temporal fascia and bevel blade parallel to the hair follicles.

- Identify the orbicularis oculi and remain in a superficial plane to this muscle.
- Neck dissection
  - Local anesthetic is administered if general anesthetic is used.
    - Infiltrate incision site with 0.5% lidocaine with epinephrine (1:200 000). Regions of subcutaneous undermining are infiltrated with 0.5% lidocaine with epinephrine (1:200 000).
  - Incise the skin through 3.5 mm submental incision 5 mm caudal to the submental crease previously marked.
  - Use Bovie cautery or scissors to begin undermining in subcutaneous tissue to connect lateral dissection subcutaneous planes with that of the lower face.
  - Defat submental region above the platysma in the midline.
  - Incise platysma in midline to level of the thyroid cartilage.
  - Remove interplatysmal and subplatysmal fat.
  - Fat is resected flush with the anterior bellies of the digastric muscles.
    - Subplatysmal fat is excised flush with the digastric muscles to avoid creation of a cavity between the muscles.
    - Digastric muscles may be plicated in the midline or partially resected if bulging prominent.
  - Dissection extends inferiorly to the thyroid cartilage inferiorly and laterally to the anterior belly of the digastric. Lateral dissection is strictly in a preplatysmal plane.
  - Platysmaplasty
    - 3-0 PDS suture used in running fashion to sew cut edges of platysma to midline from chin to thyroid cartilage and back to the chin (corset platysmaplasty).
  - Close incision with subdermal 4-0 Monocryl suture and running 5-0 subcutaneous fast-absorbing suture.

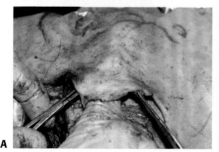 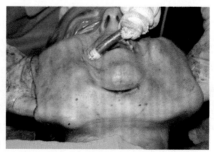

TECH FIG 1 • A. Skin flaps elevated. **B.** Extent of cheek and neck dissection

- Skin redraping
  - Goal: Skin shifted along vector perpendicular to the nasolabial fold. In postauricular region, skin should be shifted along vector parallel to mandibular border for optimal improvement of the anterior neck.
  - Suspend skin flap first at the cranial most aspect of the helix with vector perpendicular to nasolabial fold.
  - Use a face-lift marker and incise in a T-shaped incision in flap.
  - Suspend flap with a 4-0 Prolene suture.
  - A third suture is placed high in the postauricular region.
  - Second point of suspension is at the lobular region where 4-0 Monocryl suture suspends flap at inferior lobule.
  - Flap is divided at the lobule and exteriorized.
- Skin flap tailoring
  - Preauricular trimming/closure
    - Mark skin flap redundancy and trim skin flap. Preauricular portion of flap is trimmed to match preauricular curves.
    - Care must be taken over tragal region to avoid tragal retraction from tension on skin flap and tragus.
  - Defat pretragal portion of skin flap for pleasing contour.
  - Affix skin flap to cranial preauricular skin with 4-0 Monocryl subdermal sutures.
  - Run 6-0 fast-absorbing sutures for preauricular closure taking care to evert skin edges.
  - Postauricular trimming/closure
    - Trim anterior border of the postauricular skin flap to match curve of incision in auriculomastoid sulcus.
    - Excise skin along posterior border of the postauricular skin flap using face-lift marker as guide. Wound edges should touch one another without gaps (ie, no tension on postauricular skin flaps).
    - Run 5-0 fast-absorbing gut suture for single-layer closure.

PEARLS AND PITFALLS

Tension	Preauricular incision under moderate tension. Postauricular incision should be under no tension. Tension in the postauricular region leads to a hypertrophic scar at best or skin slough at the worst.
Release of ligaments	Subcutaneous dissection over the cheek over the region of the major zygomatic ligament must be done carefully as nerve injury can occur in a deep dissection.
Dissection plane	In the cheek, the dissection of the skin-only face-lift is more superficial than the deeper dissection over the platysma.
Excellent results	Excellent results in skin-only face-lift are predicated on the release of mandibular ligaments, zygomatic ligaments, and masseteric ligaments.
Neck	Patients with platysmal banding require an anterior neck approach platysmaplasty in addition to the skin-only face-lift.
Cautery	Bipolar cautery use rather than unipolar cautery use reduces both the incidence of neuropraxia and neck drainage.

POSTOPERATIVE CARE

- Patient discharged form postoperative unit after procedure.
- A head dressing is not essential, but a soft dressing prevents unsightly blood leakage and is removed the following morning.
- Patients are provided with analgesics only.
- Patients are examined 1 day after surgery with care to examine suture lines and skin flaps.

- Patient drains are removed 1 day after surgery regardless of output unless drainage is significant, ie, greater than 30 cc.
- Patients begin showering 1 day after surgery following removal of dressings.
- Residual sutures are removed 7 days after surgery.

OUTCOMES

- See **FIGS 2** and **3**.

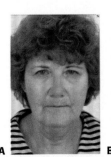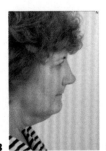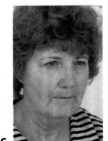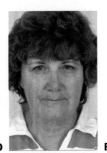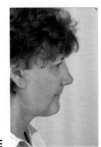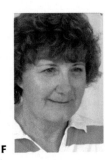

FIG 2 • A–C. Preoperative. **D–F.** Postoperative 1 year—Skin-only face-lift with neck lift

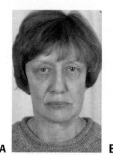 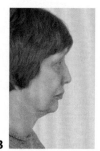 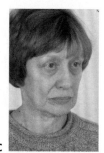 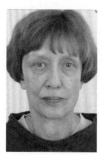 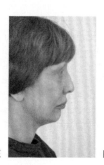 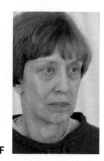

A   **B**   **C**   **D**   **E**   **F**

FIG 3 • **A–C.** Preoperative. **D–F.** Postoperative 1 year—Skin-only face-lift and neck lift

COMPLICATIONS

- Early complications
  - Hematoma: The incidence of hematoma formation is variable ranging from 1% to 10%. One should maintain blood pressure at preoperative levels during closure to detect bleeding once epinephrine effect wanes. Small hematomas are dealt with in a conservative fashion. Large hematomas must be drained in the operating room and cleared through (milking out through drains or aspirated with needle).
  - Seromas: Occur in the neck region and lower face. If seroma forms after drain removal, aspirations with a needle and syringe in clinic are required. Undrained seromas lead to neck irregularities that can be difficult or impossible to correct.
  - Sialoma: Rarely occur, caused by parotid gland injury. This is diagnosed with high amylase levels. Leaks resolve with conservative treatment in the absence of distal obstruction.
  - Facial nerve injury: Permanent injury incidence is 0.4% to 2.6%. Most common branches injured are injuries include buccal branches. Buccal branch injury is not apparent as there are many interconnections between the buccal branch and other facial nerve branches. Marginal mandibular nerve injury is the second most common but is apparent due to it being single nerve without interconnections with other branches. Early nerve defects are neuropraxic rather than axonotmesis and usually resolve.

The marginal mandibular and cervical nerves are differentiated as the marginal mandibular gives innervation to the mentalis, which results in the lack of lip eversion when injured.

- Late complications
  - Contour irregularities: Occur as a result of asymmetric fat excision
  - Pixie ears: Caused by tension on the lobule during closure
  - Unsatisfactory scars: Widened misplaced scars, hypertrophic scars, or skin slough
  - Alopecia
  - Loss of tragal definition

REFERENCES

1. Stuzin JM, Baker TJ, Gordon HL. The relationship of the superficial and deep facial fascias: relevance to rhytidectomy and aging. *Plast Reconstr Surg.* 1992;89(3):441-449.
2. Huettner F, Rueda S, Ozturk CN, et al. The relationship of the marginal mandibular nerve to the mandibular osseocutaneous ligament and lesser ligaments of the lower face. *Aesthet Surg J.* 2015;35(2): 111-120.
3. Alghoul M, Bitik O, McBride J, Zins JE. Relationship of the zygomatic facial nerve to the retaining ligaments of the face: the Sub-SMAS danger zone. *Plast Reconstr Surg.* 2013;131:245e-252e.
4. Pitanguy I, Ramos AS. The frontal branch of the facial nerve: the importance of its variations in face lifting. *Plast Reconstr Surg.* 1966;38(4):352-356.
5. Lambros V. Observations on periorbital and midface aging. *Plast Reconstr Surg.* 2007;120(5):1367-1376.

Indications and Techniques for Face-Lifting and Neck Lifting

David A. Hidalgo and Sammy Sinno

GENERAL CONCEPTS

- Facial aging is a result of progressive degenerative changes in the skin, deeper soft tissues, and underlying skeletal structures, often occurring independently and each to variable degrees.
- Although new nonsurgical techniques that attempt to restore a more youthful facial appearance continue to develop, surgical rejuvenation remains the most powerful approach.
- Face-lifting and neck lifting involves dissection and manipulation of facial skin and deeper soft tissues to create an aesthetically rejuvenated facial appearance and youthful contour in the neck.
- The superficial musculoaponeurotic system (SMAS) layer of the face can be manipulated independent of facial skin in several ways to provide more natural and long-lasting results.
- SMAS technique options include SMAS flap, SMASectomy, and SMAS plication.[1-3] Facial contour, skin quality, soft tissue volume, and bone structure all influence the choice of technique.
- There are various strategies applicable to treating aging changes in the neck that address visible muscle banding, skin laxity, and general neck contour.
- Adjunctive procedures involving periorbital surgery, regional resurfacing, soft tissue volume augmentation, skeletal augmentation, and others enhance the results of face-lifting and neck lifting.

ANATOMY

- The face is a lamellar structure that, from superficial to deep, consists of skin, subcutaneous fat, SMAS, deep fascia (parotidomasseteric fascia), the mimetic muscles, facial nerve branches and the parotid gland, muscles of mastication, deep fat compartments, and bone.
- The facial nerve innervates most muscles of facial expression on their deep surface and is protected in the area over the parotid by the parotidomasseteric fascia.[4]
- The SMAS is contiguous with the platysma muscle inferiorly and the galea aponeurotica superiorly.[5] Tightening of this layer repositions ptotic facial tissues and is a key component of restoring youthful facial contour.
- The platysma muscle in the neck typically develops ligamentous laxity with aging. This commonly results in the development of visible medial muscle edges (bands) anteriorly that exhibit variable thickness, length, and spacing between them. Excess subcutaneous fat superficial to the muscle can also contribute to the appearance of an aging neck.

- Structures deep to the platysma including subplatysmal fat, submandibular glands, digastric muscles, and the hyoid bone can also contribute to contour problems independent of the aging process, as can skeletal conditions such as microgenia.

PATIENT HISTORY AND PHYSICAL FINDINGS

- Patients typically present for surgical rejuvenation of the face and neck over the age of 50, but some seeking correction of minimal deformities can present in their early 40s.
- Patients presenting for the first time in their 70s are also reasonable candidates provided there are no prohibitive medical conditions.
- The best candidates for surgery are those with significant aging changes who are motivated for the right reasons; good candidates should be psychologically stable and have realistic expectations.
- Characteristic signs of facial aging include deepening of the nasolabial folds with associated midface ptosis and deflation; progressive actinic skin damage and laxity; subcutaneous atrophy; development of jowls, "marionette lines," and adjacent prejowl hollowing; and platysma laxity leading to anterior bands and an obtuse cervicomental angle laterally.
- Smoking increases the risk of wound complications, particularly in the setting of wide skin undermining. Therefore, complete cessation of smoking is required for at least 3 weeks prior to surgery. Nicotine substitutes of all types are also prohibited.
  - Strategies to minimize complications when uncertainty exists regarding compliance include avoiding retrotragal incisions, limiting the extent of the retroauricular incision design (short-scar option if appropriate), avoiding opening the anterior neck, and limiting skin undermining.
- Patients with a BMI over 30 and significant medical conditions such as obstructive sleep apnea, severe diabetes, or cardiovascular disease are unfavorable candidates for surgery in an office-based setting. Men with a history of obstructive urinary symptoms should have a urology consultation prior to surgery.

IMAGING

- Although 3D scanning is available today, it does not significantly enhance communication between the surgeon and patient beyond what high-quality facial photographs and mirror examination can achieve.

SURGICAL MANAGEMENT

Preoperative Planning

- Skin quality is assessed including thickness, elasticity, and degree of actinic damage.
  - Many patients will benefit from simultaneous regional skin resurfacing with a chemical peel such as 30% trichloroacetic acid for the thinner periorbital skin or dermabrasion for the thicker perioral skin.
  - Lasers are an alternative resurfacing modality, perhaps best suited to full face treatment with fractionated laser-based technology subsequent to surgery.
- Patients with high sideburns are advised that their hairline may move slightly or that a subsideburn incision may be necessary to prevent excessive movement. The latter is more common in secondary or tertiary cases.
  - Pretrichial temporal incisions are another option but can cause variable scar quality and generally are not well accepted by patients.
- The choice between a pretragal and retrotragal incision is influenced by tragal anatomy, its overlying skin quality, and adjacent preauricular skin thickness and texture.
  - Retrotragal incisions effectively break up the continuity of the preauricular incision but must be carefully crafted to avoid an unnatural-appearing tragus.
  - Women who have a large, projecting tragus with thin, delicate overlying skin and adjacent thick cheek skin are better suited to a pretragal incision.
  - Most men are also good candidates for pretragal incisions to avoid the transposition of thicker, hair-bearing skin over the tragus and to avoid a more feminized appearance in this area.
- Women under 60 years with minimal neck changes seeking improvement for early jowls and nascent lateral cheek laxity are often good candidates for a posterior incision pattern limited to the postauricular sulcus (short-scar technique).[6] This is particularly advantageous in those who habitually expose this area due to hairstyle preferences.
  - Nevertheless, well-designed and expertly executed full postauricular scar patterns are preferred to a more limited incision approach that fails to correct cervical skin laxity.
  - Most women and even men with complete alopecia are best served with a complete postauricular scar pattern.
- Individual bone structure, soft tissue volume, and surgical timing (primary or secondary, tertiary) are all influential in selecting the optimal SMAS technique for each patient. Those with strong mandibular or maxillary bone contours generally require less SMAS manipulation, as do those with lighter soft tissue volumes. The opposite scenarios argue for more extensive SMAS manipulation.
  - For patients with prominent facial bone structure and light or medium thickness soft tissues, a SMASectomy is indicated.
  - For patients with normal or small facial bone structure who require more extensive repositioning of heavier facial soft tissues, an extended SMAS flap is more effective.
  - For patients with thin, minimally ptotic soft tissues, or in secondary or tertiary cases, a SMAS plication is appropriate.

- Facial fat volume and distribution are assessed.
  - If significant hollowing in the prejowl sulcus or deflation of the malar compartment is observed, adjunctive fat grafting of these areas should be considered at the time of the primary procedure.
  - Prominent lateral cheek hollowing, seen less commonly, is best treated with a separate fat grafting procedure at a later procedure.
- The extent of cervical skin laxity and the underlying neck contour are evaluated.
  - Older patients with very loose skin of poor quality that extends to the base of the neck are always counseled that they may need a limited secondary procedure at 1 year to obtain an optimal, durable result. This also applies to younger patients having a single strong midline submental skin band.
  - It is important to discuss this preoperatively with those having either of these characteristics.
- Anterior neck surgery is indicated for platysmal bands that are prominent and generally no further apart than 2.5 cm. Patients are advised that a 2.5- to 3-cm submental incision will be necessary to accomplish this.
  - Subplatysmal fat excision is a helpful adjunct for improving an obtuse cervicomental angle and can be an indication alone for opening the neck in the absence of platysmal bands.
  - Partial excision of the submandibular glands and digastric muscles is a much more aggressive and controversial approach for contour improvement and is not routinely recommended.
- Patients are counseled on the option of having a chin implant placed when microgenia is present. Even in subtle cases, an extra small implant is often beneficial.
  - Ptotic chin pads (witch's chin deformity) and more subtle chin/neck junction depressions should be noted and addressed in the surgical plan.
- Perioral resurfacing is often indicated in conjunction with face-lifting and neck lifting.
  - Upper lip rhytides are usually the first to appear and tend to be the deepest. The oral commissures, prejowl sulcus, and chin are also affected to variable degrees but usually much less than the upper lip.
  - Chemical peels, laser resurfacing, and mechanical dermabrasion are all effective at improving rhytides but also can cause depigmentation of the treated areas.
  - Nevertheless, even conservative rhytide ablation significantly enhances the overall result of surgery. Dermabrasion, perhaps the least technically sophisticated and oldest tool, allows precise depth control of treatment in experienced hands.
- Simultaneous periorbital rejuvenation is frequently requested and discussed and, less commonly, a nasal tip plasty to address concerns regarding a bulbous or drooping tip.
  - Earlobe reductions or repair of elongated or lacerated earlobe piercings are also sometimes requested during the preoperative evaluation.

Patient Preparation

- All patients have standardized multiview facial photographs taken, with additional views of areas where adjunctive treatment is planned.

- These photographs are used for preoperative planning and communication, intraoperative reference, and postoperative outcome discussions.
- Medical clearance is routinely obtained in patients over 60 or in younger patients with specific medical conditions of concern.
- Patients taking blood-thinning medications for cardiac stents or arrhythmias must be evaluated by their cardiologist to determine the safety of discontinuance for a suitable interval both before and after surgery. The same applies to patients on prophylactic low-dose aspirin.
- Strict blood pressure control is necessary perioperatively to facilitate surgery and minimize the potential for a postoperative hematoma. Therefore, patients with hypertension must optimize their medical regimen for blood pressure control prior to surgery.
  - Clonidine can be administered from either an oral or transdermal route immediately prior to surgery to manage blood pressure that remains refractory to tight control.
- Hospital employees, such as anesthesiologists and nurses, or others with a prior history of MRSA should be screened with a nasal swab culture.
  - Patients who test positive should be treated with Bactroban (mupirocin) prior to surgery to eliminate their carrier status.
- The benefits of perioperative homeopathic use such as *Arnica montana* for ecchymosis and bromelain for edema are unproven but can be safely employed at the surgeon's discretion.
  - Excessive doses of *Arnica* may increase the risk of hemorrhage.

- Patients are instructed to wash their face and hair thoroughly the night before surgery, remain nothing by mouth (NPO) after midnight, and take their blood pressure medication on the morning of surgery.

Patient Positioning

- The patient is positioned supine on the operative table with the knees slightly bent to optimize lower extremity venous return.
  - The arms are carefully immobilized and a warming blanket is placed.
  - A triangular headpiece facilitates performing the procedure.
- Anesthesia is induced, either an oral airway or laryngeal mask airway (LMA) placed, and the patient typically maintained on propofol for the duration of the procedure.
  - Normotensive anesthesia is preferred throughout the procedure in order to minimize the prospect of hematoma development.
- Consideration should be given for placement of a urinary catheter for long procedures and for men with a history of obstructive symptoms.
- One preoperative dose of cephalosporin is administered.
  - If the patient is a hospital employee or has a history of MRSA, vancomycin is given instead.
- The incisions and key reference points are marked, the sites of injection prepped with Betadine swabs, and the areas of dissection infiltrated with a dilute lidocaine and epinephrine solution (100-cc normal saline, 100 cc 1% lidocaine, 1 cc of epinephrine).
  - Tumescent technique is not necessary, and typically 200-cc total is used for the face and neck.
- The face is then prepped with Zephiran Chloride (benzalkonium chloride) and a head drape applied.

■ Incisions

- Incisions are all made using a no. 10 blade scalpel.
- Temporal incisions within the scalp angle back approximately 20 to 30 degrees above the ear to avoid the course of the superficial temporal artery (**TECH FIG 1A**).
  - Pretrichial incisions are avoided in the temporal area due to their inconsistent healing quality.
- Subsideburn incisions are positioned at the root of the helix and extend transversely for no more than 2 cm when needed.
  - A commitment for making subsideburn incisions is generally not necessary until skin redraping at the time of closure.
- The retrotragal incision is positioned slightly posterior to the free edge of the tragus and defines its superior and inferior borders. The inferior portion of the incision then extends anterior to the tragus for several millimeters before making a sharp angle to parallel the attached portion of lobule (see **TECH FIG 1A**).
  - Pretragal incisions parallel the curve of the helix to its root and then inflect downward with a short mirror

image curve that then straightens to parallel the tragus down to the lobule (**TECH FIG 1B**).
- Short-scar postauricular design can use the full length of the sulcus to allow for even skin distribution when closing, thereby minimizing the potential for significant pleat formation (**TECH FIG 1C**).
  - Full postauricular incisions reflect posteriorly high in the sulcus, cross the mastoid skin with a gentle upward curve, and then continue into the occipital scalp parallel to and just inside the hairline, cut on a bevel to preserve hair shafts (**TECH FIG 1D**).
- The submental incision is 2.5 to 3 cm in length and can be placed either in the natural crease or slightly posterior to it, depending on surgeon preference.
- Creation of a "mesotemporalis" by deep dissection in the temporal area is not recommended as this maneuver predisposes to late (10 to 14 days) massive superficial temporal artery hemorrhage. This complication occurs suddenly and is associated with challenging patient management issues.

TECHNIQUES

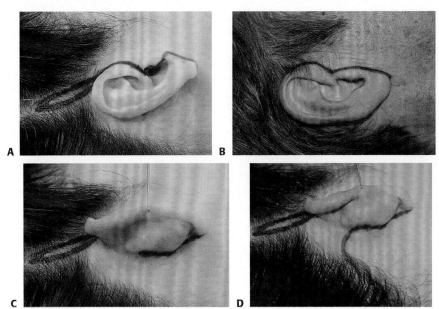

TECH FIG 1 • Incisions. **A.** The temporal scalp incision is angled backward approximately 30 degrees to avoid the superficial temporal artery. A small amount of scalp skin can be pre-excised as shown by the design. The retrotragal portion of the skin incision lies posterior to the free edge of the tragus. The incision then turns a right angle at the lower border of the tragus to parallel the lower ear and lobule. Avoid pretrichial incisions (*red line*) when possible. **B.** Pretragal incision design in a male. **C.** Short-scar postauricular incision design can use the whole length of the sulcus to facilitate an even distribution of skin during closure. **D.** Typical postauricular skin incision design. The incision reflects from the postauricular sulcus high on the mastoid bare skin before transitioning into the occipital scalp.

■ Skin Flap Elevation

- Once all incisions have been made, the no. 10 blade is used to begin the skin flap elevation 1.5 to 2 cm anteriorly in the preauricular area (**TECH FIG 2A,B**). Care is taken to maintain proper thickness when starting the flap with the knife.
  - The postauricular and upper neck skin is then raised sharply off the mastoid and origin of the sternomastoid muscle (**TECH FIG 2C**). Hemostasis is obtained in all areas raised so far.

- In the case of retrotragal incisions, soft tissue is sharply undermined at the base of the tragus and folded over anteriorly (**TECH FIG 3**).
  - It is sutured to the SMAS with a continuous 4-0 Vicryl suture.
  - This maneuver creates a "hill and valley" effect just anterior to the tragus. As the skin follows this contour during closure, tragal definition is enhanced.

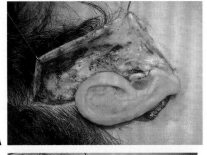

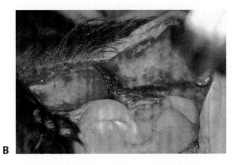

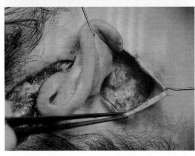

TECH FIG 2 • **A.** In temporal incisions, the temporal scalp is raised in a subcutaneous plane. **B.** Raising this area in a deep plane with a transition zone to the subcutaneous plane inferiorly over the cheek should be avoided. **C.** The skin flap is shown raised over the mastoid and sternomastoid muscle origin in this short-scar example. This is a good time to obtain hemostasis of all areas prior to raising the skin flap over the cheek and neck.

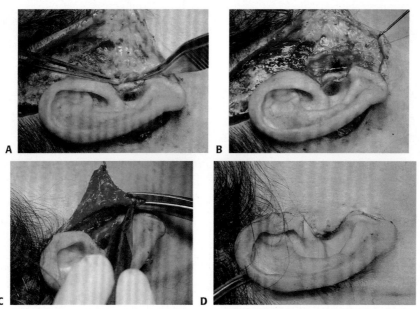

TECH FIG 3 • **A.** In retrotragal incisions, the soft tissue over the tragus is raised as a flap. **B.** The flap is then reflected anteriorly and sutured to the preauricular SMA. The skin that will overlie the tragus at closure is thinned inferiorly where the incision pattern transitions to parallel the lower ear and also along its superior edge. **C.** The central portion is not thinned in order to avoid vascular compromise. **D.** Final closure.

- Curved Mayo or similar scissors with "tips down" are used to raise the skin flap under direct vision with trans-illumination, except in the region of the great auricular nerve where "tips up" aids in avoiding injury.
- The proper plane of subcutaneous elevation is most readily identified in the temporal area, which is then extended over the orbicularis oculi and the malar eminence.
  - A cobblestone appearance of the subcutaneous flap fat over the lateral zygoma verifies the correct plane.
- Dissection of the neck in a subcutaneous plane is next performed.
  - The platysma should not be directly exposed until at least several centimeters below the mandibular border. Observing this principle prevents platysma denuded of fat from being repositioned above the mandibular border when the SMAS is tightened.
  - The skin flap is dissected for a short distance above the mandibular border in the jowl region, tapering closer to the mandible border as the mentum is approached.

- Release of the mandibular ligaments adjacent to the mentum is not critical although some would disagree.
- The extent of medial neck dissection is variable depending on conditions and goals. It can be extended almost to the midline to anticipate dissection of the anterior neck through a submental incision if that is planned later.
- It is easiest to raise the skin flap from above to below as described and then perform the midcheek skin elevation only to the extent necessary for adequate SMAS exposure.
  - Undermining rarely proceeds within 2 cm of the nasolabial fold.
  - Excessive release of the skin flap is avoided in this area to allow maximum skin movement with SMAS tightening.

■ SMAS Treatment Options

SMAS Flap

- A line is drawn over the zygomatic arch to establish the superior border of the SMAS flap.
- The SMAS is incised with a no. 10 blade in the preauricular area. Sharp elevation continues over the surface of the parotid gland and then switches to scissors.
- The SMAS is then bluntly dissected anterior to the gland with delicate vertical spreading of the scissor tips to expose and release the masseteric-cutaneous ligaments and then the zygomatic-cutaneous ligaments superiorly (McGregor patch) (**TECH FIG 4**).
  - The latter usually includes cauterization of a small branch of the transverse facial artery.

- The medial extent of SMAS flap elevation can either cease once the border of the zygomaticus major muscle is identified or can proceed beyond it and over the zygomaticus minor muscle (extended SMAS dissection) to achieve greater midface correction.
  - The lateral border of the platysma is then elevated over the tail of the parotid gland with careful sharp and blunt dissection.
- The muscle border is mobilized inferiorly for several centimeters with care taken to identify and avoid both the great auricular nerve and external jugular vein.
- The SMAS is then elevated vertically and slightly posteriorly.

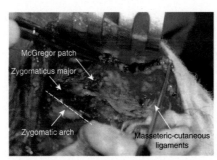

TECH FIG 4 • A SMAS flap is shown on the right side. It is initially incised along the zygomatic arch, elevated rapidly over the parotid gland, and then dissection carefully extended medially to expose the zygomaticus major and the masseteric-cutaneous ligaments. Small vessels are usually encountered anterior to the parotid gland (McGregor patch).

- After initial fixation in the preauricular area with a 4-0 Mersilene suture, the excess is either folded over superiorly to add volume or excised.
  - The flap is then sutured at the level of the zygomatic arch with interrupted 4-0 Mersilene sutures.
- The immediate preauricular portion of the SMAS flap is incised inferiorly while pulling on the cut end in a posterolateral direction in order to transpose the split portion of the flap behind the ear.
  - It is sutured to the mastoid fascia with 2-0 Maxon (polyglyconate) sutures chosen for their considerable strength, allowing maximum traction on the platysma component to improve cervical contour.
- The SMAS flap suture line is then oversewn with a running 4-0 PDS (polydioxanone) suture along the zygomatic arch and preauricular area.
  - The suture line is made smooth and isolates the parotid gland from the subcutaneous plane to help insure against fistula formation.

SMASectomy

- A line is first drawn over the zygomatic arch to properly orient SMASectomy design.
- A second line is drawn between the malar eminence and just above the angle of the mandible where the preparotid SMAS is still fixed to the gland.
- The SMAS is placed on traction below this line with Cushing forceps to assess the degree of soft tissue laxity and the amount of SMAS movement possible.
  - This is typically 1.5 to 2 cm at the angle of the mandible (less in secondary or tertiary face-lifts) with somewhat less as the malar area is approached.

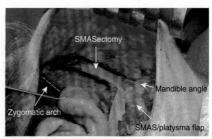

TECH FIG 5 • A SMASectomy excision is shown on the right side. The relation of the excisional design pattern to the zygomatic arch and angle of the mandible is illustrated, as is the SMAS/platysma transposition flap.

- A second parallel line is then drawn based on this maneuver to indicate the inferior border of the excision design.
- The area of SMAS between the two lines is then excised in portions, carefully observing the depth of the excision as this is done (**TECH FIG 5**).
  - Medially, where distal facial nerve branches become more superficial, the excision depth is more conservative.
- The lateral platysma is then mobilized as described for the SMAS flap and sutured in the mastoid area with 2-0 Maxon sutures.
- The cut edges of the SMAS are sutured with 4-0 Mersilene in interrupted fashion.
- A 4-0 PDS continuous suture is then placed to smooth contour over the suture line.

SMAS Plication

- The SMAS is marked identical to a SMASectomy design.
  - The SMAS within the marked pattern is plicated with interrupted 4-0 Mersilene sutures.
  - The lateral platysma is treated in the same fashion as described with SMASectomy.
- A 4-0 PDS continuous suture is then placed to contour smoothly over the suture line.
- After all SMAS techniques, the skin is examined to identify dimpling due to SMAS traction effects, with additional skin release performed as indicated. This is typically necessary in the midcheek but also commonly over the orbicularis oculi muscle above and in the neck below.
  - The midcheek release is done very conservatively to minimize the loss of beneficial skin movement resulting from SMAS tightening.

■ Anterior Neck Treatment

- The anterior neck dissection can be done either at the beginning of the procedure or after skin flap elevation and SMAS fixation. Expert opinion is mixed on this matter, although opening the anterior neck later seems to be more popular.
  - The theoretical concern in the debate is that tightening the SMAS first will restrict medial mobilization of

the platysma for plication, whereas approximating the platysmal bands first will limit the degree of SMAS tightening possible.
- Platysma bands less than 2.5 cm apart can usually be approximated in the midline whether or not this is done initially or after SMAS tightening.
  - Platysmal plication becomes more challenging as the gap between the muscle edges increases. It should probably be deferred when bands are 3 cm apart or

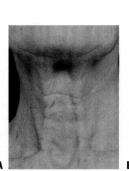
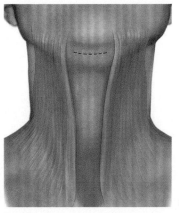
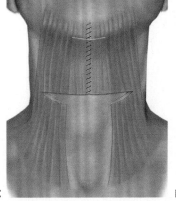
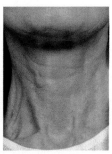

A   **B**   **C**   **D**

TECH FIG 6 • **A.** Example of full-length platysma bands. **B,C.** Repair includes approximating the free edges and dividing the muscle transversely. The muscle transection is performed low, where the muscle is thin and extends as far as 4 cm laterally. **D.** Result.

more, although dividing the muscle inferiorly improves medial mobilization considerably.

- The access incision for anterior neck dissection is placed in the submental crease although just posterior to this landmark is common practice.
- Liposuction is generally avoided although when done briefly with a small cannula can facilitate dissection.
- Subcutaneous skin elevation proceeds inferior to the cervicomental angle to the limits of visibility.
- Subcutaneous fat is conservatively removed by direct excision with care taken to leave adequate thickness and a smooth internal flap contour.
- Subplatysmal fat excision is performed following mobilization of the platysma edges in patients exhibiting an obtuse cervicomental angle.
- Submandibular gland resection and shave excision of the digastric muscles are considered only for extreme cases. The former requires considerable experience.
- The medial borders of the platysma are sutured together with interrupted 4-0 Mersilene sutures and can be reinforced with a second running layer of 4-0 Mersilene if desired (**TECH FIG 6**).
- A low transverse platysmal transection is performed bilaterally up to 4 cm, leaving at least a 2-cm lateral band of muscle intact over the sternomastoid muscle and external jugular vein.
- Correction of a "witch's chin" deformity can be performed by defatting the ptotic chin pad.
    - De-epithelializing an ellipse of skin at the submental incision and burying it can also help smooth out chin-neck junction depressions.
    - Occasionally, a conservative elliptical skin excision can aid reduction of submental skin redundancy.

Skin Redraping and Closure

- Both sides are closed at the end of the procedure, which is preferred to sequentially closing during the procedure. This allows hemostasis to be performed once after the SMAS treatment and for the second time just prior to final closure to provide two opportunities to confirm hemostasis.
    - Additionally, venous oozing on the flap undersurface will become more apparent later as the epinephrine wears off and also because each side has been

dependent while the other side is dissected. This helps prevent the development of small collections of venous blood under the flap postoperatively.

- Small-diameter closed suction drains are placed on each side if the anterior neck has not been opened. A single drain is passed all the way from one side to the opposite if the anterior neck has been opened.
- The skin is redraped in a superoposterior direction and anchored at the root of the helix with a 4-0 Vicryl suture.
    - Tension should not be excessive. Blanching of the skin flap and the appearance of traction lines should both be avoided.
- The skin is then placed on traction posteriorly and anchored with a 4-0 Vicryl suture at the highest point of the postauricular sulcus incision.
    - Excess occipital area skin is excised while maintaining the skin on tension with a hook.
    - That portion of the incision is closed with staples.
    - The remaining excess skin in the mastoid area is then conservatively trimmed so the edges appose with no gap.
    - Patients with short-scar postauricular incision design do not require any of these steps but simply a minimal trim of excess skin near the lobule (**TECH FIG 7**).
- The temporal incision is closed with clips with care taken not to raise the sideburn level. Little skin trimming is typically necessary because pre-excision has already been performed in this area.

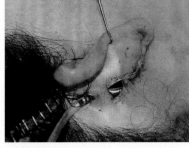

TECH FIG 7 • Closure of a short-scar postauricular incision on the right side is shown. Using the full length of the sulcus avoids creating pleats with a shorter incision.

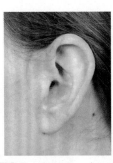 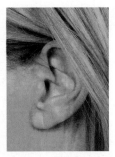

TECH FIG 8 • A,B. Examples of well-healed preauricular incisions that were properly designed and closed.

- This is the time when the need for a subsideburn incision is considered. This option prevents hairline elevation by excising a small wedge of skin. These incisions are typically short and heal inconspicuously. They are more commonly used in secondary or tertiary cases.
- Excess skin is trimmed in the preauricular area such that the edges are closely apposed with no tension required for the final closure.
  - Tragal skin defatting for retrotragal incision closure must be done conservatively and primarily at the edges in order to avoid vascular compromise of the skin.
- A 4-0 double-armed Monderm (glycolide and e-caprolactone) barbed suture is used for intracuticular closure of the preauricular and postauricular incisions.

- The suture starts at the lobule attachment point and runs anteriorly and posteriorly cephalad to complete closure.
- These incisions heal extremely well if properly designed and closed (**TECH FIG 8**).
- If indicated, a subperiosteal pocket is created over the mentum and a chin implant placed.
  - It is aligned with a midline skin marking made prior to surgery with the patient in a sitting position.
  - Curvilinear implants in small and extra small sizes are suitable for most female patients.
  - The implant is secured with several 4-0 Vicryl sutures. A running 5-0 nylon is used to close the submental incision after placement of a single 4-0 Vicryl dermal suture in the middle.

Ancillary Procedures

- Ancillary procedures such as perioral dermabrasion, periorbital (**TECH FIG 9A,B**).
  - Facial fat grafting is usually done early in the procedure, soon after fat preparation is complete.
- At the conclusion of the procedure, the skin flap color is assessed. If the skin is dusky in the preauricular or postauricular area or both, nitropaste is applied prior to placement of the dressing as a one-time treatment to reduce vascular congestion (**TECH FIG 9C,D**).
- A light head dressing is placed.

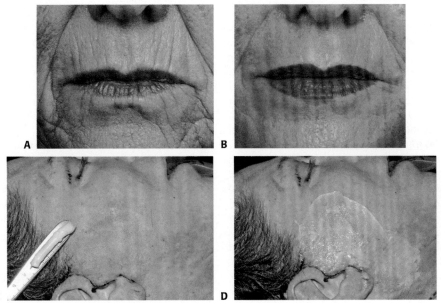

TECH FIG 9 • A,B. Resurfacing of the perioral area with dermabrasion or other modalities is commonly indicated. Care must be taken regarding depth of treatment in order to avoid causing hypopigmentation. **C,D.** Nitropaste is routinely placed on the cheeks and postauricular area to speed resolution of flap congestion.

PEARLS AND PITFALLS

Patient factors	■ Patients with BMI greater than 30, sleep apnea, or severe diabetes should have surgery in a hospital setting.
	■ Meticulous perioperative blood pressure control reduces hematoma rate.[7]
	■ Avoid operating on active smokers.
Incisions	■ Avoid pretrichial incisions and deep temporal dissection.
	■ Avoid tragal blunting with meticulous insetting technique.
	■ Use pretragal incisions for most men.
	■ Consider short-scar technique for young patients.
	■ Use subsideburn incisions to prevent hairline elevation.
Skin flap elevation	■ Avoid excessive medial cheek elevation.
	■ Perform more limited flap elevation in smokers.
SMAS technique	■ Use a SMAS flap for patients needing more midface correction.
	■ Use a SMASectomy in patients with prominent skeletal framework and lighter soft tissues.
	■ Use SMAS plication for patients with thin tissues and secondary or tertiary cases.
Neck treatment	■ Avoid opening the anterior neck when the medial platysmal borders are very widely separated and in smokers.
	■ Performing a low platysmal transection will allow the medial borders of the muscle to come together more easily.
	■ Avoid excessive subplatysmal tissue resection.
	■ Patients with severe cervical skin laxity should be advised initially that a secondary procedure may be necessary to achieve an optimal outcome.
Complications	■ Hematomas can be avoided with meticulous hemostasis and normotensive intraoperative blood pressure maintenance.
	■ Patients at high risk for MRSA infection should be cultured by nasal swab preoperatively and treated prior to surgery if positive.

POSTOPERATIVE CARE

- Ambulation is encouraged, beginning on the day of surgery.
- Cool compresses are useful for the first 24 hours.
- The head dressing is removed on the 1st postoperative day. Drains are removed on the 1st postoperative day if the anterior neck was not opened and on the 2nd day if it was.
- Aquaphor is placed on resurfaced areas until re-epithelialization has occurred, usually by 1 week.
- Oral antibiotics can be given for up to 1 week postoperatively although proof of benefit has not been established.
- Detailed written instructions are given regarding early postoperative conduct such as talking, positioning (awake and sleeping), hygiene, and activity restrictions.
  - Alcohol and excessive salt intake is discouraged for 2 weeks and smoking for 6 weeks following surgery.
- Patients are seen within 48 hours, at 6 days for suture removal, and typically at 6 weeks for further follow-up.

OUTCOMES

- Patients undergoing face-lifting and neck lifting can achieve very satisfying results when the most appropriate techniques are selected and expertly performed.
- Results in the cheek generally endure for about 10 years while ongoing aging changes in the neck become evident sooner.

COMPLICATIONS

- Massive hematomas of sudden onset require emergent evacuation.
  - Smaller or slow developing hematomas can often be managed by beside treatment with sterile catheter aspiration and irrigation with an epinephrine-containing solution.[8]

- Nerve injury
  - Great auricular nerve injuries should be immediately repaired with fine nylon sutures and the repair buried below the platysma muscle if possible.
  - Cervical branch paresis resulting from cautery or traction injury typically resolves by 6 weeks. If afflicted patients are able to purse their lips, this confirms that the mandibular branch is intact and spontaneous resolution can be expected. Neuromodulators can be helpful to disguise the injury, but their duration of effect is typically longer than the nerve recovery period.
  - Frontal branch injury is of greater concern because overlapping innervation is not typical in this area. Neuromodulator use is more applicable in this situation. Failure of the injury to resolve may be an indication for a brow lift.
- Infection
  - Patients should be routinely seen within 24 hours after surgery and by 48 hours at the latest. Significant postoperative infections become apparent early on and require aggressive treatment.
  - Early infection is typically bilateral and presents with dusky flaps and multiple small pustules in the preauricular and postauricular areas (**FIG 1**). Intravenous antibiotics should be instituted immediately. Vancomycin is the drug of choice to cover the possibility of MRSA infection. Patients can be managed with outpatient intravenous antibiotics but must be seen daily until resolution appears certain.
  - Delayed infection with *Mycobacterium fortuitum* is rare and insidious. It presents with numerous small erythematous nodules. Multiple debridements and prolonged antimicrobial therapy are typically required. Long-term outcome is generally excellent with little residual scarring evident.

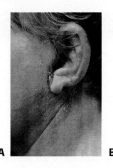 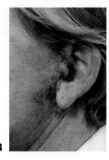 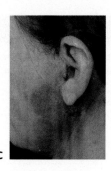

A   **B**   **C**

FIG 1 • **A.** Early appearance of infection, which is usually bilateral. **B.** Skin slough should not be debrided until sharp demarcation is evident. Ultimately, these problems usually heal well. **C.** Parotid fistulas are heralded by cheek erythema and high output of clear drainage.

- Evolving skin slough requires frequent monitoring and treatment with topical and oral antibiotics (**FIG 1B**).
  - Debridement, if necessary, is delayed until sharp demarcation is evident. Scar revision may be necessary at the appropriate time interval.
- Localized fluid masses in the cheek are usually venous collections that often not responsive to aspiration.
  - Evacuation of subcutaneous fluid collection through the preauricular incision, though seemingly an aggressive approach, offers a rapid and definitive end to the problem.
- Parotid fistula is a rare complication and is heralded by persistent high drainage output, predominantly clear, and cheek erythema (**FIG 1C**). A high amylase level in the fluid confirms the diagnosis.
  - A short trial of serial aspiration can be undertaken, but lack of response requires placement of a drain.
  - Injecting the gland with botulinum toxin is a helpful adjunct although this can result in visible gland atrophy, presumably short term.
- Excessive scarring results from either skin loss or excessive closure tension. Both are amenable to revision provided sufficient skin laxity is present.

- Hypertrophic healing tendency is a more common problem and can usually be successfully managed with serial steroid injections.

REFERENCES

1. Stuzin JM, Baker TJ, Gordon HL, Baker TM. Extended SMAS dissection as an approach to midface rejuvenation. *Clin Plast Surg.* 1995;22(2):295-311.
2. Baker DC. Lateral SMASectomy. *Plast Reconstr Surg.* 1997;100(2): 509-513.
3. Robbins LB, Brothers DB, Marshall DM. Anterior SMAS plication for the treatment of prominent nasomandibular folds and restoration of normal cheek contour. *Plast Reconstr Surg.* 1995;96(6):1279-1287.
4. Stuzin JM, Baker TJ, Gordon HL. The relationship of the superficial and deep facial fascias: relevance to rhytidectomy and aging. *Plast Reconstr Surg.* 1992;89(3):441-449.
5. Mitz V, Peyronie M. The superficial musculo-aponeurotic system (SMAS) in the parotid and cheek area. *Plast Reconstr Surg.* 1976;58(1):80-88.
6. Baker DC. Minimal incision rhytidectomy (short scar facelift) with lateral SMASectomy: evolution and application. *Aesthet Surg J.* 2001;21(1):14-26.
7. Trussler AP, Hatef DA, Rohrich RJ. Management of hypertension in the facelift patient: results of a national consensus survey. *Aesthet Surg J.* 2011;31(5):493-500.
8. Baker DC, Chiu ES. Bedside treatment of early acute rhytidectomy hematoma. *Plast Reconstr Surg.* 2005;115(7):2119-2122.

Indications and Technique for Extended SMAS Face-Lift and Necklift

James M. Stuzin and Sammy Sinno

DEFINITION

- Facial aging is the result of many changes that occur in the skin, soft tissues, fat, and facial skeleton.
- Early attempts at surgical facial rejuvenation were skin tightening procedures.
- The works of Skoog, Mitz, and Peyronie demonstrated that soft tissue repositioning of facial fat can restore a more youthful facial contour.[1]
- The primary advantage of skin and superficial musculoaponeurotic system (SMAS) flap elevation separately is greater aesthetic control in terms of repositioning facial fat independent of skin flap redraping.
- Another major advantage of an extended SMAS flap technique is the ability to restore facial shape of youth by building volumetric highlights over the anterior and lateral zygoma juxtaposed with submalar concavity.[2]

ANATOMY

- The layers of the face are skin, subcutaneous fat, SMAS, the muscles of facial expression, deep fascia or parotidomasseteric fascia, and the plane of the facial nerve, parotid duct, and facial vessels.
- The thickness of these layers, particularly the SMAS, varies region to region.
- The muscles of the face are all innervated on their deep surface except for the deepest muscles of facial expression, which are the mentalis, levator anguli oris, and buccinators.
- The parotidomasseteric fascia protects the facial nerve branches in the preparotid area (**FIG 1**).

PATIENT HISTORY AND PHYSICAL FINDINGS

- The patient presenting with facial and neck aging demonstrates volume decent, deflation, and radial expansion of facial soft tissue from the center of the face to the periphery.
  - The extended SMAS technique attempts to address these concerns by repositioning and conforming the descended facial fat to more aesthetically pleasing areas of the facial skeleton.
- On physical examination, the skin quality, elasticity, amount and location of subcutaneous fat, depth of the nasolabial fold, degree of jowling, deflation, skeletal support, malar convexity, and submalar concavity are noted.
  - Platysma position and descent are similarly examined.

SURGICAL MANAGEMENT

Preoperative Planning

- Patients are asked to bring pictures from their youth. Although patients cannot be made to look exactly like they were when younger, a similar facial shape to youth can be restored with this technique in many patients.
- Antibiotics are started 1 day before surgery and continue for 5 days afterward.
- An intertragal incision is marked along with a temporal incision and partial hairline retroauricular incision.

Positioning

- The patient is in a supine position for this procedure.
- Induction of anesthesia is achieved with midazolam and fentanyl.
- Ketamine is given for local injection, which is a mixture of lidocaine and bupivacaine.
- Propofol and valium drips are used on an as-needed basis at the discretion of the anesthesiologist.

Approach

- A submental incision just caudal to the submental crease is used for neck contouring.

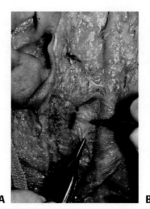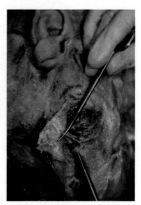

A   **B**

FIG 1 • **A.** Cadaver dissection in the parotid area showing the parotidomasseteric (or deep facial) fascia. **B.** When the parotidomasseteric fascia is reflected, the branches of the facial nerve are visualized.

■ Extended SMAS Face and Neck Lift

Incisions and Dissection

- The partial hairline retroauricular incision is made with a no. 15 blade.
- A no. 10 blade is used in the postauricular region for the adherent fascial dissection over the adherent cervical skin ligaments overlying the sternocleidomastoid (SCM).
- The other incisions are dissected with a no. 15 blade. In the temporal area, dissection is carried deep to the temporoparietal fascia. Deep dissection here protects the hair follicles and tends to be avascular. However, the superficial temporal artery must be ligated.
- The beginning of the subcutaneous dissection over the lateral fat compartment is fascial. Using facelift scissors, the interface between the SMAS and the fat can be precisely raised with transillumination.
- When extending the subcutaneous dissection inferiorly, take care to stay superficial above the cervical fascia overlying the SCM to avoid injury to the great auricular nerve.
- As the anterior subcutaneous dissection proceeds from the lateral to middle superficial fat compartment, the dissection becomes easier as proceeding distal to the ligaments overlying the parotid.
  - Skin flaps should be dissected thinner in the region overlying where the SMAS is to be dissected to leave more fat on the SMAS for subsequent SMAS flap elevation (and avoidance of tearing).
- In the neck, the dissection is carried in the interface between the preplatysma fat and the platysma. In other words, the fat is left intact on the skin flap, whereas the platysma muscle is kept down.

- Once over the zygoma, specifically where the arch and body meet, zygomatic ligaments are encountered, and it is easy to carry dissection deep to the SMAS.
- Along the inferior lateral border of the zygomatic eminence, the zygomatic cutaneous and upper masseteric ligaments emerge, as well as perforators from the transverse facial artery.
- The zygomatic branches of the facial nerve also are superficial in this region, and inadvertent dissection deep to the SMAS in this region may produce a motor branch injury.
- Avoid dissecting thick skin flaps in this region; it may be easier to work from above and below and connect in the middle in terms of defining the proper plane of dissection when working in this region of high ligamentous density within the midcheek. This region represents the transition between the middle and malar fat compartments.
- Avoid unnecessary dissection in the area of malar bags to avoid malar edema.
- After completing the subcutaneous dissection, the SMAS is injected with local anesthetic just prior to elevation.
- The incision begins along the zygomatic arch and then extends superiorly toward the lateral malar eminence at the junction where the arch and body of the zygoma intersect (**TECH FIG 1A**).
  - It then angles up toward the lateral canthus along the lateral orbital rim, then heads inferiorly toward the anterior extent of skin undermining.
  - The lateral incision follows the lateral border of the platysma inferiorly.
- SMAS elevation begins along the lateral border of the platysma using needle tip electrocautery.

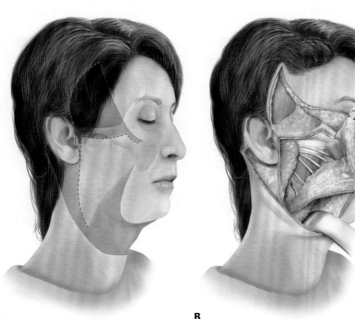

A   **B**

TECH FIG 1 • A. *Blue dashed line* shows extended SMAS flap incisions. *Pink* indicates the area of subcutaneous undermining. *Green* shows the superficial malar fat pad. **B.** The dissection is carried out past the tail of the parotid to ensure all of the retaining ligaments are released, which allows adequate SMAS mobility.

- Once sub-SMAS fat is encountered beyond the tail of the parotid, dissection can be performed bluntly, which will avoid injury to the marginal mandibular branch of the facial nerve (**TECH FIG 1B**).
  - The SMAS tends to thin over the accessory lobe of the parotid, lateral to the zygoma, and in the region of the transverse facial artery perforator; care should be taken not to tear the SMAS here.
- Once the dissection has passed the retaining ligaments,[3] dissection can stop, as further dissection will not provide additional benefit and can only serve to increase morbidity.

Redraping and Fixation

- A 3-0 Mersilene suture is placed vertically in the SMAS from the lateral incision along the zygomatic arch in front of the tragus to 5 to 6 cm below the earlobe. The exact vector of SMAS fixation will vary from patient to patient, but in most patients, a very vertical SMAS vector is utilized.
- Before definitive SMAS fixation, the skin is undermined a bit more anteriorly as necessary to avoid traction dimpling before the SMAS is fixated.
- The cephalic portion of the SMAS flap is rolled prior to fixation (**TECH FIG 2A**).
- 3-0 Mersilene is used for fixation in an interrupted fashion. Several sutures are placed. The endpoint is when malar convexity and submalar convexity is achieved.
- The lateral border of the platysma is fixated posteriorly to the mastoid fascia.
- Any fat irregularities on the SMAS are trimmed, particularly superiorly to avoid unsightly bulges.

- The submental incision is made 5 mm caudal to the submental crease.
- The crease is undermined, releasing the mandibular ligaments to obliterate the crease and optimize visualization.
- Subcutaneous undermining is performed.
- Preplatysmal fat is directly defatted. Subplatysmal fat in the midline is defatted on an as needed basis.
- The medial borders of the platysmal muscle are sutured with a 3-0 Mersilene suture in interrupted fashion. One or two sutures are placed caudal to the cervicomental angle and hyoid.
- The platysma is then divided inferiorly and laterally for approximately 5 cm (**TECH FIG 2B**). Care must be taken to avoid injuring the anterior jugular vein.
- After release of the platysma, additional Mersilene sutures are placed in the platysma to restore tension after platysma release and allow the platysma to conform to the floor of the mouth and thyroid cartilage.
- Meticulous hemostasis is obtained.
- Two drains are placed from the retroauricular incision extending to the base of the neck.
- The skin is carefully redraped and trimmed without any tension. The skin is usually redraped with a posterior lateral vector as opposed to the vertical vectoring of the SMAS flap.
- Skin incisions are closed with 4-0, 5-0, and 6-0 nylon sutures.
- Any fat injections are performed following the closure of the facial and submental incisions.
- A light head dressing is placed prior to arousal from anesthesia.

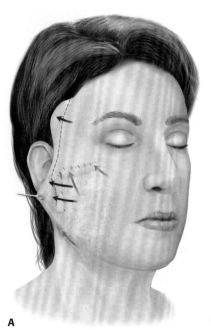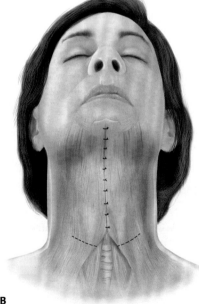

TECH FIG 2 • A. The SMAS flap is rolled then sutured with several 3-0 Mersilene sutures. **B.** The platysma is approximated from the mentum to the cricoid cartilage, followed by a horizontal cut on each side, which extends to the SCM.

A

B

PEARLS AND PITFALLS

Aesthetic considerations	■ The major advantage of the extended SMAS flap is that it allows a building of the volumetric highlights of the upper face over the lateral zygoma, restoring the malar convexity of youth; raising the skin and SMAS as separate flaps allows a greater degree of aesthetic control in terms of vector redraping. ■ Contrasting malar convexity with submalar concavity is a transition seen in youth and should be a goal in aesthetic repositioning and conforming of facial soft tissues while combating radial expansion. ■ Avoid cross-cheek depression ("joker lines"); if noted intraoperatively, fat can be added to the submalar region to ameliorate. In patients with tendency to cross-cheek depressions, vertical vectors in skin flap redraping should be avoided.
Dissection	■ The subcutaneous dissection is the most challenging portion of the procedure; use transillumination for precision. ■ By taking advantage of knowledge of the anatomy in the cheek, one can appreciate the subcutaneous dissection as it transits from lateral to medial to superficial malar cheek compartments. ■ Be careful when dissecting between the medial and malar cheek compartments; there is retaining ligamentous density, perforators from the transverse facial artery, and zygomatic facial nerve branches important for smile symmetry transiting in this area. ■ If the skin flap is raised without precision, it is often impossible to raise a substantial SMAS flap. ■ The SMAS flap must be raised beyond the accessory lobe of the parotid to ensure all retaining ligaments have been released.
Sequence	■ Perform SMAS fixation first, followed by medial platysma suturing, then platysma release and more platysma suturing as needed
Neck	■ Opening the neck offers the greatest aesthetic control in improving cervical contour.
Hematoma	■ If performing dissection deep in the temporal area and exposing the superficial temporal artery, ligation is necessary to avoid postoperative hematoma. ■ Always take time to ensure meticulous hemostasis. ■ Perioperative blood pressure control is critical to avoid a postoperative hematoma.
Drains	■ Leaving drains in longer (3–4 d) allows removal of serum that would otherwise build up and cause induration and/or bruising. ■ Place drains extending to the base of the neck.

POSTOPERATIVE CARE

- The light dressing is removed in 24 hours.
- The head remains elevated at all times, but neck flexion is not permitted.
- The drains are removed at 4 days to remove as much serous fluid as possible; this reduces induration and swelling.
- Sutures in the preauricular area removed between 5 and 7 days, with remaining sutures remove on postoperative day 10.
- If patients develop induration (commonly over the platysma plication), dilute Kenalog is injected.
- Dilute Kenalog is also injected into any persistent drain sites.

OUTCOMES

- With the extended SMAS technique, natural and hopefully long-lasting results can be obtained that restore facial shaped of youth (**FIG 2**).

COMPLICATIONS

- Hematoma (most common)
- Nerve injury
- Aggressive scarring
- Edema/ecchymosis (temporary)
- Seromas
- Infection
- Contour irregularity

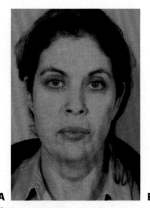 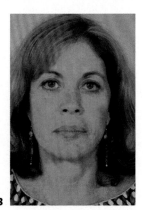

A **B**

FIG 2 • Preoperative and postoperative views of a patient who underwent an extended SMAS facelift. Notice restoration of facial shape with malar convexity, submalar concavity, a cleaner jawline, and improvement in the appearance of the neck.

REFERENCES

1. Mitz V, Peyronie M. The superficial musculo-aponeurotic system (SMAS) in the parotid and cheek area. *Plast Reconstr Surg.* 1976;58(1): 80-88.
2. Stuzin JM. Restoring facial shape in face lifting: the role of skeletal support in facial analysis and midface soft-tissue repositioning. *Plast Reconstr Surg.* 2007;119(1):362-376.
3. Furnas DW. The retaining ligaments of the cheek. *Plast Reconstr Surg.* 1989;83(1):11-16.

Lamellar High SMAS Face-Lift

Dino Elyassnia and Timothy Marten

DEFINITION

- As face-lift techniques have evolved, it has become clear that an attractive and natural appearance is not possible without diverting tension away from the skin to the superficial musculoaponeurotic system (SMAS) and platysma.
- Using the skin as the vehicle to support sagging tissue will always result in poor scars, tragal retraction, earlobe malposition, and a tight unnatural look.
- The SMAS, however, is capable of providing sustained support to facial tissues while allowing only redundant skin to be excised and wound closure under no tension. This averts a tight, "pulled" appearance and produces high-quality scars.
- A SMAS flap is a reliable and time-tested method of treating the SMAS and has been shown to provide excellent long-term outcomes. A flap is likely less destructive to the SMAS compared to various plication techniques and can be easily raised in secondary and tertiary procedures when carried out skillfully.
- The conventional "low" cheek SMAS flap elevated below the zygomatic arch suffers from the drawback that it cannot, by design, have an impact on tissues of the midface and infraorbital region. Planning the flap "higher" along the superior border of the zygomatic arch provides the biomechanical means by which a combined and simultaneous lift of the midface, lower cheek, and jowl can be obtained and avoids the need to perform a separate mid–face-lift (**FIG 1**).

ANATOMY

- The great auricular nerve is a sensory nerve derived from the cervical plexus and provides sensation to the earlobe and lateral cheek (**FIG 2**). It runs obliquely from the posterior belly of the sternocleidomastoid muscle to the earlobe. The classic external landmark to locate the nerve is at the mid-belly of the sternocleidomastoid muscle 6.5 cm inferior to bony external auditory canal.[1] The most common area of injury is where the nerve emerges from around the posterior border of sternocleidomastoid muscle.
- The facial nerve emerges through the stylomastoid foramen and is immediately protected by the parotid gland. Within the parotid, it divides into an upper and lower trunk and then into its five major branches: the frontal, zygomatic, buccal, marginal mandibular, and cervical (**FIG 3**). The branches leave the parotid gland lying on the surface of the masseter immediately deep to the parotidomasseteric fascia. Medial to the masseter, the nerve branches lie on the buccal fat pad

and at the same depth as the parotid duct and facial vessels. The nerve branches then proceed to innervate the mimetic muscles on their deep surface (except for the deep layer of muscles, mentalis, levator anguli oris, and buccinator).
- The retaining ligaments of the face (**FIG 4**) are vertically oriented fibers that penetrate the concentric horizontal layers of the face and function in a supportive role.[2,3] There seems to be two types of retaining ligaments:
  - The first type is true osteocutaneous ligaments that run from the periosteum to the dermis and are made up of the zygomatic and mandibular ligaments.
  - The second type of retaining ligaments is formed by a coalescence of superficial and deep facial fascia that form fibrous connections vertically spanning from deep structures such as the parotid gland and masseter muscle to the overlying dermis. Examples of these include parotid and masseteric cutaneous ligaments.
- The parotid cutaneous ligaments span over the entire surface of the parotid gland.
- The masseteric cutaneous ligaments are a series of fibrous bands that are found along the entire anterior border of the masseter muscle starting in the malar region down to the mandibular border.

PATIENT HISTORY AND PHYSICAL FINDINGS

- A focused history should include all previous cosmetic surgery or treatments including previous face-lifts, injectables, or laser treatments.
- To determine the proper location for the temporal portion of the face-lift incision, each patient's cheek skin redundancy must be examined, and location of temple and sideburn hair noted. Assessing cheek skin redundancy requires pinching up redundant skin over the upper cheek and measuring it. Also, the distance between the lateral orbit and anterior aspect of the temporal hairline must be measured. In youthful individuals, the distance should measure no more than 4 to 5 cm (**FIG 5**).
- If cheek skin redundancy is small and ample temple and sideburn hair is present, a temple incision can be placed within the temple scalp (**FIG 6A**).
- When the temporal hairline is predicted to shift more than 5 cm away from the lateral orbit or sideburn shifted above the junction of the ear with the scalp, a temple hairline incision should be used (**FIG 6B**). Failure to follow this plan can result in unnatural shifting or displacement of the temporal hair.

Low SMAS

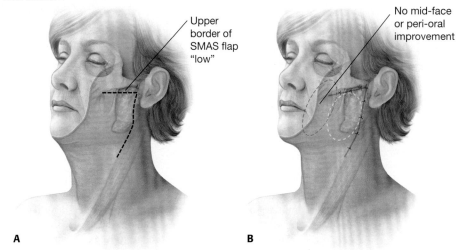

Upper border of SMAS flap "low"

No mid-face or peri-oral improvement

A   **B**

High SMAS

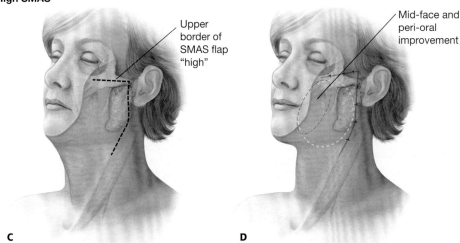

Upper border of SMAS flap "high"

Mid-face and peri-oral improvement

C   **D**

FIG 1 • "High" and "low" SMAS techniques compared. **A.** Plan for low SMAS procedure. Note that upper border of the flap lies *below* the zygomatic arch. **B.** Low SMAS flap after dissection and suspension. Area of flap effect (*green solid circle*) is limited to the lower cheek and jowl, and no improvement is obtained in the midface, infraorbital, or perioral regions (*black dashed circle*). **C.** Plan for high SMAS procedure. Note that upper border of the flap lies *over* the zygomatic arch. **D.** High SMAS flap after dissection and suspension. Area of flap effect (*green solid circle*) includes not only both the cheek and jowl but the midface, infraorbital, and perioral regions (*black dashed circle*) as well.

■ Like the temple, planning the appropriate location for the occipital incision requires examining each patient's neck skin redundancy. This is done like the cheek and entails pinching up tissue over the upper lateral neck and measuring it.

■ If 2 cm or less of excess neck skin is present, the incision can be placed transversely, high on the occipital scalp into the hair.

■ If more than 2 cm of neck skin redundancy is present, the incision should be placed along the occipital hairline but then turned into the scalp at the junction of the thick and thin hair at the nape of the neck (**FIG 7**). Failure to follow this plan can result in a visible notching of the occipital hairline.

IMAGING

■ Typically, radiographs are not necessary in facial rejuvenation surgery.

■ All patients should have standardized photographs taken preoperatively, and any markings made preoperatively on patients should be photographed as well.

■ These photos should be used intraoperatively to help guide treatment.

SURGICAL MANAGEMENT

■ A lamellar dissection for a high SMAS face-lift involves elevating the skin and SMAS as separate layers so that they can be advanced "bidirectionally" along different vectors and suspended under differential tension. Because skin and SMAS age at different rates and along somewhat different vectors, a lamellar strategy is needed to address each layer individually and to create a natural improvement.[4,5]

■ On the other hand, if a composite dissection is performed, the skin and SMAS must be advanced with the same amount in the same direction under more or less similar tension, which can result in skin overshifting, skin overtightening, and other unnatural appearances.

Preoperative Planning

■ All patients undergo a preoperative physical evaluation, and patients with significant medical problems must be cleared by their internist.

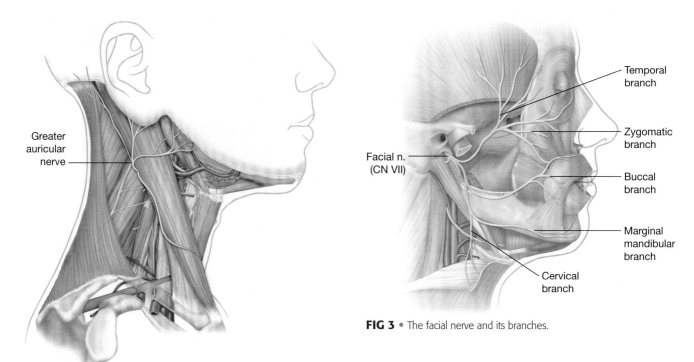

FIG 2 • The great auricular nerve can be seen lying over the midbelly of the sternocleidomastoid muscle 6.5 cm below the external auditory canal.

FIG 3 • The facial nerve and its branches.

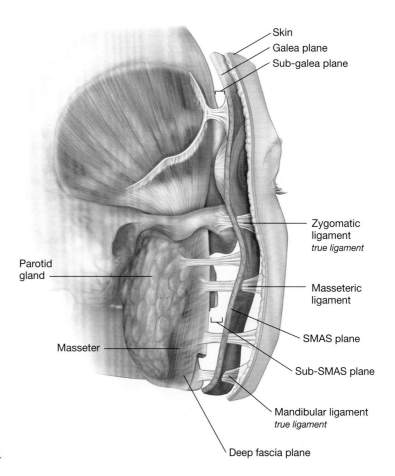

FIG 4 • The retaining ligaments of the face.

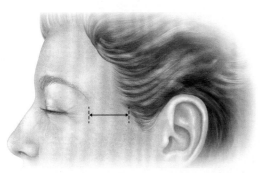

FIG 5 • Assessing "temporal skin show." The distance between the lateral orbit and the temple hairline and how it will change with skin flap shift must be considered when planning the temple portion of the face-lift incision.

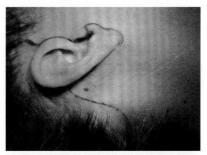

FIG 7 • Plan for incision along the occipital hairline. An incision along the occipital hairline should be considered whenever objectionable displacement of the occipital hairline is predicted. This incision plan protects the hairline and prevents hairline displacement. (Courtesy of T. J. Marten, MD, FACS.)

- Patients are required to avoid all medications or supplements that increase the risk of bleeding for 2 weeks prior to surgery.
- All patients who smoke are asked to quit 4 weeks before their procedure and are required to avoid smoking and all secondhand smoke for 2 weeks after. Patients who smoke or have a significant history of smoking are advised in writing that their risk of serious complications is significantly higher than is that of nonsmokers.
- Patients are instructed no to color, "perm," or otherwise chemically treat their hair for 2 weeks before surgery and after surgery as this can result in hair breakage and hair loss.
- It is important that adequate OR time be allotted for contemporary face-lift procedures. A high SMAS face-lift, when performed in conjunction with foreheadplasty, eyelid surgery, fat injections, or other facial procedures, will often take up to 6 to 8 hours or more. It is strongly recommended that any surgeon new to these techniques consider staging a full-face rejuvenation over 2 separate days. Typically, face-lift and neck lift are performed the first day, and the patient is then kept overnight and then returned to the OR the following day or a few days later for the remainder of the procedures.

Positioning

- The majority of our face-lifts are performed under deep sedation administered by an anesthesiologist using a laryngeal mask airway (LMA).

- The patient is placed supine on a warmed and well-padded operating table with special effort made to ensure that all pressure points are well protected.
- The patient's lower extremities are then elevated and anti-embolic pedal compression devices applied.
- Each patient receives a full surgical scrub of the entire scalp, face, ears, nose, neck, shoulders, and upper chest with full-strength (1:750) benzalkonium chloride (Zephran) solution. The head is then placed through the opening of a "split sheet" leaving the entire head and neck region including the scalp unobstructed from the clavicles up.
- The breathing circuit is draped separately from the patient by wrapping it with a sterile sheet that allows it to move during the procedure as the patient's head is turned from side to side.
- After the general prep and draping, the surface of the ear is prepped with Betadine using cotton swabs, and then Kittner "peanut" sponges are placed in each auditory meatus.

Approach

- 0.25% bupivacaine with epinephrine 1:200 000 is used for sensory nerve blocks and for infiltrating the area marked for incision. Areas of subcutaneous dissection are infiltrated with 0.1% lidocaine with epinephrine 1:1 000 000.
- All incisions on the scalp or along scalp-skin interfaces must be made precisely parallel to hair follicles to avoid injury to them that can result in peri-incisional alopecia.

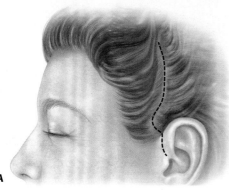
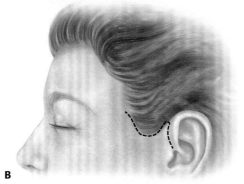

A   **B**

FIG 6 • **A.** Plan for incision on the temporal scalp. This plan is used for patients predicted to have minimal or modest shift of sideburn and temple hair after elevation of the cheek flap. It will *not* be appropriate for all patients. **B.** Plan for incision along the temporal hairline. An incision along the temporal hairline should be considered whenever objectionable displacement of the sideburn and temple hair is predicted.

- The prehelical portion of the preauricular incision should be made as a soft curve paralleling the curve of the anterior border of the helix. As the tragus is approached, the incision is carried into the depression superior to it.
- Next, the incision is carried precisely along the posterior margin of the tragus in a retrotragal position. This location provides for the best option for avoiding a color or texture mismatch in the preauricular skin and the best concealment of the scar.

- At the inferior portion of the tragus, the incision must turn anteriorly and then again inferiorly into the crease between the anterior lobule and cheek. This creates a distinct inferior tragal border.
- The incision will then continue around the lobule and then precisely within the auriculomastoid crease. The occipital and temple portions of the incision are made according to the preoperative plan (see above).

■ Skin Flap Elevation

- Cheek flap dissection is begun using Adson forceps and a small Kaye scissors or scalpel grasping only tissue edges that will later be excised. Once the edge is elevated, gentle traction is applied by the assistant with double-pronged skin hooks.
- Dissection is then carried out using medium Metzenbaum scissors with the surgeon and assistant working together using a "four-handed" technique (**TECH FIG 1A**):
  - The assistant applies gentle skin traction upon the skin flap directed toward the surgeon with one double-pronged skin hook in each hand, while the surgeon dissects and provides gentle countertraction toward the assistant with the fingertips of the nondominant hand.
  - As the dissection advances, one skin hook is exchanged for a small Deavor malleable-type retractor, and the remaining skin hook is used to drape the flap over the retractor.

- Proper assistance will require two team members scrubbed with the surgeon. One team member will need to be committed to providing retraction, while a second member is needed to manage all tasks related to passing of instruments.
- The assistant must be taught to not apply excessive force on delicate skin flaps, and the surgeon must avoid retracting for herself or himself as this invariably leads to rough handling of the flap.
- Skin flaps should be elevated sharply under direct vision and blind dissections avoided. This is especially important in the preauricular area and over the cheek where a deep dissection can injure the underlying superficial musculoaponeurotic system (SMAS) and compromise its use as a flap. However, dissection too close to the posterior surface of the skin flap can result in injury to the subdermal microcirculation.

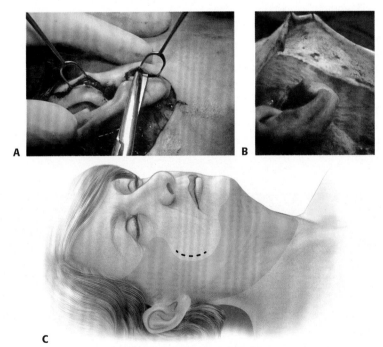

TECH FIG 1 • "Four-handed" technique. **A.** The assistant applies gentle traction upon the skin flap toward the surgeon with two large double-pronged skin hooks with one retractor held in each hand. The surgeon then dissects while providing gentle countertraction toward the assistant with the fingertips of the opposite hand. **B.** Appearance of a transilluminated skin flap in the cheek. If dissection is in the proper plane as in this case, the undersurface of the flap will have a rough, "cobblestone" appearance to the fat. **C.** Extent of subcutaneous undermining. *Shaded area* shows area of subcutaneous undermining. Note that the platysma-cutaneous ligaments (*black dots*) are not undermined and are preserved. Preservation of platysma-cutaneous ligaments and proper elevation and fixation of the SMAS will provide support of lateral perioral tissues.

T E C H N I Q U E S

- Some visual clues can be helpful in determining the proper plane for dissection. This will require proper lighting and transillumination of skin flaps. If dissection is too deep, the underside of the flap will appear smooth and cloudy when transilluminated. If dissection is in the proper plane, however, transilluminated flaps will have a rough, "pebbled," or "cobblestone" appearance (**TECH FIG 1B**).
- Postauricular skin flap undermining is most easily begun inferiorly if the occipital incision is made along the occipital hairline as more subcutaneous fat is usually present and the proper plane is easier to identify compared to more superiorly where less subcutaneous fat is present and the skin and fascia lie in close proximity. Once the proper plane is established, two large double-pronged skin hooks are placed by the assistant, and the dissection continues posterior to anterior rather than superior to inferior.
- As the dissection progresses toward the upper lateral neck, care must be taken to avoid injury to the greater auricular nerve.
- As dissection is continued further anteriorly into the cervical region, subcutaneous fat becomes more abundant, and the flap is easier to dissect; however, care should be taken to remain in a subcutaneous plane. Compared to the cheek skin flap that must be kept thin, a thicker layer of fat can be kept on the undersurface of the cervical flap. However, the majority of preplatysmal fat should be kept on the platysmal surface as this makes fat sculpting easier later in the procedure.
- If a submental incision is planned, completing dissection of the anterior neck skin flap will be more easily performed through it rather than the postauricular incisions. (For planning the submental incision, see "Neck Lift" chapter).
- The neck should be undermined completely in most cases, but it should not arbitrarily include the entire face (**TECH FIG 1C**). Preservation of the anterior platysma-cutaneous ligaments will create attractive and youthful appearing elevation of perioral tissue that cannot be obtained with wide undermining. If these platysma-cutaneous ligaments are divided in the perioral cheek, the SMAS effect on this area will be negated, and the benefit of SMAS elevation will be lost.

■ Temple Dissection

- The temple incision is made either on the temporal scalp or along the anterior hairline based on the preoperative plan.
- When on the temporal scalp, the incision is taken down to the deep temporal fascia, and the temporal hair-bearing flap is undermined in the subgaleal plane anteriorly to the lateral brow, inferiorly to the mid temple, and superiorly to the temporal line.
- The bridge of fascia (mesotemporalis) between the deep dissection in the temple and the subcutaneous dissection in the cheek can be partially divided posterior to the temporal hairline (**TECH FIG 2A**). Usually, this bridge of tissue contains the anterior branch of the superficial temporal artery and must be ligated. The frontal branch

of the facial nerve lies anterior and inferior to this vessel and is safe.
- This method of dissection promotes the two planes of dissection to be joined to improve exposure.
- When an incision along the temporal portion of the anterior hairline is indicated, it is made a few millimeters within it with a slight bevel or parallel to the hair follicles.
- The incision should be made no higher than the junction of the temporal hairline with the frontotemporal hairline. If carried any higher, the scar can be visible as hair tends to grow posteriorly in this area.
- After the incision is made along the hairline, the skin flap is raised in the subcutaneous plane connecting with the cheek skin flap dissection, and no transition between planes is necessary (**TECH FIG 2B**).

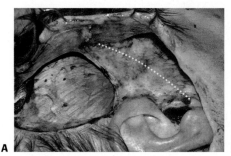
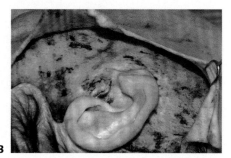

TECH FIG 2 • A. Dividing the mesotemporalis. The bridge of tissue situated between the subfascial (subgaleal) dissection in the temple and the subcutaneous dissection in the cheek can safely be divided posterior to the course of the frontal branch of the facial nerve (*white dotted line*). This bridge of tissue usually contains the anterior branch of the superficial temporal artery which must be divided and cauterized or ligated (*black arrows*). **B.** Flap dissection with hairline incision. When an incision along the temporal hairline is used, all dissection will be in a subcutaneous plane, no transition between planes will be necessary, and the superficial temporal vessels are left undisturbed, beneath the superficial temporal fascia.

■ SMAS Dissection

- To begin, markings are made for the SMAS flap. A line is marked "high" over the midportion of the zygomatic arch from the infraorbital rim to a point 1 centimeter anterior to the superior portion of the tragus. The marking is then turned inferiorly and carried over the preauricular portion of the parotid 1 to 2 cm anterior to the ear and continued inferiorly and posteriorly to the anterior border of the sternocleidomastoid (**TECH FIG 3A**).

- Flap elevation is begun by incising the SMAS over the zygomatic arch. This is done by grasping the preauricular tissue overlying the lateral arch with an Allis clamp on each side of the marked line. Metzenbaum scissors are then used to incise along the marking medially for a few centimeters. Allis clamps are then released and reapplied incrementally as the incision proceeds medially along the marked line. A considerable amount of tissue lies over the arch, and the frontal branch will be safely beneath half a centimeter or more of fibrous fat.

- The preauricular limb of the SMAS incision is then made using the same technique, and these two incisions define the "high" SMAS flap to be elevated.

- Next, the corner of the flap is grasped with Allis clamps, and elevation is begun with scissors. Undermining should be limited in the preparotid cheek, more extensive over the zygoma and upper midface (**TECH FIG 3B**).

- Sharp scissors dissection of the flap is usually required posteriorly over the parotid where the plane between parotid fascia and SMAS is often indistinct. If a portion of the parotid fascia is incidentally raised with the SMAS flap in exposing the lobular surface of the gland, this is of no clinical significance and should be used by the surgeon as an aid in identifying the proper plane slightly more superficial.

- A distinct plane does exist, however, medial to the parotid between the SMAS-platysma and the parotidomasseteric fascia. This plane is most easily identified in the lower cheek where it can be entered by gentle blunt dissection. The parotidomasseteric fascia will be seen as a thin, shiny transparent layer covering the masseter, buccal fat, and facial nerve branches. Blunt dissection on top of this layer is safe; however, care must be taken to not violate this layer as it can result in a facial nerve injury. Sub-SMAS dissection must be carried over the anterior border of the parotid in the lower cheek to ensure the parotidomasseteric ligaments are released; otherwise, an optimal SMAS effect will not be obtained.

- As SMAS flap dissection is made medially in the upper cheek over the superior portion of the parotid and its accessory lobe, the SMAS will be seen to thin and invest the lip elevators. At this point, the dissection must be taken superficial to the superior portion of the zygomaticus major muscle. Just at the malar origin of this muscle, the zygomatic ligaments will be found. These fibrous connections between periosteum and skin must be divided, and when completely released, a dramatic liberation of the flap will be obtained.

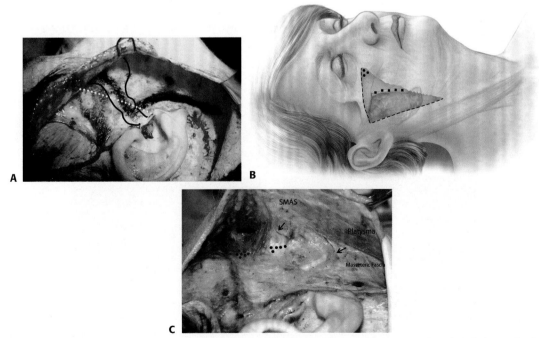

TECH FIG 3 • Plan for "high SMAS" flap. **A.** The superior margin of flap is planned over the zygomatic arch and not below it. The frontal branch of the facial nerve (*dashed line*) lies safely posterior and deep to the majority of the dissection. **B.** Approximate extent of SMAS undermining. Complete release of the SMAS flap will require that both the parotidomasseteric ligaments (*squares*) and the zygomatic ligaments (*circles*) be released. **C.** Completed SMAS flap elevation. Inferior to the origin of the zygomaticus major muscle (*large arrow*), and superomedial to the accessory lobe of the parotid, lies the zone of transition between the zygomatic (*blue dots*) and masseteric-cutaneous ligaments (*black dots*) and the most potentially dangerous part of the SMAS dissection. Proper liberation and release of the SMAS flap usually require at least partial division of restraining attachments in this area but move the dissection into very close proximity to the zygomatic branch of the facial nerve (*small arrow*).

■ Directly inferomedial to the origin of the zygomaticus major muscle, and superomedial to the accessory lobe of the parotid, lies the zone of transition between the zygomatic and masseteric-cutaneous ligaments and the most dangerous part of the SMAS dissection. Proper liberation of the SMAS flap usually requires at least partial division of restraining ligaments in this area but moves the dissection into very close proximity to the zygomatic branches of the facial nerve (**TECH FIG 3C**).

■ In this area, it can be difficult to distinguish between nerve branches and ligamentous attachments. The inexperienced surgeon should consider using loupe magnification and the use of a disposable nerve stimulator to aid in the dissection. If confusion is encountered or the anatomy is unclear, it is better to limit dissection in this area until additional experience is gained as no amount of improvement in SMAS release is worth a facial nerve injury.

■ The endpoint to the SMAS dissection is ultimately clinical and not anatomic. Gentle traction on the superior margin of the flap should produce motion at the nasal ala, philtrum and stomal angle, and elevation of infraorbital and lower eyelid tissue. If there is limited movement with this traction test, then residual tethering fibers are identified and released and the traction test repeated.

■ SMAS Suspension

■ Once the SMAS flap has been properly released, it should be shifted in a posterior-superior vector parallel to the long axis of the zygomaticus major muscle. If a more vertical or posterior vector is used, the function of the zygomatic major muscle will be corrupted, and abnormal appearances during animation may result.

■ The technique of flap suspension will vary depending on overall facial morphology. In most cases, no trimming of the superior margin of the flap is performed as the overlapping tissue segments of SMAS add volume to the zygomatic arch. In cases where a temporal scalp incision is used, the superior edge of the flap is anchored well over the zygomatic arch directly to the deep temporal fascia using 3-0 Vicryl or Mersilene (**TECH FIG 4A**). Suspension in this manner is greatly facilitated if the mesotemporalis is gently pushed inferiorly as sutures are placed. No suturing is needed more medially over the zygoma or along the infraorbital rim as this can result in unnatural tissue tethering and dimpling.

■ When an incision along the temporal hairline is used, the deep temporal fascia will not be exposed. In these cases, the galea can be incised just inferior to the sideburn to expose the deep temporal fascia. The SMAS can then be anchored as described above (**TECH FIG 4B–E**).

■ In patients with a wide midface (ie, Asian or Slavic ancestry) or in many men, overlapping the SMAS may not be artistically appropriate. In such cases, the redundant tissue along the superior edge of the flap can be excised, and the flap margin sutured edge to edge to the superior margin of the initial incision made in the SMAS over the zygomatic arch.

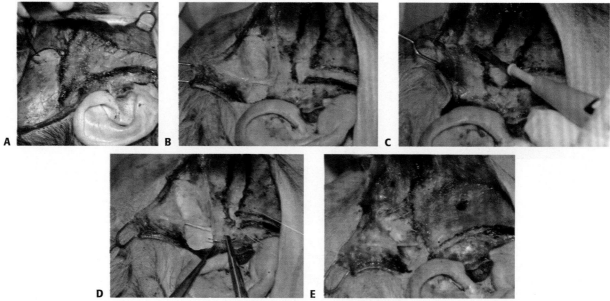

TECH FIG 4 • High SMAS flap suspension with a temporal scalp incision. **A.** The SMAS flap has been advanced superiorly, the mesotemporalis pushed inferiorly, and the flap secured to the temporalis muscle fascia. **B–E.** High SMAS flap suspension with temporal hairline incision. To gain access to the temporalis muscle fascia to suspend the SMAS, the sideburn is retracted and the galea incised **(B)**. Completed incision of the galea under the sideburn exposing the temporalis muscle fascia. Once incised, a "mesotemporalis" (transition from subcutaneous plane of cheek to subgaleal plane in temple) is created **(C)**. The suture has been placed through the corner of the SMAS flap. Note that the mesotemporalis is being pushed inferiorly as the suture is placed **(D)**. Additional sutures have been placed between the superior margin of the SMAS flap and the temporalis muscle fascia, securely anchoring the flap. Once suspension of the SMAS is complete, the sideburn is placed back in a proper anatomic place and anchored down **(E)**.

- Regardless of how the superior margin of the flap is secured, some trimming of the posterior margin of the flap is needed to facilitate edge-to-edge approximation to the posterior flap incision as overlapping here is artistically inappropriate. This should be done after the superior margin of the flap is secured.
- Unlike the superior margin of the flap, it is counterproductive to place tension on the posterior margin of the flap. Thus, the posterior margin should be trimmed conservatively to avoid a tight closure.
- To provide additional support to the anterior neck and improve contour, the excess tissue along the posterior margin of the SMAS flap can be trimmed but left attached inferiorly to the platysma and used as a postauricular transposition flap (see **FIG 1C**).

- Due to the increased length obtained with this transposition flap, it can be sutured to the immobile mastoid fascia by creating a dynamic sling that tightens the submental region when the patient looks down. This tightening is obtained because the mastoid moves superiorly with neck flexion pulling the flap up with it.
- When designing the postauricular transposition flap, the SMAS must be incised low enough so that this flap exerts its effect on the platysma below the mandibular border so as to improve submental contour.
- When using the postauricular transposition flap in conjunction with anterior platysmaplasty, the transposition flap should be secured after anterior platysmaplasty is completed or else it may not be possible to approximate the platysma anteriorly.

■ Skin Flap Repositioning, Trimming, and Closure

- Skin flap repositioning should be performed with the patient's head in a neutral position. To avoid unnatural appearances, the skin flaps must be shifted in a slightly more posterior direction than that of the SMAS. Also, it is critical to remember that the goal of skin excision is to remove redundancy and not tighten the skin flap.
- Cheek skin flaps should be shifted along a vector roughly perpendicular to the nasolabial fold, while neck skin should be shifted along a vector parallel to the mandibular border.
- There are two points of skin flap suspension that set the stage for the remainder of the closure. The first point is located just above the ear where the anterior-superior most part of the ear joins the scalp. The cheek flap is shifted and the redundancy gauged with a face-lift marker (**TECH FIG 5A**). The flap should be held under just greater than normal skin tension when the mark is made and a small "T" shaped incision made into the flap at the marked point. The flap is then anchored at this point with a half-buried vertical mattress suture of 4-0 nylon with the knot on the scalp side.
- The second key point of suspension is in the postauricular area at the superior aspect of the occipitomastoid incision. The flap is shifted roughly parallel to the mandibular border so that skin is suspended under minimal or no tension and that little or no skin needs to be trimmed from the anterior flap border that will be sutured to the postauricular incision. The flap is secured with a simple suture of 4-0 nylon; no incision into the flap is necessary.
- Once these two key sutures are placed, the flap overlying the inferior portion of the ear should be carefully divided and the lobule exteriorized. This is a key step and must be performed incrementally and with great care to avoid earlobe malposition. If this is done properly, the apex of the incision should sit snugly against the inferior most portion of the conchal cartilage.
- Skin flap trimming and incision closure should begin in the postauricular area along the auriculomastoid sulcus. Little to no skin needs to be trimmed from the anterior border of the postauricular flap, and the incision is

closed with several interrupted sutures of 4-0 nylon. If it appears that a large amount of skin needs to be excised from this area, the flap has been shifted too far anteriorly and superiorly and should be adjusted.
- Next, trimming and closure of the occipital portion of the incision are performed. If the occipital incision has been made along the occipital hairline as usually most appropriate, skin will only be excised along the posterior border of the postauricular skin flap. It is incorrect to excise any skin over the apex of the occipitomastoid incision as this will lead to a wide scar (**TECH FIG 5B**). A face-lift marker is used to gauge redundancy, and the flap is trimmed so that closure is performed under no skin tension and the wound edges about one another before sutures are placed. Closure is then performed with multiple half-buried vertical mattress sutures of 4-0 nylon and simple interrupted sutures of 6-0 nylon.
- The preauricular area is closed next. Skin flap redundancy should be carefully gauged using a face-lift marker, whereas the pretragal portion of the skin flap is held down into the pretragal hollow with an instrument by the assistant. This ensures that enough skin is present to fill the pretragal sulcus and provide natural preauricular contours. The prehelical portion of the flap is trimmed to fill in the prehelical incision without any skin tension. This is closed in one layer using interrupted 6-0 nylon or running 6-0 polypropylene.
- The prelobular (subtragal) portion of the cheek skin flap is trimmed next using a similar technique of marking excess with the face-lift marker and closed under no tension in a single layer with several interrupted 6-0 nylon sutures.
- Once the prehelical and prelobular areas have been closed, the tragal flap is trimmed. As elsewhere in the preauricular closure, the tragal flap must be trimmed with slight redundancy with the assistant holding the pretragal portion of the skin flap down into the pretragal hollow. Trimming the tragal skin flap too short is an error that will result in tragal retraction and an unnatural "chopped off" appearance. The tragal flap does not need to be thinned except at its posterior margin, and closure is done in one layer as above.

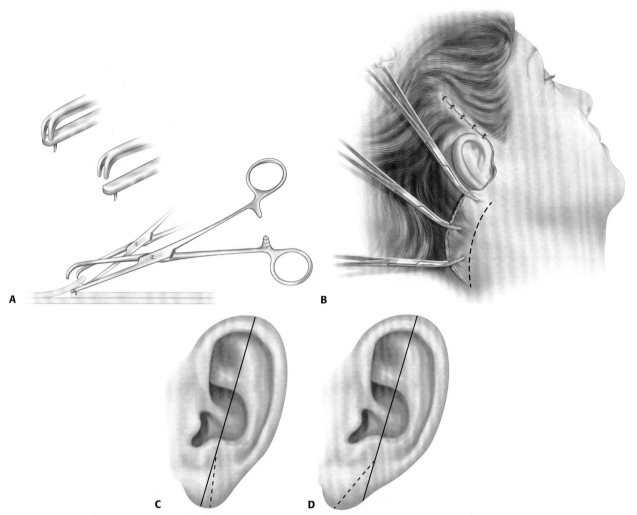

TECH FIG 5 • A. The face-lift marker. The use of a flap marker provides a reliable means for appropriate excisions of skin to be made. The pin on the lower jaw of the marker is placed near the edge of the incision. The skin flap is then draped over the lower jaw of the instrument, and the instrument is closed. On closing, the upper jaw of the instrument marks the precise position of the edge of the scalp flap beneath it. **B.** *Incorrect* trimming of postauricular skin flap. It is an error to excise any skin over (superior to) the apex of the occipitomastoid incision and shorten the post-auricular flap along the long axis of the sternocleidomastoid muscle. There is no true excess of skin along this vector nor any aesthetic benefit from shifting skin in this direction. **C,D.** Proper insetting of the earlobe. In the artistically ideal "nonsurgical" appearing ear, the long axis of the earlobe (*dotted line*) sits approximately 15 degrees *posterior* to the long axis of the ear itself (*solid line*) in the lateral view **(C)**. As this angle is reduced, or the axis of the lobule shifted anterior to the long axis of the ear, an old, unnatural, and "face-lift look" is produced **(D)**.

- There is nothing as telltale as an abnormal position of the earlobe, and for this reason, the lobule should be inset as the last step in the preauricular closure. The cheek flap should be trimmed and the earlobe inset so that the lobule ends up situated in a posterior and somewhat superior position even if it was in a more anterior and inferior position before surgery. This is because the long axis of a natural appearing earlobe ideally sits approximately 15 degrees posterior to the long axis of the ear itself (**TECH FIG 5C,D**). As this shifts anteriorly or too far inferiorly, an unnatural "face-lift look" is produced. Insetting the lobule in the proper position often requires the lobule be released from tethering tissue. It is then secured in two layers to protect the incision in the first few weeks from disruption when patients pull clothing, jewelry, and other items off over their heads. If the lobule is inset

correctly, often skin redundancy will be present on the posterior surface of the ear. This can be easily treated by excising a triangle of skin in this area.

- If the temporal portion of the face-lift incision has been made on the temporal scalp, the incision is closed in one layer without excision of any hair-bearing temporal tissue. A small amount of cheek skin and scalp only will be excised immediately above the ear. If the temporal incision has been made along the hairline, skin only will be conservatively trimmed and closure performed in one layer without any skin tension using a combination of half-buried vertical mattress 4-0 nylon sutures and simple interrupted 6-0 nylon sutures.

- After all planned procedures have been completed, the patient's hair is shampooed, rinsed, and detangled, and no dressings are required or applied.

PEARLS AND PITFALLS

Incision planning	■ Proper analysis, careful planning, and the use of an incision along the hairline when indicated can avert hairline notching and displacement without compromising the overall outcome. ■ This is particularly true of patients with marked skin redundancy and those presenting for secondary problems.
Skin tension	■ Skin was not meant to support sagging tissues, only redundant tissue is removed, and closure must be made under normal skin tension.
SMAS design	■ Planning the SMAS flap "high" over the zygomatic arch provides an improvement to the midface in addition to the jawline.
SMAS elevation	■ Key zygomatic and masseteric cutaneous ligaments must be released, but the endpoint of the dissection is clinical and not anatomic.
SMAS suspension	■ A lamellar dissection allows the SMAS to be suspended in a more superior vector compared to the skin.
Skin trimming	■ Inappropriate excision of the skin over the apex of the occipitomastoid defect is the cause of hypertrophic healing in the postauricular area.

POSTOPERATIVE CARE

■ Most patients are discharged to an aftercare specialist for the first night with specific instructions. Patients are asked to rest quietly and apply ice compresses to their eyes for 15 to 20 minutes every hour they are awake for the first 3 days.

■ All patients are provided oral analgesics, sleeping pills, antiemetics, ophthalmic ointment, and eye drops.

■ All patients are instructed to sleep flat on their backs without a pillow or with a small cylindrical neck roll. This posture assures an open cervicomental angle and averts folding of the neck skin flap. Patients are also shown an "elbow on knees" position to ensure an open cervicomental angle while sitting.

■ Patients begin a daily routine of showering and shampooing no later than 3 days after their procedure to help remove crusting at suture lines, keep bacteria count down, and improve overall well-being. Patients should be warned that their scalp and parts of their face may be partially numb and should be careful when showering that water is not too hot and that hairdryers are not on high settings.

■ Drains are usually left in the neck until the first postoperative visit 4 to 5 days after surgery. Sutures are removed in two visits over a period of 7 days.

■ Patients are asked to set aside 2 to 3 weeks to recover from surgery. If the patient is doing well, they can return to light office work and casual social activity 9 to 10 days after surgery. Patients are advised to avoid all strenuous activity during the first 2 weeks after surgery. Two to three weeks after surgery, they are allowed to begin light exercise and gradually work up their activity as tolerated by 6 weeks.

■ Patients are informed that it will often take 2 to 3 months to look good in a photo or to be seen at an important social function.

OUTCOMES

■ See **FIGS 8** to **10**

COMPLICATIONS

■ The most common complication is a hematoma. The incidence ranges from 2% to as high as 10%. The incidence is higher in men and patients with a history of hypertension. Preoperative measures to reduce the risk include control of blood pressure and avoidance of medications and supplements that may affect bleeding. Intraoperative maneuvers include close cooperation with the anesthesiologist to rigorously control blood pressure along with meticulous hemostasis.

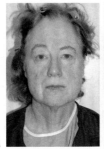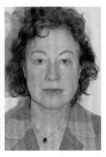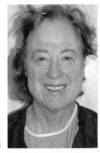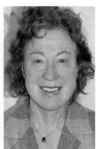

A   **B**

FIG 8 • A. AP view. On the left, preoperative view of a woman, age 65. She has had previous upper and lower eyelifts performed by another surgeon. Note midface, cheek, and jawline laxity and poor transition from lower eyelid to malar area. On the right, same patient, 13 months after high SMAS face-lift, neck lift, hairline lowering forehead lift, upper and lower eyelifts, perioral dermabrasion, and fat transfer to the cheeks and lips. No skin resurfacing, facial implants, or other ancillary procedures were performed. The midface, cheek, and jowl have been repositioned harmoniously and in a uniform and balanced manner. Note smooth facial contours, more youthful facial shape, and absence of a pulled or a "face-lifted" appearance. **B.** AP view smiling. On the left, preoperative view of a woman, age 65. She has had previous upper and lower eyelifts performed by another surgeon. Note that but improvement along the jawline can be seen when the patient smiles, but midface ptosis and cheek laxity are accentuated. On the right, same patient, 13 months after high SMAS face-lift, neck lift, hairline lowering forehead lift, upper and lower eyelifts, perioral dermabrasion, and fat transfer to the cheeks and lips. The midface, cheek, and jowl have been repositioned harmoniously and in a uniform and balanced manner. Note soft, natural facial contours and the absence of a tight, pulled, or "face-lifted" appearance.

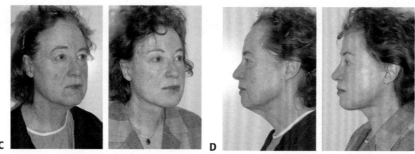

FIG 8 (Continued) • **C.** Oblique. On the left, preoperative view of a woman, age 65. She has had previous upper and lower eyelifts performed by another surgeon. Note sagging midface, cheeks, and jowl, and infraorbital hollowness. On the right, same patient, 13 months after high SMAS face-lift, neck lift, hairline lowering forehead lift, upper and lower eyelifts, preoral dermabrasion, and fat transfer to the cheeks and lips. The midface, cheeks, and jawline have been repositioned in a balanced and harmonious fashion. Note also the improved transition from lower eyelid to malar region. **D.** Lateral view. Preoperative view of a woman, age 65. She has had previous upper and lower eyelifts performed by another surgeon. Note sagging mid-face, cheek and jowl, and poor transition from lower eyelid to malar area. Same patient, 13 months after high SMAS face-lift, neck lift, hairline lowering forehead lift, upper and lower eyelifts, perioral dermabrasion, and fat transfer to cheeks and lips. The midface, cheek, and jowl have been repositioned harmoniously and in a balanced manner. Note also improved transition from lower eyelid to cheek.

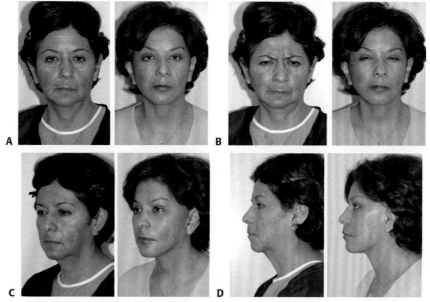

FIG 9 • **A.** AP view. On the left, preoperative view of a woman, age 55. Note midface ptosis, heavy jowls, deep nasolabial lines, and poor jawline contour. She has had no prior plastic surgery. On the right, same patient, 1 year 6 months after high SMAS face-lift, neck lift, limited incision forehead lift, and upper lower eyelifts, chin augmentation, and fat transfer to the lips and cheeks. No skin resurfacing or other ancillary procedures were performed. Midface, cheek, and jowl have been repositioned harmoniously and in a uniform and balanced manner. Note smooth facial contours, more youthful facial shape and absence of a pulled or a "face-lifted" appearance. **B.** AP Frowning. On the left, preoperative view of a woman, age 55 frowning. She has had no prior plastic surgery. On the right, the same patient, 1 year 6 months after High SMAS face-lift, neck lift, limited incision forehead lift, upper and lower eye blepharoplasties, chin augmentation, and fat transfer to the cheeks and lips. She is trying to frown in this photograph but is no longer able to do so due to muscle modification performed as part of the forehead lift procedure. **C.** Oblique view. On the left, preoperative view of a woman, age 55. Note midface ptosis, sagging cheek, and jowl, and perioral laxity. She has had no prior plastic surgery. On the right, same patient, 1 year 6 months after High SMAS face-lift, neck lift, limited incision forehead lift, upper and lower blepharoplasties, chin augmentation, and fat transfer to the cheek and lips. The midface, cheek, and jowl have been repositioned harmoniously in a balanced manner. Note smooth facial contours, more youthful facial shape. **D.** Lateral view. On the left, preoperative view of a woman, age 55. Note midface ptosis, sagging cheek, and jowl and poor transition from lower eyelid to malar area. She has had no prior plastic surgery. On the right, same patient, 1 year 6 months after High SMAS face-lift, neck lift, limited incision forehead lift, upper and lower eyelifts, chin augmentation, and fat transfer to cheeks and lips. Note restoration of attractive malar contour, improved transition from lower eyelid to cheek, elevation of perioral area, and well-defined jawline.

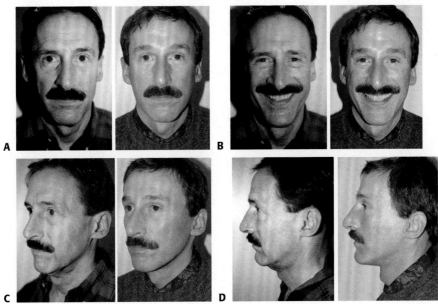

FIG 10 • A. AP view. On the left, preoperative view of patient, age 60. Atrophy in the infraorbital, perioral, and upper midface regions is evident. Loss of attractive facial contour due to deep tissue ptosis can be seen in the cheek, jowl and perioral regions. On the right, the same patient, 14 months after high SMAS face-lift, neck lift, closed foreheadplasty, conservative upper and lower blepharoplasty and partial facial fat injections. Fat injections have provided filling of the infra-orbital and per-oral areas. Note restoration of youthful facial shape without a tight or pulled appearance. **B.** AP smiling view. On the left, preoperative view of patient, age 60. On the right, the same patient, 14 months after high SMAS face-lift, neck lift, closed foreheadplasty, conservative upper and lower blepharoplasty, and partial facial fat injections. Note natural contour is present, even in animation. **C.** Oblique view. On the left, preoperative view of patient age 60. Note lateral brow ptosis, mid-face ptosis and loss of youthful malar, perioral and mandibular contour. On the right, the same patient, 14 months after high SMAS face-lift, neck lift, closed foreheadplasty, conservative upper and lower blepharoplasty and partial facial fat injections. Note improved brow position, restoration of cheek fullness, improved transition from lower lid to cheek, elevation of ptotic perioral tissue, smooth jawline and improved submental contour. **D.** Lateral view. On the left, preoperative view of patient age 60. Note malar flattening, perioral laxity, ptotic jowl and cervicosubmental laxity. A prominent submandibular gland can also be seen. On the right, the same patient, 14 months after high SMAS face-lift, neck lift, closed foreheadplasty, conservative upper and lower blepharoplasty and partial facial fat injections. The protruding portion of the submandibular gland has also been excised. Note the restoration of cheek fullness, elevation of ptotic perioral tissue, smooth jawline and improved cervicosubmental contour. The face has a natural appearance, and all scars are well concealed (Courtesy of T. J. Marten, MD, FACS).

Most hematomas will occur in the first 12 hours postoperatively so close monitoring in the recovery and over the first evening is critical. This includes proper management of pain, anxiety, blood pressure, and nausea.

- A less common complication is skin slough which is most commonly the result of tension. Skin slough resulting from underlying circulatory problems includes smoking, acne scarring, and diabetes.
- One of the most devastating complications after a face-lift is facial nerve injury. Fortunately, the incidence is less than 1%. The facial nerve branches most at risk include the buccal, frontal, and marginal mandibular.

REFERENCES

1. McKinney P, Katrana DJ. Prevention of injury to the great auricular nerve during rhytidectomy. *Plast Reconstr Surg* 1980;66:675-679.
2. Furnas DW. The retaining ligaments of the cheek. *Plast Reconstr Surg* 1989;83:11.
3. Stuzin JM, Baker TJ, Gordon HL. The relationship of the superficial and deep facial fascias: relevance to rhytidectomy and aging. *Plast Reconstr Surg* 1992;89:441-449.
4. Marten TJ. Face lift planning and technique. *Clin Plast Surg* 1997;24: 269-308.
5. Marten TJ. Lamellar high SMAS face and midface lift. In: Nahai F, ed. *The Art of Aesthetic Surgery.* St. Louis, MO: Quality Medical Publishing; 2005:1110-1192.

45
CHAPTER

SMASectomy Face-Lift

Steven M. Levine and Daniel C. Baker

DEFINITION

- Surgery is the standard for addressing descent and laxity in the aging face.
- SMASectomy refers to the removal of a strip of superficial musculoaponeurotic system (SMAS) at the junction of the fixed and mobile SMAS.

ANATOMY

- Relevant anatomy is the recognition of the difference between fixed and mobile SMAS. The location of this intersection varies between patients but is roughly found on a diagonal line connected the earlobe to the lateral canthus (**FIG 1**).

PATIENT HISTORY AND PHYSICAL FINDINGS

- Beyond usual history and physical findings to indicate a patient for a face and neck lift, the specific question to note is whether the patient has a full, wide face or a thinner face that could benefit from SMAS being "stacked" on itself to add volume.
- The authors refrain from providing specific guidelines or measurements as the ultimate decision is a function of the aesthetic sense of the surgeon.

SURGICAL MANAGEMENT

- Surgery should be performed in an accredited operating room.
- SMASectomy can be performed under local anesthesia with or without sedation or general anesthesia.

Preoperative Planning

- Consideration should be given as to whether the surgeon believes the patient will benefit from an SMASectomy (removal of tissue) or a plication (imbrication of tissue); however, this decision can also be made intraoperatively.
- The rest of the surgery is planned like any other biplanar face-lift.

Positioning

- The patient is supine on the procedure table.
- Usually, the head of bed is slightly elevated.
- The authors prefer to sit for maximum stability.

Approach

- An incision pattern is chosen (either preauricular or intratragal).
- The skin is elevated in the subcutaneous plane after infiltration with local anesthesia with epinephrine.
- The SMAS is identified, and a plan is created.

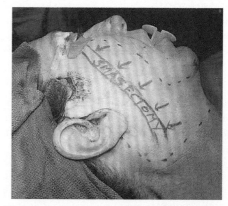

FIG 1 • Although the junction of the fixed and mobile SMAS may vary from patient to patient, it is generally found near a line from the lobule of the ear to the lateral canthus.

SMASectomy

- The area of superficial musculoaponeurotic system (SMAS) to be removed is best visualized after performing a lateral platysmaplasty.[1]
- A lateral platysmaplasty is performed by elevating the SMAS/platysma flap just in front of the sternocleidomastoid (SCM) muscle.
  - The author prefers to do this with a Bovie electrocautery, though any means is acceptable.
  - The flap should be elevated to allow the SMAS/platysma to freely rotate in a chosen vector cephalad and lateral to the surgeon's desires.
- The flap is then fixed to mastoid fascia with 3-0 PDS sutures and can be reinforced to the fascia of the SCM.
- Once this flap is secured, a bunching of tissue can be noted, usually near the angle of the mandible.

- This bunching is the most proximal component of the SMAS to be removed as a dog-ear, which is in effect the SMASectomy (**TECH FIG 1A**).
  - Scissors can be used to spread beneath the SMAS to safely develop the plane over the parotid fascia.
  - Care must be taken to protect the facial nerve until the distal portion of parotid fascia.
- To achieve a midface elevation, the SMASectomy must be carried out to the midface, beyond the parotid fascia (**TECH FIG 1B**).
- The edges of fixed and mobile SMAS are reapproximated using buried interrupted 3-0 PDS sutures (**TECH FIG 1C**).
- The SMAS is trimmed of irregularities.
- The skin flap is redraped, trimmed, and sewn under no tension.
- The authors prefer to leave drains, but this understandably varies between surgeons.

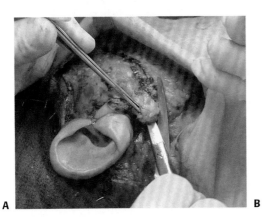

A

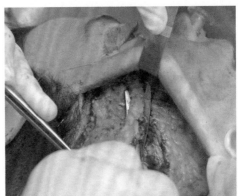

B

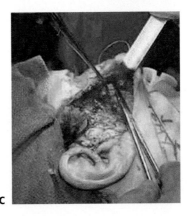

C

TECH FIG 1 • **A.** Tissue bunching near the angle of the mandible indicates a common starting point for the SMASectomy. **B.** The SMASectomy is carried anteriorly past the parotid tail to achieve midface elevation. **C.** The edges of the SMAS are reapproximated.

PEARLS AND PITFALLS

Technique	▪ Doing lateral platysmaplasty prior to SMASectomy will set up the exact starting point for the SMASectomy.
Facial nerve	▪ Facial nerve is protected over the parotid gland. Beyond the parotid gland, it is important to note the depth of your excision and take extra caution.
Suturing	▪ Always bury knots to avoid seeing or feeling bumps through the facial flap. ▪ Always check the facial surface after each SMAS suture. If too much or too little movement, remove suture and replace.

POSTOPERATIVE CARE

- Cool packs are also used to reduce swelling.
- Strict blood pressure control is enforced postoperatively.
- Patients are instructed to avoid lifting or bending for 2 weeks.
- The authors prefer to place patients in a face and/or neck compressive dressing for at least 4 to 6 hours after surgery but up to 24 hours.
- Drains are usually removed at 48 hours.
- All patients are seen by the surgeon the following morning and then again multiple times over the following week.
- Sutures are usually removed at 1 week.

OUTCOMES

- SMASectomy can achieve excellent jawline contour and midface elevation.

- The amount of midface elevation is dependent on how high the SMAS is operated on during the procedure.

COMPLICATIONS

- Bruising and hematoma are the most common complications.
- Hematomas in males are twice as common as they are in females.
- Facial nerve injury should be exceedingly rare with these techniques and should only be temporary when observed.

REFERENCE

1. Baker DC. Lateral SMASectomy, plication and short scar facelifts: indications and techniques. *Clin Plast Surg.* 2008;35(4):533–550, vi. doi:10.1016/j.cps.2008.06.003.

Indications and Technique for Deep Plane Face-Lift

Thomas A. Mustoe

DEFINITION

- Facial aging is caused by relaxation and descent of the deeper layers of the face, including the subcutaneous fat, and the underlying superficial fascial layer that encompasses the superficial muscles as well as the skin.
- Because these layers are closely adherent, the deep plane face-lift recognizes the principles that in order to properly correct the relaxation and descent, all layers must be addressed with complete release, even tension, and avoidance of excess tension on the skin to achieve reliably a natural appearance.

ANATOMY

- The critical anatomy to understand is the makeup of the superficial musculoaponeurotic system (SMAS) or fascia, which is a thin fascia layer just deep to the subcutaneous fat. It is contiguous with the platysma muscle and is continuous to the inferior surface of the orbicularis oculi muscle.
- There are retaining ligaments that are collagen attachments passing from the SMAS to the deeper tissues, which in the midface region are just lateral to the origin of the zygomaticus major muscle (the zygomatic retaining ligaments) and in the region of the superior most portion of the platysma muscle (masseteric retaining ligaments).
- In the neck, the retaining ligaments or deep attachments are along the posterior border of the SMAS, just anterior to the greater auricular nerve, and run obliquely down the neck where they have attachments to the sternocleidomastoid muscle. There are also attachments in the region of the anteroinferior portion of the parotid gland.
  - For the SMAS to be completely mobile, all of these attachments must be divided.[1]
- Immediately underneath the SMAS are the branches to the facial nerve.
- In the neck, the cervical branch comes out from the parotid and up into the platysma anterior to the retaining ligaments at the anteroinferior edge of the platysma and can be safely preserved while fully releasing the SMAS.[1]
- The marginal mandibular branch is well protected underneath the masseteric fascia.
- The major buccal branch runs just above the Stensen duct and is underneath the very thin deep fascia overlying the buccal fat pad, which is more easily penetrated, meaning that nerve is less well protected but easily seen.
- The zygomatic branch runs underneath the zygomaticus major muscle and thus is protected.
- Finally, the frontal branch becomes more superficial above the zygomatic arch. Dividing the SMAS at the level of the arch protects the frontal branch while still allowing elevation of the malar fat pad with the SMAS if the dissection extends below the inferior edge of the orbicularis oculi muscle to preserve innervation to that muscle.

NATURAL HISTORY

- The aging process with relaxation of the SMAS and fat as well as overlying skin is progressive, with loss of collagen fibers and increasing viscoelasticity of the overlying skin.[2,3]
- However, the aging process is genetically highly variable. In patients of Asian background, for instance, the skin is somewhat thicker, and the retaining ligaments are stronger, and so development of jowls and malar descent is less pronounced with age.
- In addition, there is loss of facial fat with age particularly around the mouth, and to a variable degree in the cheeks, so that facial rejuvenation usually includes some degree of volume restoration, particularly around the mouth.
- Fat also accumulates in the submental region, and in some patients (small percentage), a true excess accumulates in the jowl region, which when combined with loss of fat in the prejowl perioral area accentuates the loss of a firm jawline.

PATIENT HISTORY AND PHYSICAL FINDINGS

- The characteristic features of the aging face are development of jowls, malar descent, loss of facial fat, accumulation of submental fat, relaxation of the orbicularis muscle and overlying skin, and relaxation of the platysma muscle and overlying skin.
- In many patients, the relaxation of tissues is more pronounced in one region than another.

NONOPERATIVE MANAGEMENT

- Although nonoperative management of the aging face with fillers and fat, as well as noninvasive and minimally invasive techniques using laser, focused ultrasound, and radiofrequency, has increased greatly, there are limitations.
- More advanced relaxation of the skin and deeper tissues can only be corrected with a face-lift.

SURGICAL MANAGEMENT

- The author performs a deep plane rhytidectomy in all patients who are candidates for face-lift, even those with changes limited to the neck and/or jowls, without significant changes in the midface.
- What does vary is the extent of the dissection. In patients who are mainly concerned about the neck and jowls with

early aging changes, undermining and release of the SMAS in the midface can be quite limited without extending out to the masseteric and zygomatic retaining ligaments, but a deep plane dissection is still done in the neck.

- The incisions can also be limited with a postauricular incision limited to the sulcus, and the preauricular retrotragal incision also limited. With a more limited dissection, the recovery period is accelerated.
- Although the submental fat, including subplatysmal fat, and superficial release of skin attachments is always addressed with fine handheld cannulas through two or three 2-mm incisions, as the author's experience has increased, a submental incision is never done except in the occasional patient 6 months postoperatively who is bothered by persistent platysmal bands in the postoperative period.
- The main steps of the procedure are as follows:
  - Make a retrotragal incision with superior and postauricular extensions.
  - Raise a superficial skin flap, which is elevated above the zygomatic arch to the lateral border of the orbicularis oculi muscle, and below that over the lateral cheek over several centimeters.
  - Incise the SMAS at the level of the zygomatic arch, extending out to the orbicularis oculi muscle and in front of the ear. A portion of the SMAS is then elevated lateral to the retaining ligaments.
  - The postauricular dissection is carried out deep to the superficial fascia over the investing fascia of the sternocleidomastoid muscle.
  - The sub-SMAS dissection is then extended in a wide arc in front of and inferior to the ear until all of the retaining ligaments are released, and the SMAS slides easily along with the overlying skin.
  - Deep sutures are placed anchoring and repositioning the SMAS.
  - Excess skin and SMAS are cut, and final skin suturing is complete.

- The neck is addressed as described above with blunt undermining and liposuction with the use of fine cannulas.
- The other side is performed in identical fashion.

Preoperative Planning

- The patient should be medically cleared for surgery, including a recent normal electrocardiogram.
  - If the electrocardiogram is abnormal, consideration of specific cardiac clearance may be indicated including other studies such as a stress test.
- Hypertension must be well controlled, and clonidine is routinely given as a preoperative dose of 0.1 to 0.3 mg to minimize postoperative hypertension, which is a major risk factor for postoperative hematoma.
- Smoking must be stopped at least 3 weeks prior to surgery, and if there is any concern about smoking cessation, strong consideration should be given to measuring nicotine levels.
- The risks are discussed prior to surgery including hematoma, infection, skin necrosis, facial nerve injury, and the limitations of loss of elasticity, which means that some relaxation of tissues is inevitable in the postoperative period and must be viewed as a limitation rather than a failure of the procedure.

Positioning

- Positioning is straightforward in the supine position, with the head slightly elevated (10 degrees is sufficient) to enhance venous return.
- The head should be placed on a flat surface for easy turning.

Approach

- Usually, a full-length incision as described below is used, but when aging changes are early, the incision can be limited behind the ear to the postauricular sulcus and in front of the ear to the level of the superior edge of the tragus and to the top of the ear without extending underneath the sideburn.

T E C H N I Q U E S

■ Modified Deep Plane Rhytidectomy with Midface Elevation and Elimination of Submental Incision

Markings and Incisions

- The markings are consistent whether male or female and can be shortened for short scar technique or face-lifts with more limited dissection and less tissue rearrangement.
- The essential steps are an extension above the helix into the hair directly vertically; a V-shaped extension along the sideburn, stopping at the anterior point where the hair is no longer growing down to hide the incision; a retrotragal incision, taking care to have sharp angles rather than curves at the superior edge and incision of the tragus; and a postauricular incision that curves up high on the mastoid and into the hairline at approximately the superior edge of the tragus (**TECH FIG 1A**).
- In a subcutaneous plane, the cheek skin is elevated to the lateral edge of the orbicularis oculi muscle (**TECH FIG 1B**).
- An incision is made through the SMAS at the level of the zygomatic arch (high enough to allow the midface

to come up as part of the SMAS) and in front of the ear, and the SMAS elevation is begun extending to the extent of the previous subcutaneous dissection (**TECH FIG 1C**).

SMAS Dissection

- The dissection is begun behind the ear below the level of the superficial fascia and further inferior with exposure of the vestigial postauricular muscle, the greater auricular nerve, and the investing fascia of the sternocleidomastoid muscle (**TECH FIG 2A**).
- Sharp dissection is carried around the ear lobule, connecting the anterior sub-SMAS dissection with the posterior dissection and taking care to elevate the entire SMAS, which extends to the greater auricular nerve.
  - The parotid fascia is exposed, and the SMAS is clearly demarcated by its dense collagen content (**TECH FIG 2B,C**).
- The sub-SMAS dissection is then extended beyond the parotid gland anteriorly to expose the masseteric fascia. This is easily done and is avascular except for an occasional perforating vessel (**TECH FIG 2D,E**).

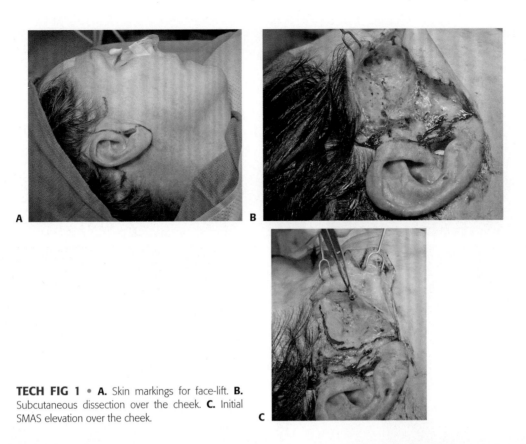

TECH FIG 1 • **A.** Skin markings for face-lift. **B.** Subcutaneous dissection over the cheek. **C.** Initial SMAS elevation over the cheek.

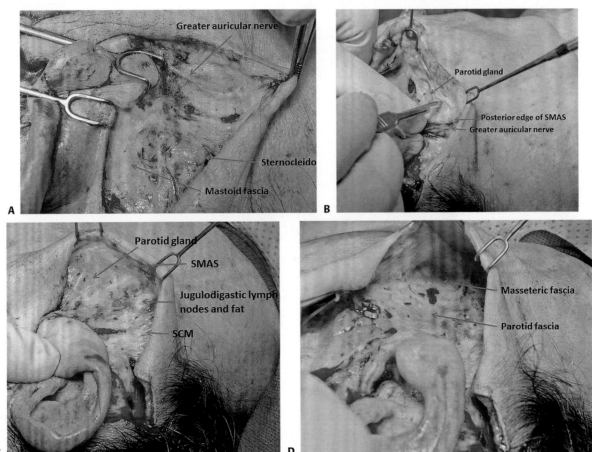

TECH FIG 2 • **A.** Initial dissection in the neck with exposure of greater auricular nerve. **B.** Initial elevation of SMAS over parotid and extending posteriorly. **C.** Exposure of parotid fascia with transition zone between parotid and SCM. **D.** Completion of dissection over parotid with exposure of masseteric fascia.

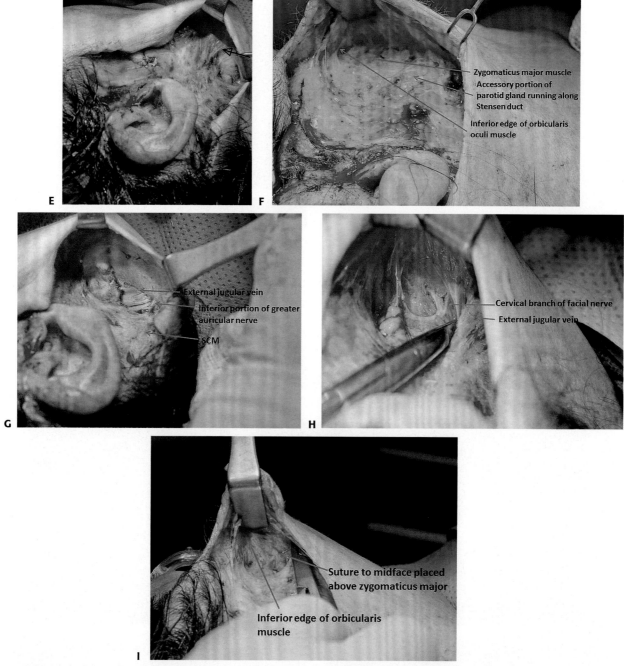

TECH FIG 2 (Continued) • **E.** Inferior view of completion of dissection over parotid extending posteriorly. The *arrow* is indicating the retaining ligament at the anterior border of the parotid gland. **F.** Extension of sub-SMAS dissection over the midface with exposure of zygomaticus major and inferior edge of orbicularis oculi. **G.** Extension of sub-SMAS dissection in the neck with inferior release of posterior edge of SMAS and exposure of external jugular vein and inferior course of greater auricular nerve. **H.** Another view of extension of sub-SMAS dissection in the neck with visible collagen attachments (retaining ligaments) at anteroinferior edge of the parotid. **I.** Exposure of cervical branch of facial nerve coming out of anteroinferior edge of parotid and coursing superficially up into deep surface of platysma.

- The dissection is carried superiorly over the midface, with release of the zygomatic and masseteric retaining ligaments, exposure of the zygomaticus major muscle, and extending under the inferior edge of the orbicularis oculi muscle so that elevation of the SMAS includes the cheek mass and tightens the orbicularis muscle (**TECH FIG 1F**).

- The dissection is then extended beyond the anteroinferior edge of the parotid with release of the neck retaining ligaments, and exposure of the external jugular vein, and inferior path of the greater auricular nerve (**TECH FIG 1G,H**).
  - With release of the attachments beyond the parotid that allow full mobilization of the neck, the cervical

branch of the facial nerve can sometimes be seen coursing up into the platysma (**TECH FIG 1I**).

■ Inferiorly, the dissection is variable, depending on the extent of neck mobilization, but generally goes to where the greater auricular nerve crosses the posterior border of the SCM and over the investing fascia of the entire SCM posteriorly.

Closure and Completion

■ The closure begins with placing two 3-0 PDS sutures from the midface area (above the zygomaticus major into inferior edge of orbicularis muscle and then back to temple) (**TECH FIG 3A**).

■ Next, the corner of the SMAS is sutured in a posterosuperior direction into deep tissues just above the anterior helical rim (**TECH FIG 3B,C**).

■ The skin is rotated superiorly and, depending on skin laxity, may have a more posterior vector than the SMAS that is rotated primarily in a superior direction.

■ Excess skin is excised avoiding a dog-ear at the anterior edge of the sideburn, and closure is begun (**TECH FIG 3D**).

■ Posteriorly, two or more sutures are placed from the SMAS-skin composite flap up to the mastoid (**TECH FIG 3E**).

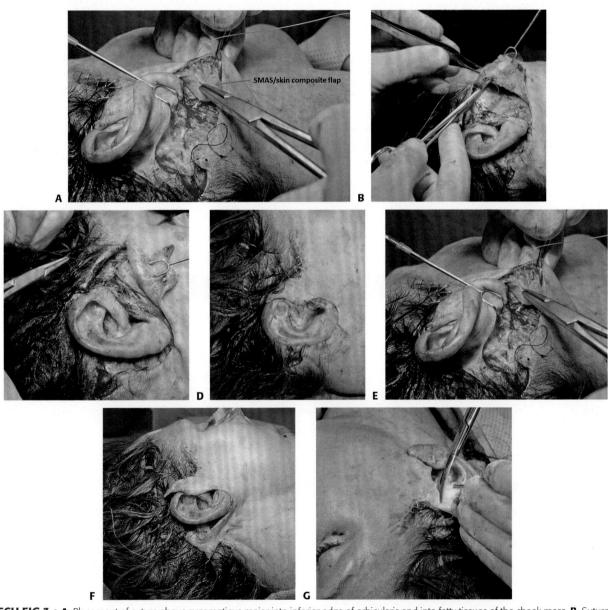

TECH FIG 3 • A. Placement of suture above zygomaticus major into inferior edge of orbicularis and into fatty tissues of the cheek mass. **B.** Suture placed into superolateral corner of elevated SMAS, which will be elevated in a primarily superior vector. **C.** Suture from corner of SMAS being tied down to deep tissues at superoanterior edge of the ear. **D.** Closure at sideburn after trimming of excess skin, which has been rotated in a superoposterior direction. **E.** Posterior suture behind the ear grasping SMAS as part of SMAS-skin composite layer, which will be tied posterosuperiorly to mastoid fascia. **F.** View after suturing of SMAS is complete and initiation of postauricular suture line along the hairline with separate cut into the hairline. **G.** Trimming skin anteriorly along helix and tragus. Skin is under no tension.

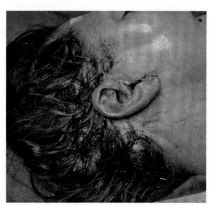
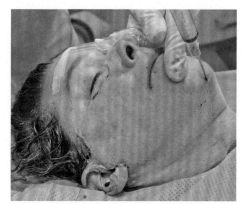

H   **I**

TECH FIG 3 (Continued) • **H.** Completed skin closure. **I.** Submental liposuction being performed after the first side of the face is closed, through stab incision.

- Skin closure is initiated posteriorly. The length of the incisions is controlled by cuts into the hair with superior rotation and an extension of variable length along the edge of the hairline (**TECH FIG 3F**).
  - In selected patients with minimal neck laxity, a short scar technique is utilized by confining the scar to the postauricular sulcus and accepting some pleating.
- The skin is then trimmed and defatted along the tragus, and the posterior skin is excised (**TECH FIG 3G,H**).

- Submental liposuction is carried out with a handheld fine cannula, and subplatysmal liposuction is also performed when there is significant subplatysmal fat.
  - The cannula is used to undermine the entire neck down to the sternal notch and separate skin-platysma attachments. This step is always performed even if there is no submental fat (**TECH FIG 3I**).
- The same procedure is then carried out on the contralateral neck and face.

PEARLS AND PITFALLS

Skin elevation over the cheek	■ When there are significant crow's-feet, extending dissection over orbicularis to orbital rim will reduce wrinkles.
SMAS dissection, midface	■ In patients with minimal midface descent, the dissection can be limited to the posterior edge of the zygoma to minimize swelling and avoid more dangerous parts of the dissection.
SMAS dissection of the neck	■ The extent of the dissection is dictated by the amount of neck laxity, but it is important to capture all of SMAS in the region of the ear lobule to aid in closure.
Hemostasis	■ It is important to get hemostasis several times prior to closure to minimize hematoma risk.
Closure	■ All tension should be borne through the SMAS. Skin closure should be absolutely tension-free.

POSTOPERATIVE CARE

- Drains can be used, though the author does not find them necessary. The area of potential concern for the accumulation of fluid is behind the ear, and this problem is minimized by the use of several sutures behind the ear from the neck flap to the mastoid area to help in fixation and minimize dead space (ie, they serve as quilting sutures).
- The head is elevated with an extra pillow or by placing a cushion underneath the mattress at the head of the bed.
- The head is wrapped overnight as a convenience to absorb fluid and blood leaking through the incision line, and then the patient is instructed to shampoo and wash the area. The incisions have ointment applied to them twice daily until the sutures are removed 7 days after surgery. The preauricular sutures are absorbable.

OUTCOMES

- The final outcome is about 3 months after surgery, when virtually all swelling is resolved and tissue relaxation has occurred. The aging process of course continues but at its normal, gradual pace.
- An estimate to patients is that the tissue relaxation that existed preoperatively in the neck and face will be corrected by 80%, which of course varies depending on the intrinsic viscoelastic properties of the individual patient's skin and SMAS.
- Some patients (5% to 10%, skewed toward older patients with more advanced tissue relaxation and greater viscoelastic properties) will not be fully satisfied with the results and elect to undergo an early second face-lift (less than 2 years after the first one).[3]

COMPLICATIONS

- Hematoma is the most common complication and occurs about 1% of the time, virtually always within the first 24 hours and usually due to labile blood pressure in the postoperative period that is more common in the elderly, and is minimized but not completely prevented by the use of clonidine preoperatively.
- Infection is very rare and has been localized to an area of wound breakdown. This has been minimized by postoperative wound hygiene.
- Marginal skin necrosis behind the ear has been a rare occurrence, easily treated with local wound care, due to the enhanced blood supply of the dissection deep to the superficial fascia and preservation of SMAS skin attachments (composite dissection).
- Although the facial nerve is at risk, I have had no permanent injuries. Neuropraxia of the cervical branch of the facial nerve (pseudomarginal mandibular paralysis) has occurred in 1 of 200 patients earlier in my experience but with much less frequency in the last 10 years with full understanding of the anatomy of the cervical branch. I have had one incidence of neuropraxia of the buccal branch due to thermal injury and one case of frontal branch neuropraxia in my personal series of more than 1500 cases. All cases of neuropraxia have resolved within 2 to 3 months.

REFERENCES

1. Saulis AS, Lautenschlager EP, Mustoe TA. Biomechanical and viscoelastic properties of skin, SMAS, and composite flaps as they pertain to rhytidectomy. *Plast Reconstr Surg.* 2002;110:590-598.
2. Mustoe TA, Rawlani V, Zimmerman H. Modified deep plane rhytidectomy with lateral approach to the neck: an alternative to submental incision and dissection. *Plast Reconstr Surg.* 2011;127:357-370.
3. Rawlani V, Mustoe TA. The staged facelift: addressing the biomechanical limitations of the primary facelift. *Plast Reconstr Surg.* 2012; 130(6):1305-1314.

CHAPTER

Isolated Neck Lift

Alan Matarasso and Sammy Sinno

DEFINITION

- The appearance of neck aging can occur as early as the late 30s.
- Differences in the quality of skin above and below the mandible can contribute to neck aging independently. The neck changes may occur prior to facial aging, which can be particularly disconcerting to patients.
- Recent advances allow the neck to be rejuvenated in a spectrum of methods that include neck lift, minimally invasive surgical procedures (submentalplasty and liposuction), and nonsurgical methods depending upon the indications and goals.
- The most comprehensive treatment of the aging neck requires an isolated neck lift.

ANATOMY

- The youthful neck is characterized by a distinct mandibular border with the relative absence of jowls, subhyoid depression, visible thyroid cartilage bulge, distinct border to the sternocleidomastoid (SCM) muscle, and a cervicomental angle between 105 and 120 degrees (**FIG 1**).[1]
- The aging neck is manifested by attenuation of retaining ligaments from the medial platysma, which leads to platysma edge shortening and banding. Additionally, there can be accentuation of preplatysmal or subplatysmal fat, laxity of skin with texture changes, hypertrophy of the

digastric muscles, and hypertrophied and/or ptotic submandibular glands.
- Treatment options vary based on individualized patient assessment of key anatomic landmarks and treatment goals.

PATIENT HISTORY AND PHYSICAL FINDINGS

- Ideal candidates for an isolated neck surgery procedure are those who want to address neck rejuvenation without the need to concomitantly treat the midface with a face-lift.
- During the initial consultation, it is essential to evaluate the patient's goals and expectations and to reconcile them with the surgeon's evaluation and treatment plan. Furthermore, it is important to discuss relevant procedures that may play a role in enhancing the result of neck surgery, such as chin augmentation, buccal fat pad removal, salivary gland treatment, skin quality enhancement, or midface treatments.[2,3]
- When evaluating the patient and discussing the surgical options, the patient should be educated on the algorithm to discuss the surgical treatments available to treat the various soft tissue components of the aging neck.
- More advanced cases of the aging neck are treated with a neck lift that encompasses liposuction as indicated and submentalplasty along with wide skin flap undermining, elevation, and skin excision.
- Less severe cases can be treated with minimally invasive surgical procedures, including liposuction for fatty necks or submentalplasty that applies liposuction and midline platysma muscle treatment.
- Nonsurgical methods including Ultherapy (Ulthera, Mesa, AZ), among other "tightening" energy-based systems, Kybella (Allergan, Weston, FL), and Botox (Allergan, Weston, FL) can be used to improve the appearance of the neck skin, fat, and muscle, respectively, albeit with a different result than a surgical procedure.

IMAGING

- No imaging other than routine preoperative clearance imaging is needed.

SURGICAL MANAGEMENT: NECK LIFT

Preoperative Planning

- A traditional neck lift encompasses improvement in the area from the jawline down to the clavicle.
- The quality and quantity of skin are noted.

FIG 1 • Relevant neck anatomy.

Labels on figure: Digastric muscle; Submandibular gland; Platysma muscle; Sternocleidomastoid muscle

- If patients desire improvement in the jowls as well as the neck, an "extended" neck lift can be considered, which addresses the same areas as neck surgery and incorporates improvement in the jowl region. This is accomplished by extending the neck lift incision slightly cephalically toward the tragus, which allows jawline skin advancement, SMAS tightening, and jowl liposuction.

Positioning

- The patient is placed in the supine position for this procedure.

Approach

- The isolated neck lift procedure is performed under general anesthesia administered by an anesthesiologist.
- Perioperative antibiotics are used, and TED stockings or sequential compression devices are placed for the entirety of the case.
- Antibiotic ointment is placed in the nostrils and cotton soaked in Betadine is placed in each ear canal.

■ Isolated Neck Lift

- The surgical field is infiltrated with local anesthetic solution containing 1 mL of 1:1000 epinephrine, 100 mL of 1% lidocaine, and 200 mL of normal saline.
- After waiting for the effect of the local anesthetic, we begin with liposuction of the subcutaneous fat as indicated. A 2.4-mm Mercedes cannula is used for the neck liposuction, and a 1-8 mm Mercedes cannula is used for the jowl area. Additional liposuction is conducted with a spatula tip cannula.
- After completion of liposuction, a submental incision is made just above or below the natural submental crease if treatment of the platysmal muscle is indicated (submentalplasty).
- Wide undermining of the neck skin is performed with the aid of a lighted fiber-optic retractor and the assistant placing countertraction on the skin.
- Medial platysmal bands are identified. In patients who have loose redundant or hypertrophic anterior platysmal bands, a strip of excess platysmal muscle is excised.
- After the platysmal band is resected, submuscular fat can be identified and treated in patients who will benefit from a reduction. This is carried out by directly excising small amounts of fat and melting the remainder with a ball tip electrocautery.

- Attention is then returned to the platysmal muscle. Various options for the repair of the midline platysmal muscle repair have been described.[4] The muscle is approximated with interrupted 3-0 Mersilene (Ethicon, San Lorenzo, PR) sutures (**TECH FIG 1A**).
- Once the anterior neck treatment is completed, the patient's head is turned and the surgery continues on the right side of the neck where the incisions are made. The skin flaps are incised and undermined under direct vision sharply and with face-lift scissors. The neck is completely undermined from side to side by connecting the dissection with the prior submental plane.
- The lateral border of the platysma is located and evaluated.
  - If the platysma is lax or redundant, it is undermined with sharp and blunt dissection at least 3 to 4 cm below the angle of the mandible, back cut, and sutured to the sternocleidomastoid (SCM) fascia with 3-0 Mersilene suture (Ethicon, San Lorenzo, PR) while avoiding placing excessive tension on the midline repair.
  - In other cases, the platysma is plicated to the SCM at 3 to 4 points including the lower superficial musculoaponeurotic system (SMAS) for jowl improvement (**TECH FIG 1B**).

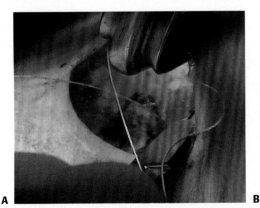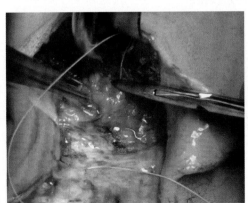

A   **B**

TECH FIG 1 • A. Plication of medial platysma borders. **B.** Suturing of the lateral border of the platysma to sternocleidomastoid fascia.

T E C H N I Q U E S

- Final hemostasis is achieved by electrocautery, and Jackson-Pratt drains (Cardinal Health, Dublin, OH) soaked in Betadine are placed and brought out through the wound and sutured.
- Excess skin is elevated, advanced, redraped, and excised so as to optimize the result and preserve the integrity of the hairline.
- The hair-bearing region is closed with staples, and the area between the hair-bearing region and postauricular incision is closed with half-buried absorbable sutures.

- The postauricular crease is closed with 3-0 nylon sutures; the lower preauricular area, if opened for an extended neck lift, is closed with a 5-0 nylon suture.
- The submental region is the last area inspected for hemostasis after closing both sides of the neck incision. The submental incision is closed with a subcuticular 5-0 Prolene and 5-0 interrupted nylon (Ethicon, San Lorenzo, PR).
- Antibiotic ointment is placed on the wounds. A three-layer face-lift dressing consisting of gauze and SurgiNet (Won Industry, Gyeonggi-do, Korea) is placed on the patient.

PEARLS AND PITFALLS

Neck aging	▪ Occurs in conjunction and often more rapidly or can be more apparent than facial aging. ▪ It is a result of changes in the skin, platysma, and fat of the neck. Other structures such as the digastric muscle and submandibular glands can also contribute to neck aging. ▪ Nonsurgical treatments offer improvement when directed at the appropriate layer of tissue. ▪ Liposuction and submentalplasty can produce significant results in patients with appropriate skin. ▪ The most comprehensive treatment of the aging neck is a surgical neck lift.
Medial platysma treatment	▪ After any platysma redundancy is removed, it is repaired in the midline, which, when completed, resembles the Eiffel Tower. ▪ The platysma is back cut at the level of the cricoid cartilage. ▪ The hyoid fascia can be incorporated as a potential means of reducing recurrent platysma banding, which can be a formidable issue.
Lateral platysma treatment	▪ If the platysma is lax or redundant, it is undermined at least 3 to 4 cm below the angle of the mandible, back cut, and sutured to the SCM fascia. ▪ In other cases, the platysma is plicated to the SCM at three points including the lower SMAS for jowl improvement.

POSTOPERATIVE CARE

- Attempts should be made to keep the neck extended in a semisniffing position to avoid skin flap ischemia.
- Dressing and drains are removed on the first postoperative day, and suture lines are treated with antibiotic ointment. The drain tracts are "milked" of excess fluid.
- Staples and sutures are removed within the first 10 days.
- Return to normal activities usually occurs progressively from 2 to 6 weeks. During that time, patients should avoid excessive sun exposure or nonsurgical facial treatments.
- Firm scars are treated with massage and occasionally ultrasound therapy, as these tend to resolve with time.

OUTCOMES

- Isolated surgical treatment for the aging neck is a viable option for a subset of patients who either do not require or may not wish to have a concurrent treatment of the midface. Optimal aesthetic

results can be achieved by tailoring the procedure to the underlying anatomy and expectations of the patient (**FIG 2**). Ultimately, judicious patient selection and education will provide for the greatest satisfaction in patients undergoing isolated neck lift surgery.

COMPLICATIONS

- Complications can vary depending on the extent of the procedure that is performed. Most frequent complications include seroma and hematoma.
- Although skin necrosis is infrequent, it can be a significant complication when it occurs. We use dimethyl sulfoxide or nitroglycerin ointment for these issues.
- Facial nerve injuries are less common than in face-lifts but can occur. Most often, the marginal mandibular branch and the cervical branch are placed at risk during the procedure if the overlying platysma muscle is breached; this is more frequent in secondary surgery. It has a tendency to occur when defatting just lateral to the submental incision caudal to the mandible.

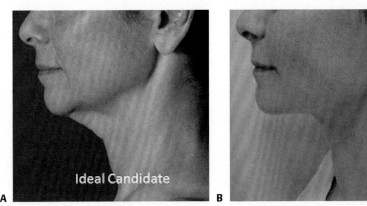

FIG 2 • Preoperative **(A)** and postoperative **(B)** views of patient who underwent isolated neck lift. Note the drastic improvement in cervical contour.

REFERENCES

1. Matarasso A. Managing the components of the aging neck: from liposuction to submentalplasty, to neck lift. *Clin Plast Surg.* 2014;41(1):85-98.
2. de Castro CC, Aboudib JH Jr, Roxo AC. Updating the concepts on neck lift and lower third of the face. *Plast Reconstr Surg.* 2012;130(1):199-205.
3. Feldman JJ. Neck lift my way: an update. *Plast Reconstr Surg.* 2014; 134(6):1173-1183.
4. de Souza Pinto EB. Importance of cervicomental complex treatment in rhytidoplasty. *Aesthetic Plastic Surg.* 1981;5(1):69-75.

48

CHAPTER

Subplatysmal Neck Lifting

Dino Elyassnia and Timothy Marten

DEFINITION

- A well-contoured neck is an artistic imperative to an attractive appearance.
- A good neckline conveys a sense of youth, health, and vitality and lends an appearance of sensuality and beauty (**FIG 1**).
- Neck improvement is of high importance to almost every patient seeking facial rejuvenation, and the results of our face-lift procedures are largely judged by the outcome of the neck.
- Traditional neck lift techniques do not adequately address many aspects of aging in the submental region, and it is not enough in most situations to limit treatment to preplatysmal lipectomy alone or with postauricular skin excision. Subplatysmal problems will contribute significantly to aging and require treatment in most cases if optimal results are to be obtained (**FIG 2**).

ANATOMY

- It is critical to understand the distribution of fat in the cervicosubmental region. Cervical fat is present in three distinct layers—preplatysmal, subplatysmal, and deep interdigastric fat.
- Subplatysmal fat will be evident as a centrally situated triangular shaped fat pad with its base lying at the hyoid and tip near the mentum (see **TECH FIG 1A**). The two sides of the triangle will lie along each digastric muscle. Deeper interdigastric fat is situated in between and deep to the plane tangent to the anterior bellies of the digastric muscles.
- The submandibular gland (SMG) is a lobulated, pink to tan-colored structure covered by a smooth capsule. It sits in confined space with the anterior belly of the digastric muscle lying medial, the mandibular border lateral, and the mylohyoid muscle deep (see **TECH FIG 2A**). The superficial and deep lobes are separated by the mylohyoid muscle.
- Important neurovascular structures will all lie extracapsular to the gland, so intracapsular dissection is safe. The marginal mandibular nerve will lie superior and lateral to

the SMG. The facial artery and vein will lie in close proximity with the vein passing superficial and the artery deep to the gland. An intraglandular perforator artery arising from a branch of the facial artery will be found within the posterior portion of the superficial lobe in a central location.

PATIENT HISTORY AND PHYSICAL FINDINGS

- Success or failure in treating the neck lies in the ability of the surgeon to identify the anatomic basis of patient problems and to form a sound surgical plan for their correction.
- A focused history should include all previous cosmetic treatments for the neck including previous neck lift or noninvasive treatments like Thermage, Ulthera, Kybella, etc.
- Obtain any history of dry mouth or Sjogren syndrome as this is a relative contraindication to reduction of the prominent SMG.
- The cervicosubmental region of each patient must be carefully examined both at rest and during platysmal activation to distinguish between soft adynamic cervical bands and dynamic hard bands. This is best accomplished by asking the patient to "push the jaw forward and tighten the neck." Soft bands change little during activation and are predominantly a problem of loose skin or platysmal laxity, whereas hard bands become tight or exaggerated and indicate a problem of platysma hyperfunction (**FIG 3**).
- Evaluating the location of fat in the neck is also made easier by palpating the neck with and without platysmal activation. Fat lying predominantly in a preplatysmal position will generally feel "soft" and remain in the examiner's grasp upon platysmal activation. However, fat in a subplatysmal location will have a firmer feel and will tend to be pulled superiorly out of the examiner's grasp when the platysma is contracted (**FIG 4**).
- SMGs are usually palpable as firm, smooth, discrete, mobile masses in the lateral submental triangle. Large glands

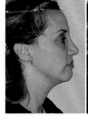
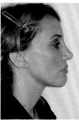
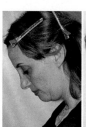
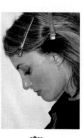
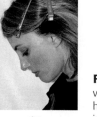

before   after   before   after

FIG 1 • Patient seen before and after neck lift. A good neckline conveys a sense of youth, health, fitness, sensuality, and beauty. The patient has also undergone a face-lift, foreheadplasty, eyelid surgery, and fat injections.

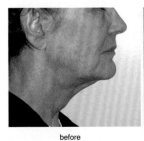
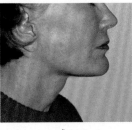
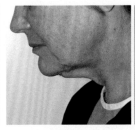
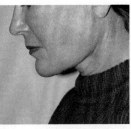

before   after   before   after

FIG 2 • Patient seen before and after neck lift. A careful evaluation of the preoperative photo shows platysmal laxity, excess subplatysmal fat, large submandibular glands, and digastric muscle hypertrophy. Removing subcutaneous fat and tightening skin over these anatomic problems do not correct them and cannot produce the type of improvement shown here.

requiring treatment are most readily visible in the secondary face-lift patient who has had prior aggressive lipectomy; however, they can be more hidden in the primary patient with a full neck and must be palpated to ascertain their size and need for treatment (**FIG 5**).

- A small subgroup of patients will present with large, bulky anterior bellies of their digastric muscles that are evident on visual exam as linear paramedian submental fullness. These are most often seen in the secondary face-lift patient who has had prior aggressive lipectomy (**FIG 6**). However, in the typical primary patient, it is difficult to assess their size; thus, the decision to treat these muscles is usually made intraoperatively.

IMAGING

- Typically, radiographs are not necessary in facial rejuvenation surgery.
- All patients should have standardized photographs taken preoperatively, and any markings made preoperatively on patients should be photographed as well.
- These photos should be used intraoperatively to help guide treatment.

NONOPERATIVE MANAGEMENT

- Some limited options exist to treat isolated problems in the neck.
- Neuromodulators can be used to treat dynamic platysmal bands. Some have reported success using neuromodulators to partially reduce the size of SMGs, but results have been mixed at best.
- Deoxycholic acid (Kybella) is an injectable medication recently approved for reduction of submental fat. Also,

CoolSculpting has been approved for the same treatment. At this point, it is unclear if these treatments are only affecting the subcutaneous fat or also having an impact on subplatysmal fat. Significant reduction of subcutaneous fat is likely not appropriate for most patients in the typical face and neck lift age group. Thus, like submental liposuction, use of these newer treatments should probably be limited to younger patients with discrete subcutaneous fat excess in the submental area.

SURGICAL MANAGEMENT

- Traditional neck lift techniques that focus on preplatysmal lipectomy, skin excision, and platysmaplasty do not adequately address many aspects of aging in the submental region. For many patients, subplatysmal fat accumulation, SMG enlargement, and digastric muscle hypertrophy will contribute significantly to the neck deformity and necessitate additional treatment.[1,2]
- In all but the unusual or young patient, the majority of cervical fat accumulates in a subplatysmal location, and little if any will need to be removed from the preplatysmal layer. As patients age, fat stores generally shift from a preplatysmal location to a subplatysmal one. The small amount of subcutaneous fat present must be preserved to maintain a soft appearance to the neck.
- Large SMGs often contribute to the appearance of a full, "obtuse," and "lumpy" neck. Glands protruding inferiorly to a plane tangent to the ipsilateral digastric and the mandibular border are likely to be problematic if excess cervical

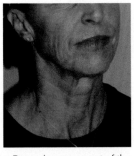
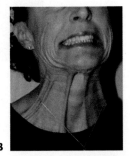

FIG 3 • Dynamic assessment of the cervicosubmental region. The neck is examined in repose (**A**) and as the platysma is contracted (**B**). Dynamic platysma muscle irregularities are often referred to as "platysma bands."

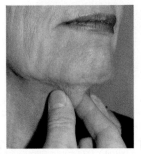
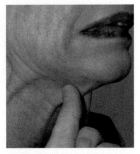

A   B

FIG 4 • Assessing the location of cervicosubmental fat. **A.** Submental "waddle" is grasped with the face and neck in repose. **B.** The patient is then asked to activate the platysma muscle. In this example, fat is pulled superiorly from the examiner's grasp indicating a predominantly *sub* platysmal position. Fat lying predominantly in a subcutaneous, preplatysmal position would tend to remain within the examiner's grasp when the platysma is activated.

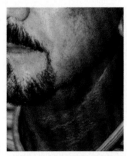 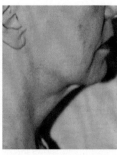

FIG 5 • Prominent submandibular glands. Submandibular glands are usually evident as protruding masses in the lateral submental triangle, lateral to the anterior belly of the ipsilateral digastric muscle. **A.** Patient with residual prominent submandibular gland after face-lift and submental liposuction. His prior procedure has made the prominent glands more obvious. **B.** Patient with residual prominent submandibular gland after "weekend neck lift." Aggressive resection of subcutaneous fat has exposed the prominent gland.

fat is removed, platysma is tightened, and excess skin is removed. These glands warrant reduction, and the protruding portion can be incrementally resected through the submental incision.

- The decision to perform SMG reduction should be made in conjunction with the patient after appropriate discussion of the benefits versus risks. Patients should know that the procedure may prolong submental induration and carries a small but unlikely risk of bleeding, sialoma, salivary fistula, and dry mouth. Patients should also be informed, however, that only the protruding portion is excised and the majority of the gland is left in place.
- Once treatment of subplatysmal fat and SMGs has been performed, the anterior bellies of the digastric muscles should be evaluated. If the muscle bellies are deemed to be prominent intraoperatively, subtotal digastric myectomy should be performed. Failure to evaluate bulging of these muscles after other modifications of the submental region can lead to an unexpected and objectionable submental bulge postoperatively.

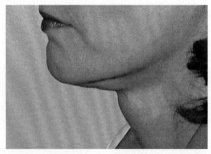

FIG 6 • Prominent anterior belly of the digastric muscle. The patient has had prior face and neck lift. The anterior belly of the digastric muscle can be seen as objectionable linear paramedian fullness in the submental region that spoils an otherwise good result. Prominent digastric muscles often go unnoticed at the time of the primary procedure due to the fact that they are frequently hidden by cervical fat and lax platysma muscle. (Courtesy of T. J. Marten, MD, FACS.)

Preoperative Planning

- All patients undergo a preoperative physical evaluation, and patients with significant medical problems must be cleared by their internist.
- Patients are required to avoid all medications or supplements that increase the risk of bleeding for 2 weeks prior to surgery.
- The majority of our neck lifts are performed under deep sedation administered by an anesthesiologist using a laryngeal mask airway (LMA). This allows the patient to be heavily sedated but still maintains spontaneous breathing without compromise of the airway.
- The flexible LMA is also particularly useful in neck surgery. When this device along with the breathing circuit is draped separately, it can be moved side to side during surgery giving unobstructed access to the submental region.

Positioning

- The patient is placed in the supine position, and a surgical scrub of the entire scalp, face, ears, nose, neck, shoulders, and upper chest is performed with full-strength (1:750) benzalkonium chloride. The patient's head is then placed through the opening of a split sheet leaving the entire head and neck region unobstructed from the clavices up. No "turban" or "head wrap" is used to allow total access.
- In addition, the breathing circuit is draped separately from the patient as described above.

Approach

- Whether performing a neck lift alone or in combination with a face-lift, a submental incision is used to access the subplatysmal space.
- This incision should be placed posterior to the submental crease at a point roughly half the distance between the mentum and hyoid. This is usually 1 to 2 cm posterior to the submental crease and measures 3 to 3.5 cm in length (**FIG 7**). It can be longer as long as it remains concealed under the mandible after skin flaps are shifted superiorly.
- Placing the incision posterior to the submental crease provides better access to the submental region, prevents accentuating a "witch's chin," and still heals in an inconspicuous scar.

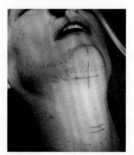

FIG 7 • Plan for the submental incision. The submental portion of the face-lift incision (*solid line*) should be placed posterior to the submental crease (*dotted line*), approximately one-half the distance between the mentum and hyoid (*arrows*). Usually, this corresponds to a point about 1.5 cm posterior to the submental crease.

■ Skin Flap Elevation

- First, sensory nerve blocks are performed using 0.25% bupivacaine with epinephrine 1:200 000. This allows the neck to be injected with a reduced degree of stimulation. This same solution is used to infiltrate the submental incision.
- Next, areas of subcutaneous dissection are generously infiltrated with 0.1% lidocaine with epinephrine 1:1 000 000. Infiltration of the neck and submental region is carried out with a 1.6-mm multihole blunt-tipped infiltration cannula via a stab incision at the earlobe or jawline. No direct infiltration is needed beneath the platysma if the subcutaneous tissues are infiltrated generously.
- The submental incision is made as described above (see Approach). The surgeon should stand at the head of the table, and with the assistant retracting the skin edges with a pair of 10-mm double-pronged skin hooks, skin undermining is done using Metzenbaum scissors.

- Subcutaneous dissection is carried out leaving the majority of preplatysmal fat on the platysma surface so that fat excision and sculpting will be easier to perform if needed at the end of the procedure. However, in contrast to the face-lift skin flap, a slightly thicker layer of fat should be preserved on the cervical skin flap to help avoid a hard or over-resected appearance to the submental area.
- A retrograde dissection should be made subcutaneously up onto the inferior chin to ensure release of the submental crease and mandibular retaining ligaments. Some bleeding should be expected with this necessary maneuver. Subcutaneous dissection is continued inferiorly and laterally, and if an "extended neck lift" or face lift is being performed, the submental dissection will join the lateral skin flap dissection from a postauricular incision. If this lateral dissection is being performed, care must be taken to avoid injury to the greater auricular nerve.

■ Cervical Lipectomy

- The focus of cervical lipectomy in most cases should be subplatysmal fat (**TECH FIG 1**). The subplatysmal space is entered by incising the superficially situated fascia between the medial platysma muscle borders using a Metzenbaum scissors. A combination of blunt and sharp scissors technique is used to isolate each muscle edge. The muscle edge is then grasped and retracted by the assistant using a skin hook or Allis forceps.

- The dissection is then carried laterally over the anterior belly of the digastric muscle hugging the undersurface of the platysma in a relatively avascular plane. Subplatysmal fat should be left on the deep surface of the neck and not raised with the platysma flap to facilitate fat removal as it is technically more difficult to resect fat from the undersurface of the platysma muscle.
- The plane tangent to the anterior bellies of the digastric muscles with the neck neutral or slightly flexed should be used

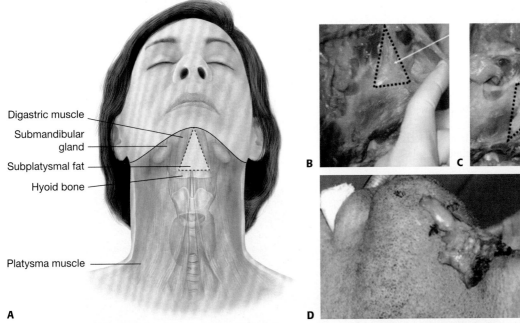

TECH FIG 1 • Subplatysmal fat. **A.** Illustration of the triangular shaped subplatysmal fat located in the submental space with its tip near the mentum and base at the hyoid bone. **B.** Cadaveric demonstration of subplatysmal fat. The *arrow* is pointing to the subplatysmal fat. The right and left borders of the platysma have been elevated clearly displaying the submental space. The subplatysmal fat pad can be seen overlying the digastric muscles to the upper right and left of the triangle with the hyoid bone at the base of the triangle. **C.** Cadaveric demonstration of subplatysmal fat. The two *upper arrows* point to the anterior bellies of the right and left digastric muscles and the *lower arrow* points to the subplatysmal fat pad. In this photo, the fat pad has been reflected downward but still attached at its base. The hyoid is now visible along with the interdigastric space. There is a small amount of deep cervical fat visible between the two *upper arrows*. **D.** Intraoperative demonstration of the subplatysmal fat specimen lying over the submental space from which it was removed. The patient's chin is pointing superiorly with the neck to the right of the photo.

as the landmark for subplatysmal fat removal. All fat lying superficial to this plane should be removed theoretically. If fat excision is made with the neck extended, inadvertent overexcision can occur. Any fat situated deep to this plane (interdigastric fat) should not be removed and the temptation to totally "clean out" the deep cervical space resisted, or else a significant submental depression will result.

- If large SMGs or anterior bellies of the digastric muscles are present and it is elected that they not be treated, subplatysmal fat removal should be more conservative if accentuation of these problems is to be avoided. Also, fibrous fat in the prehyoid region should not be arbitrarily removed, especially in women, as accentuation and masculinization of the larynx can occur.

- Subplatysmal fat should be removed incrementally by paying close attention to the new contours created. This is typically carried out with an extended Bovie and suction to evacuate smoke.

- In almost all cases, it is best to leave the subcutaneous fat layer untouched until all other maneuvers are completed including advancement of SMAS flaps (if concomitant face-lift is being performed). Little if any subcutaneous fat will require excision in most cases for patients in the typical face or neck lift age group. When necessary, this can be completed under direct vision using Metzenbaum scissors or a small suction cannula ("open" liposuction) once correction of deep layer neck problems has been made and prior to closure.

■ Submandibular Gland Reduction

- Prominent SMGs will be encountered as subplatysmal dissection is carried over the anterior belly of the digastric muscle. The prominent gland will appear as a smooth pink to tan-colored mass covered by a smooth capsule (**TECH FIG 2**).

- Reduction is begun by incising the capsule overlying the gland inferomedially just lateral to the anterior belly of the digastric muscle. The gland will be evident once exposed in this manner due to its distinctive lobulated appearance. Its inferior portion can be grasped and easily separated from adjacent tissue inside its capsule using a gentle blunt scissors spreading technique.

- A key step in the safe performance of the procedure is adequate mobilization of the gland, which will make both gland resection and the control of any intraglandular bleeding easier. Although all vital structures are outside the capsule, care should be taken when mobilizing the gland superolaterally as both the facial vein and marginal mandibular branch of the facial nerve and in close proximity.

- Once adequately mobilized, the inferior portion of the gland is grasped and pulled gently inferiorly and medially out of its fossa and away from adjacent structures. The redundant portion is subsequently incised incrementally

under direct vision in a medial to lateral direction using an extended cautery. Excision of the excess part of the gland should be performed in such a manner that the portion protruding inferior to the plane tangent to the ipsilateral mandibular border and the anterior belly of the digastric muscle will be removed. It is usually best that the initial resection is conservative and that the gland is incrementally reduced as needed. Never is it necessary or appropriate to remove an entire gland, which will result in a depression or other contour deformity and could precipitate dry mouth.

- Proper instrumentation and personnel are needed to perform this procedure. An extended cautery along with long insulated forceps is necessary along with a fiberoptic headlight (our preference) or retractor and suction. Also, two assistants will be needed for retraction, passing of instruments, etc. If a smoke evacuator is used, a second suction should be set up in the event that bleeding is encountered.

- SMG reduction must not be performed without proper preparation as mentioned above, and considerable caution as intraglandular vessels is often encountered and can produce brisk bleeding. These vessels are more commonly encountered when larger resections are made. Typically, bleeding will occur from both the gland and the specimen side, and this is usually best controlled by

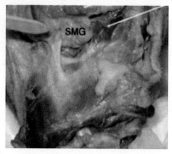
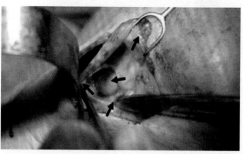

TECH FIG 2 • Surgical approach to submandibular gland reduction. **A.** Cadaveric demonstration of submandibular triangle. The excessive portion of the submandibular gland (SMG) is found protruding inferiorly to a plane tangent to the digastric (*lower arrow*) and the mandibular border (*small upper arrow*). **B.** Intraoperative photo demonstrating exposure of the submandibular gland. A submental incision has been made approximately 1 cm posterior to the submental crease and the neck subcutaneously undermined. The right platysma muscle has been elevated and is retracted with a double-pronged skin hook and a malleable retractor. The gland will be seen as a distinct bulge just lateral to the ipsilateral anterior belly of the digastric (scissors tips rest on digastric). The capsule has been incised inferiorly and medially and the submandibular gland isolated using blunt dissection.

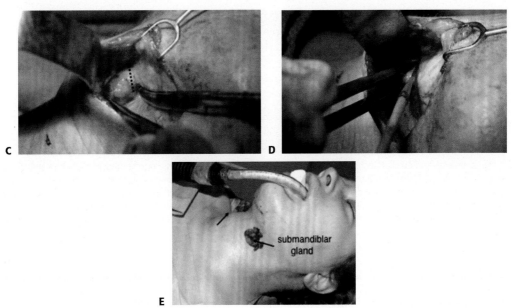

TECH FIG 2 (Continued) • **C.** Intraoperative photo prior to resection of the excess portion of the gland. The gland has been mobilized and gently pulled inferiorly. The *dotted line* represents the level at which the inferior portion of the gland will be excised. **D.** Intraoperative photo just prior to partial gland excision. This should be performed in such a manner that the portion protruding inferior to the plane tangent to the ipsilateral anterior belly of the digastric muscle and the ipsilateral mandibular border will be resected incrementally with electrocautery. **E.** Patient seen immediately after neck lift that included submandibular reduction. The excised portions of the glands are also demonstrated on both the right and left sides.

quickly moving the cautery back and forth between each end of the cut vessel. If bleeding is brisk and not easily controlled with simple cautery, the cut edge of the gland should be compressed with forceps and the vessel isolated and cauterized. In the unlikely event that bleeding cannot be controlled by these means, the submandibular fossae should be packed with gauze and digital pressure applied firmly for several minutes.

- Once the excision is complete, it is not necessary to oversew the cut edge of the gland or close the gland

capsule. It is also not necessary to overcauterize the cut edge of the gland as this will result in more prolonged edema.

- A drain should be placed in the subplatysmal space with this procedure and left in place for several days. It is safest to perform the platysmaplasty before drain placement and then to perforate the platysma and thread the drain into place. This is to avoid the drain being caught with a suture during platysmaplasty.

■ Partial Digastric Myectomy

- Superficial, subtotal anterior digastric myectomy is performed under direct vision through the submental incision after the subplatysmal space has been opened, the platysma muscle has been mobilized, and subplatysmal fat and protruding portions of the SMG have been excised as needed.
- The redundant portion of the muscle can be excised by either a tangential strip excision technique or by a partial division and excision technique. Although both are reliable and effective, in most cases, tangential strip excision provides the simplest method of reducing the muscle.
- Tangential strip excision is performed by grasping the superficial redundant portion of the muscle belly with a forceps and excising a strip of muscle longitudinally with

Metzenbaum scissors or cautery. Excision is begun near the muscle origin at the mentum and continues toward the lateral hyoid. The muscle is then reassessed and the action repeated until the protruding portion is fully removed and optimal contour obtained.

- In the partial division and excision technique, the excess muscle is gauged and isolated on a tonsil forceps by pushing the tips of the instrument through the mid-muscle belly at the level of optimal contour and spreading to split the muscle along the length of its fibers. The isolated muscle segment resting on the instrument consisting of the superficial, protruding portion of it is then excised with scissors or cautery by dividing it at the mentum and hyoid (**TECH FIG 3**). Usually, this entails the excision of the superficial most half or less of each muscle.

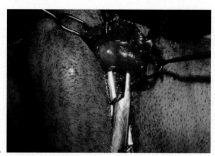
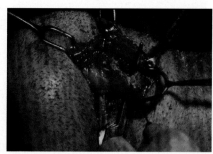

TECH FIG 3 • Partial division and excision technique of digastric muscle reduction. **A.** Excess muscle present is gauged and isolated on a tonsil forceps by pushing the tips of the instrument through the midmuscle belly at the level of optimal contour and spreading to split the muscle along the length of its fibers (view from patient's right digastric muscle through submental incision. Patient's chin is at the left upper corner of the photo and the neck is on the right). **B.** The isolated muscle segment resting on the instrument consisting of the superficial, protruding portion of it is then excised with scissors or cautery by dividing it near the mandible and the hyoid. The neck is then re-examined and the maneuver repeated if necessary until an improved contour is obtained.

■ Anterior Platysmaplasty and Myotomy

- Platysmaplasty consists of suturing the medial muscle borders together from mentum to thyroid cartilage in one or two layers. If redundant muscle is present, it is excised medially before suturing is performed so that a smooth, edge-to-edge approximation can be made (**TECH FIG 4**).
- This is usually performed using simple interrupted sutures of 3-0 Vicryl or Mersilene on a medium tapered needle. A running suture is not recommended as this can cause a "purse string" effect potentially leading to the formation of a midline band postoperatively. Once initial approximation is made with interrupted sutures, the line of repair can be oversewn with a simple running suture if desired. The repair should be snug but not tight.
- When performing a face and neck lift together, cheek SMAS flaps should be suspended prior to anterior platysmaplasty to allow optimal treatment of the jowl. If postauricular transposition flaps are planned, this should be performed after anterior platysmaplasty to prevent difficulty in joining the medial borders of the platysma anteriorly.
- Platysma myotomy should be performed after anterior platysmaplasty if indicated (**TECH FIG 5**).
- This should be done low in the neck at the level of the cricoid cartilage. At this level, the muscle is thin and will bleed less, and the cut edges are less likely to be visible postoperatively. In addition, a smooth transition across the cervicomental angle is maintained and lower lip dysfunction is avoided.
- Platysma myotomy is best begun through the submental incision just below the inferiormost suture from the platysmaplasty. The medial muscle border is grasped and lifted away from the deep cervical fascia with forceps. Myotomy is then made by nibbling though the muscle in small increments with Metzenbaum scissors. As the muscle is divided, it usually separates a centimeter or more exposing the fascia beneath it. Gentle spreading with scissor tips before each cut is made helps separate the muscle from the underlying cervical fascia and

facilitates dissection. The myotomy is continued laterally and slightly superiorly.
- If full-width division of the platysma is planned, the lateral most portion of the transection is completed through the postauricular incision. The lateral transection is complete when brought into continuity with the myotomy from the anterior approach.
- Prior to skin closure, usually one drain is placed in the subplatysmal space if deep layer problems have been treated, and a second drain is placed subcutaneously. If significant oozing is encountered at the end of the procedure or in male patients, an additional drain can be considered for the subcutaneous space.

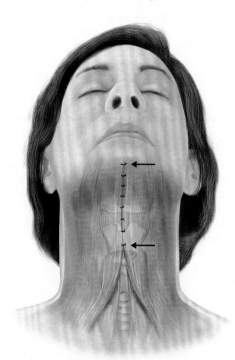

TECH FIG 4 • Anterior platysmaplasty. Repair of platysma diastasis from mentum to thyroid cartilage (*arrows*) improves submental support and helps consolidate the neck. It is not an adequate or effective treatment of platysma bands, however.

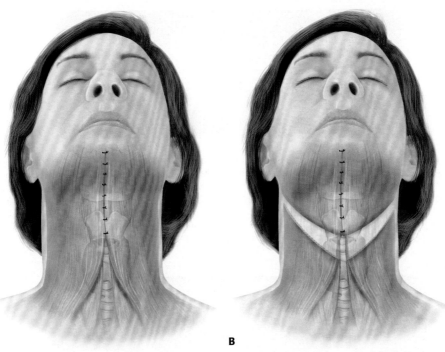

A   **B**

TECH FIG 5 • Plan for "full-width" platysma transection. Full-width myotomy not only corrects anterior and lateral bands but provides improved definition over the lateral mandibular border. However, for patients with only anterior bands, a partial-width transection beginning medially may be adequate. **A.** Anterior neck after platysmaplasty but before full-width platysma myotomy. **B.** After full-width platysma myotomy (note: myotomy is most easily and effectively performed after platysmaplasty has been completed).

PEARLS AND PITFALLS

Subcutaneous fat	■ This layer of fat is essential to maintaining a soft smooth contour to the neck. In most cases, very little subcutaneous fat needs to be removed if proper attention is paid to deep layer problems.
Subplatysmal fat	■ Aggressive treatment of subplatysmal fat can make submandibular glands and digastric muscles much more visible; thus, a surgeon should be prepared to treat all three problems in such cases.
Submandibular gland reduction	■ It is critical to adequately mobilize the gland prior to resection. This will greatly simplify both resection and control of any significant bleeding.
Digastric muscle hypertrophy	■ In most cases, the decision to treat digastric muscles is made intraoperatively after treating other deep layer problems.
Anterior platysmaplasty	■ There is no need to suture the platysma under great tension when deep layer problems are adequately addressed. A snug one-layer edge-to-edge closure after excision of any redundant platysma is adequate.
Recovery	■ Subplatysmal maneuvers will lead to a longer period of swelling and induration, and surgeons using these techniques should be prepared to counsel patients.

POSTOPERATIVE CARE

- No dressings are required or used. They are arguably dangerous for tenuous skin flaps and uncomfortable for patients and preclude inspection and monitoring of the operative site.
- All patients are instructed to sleep flat on their backs without a pillow or with a small cylindrical neck roll. This posture assures an open cervicomental angle and averts dangerous folding of the neck skin flap and obstruction of regional cervical lymphatics. Patients are also shown an "elbow on knees" position that accomplishes this open cervicomental angle while sitting.
- Patients are allowed to take their usual diet after surgery but to avoid overly sweet, salty, sour, or dry foods for several

weeks. This in particular is important if the SMGs have been treated.
- The neck drains are usually left in place for 4 to 5 days. This will help speed the overall resolution of edema, ecchymosis, and induration.
- Patients are asked to set aside 7 to 10 days to recover depending on the extent of their surgery, and additional time off is recommended if a face-lift or related procedure is simultaneously performed.

OUTCOMES

- See before and after examples (**FIGS 8** to **10**).
- See case examples of before and after photos.

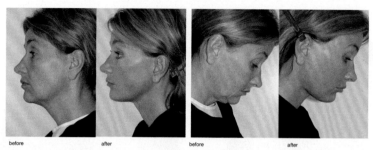

before   after   before   after

FIG 8 • Before and after surgery views of a woman, age 46 who has had no prior surgery. Note full neck, obtuse cervicosubmental contour and "double chin" appearance when the patient looks down in before views. Palpation of the lateral submental triangle revealed a firm mobile mass consistent with an enlarged submandibular gland. Her preoperative appearance suggests the presence of a "low hyoid." The same patient 11 months after face-lift, neck lift, forehead lift, lower eyelift, and facial fat grafting. The neck lift procedure included excision of subplatysmal fat, submandibular gland reduction, superficial digastric myectomy, anterior platysmaplasty, and full-width platysma myotomy. Note attractive, youthful-appearing neckline even when the patient looks down. Comprehensive neck surgery has corrected problems that are commonly misinterpreted as a low hyoid position. The double chin deformity has also been corrected. (Surgical procedures performed by Timonthy J. Marten, MD, FACS.)

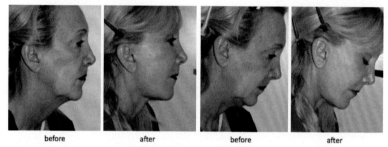

before   after   before   after

FIG 9 • Before and after surgery views of a woman age 55 who has had prior eyelifts and a perioral chemical peel by another surgeon. Note full neck, obtuse cervicosubmental contour and "double chin" appearance. Palpation of the lateral submental triangle revealed a firm mobile mass consistent with an enlarged submandibular gland. Note paucity of subcutaneous neck fat. The same patient 1 year and 4 months after face-lift, neck lift, forehead lift, upper and lower eyelid lifts, perioral dermabrasion, and facial fat grafting. The neck lift included excision of a large amount of subplatysmal fat, submandibular gland reduction, superficial digastric myectomy, anterior platysmaplasty, and full-width platysma myotomy. Note the youthful neckline. The double chin deformity has been corrected by releasing the submental retaining ligaments and blending the fat of the chin and the submental area. (Surgical procedures performed by Timonthy J. Marten, MD, FACS.)

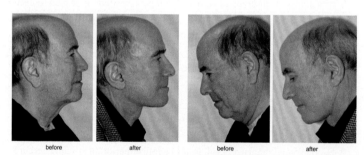

before   after   before   after

FIG 10 • Before and after surgery views of a man, age 68 who has had no prior plastic surgery. Note poor cervicosubmental contour and "double chin" appearance when the patient looks down in before views. An enlarged submandibular gland can be seen. Note paucity of subcutaneous fat that is typical for patients in older age groups. Platysmal bands are visible in the anterior neck. The same patient 1 year and 9 months after face-lift, neck lift, forehead lift, upper and lower eyelifts, facial fat grafting, and ear lobe reduction. The neck lift procedure included excision of a large amount of subplatysmal fat, submandibular gland reduction, superficial digastric myectomy, anterior platysmaplasty, and full-width platysma myotomy. Note well-defined jaw line and masculine-appearing neckline even when he looks down.

COMPLICATIONS

■ Complications associated with subplatysmal neck lifting are similar to other face and neck lift techniques (see High SMAS flap chapter).

■ Subplatysmal neck lifting in particular can lead to temporary platysmal dysfunction likely related to injury to cervical branches. This will manifest as asymmetric lip depressor function that should resolve within 3 months.

■ No major complications attributable to SMG excision, including seroma formation, salivary fistula, or gustatory sweating, have been encountered in our clinic over the last 20 years.

REFERENCES

1. Marten TJ. Treatment of the full, obtuse neck. *Aesthet Surg J*. 2005; 25(4 suppl):387-397.
2. Marten TJ. Cervical contouring in facelift. *Aesthet Surg J*. 2002; 22(6 suppl):541-548.

Indications and Techniques for Short-Scar Face-Lift

Steven M. Levine and Daniel C. Baker

DEFINITION

- Surgery is the standard treatment to address descent and laxity in the aging face.
- Short-scar face-lift is defined as an incision that remains completely preauricular.
- Most also apply that definition to face-lift incisions the extend behind the lobe and into the retroauricular sulcus, but that do not have a transverse component or cross into the hairline at any point.

ANATOMY

- Relevant anatomy is the earlobe and retroauricular sulcus.

PATIENT HISTORY AND PHYSICAL FINDINGS

- Beyond usual history and physical findings to indicate a patient for a face-lift and neck lift, the question is, "Does the patient have a significant amount of cervical laxity?"
- Short-scar face-lifts compromise on the ability to address neck laxity, specifically, inferior neck laxity. Better stated, the short-scar face-lift is ideal for a patient with minimal neck laxity who desires improvement along the jawline and midface.

SURGICAL MANAGEMENT

- Surgery should be performed in an accredited operating room.
- A short-scar face-lift can be performed under local anesthesia with or without sedation or general anesthesia.

Preoperative Planning

- Consideration should be given as to whether the surgeon believes the patient will be satisfied from the limited neck lift provided by the short-scar approach.

Positioning

- The patient is supine on the procedure table.
- Usually, the head of the bed is slightly elevated.
- The authors prefer to sit for maximum stability.

Approach

- An incision pattern is chosen, either preauricular or intratragal.
- The skin is elevated in the subcutaneous plane after infiltration with local anesthesia with epinephrine.
- The superficial musculoaponeurotic system (SMAS) is addressed by any number of acceptable means.

■ True Short-Scar Face-Lift

- The skin incision stops at the base of the earlobe without separating the neck skin from lobe.[1]
- The skin flap is undermined (**TECH FIG 1A**).
- The superficial musculoaponeurotic system (SMAS) is addressed via a flap, SMASectomy, or plication procedure.

- The skin flap is redraped, trimmed, and sewn under no tension (**TECH FIG 1B**).
- The authors prefer to leave drains, but this understandably varies between surgeons.

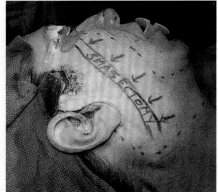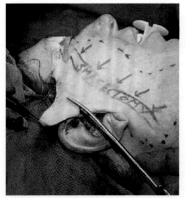

TECH FIG 1 • **A.** The pretragal incision and extent of skin undermining. The incision may extend into the retroauricular sulcus. In this patient, a SMASectomy is planned. **B.** After the SMAS has been addressed, the flap is rotated into position and excess skin is trimmed.

TECHNIQUES

Extended Short-Scar Face-Lift

- The skin incision continues to the retroauricular sulcus.
- This allows the neck to be addressed more adequately than with a true short-scar procedure.
- The skin flap is undermined.
- The SMAS is addressed via a flap, SMASectomy, or plication procedure.
- The skin flap is redraped, trimmed, and sewn under no tension.
- When sewing the skin flap, a three-point stitch is placed from the lobe, the neck skin, and deep to the fascia. This suture anchors the lobe in place to prevent a pixie ear.
  - The traditional tension-bearing retroauricular suture at the cranial end of the sulcus does not exist.
- If there was neck laxity to address, the retroauricular closure will require bunching or pleating of tissue (**TECH FIG 2**).
- The wound should be closed carefully with interrupted suture.

- This pleating settles out within 6 weeks.
- The authors prefer to leave drains, but this understandably varies between surgeons.

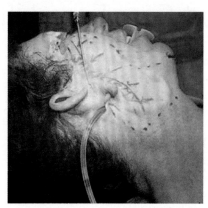

TECH FIG 2 • In a patient with mild to moderate amounts of cervical skin laxity, there may be pleating around the incisions; this will settle with time.

PEARLS AND PITFALLS

Approach	■ Do not hesitate to convert a short scar to a traditional scar for a better result.
	■ This needs to be discussed with patients preoperatively.
Flap	■ Do not overtrim the flap beneath the lobe. There should be no tension on the skin beneath the earlobe. This is more important in a short-scar operation than a traditional scar.

POSTOPERATIVE CARE

- Cool packs are also used to reduce swelling.
- Strict blood pressure control is enforced postoperatively.
- Patients are instructed to do no lifting or bending for 2 weeks.
- The authors prefer to place patients in a face and/or neck compressive dressing for at least 4 to 6 hours after surgery, but up to 24 hours.
- Drains are usually removed at 48 hours.
- All patients are seen by the surgeon the following morning and then again multiple times over the following week.

- Sutures are usually removed at 1 week.
- If needed, a low-dose steroid injection can be delivered to the subcutaneous tissue behind the ear to help soften the pleated tissue.

OUTCOMES

- Short-scar face-lifts in carefully selected patients can achieve excellent jawline contour and midface elevation, as well as some neck tightening (**FIG 1**).

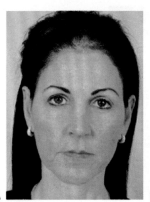 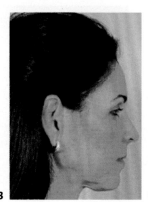 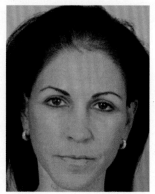 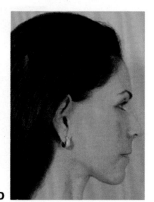

FIG 1 • Preoperative **(A,B)** and postoperative **(C,D)** views of a patient who underwent a short-scar face-lift. Note the improvement of the jowls and jawline.

COMPLICATIONS

- Bruising and hematomas are the most common complications.
- Hematomas in males are twice as common as they are in females.
- Pixie ear creation is a problem if the flap is overtrimmed or inadequately secured to the lobe and fascia.

REFERENCE

1. Baker DC. Lateral SMASectomy, plication and short scar facelifts: indications and techniques. *Clin Plast Surg.* 2008;35(4):533–550, vi. doi:10.1016/j.cps.2008.06.003.

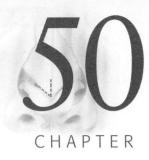

50

CHAPTER

Indications and Techniques for Buccal Fat Pad Excision

Alan Matarasso and Sammy Sinno

DEFINITION

- The buccal fat pad is prominent in the infant face, where it contributes to the suckling function of the cheek.[1]
- Typically, as the face matures, the buccal fat pad becomes less noticeable, but in some patients, it persists and serves as a primary contributor to a "round" face.
- An attractive, angular, and youthful appearing face is characterized by malar convexity juxtaposed with submalar concavity.
- Additionally, due to its intermuscular location, the buccal fat is typically spared from atrophy.[2]

ANATOMY

- The buccal fat pad is a stellate-shaped structure with four extensions.
- It is located deep to the masseter muscle and superficial to the buccinators in the buccopharyngeal membrane.
- The parotid duct pierces the fat pad as it courses to the papilla across the second maxillary molar (**FIG 1**).
- The fat pad extends to the anterior edge of the masseter muscle; it is at this location where the gland can protrude from overaggressive liposuction or facelift dissection among other causes, a phenomenon known as *buccal fat pad pseudoherniation*.[3,4]

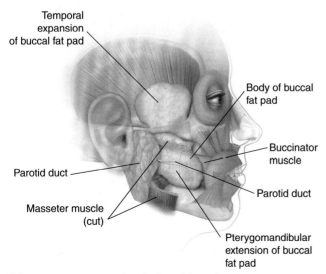

Temporal expansion of buccal fat pad

Body of buccal fat pad

Buccinator muscle

Parotid duct

Parotid duct

Masseter muscle (cut)

Pterygomandibular extension of buccal fat pad

FIG 1 • Anatomy surrounding the buccal fat pad.

- Posteriorly, the fat pad extends deep to the angle of the mandible.
- Superiorly, the fat pad extends to the temporalis muscle and deep to its fascia.
- Another superior extension continues along the zygomatic bone's contribution to the lateral orbital wall.

PATIENT HISTORY AND PHYSICAL FINDINGS

- The buccal fat pad can contribute to a "rounded" facial appearance, obliterating submalar concavity in certain patients. This feature is seen most prominently in the anterocaudal quadrant of the cheek, which is typically targeted by excision of the gland.
- The buccal fat pad is above the mandible and posterior to the nasolabial fold, an area distinct from the jowl.
- In contrast to a normally situated buccal fat pad, pseudoherniated fat can be reduced with gentle pressure.

IMAGING

- When attempting to palpate the buccal fat pad, a firm, pulsatile, or subtly pigmented palpable mass warrants further workup with an MRI.

SURGICAL MANAGEMENT

Preoperative Planning

- Patients undergoing buccal fat pad excision can have it as an isolated procedure or more commonly undergo other facial surgical procedures simultaneously.
- Indications for excision include patients with a full, round face.
- Excision is typically performed intraorally before other procedures (ie, facelift) under nonsterile conditions, to decrease the incidence of infection and risk of facial nerve injury.[5]

Positioning

- The patient is placed in a supine position and the head positioned to gain maximum exposure.

Approach

- To avoid an external incision on the face or injury to the facial nerve, the buccal fat pad is accessed through a minimal intraoral incision.

■ Buccal Fat Pad Excision

- A total of 2 to 3 cc of 1% lidocaine with 1:100 000 epinephrine is injected into the buccal mucosa across from the first and second maxillary molars (**TECH FIG 1A**).
- The cheek is retracted with a Caldwell-Luc retractor.
- A 2.5-cm incision is made between the upper first and second maxillary molar (**TECH FIG 1B**).
- A cuff of mucosa below the gingivobuccal sulcus is maintained for adequate wound closure (**TECH FIG 1C**).
  - Care is taken to visualize the papilla to avoid injury. The papilla with the cheeks are retracted laterally.
- External pressure is applied to guide the fat pad into the wound.
- The buccopharyngeal membrane is pierced with a scalpel and then entered with scissors.
- The fat pad is grasped with Adson-Brown forceps and gently teased with a hemostat (**TECH FIG 1D**).

- The exposed portion of the fat pad is clamped with traction and the excess excised. Only fat that protrudes easily is excised; overresection can cause unattractive cheek hollowing. Extreme caution to avoid hollowing should be exercised in patients with pseudoherniation.
- Avoid excess traction that can distort the anatomy.
- Care is taken to avoid accidental cautery injury to the lips by retracting with a finger and electrocoagulating the stump.
- The incision is packed with gauze soaked with lidocaine and epinephrine while the same procedure is performed on the contralateral side.
- Resections are performed on each side to maintain symmetry (**TECH FIG 1E**).
- Electrocautery is used for hemostasis (**TECH FIG 1F**).
- The incisions are closed with one interrupted 5-0 chromic suture.

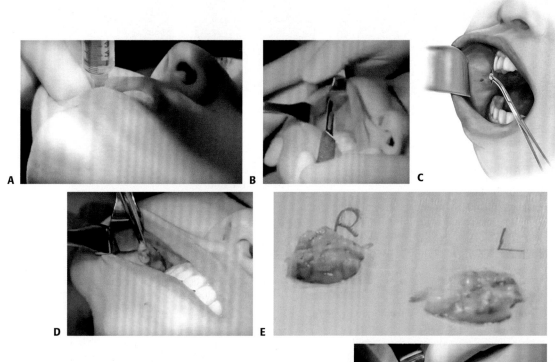

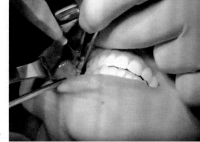

TECH FIG 1 • **A.** Injection of local anesthesia. **B.** Exposure and incision. **C.** Access for buccal fat pad excision. **D.** Buccal fat pad retrieved from incision. **E.** The specimens from each side are compared for symmetry. **F.** Meticulous hemostasis is obtained.

PEARLS AND PITFALLS

Aesthetic considerations	■ The buccal fat pad can contribute to a "rounded" facial appearance, obliterating submalar concavity in certain patients. ■ In contrast to normally situated buccal fat pad, pseudoherniated fat can be reduced with gentle pressure.
Operative sequence	■ Excision is typically performed before other procedures (ie, facelift) under nonsterile conditions, to decrease the incidence of infection and risk of facial nerve injury.
Technical considerations	■ Take care to avoid injury to the papilla; always keep this landmark visualized. ■ Avoid over-resection because this will hollow the cheek area. ■ Excess traction while grasping the fat pad can distort local anatomy. Avoid excess manipulation.
Untoward sequelae	■ A small hematoma in the recess can result in an indurated cheek mass that gradually resolves over time. ■ Prolonged cheek firmness and fullness can be caused by excessive intraoperative manipulation, exploration, or hemostasis (not a fluid collection or infection); this can be managed by external massage and/or ultrasound treatments.

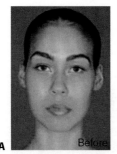 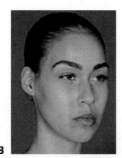 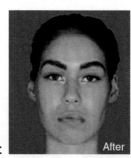 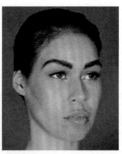

FIG 2 • **(A,B)** Preoperative and **(C,D)** postoperative views of a patient who underwent buccal fat pat excision.

POSTOPERATIVE CARE

■ The chromic sutures will dissolve.
■ Patients are encouraged to maintain adequate oral hygiene while incisions are healing by rinsing with dilute hydrogen peroxide.
■ Excessive opening and closing of the mouth ("exercising") is encouraged.

OUTCOMES

■ Buccal fat pad excision is a safe and effective technique that can restore proportion to the midface (**FIG 2**).
■ It can complement other surgical procedures such as facelifting to restore a more youthful aesthetic contour to the entire face.
■ Even as an isolated procedure, it can produce a more angular and sculpted facial appearance.

COMPLICATIONS

■ Over-resection
■ Inadequate treatment

■ Injury to the papilla
■ Facial nerve injury
■ Wound dehiscence

REFERENCES

1. Matarasso A. Buccal fat pad excision: aesthetic improvement of the midface. *Ann Plast Surg.* 1991;26(5):413-418.
2. Bansal V, Bansal A, Mowar A, Gupta S. Ultrasonography for the volumetric analysis of the buccal fat pad as an interposition material for the management of ankylosis of the temporomandibular joint in adolescent patients. *Br J Oral Maxillofac Surg.* 2015;53(9): 820-825.
3. Matarasso A. Pseudoherniation of the buccal fat pad: a new clinical syndrome. *Plast Reconstr Surg.* 2003;112(6):1716-1718.
4. Matarasso A. Pseudoherniation of the buccal fat pad: a new clinical syndrome. *Plast Reconstr Surg.* 1997;100(3):723-730.
5. Matarasso A. Managing the buccal fat pad. *Aesthet Surg J.* 2006;26(3): 330-336.

Nonsurgical Neck Contouring Using Deoxycholic Acid or Microfocused Ultrasound

Lawrence S. Bass

DEFINITION

- Submental fullness is the result of excess fat contributing to a convex surface contour.
- Skin laxity manifests as visible redundancy of skin.
- Deoxycholic acid (DOCA) is a bile salt that destabilizes cell membranes and emulsifies fat. A synthetically prepared DOCA is Food and Drug Administration (FDA) approved for the reduction of submental fat and fullness.[1]
- Microfocused ultrasound (MFUS) is a technology that uses ultrasound to image the target tissues (diagnostic ultrasound) mated with therapeutic ultrasound that produces zones of coagulation. These zones are fractionated spots of coagulation at a predetermined depth under the skin. Sound energy is delivered in a beam that transits the skin at a low energy density converging at a predetermined depth under the skin by creating a high energy density zone of defined shape and size. A line of 25 fractional zones of coagulation is produced each time the device is fired.
- Ultrasound transducers of different frequencies are selected for the desired depth of treatment. Total energy in each spot in the line can be varied on the device.

ANATOMY

- The submental area is bounded by the inferior border of the mandible (mentum) anteriorly, the hyoid bone posteriorly, and the inferior border or the mandibular bodies laterally.
- Fat in this area can be subcutaneous or subplatysmal.
- Aging changes in the neck include visible skin laxity or redundancy, prominence of visible platysmal bands, and skin surface changes.
- Laxity may manifest as a visible jowl, loss of jawline definition, and hanging festoons of skin in the neck independent of any platysmal banding.
- Transverse rhytides; crepey, rough skin texture; and solar elastosis are surface aging changes that can be treated with MFUS.

PATIENT HISTORY AND PHYSICAL FINDINGS

- Due to the focused nature of the results obtained with DOCA and MFUS, a detailed history of aesthetic issues and goals is essential to ensure that the correct therapies are selected.
- Previous aesthetic therapies and surgeries should be carefully documented. Although these treatments are frequently performed in individuals who have previously undergone some form of treatment, safety and outcomes after extensive or multiply recurrent treatments have not been formally studied or reported at this time.
- Examination should catalogue the location and magnitude of changes in each clinically pertinent tissue layer.
- The degree and location of skin laxity in the jowl, jawline, and submental area are determined along with laxity changes inferior to the thyroid cartilage, which must be addressed separately.
- Presence of visible excesses in subcutaneous fat in the jowl and submental and lateral neck areas should be recorded.
- Platysmal diastasis is an important finding both for procedure selection and patient counseling. The distance of separation and vertical extent of separation should be noted.
- Although it is not routinely possible to determine the amount of excess fat present in the subplatysmal plane on physical examination, this may limit the amount of improvement obtained with DOCA injection that addresses the subcutaneous plane only.

IMAGING

- Radiologic and diagnostic studies are not customarily used.

DIFFERENTIAL DIAGNOSIS

- Skin laxity
- Excess subcutaneous fat
- Excess subplatysmal fat
- Platysmal diastasis
- Dermal rhytids

SURGICAL MANAGEMENT

- Excess fat in the neck, in the absence of skin redundancy, has traditionally been treated with suction-assisted lipectomy. Increasingly, energy-based devices have been mated with the liposuction procedure to amplify skin tightening or lifting in patients with mild laxity resulting from aging changes.
- For more advanced aging changes with skin laxity in the jowl and neck area, surgical lifting procedures such as facialplasty, neck lift, and submentalplasty are the standard for providing the most complete correction, albeit with greater incisions, recovery time, and cost.
- More recently, minimally invasive treatments utilizing sutures that suspend facial and neck tissues and stimulate neocollagenesis are occasionally utilized.

NONSURGICAL MANAGEMENT

- DOCA injection is indicated for the treatment of subcutaneous fat in the submental area. Treatment of fat in the neck inferior to the mandible and anterior to the sternocleidomastoid muscle is also commonly performed.
- Two to six treatments are required depending on the degree of excess fat. Each treatment has up to 50 injections of a fixed dose of medicine placed at a fixed distance apart.
- The amount of fat present determines the number of treatments required. Retreatment is performed at interval of at least 1 month between treatments.
- Although larger necks can be treated, the ideal patient has modest to moderate amounts of fat and is typically treated in two to three sessions of 20 injections each.
- Treatment of jowl fat is specifically contraindicated due to concerns of injury to the marginal mandibular branch of the facial nerve. Theoretically, this may not be rational on an anatomic basis given the typical submandibular location of the nerve as it courses past the jowl area and due to the subplatysmal location of the nerve. But as of this writing, there is no published clinical experience demonstrating the safety or lack thereof for treatment of the jowl.
- MFUS has a specific FDA indication for the noninvasive lifting of skin in the jowl and neck region. Surface features such as transverse neck rhytides and laxity below the level of the thyroid cartilage can also be addressed.
- The ideal patient has good skin quality with only modest skin excess and is not substantially overweight.
- A single treatment is performed to produce neocollagenesis and skin lifting over a 3- to 6-month period, although repeat treatments may be performed for more improvement if the patient is a responder.
- The combination of DOCA injection and MFUS may provide a noninvasive means to correct many of the changes seen in the aging neck if they are mild to moderate in severity. There is currently no published literature reporting results using this combined approach.

Preoperative Planning

- The size of the treatment area for DOCA injection must be determined so the amount of medicine needed can be calculated and the patient advised of treatment cost. The patient also should be advised of the likely number of treatments to provide a complete or near-complete correction.
- Patient counseling about expected recovery after DOCA injections is essential to avoid unexpected disruption of work and social activities.
- MFUS treatment planning involves assessment of the area requiring treatment at each depth and the amount of treatment at each depth (number of lines to be placed). Although there is a theoretical standard 3-mm advancement of the transducer between lines, in practice, most providers will put a greater or fewer number of lines in a given area depending on the severity of the features being treated.

Positioning

- Patients are typically treated on a conventional examination table or chair in an examination room in the supine or partially reclining or upright position depending on provider preference. Treatment of the submental area in the upright position can be difficult with MFUS due to runoff of the fluid within the transducer when it is upside down.

Approach

- DOCA is injected in the midlevel of the subcutaneous fat with a 30-gauge needle.
- MFUS is delivered transcutaneously using ultrasound gel to couple the energy efficiently into the skin.

■ Deoxycholic Acid Injection

- Marking starts with an outline of the inferior border of the mandible. A boundary marking is placed one centimeter below the inferior border of the mandible to keep the treatment away from the marginal mandibular branch of the facial nerve. The anterior border of the sternocleidomastoid muscle may be marked. Next, the thyroid cartilage is palpated and marked followed by the location of the hyoid bone. The submental crease is outlined. These are all simple anatomic landmarks (**TECH FIG 1**).
- The fat is again palpated and lateral markings are made to delimit the intended treatment zone.
- The anterosuperior border of the treatment zone will be the submental crease. The posteroinferior border will be the hyoid bone. Assessment and selection of the lateral border markings is an important judgment for the clinician, ensuring a complete treatment in an efficient fashion.
- Local anesthesia is injected into the subcutaneous fat of the treatment area to minimize patient discomfort during and immediately after the treatment. Typically, 5 mL of 1% lidocaine with epinephrine or less is required.

- A temporary marking grid is applied to guide appropriate spacing of injections. After removing the protective plastic backing, the sheet is held against the skin and moistened. Following 15 seconds of continuous gentle pressure, the application sheet is removed leaving the treatment grid markings on the skin. Use of the grid is essential to ensure appropriate dosing and density that would be difficult to produce freehand.
- Unwanted injection dots are removed with isopropyl alcohol for clarity during treatment. The remaining dots can be counted and the necessary amount of medication drawn up.
- Each 1-mL syringe holds 5 injections. Using a 30-gauge needle, 0.2 mL is injected at each point just adjacent to the grid dot to avoid tattooing the skin. The medication is placed in the center of the subcutaneous fat, *not* intradermal or subplatysmal. Pinching up the skin at each injection site prior to insertion of the needle facilitates accurate placement of the medication.
- Once all treatment dots have been injected, the grid is removed with isopropyl alcohol and a cool compress applied.

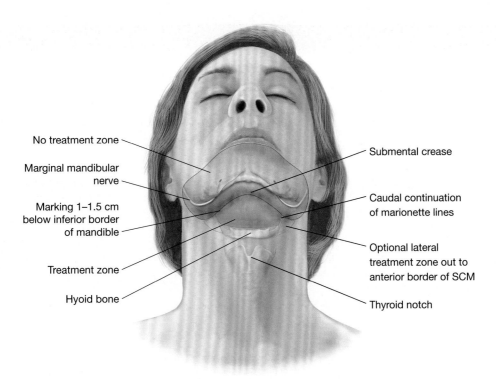

No treatment zone

Marginal mandibular nerve

Marking 1–1.5 cm below inferior border of mandible

Treatment zone

Hyoid bone

Submental crease

Caudal continuation of marionette lines

Optional lateral treatment zone out to anterior border of SCM

Thyroid notch

TECH FIG 1 • A diagrammatic illustration of typical pretreatment markings for DOCA injection.

■ Microfocused Ultrasound

- Columns of treatment are designed to cover the treatment area. These columns can be marked for clarity during the treatment.
- Ultrasound gel is placed on the selected treatment transducer. The deepest focal point transducer is used first, followed by successively more superficial transducers.
- The transducer is placed at one end of a treatment column and the ultrasound image reviewed. The image must confirm adequate contact. The firing line indicates where energy will be delivered that must be aligned with appropriate target tissues such as SMAS, platysma, or deep dermis (**TECH FIG 2**).
- Once appropriate positioning and contact is confirmed, the transducer is fired, delivering the therapeutic ultrasound and placing a line of microthermal zones (MTZ) at the selected depth.
- The transducer is then advanced 3 mm or the desired distance to place the next line. This process is continued until the column of treatment is completed followed by treatment of any adjacent columns.
- After exposure of the full treatment area with the first transducer, the process is completed again with the next (more superficial) transducer. Treatments are typically bilayer and occasionally trilayer. Skin is lifted using exposures at the SMAS/platysma level with 4.5-mm focal point depth transducers and at the dermal subcutaneous junction using 3-mm focal point depth transducers. More superficial features, like transverse neck lines, can be treated using the 1.5-mm transducers.

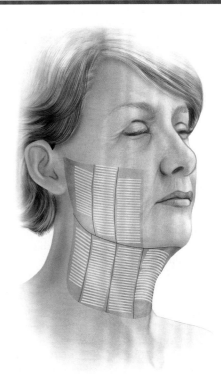

TECH FIG 2 • Application of sound energy in a clinical MFUS treatment.

PEARLS AND PITFALLS

Injection technique	▪ The needle should be placed into the middle of the subcutaneous fat. This minimizes the risk of exposure of skin or deep anatomy to effects of the medication. Pinching up the skin in the fingers of the noninjection hand facilitates precision in needle placement at the appropriate depth.
Lateral jawline	▪ Injection to fat in the lateral portion of the neck must avoid exposure of the marginal mandibular branch of the facial nerve. A buffer zone of 1 cm from the inferior border of the mandible is commonly used. ▪ Patients who have undergone previous surgery such as facialplasty deserve extra caution due to the greater potential variation in nerve position.
Jowl	▪ Although direct injection of the jowl fat is tempting, product labeling forbids injection due to concern over the marginal mandibular branch. Of course, the injection is supposed to be superficial to the platysma, and it is unclear how often the nerve even transits the jowl area en route to its muscular insertions. As of this writing, it is unknown whether this is a real or merely theoretical concern.
Injection spacing	▪ DOCA should be injected using the manufacturer supplied marking grid to insure proper spacing of doses. Closer spacing can result in tissue necrosis, and wider spacing can result in loss of efficacy.[2]
Medication dilution	▪ DOCA should be injected as supplied (10 mg/mL) without adulteration or dilution. 0.2 mL (2 mg) should be injected at each injection site. An attempt to "stretch" the medication by diluting or underdosing will result in loss of efficacy.
MFUS skin prep	▪ To facilitate gliding the handpiece, avoid heavy makeup. Men should be close shaved.
Pattern planning	▪ Modify standardized templates to adjust for size of the patient's face. Select number of lines based on severity of findings.
Transducer selection	▪ Transducers are selected for the anatomic structures requiring correction. Usually, this is a bilayer treatment with 3-mm and 4.5-mm depth transducers to target the dermal/subcutaneous junction and the SMAS and platysma, respectively.
Number of treatment lines	▪ To create observable lifting, treatments usually deliver 400 to 700 lines to the cheek and neck areas. 200 to 300 line treatments are sometimes employed for maintenance or follow-up treatments.
Maintaining/restoring gel contact	▪ Moderate pressure avoids excess thinning of the gel layer between the transducer and skin. Reapplication of gel to the transducer is usually more expedient than manipulation of the transducer against the skin in an effort to restore contact.
Convexities	▪ Convex areas such as just medial to the sternocleidomastoid muscle are particularly prone to loss of transducer contact with the skin resulting in blistering and potential scarring.
Periocular area	▪ Treatment should not be delivered within the orbital rim to avoid unintended exposure and damage to the globe.

POSTOPERATIVE CARE

▪ Both treatments benefit from cool compresses and nonsteroidal anti-inflammatory drugs (NSAIDs) to help minimize discomfort on the day of treatment.

▪ In an attempt to minimize the pronounced edema after DOCA injection, antihistamines, NSAIDs, and compression garments have been used, but formal study of this did not demonstrate any benefit.[3]

OUTCOMES

▪ Improvement in submental contour can be seen with a typical 20-injection DOCA treatment (**FIG 1**). In patients with a larger collection of submental fat, a greater number of treatments with more injections covering a larger area can be used. This provides a greater degree of improvement with durable results (**FIG 2**). Although skin laxity is generally no worse after treatment, occasional significant reduction in laxity is seen. This has not been formally studied making the degree and consistency of improvement unknown at this time (**FIG 3**).

▪ Fifty-five percent of subjects in one study reported a one-grade improvement in submental contour after two DOCA

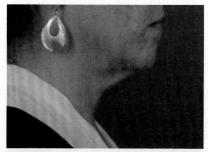

A

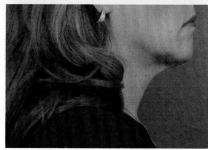

B

FIG 1 ▪ A 52-year-old woman who underwent a single DOCA treatment of 20 injections. **A.** Pretreatment. **B.** 2 months post treatment.

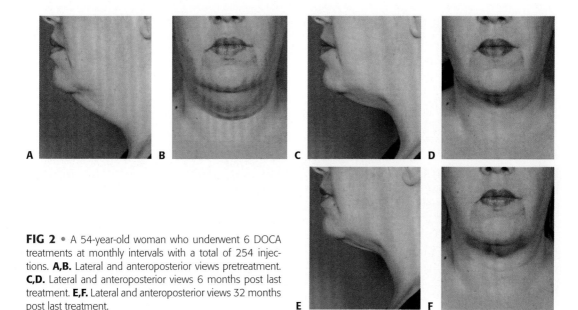

FIG 2 • A 54-year-old woman who underwent 6 DOCA treatments at monthly intervals with a total of 254 injections. **A,B.** Lateral and anteroposterior views pretreatment. **C,D.** Lateral and anteroposterior views 6 months post last treatment. **E,F.** Lateral and anteroposterior views 32 months post last treatment.

treatments and 75% after four treatments.[4] Marginal mandibular paresis was reported in 4.3%, which can take several months to resolve.

- MFUS typically reduces laxity in the neck area and sharpens the contour of the jowl/jawline area (**FIG 4**). In patients who are responders, additional treatments can be used to obtain additional improvement or to maintain the result (**FIG 5**).
- A prospective study of 93 patients treated with MFUS using the original treatment protocols (approximately 250 to 300 lines) using objective and subjective measures of response showed laxity improvement in 63.6% and 58.1%

of patients at 90 days. More than half of the patients with a BMI greater than 30 did not respond.[5]

- In another study, 67% of subjects showed improvement at 180 days post MFUS treatment. This nonresponder rate seems consistent across the available studies to date.[6]

COMPLICATIONS

DOCA

- Ecchymosis
- Edema
- Pain
- Numbness
- Erythema

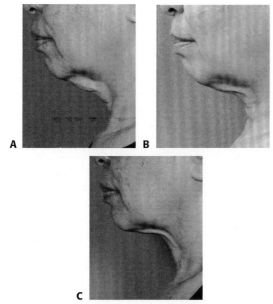

FIG 3 • A 64-year-old woman who underwent 6 DOCA treatments at monthly intervals with a total of 139 injections. **A.** Lateral view pretreatment. **B.** Lateral view 6 months post last treatment. **C.** Lateral view 32 months post last treatment.

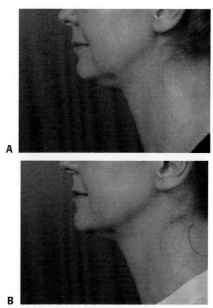

FIG 4 • A 41-year-old woman. **A.** Pretreatment. **B.** Thirteen months post a single MFUS treatment.

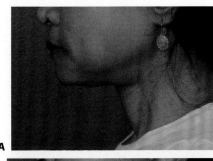

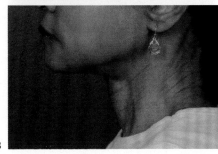

FIG 5 • A 53-year-old woman. **A.** Pretreatment age 53. **B.** Thirty months after first and 16 months after second MFUS treatment, now age 55.

- Induration
- Paresthesia
- Nodule
- Pruritus
- Dysphagia
- Facial nerve injury
- Skin loss

- Scarring
- Induration
- Nodule formation
- Facial nerve injury

MFUS
- Erythema
- Ecchymosis
- White or red wheals
- Blistering
- Scarring
- Numbness
- Facial nerve injury

REFERENCES

1. Rotunda AM. Injectable treatments for adipose tissue: terminology, mechanism, and tissue interaction. *Lasers Surg Med.* 2009;41:714-720.
2. Dayan SH, Humphrey S, Jones DH, et al. Overview of ATX0191 (deoxycholic acid injection): a nonsurgical approach for reduction of submental fat. *Dermatol Surg.* 2016;42:S263-S270.
3. Dover JS, Kenkel JM, Carruthers A, et al. Management of patient experience with ATX-101 (deoxycholic acid injection) for reduction of submental fat. *Dermatol Surg.* 2016;42:S288-S299.
4. Jones DH, Carruthers J, Joseph JH, et al. Refine-1, a multicenter, randomized, double-blind, placebo-controlled, phase 3 trial with ATX-101, an injectable drug for submental fat reduction. *Dermatol Surg.* 2016;42:38-49.
5. Oni G, Hoxworth R, Teotia S, et al. Evaluation of a microfocused ultrasound system for improving skin laxity and tightening in the lower face. *Aesthet Surg J.* 2014;34:1099-1110.
6. Fabi SG, Goldman MP. Retrospective evaluation of micro-focused ultrasound for lifting and tightening the face and neck. *Dermatol Surg.* 2014;40:569-575.

Indications and Technique for Closed Rhinoplasty in Patients With Dorsal Hump and Wide Tip

Barış Çakır and Ali Teoman Tellioğlu

DEFINITION

- The reason for a wide nasal tip is that the dome and lateral crura are wider than normal.
- The distance between the nostrils and the lateral crura is generally narrow.
- An excessively enlarged dorsal cartilage and nasal bone result in a nose with a prominent bridge that is aesthetically unacceptable.

ANATOMY

- The nose consists of mobile and immobile areas.
- The mobile part of the tip consists of the lower lateral cartilages.
- The immobile part of the nose consists of the septum, the upper lateral cartilages, the maxilla, and the nasal bones (**FIG 1**).
- The mobile nose tip is connected to the septum and the upper lateral cartilages by means of the Pitanguy and scroll ligaments. The nose tip moves up and down along these ligaments.
- The scroll and Pitanguy ligaments are formed by a thickening of the superficial musculoaponeurotic system (SMAS) at the supratip; they are functionally significant because they constitute a part of the SMAS.
- Protection and repair of these ligaments are crucial for the projection, mobility and definition of the nose.

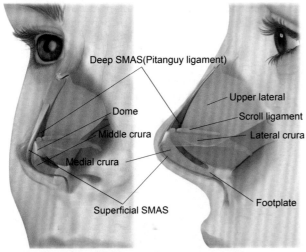

Deep SMAS(Pitanguy ligament)

Dome

Middle crura

Medial crura

Superficial SMAS

Upper lateral

Scroll ligament

Lateral crura

Footplate

FIG 1 • The nose consists of mobile and immobile areas. The mobile part of the tip consists of the lower lateral cartilage. The immobile part of the nose consists of the septum, the upper lateral cartilages, the maxilla, and the nasal bones.

PATHOGENESIS

- The cartilages and bones that form the skeleton of the nose stand in close relation to each other.
- Many patients present with a history of trauma to the nose. Generally, one can observe a large and deviated vomer.
- Our theory is that a greatly enlarged septum pushes the upper lateral cartilages anteriorly and the medial crura caudally.
- The upper lateral cartilages pull the cephalic edge of the lateral crus anteriorly and therefore distort the resting angle of the lateral crura.
- A septal cartilage that projects anterocaudally results in the domes being formed more caudal than normal.
- The lobule is formed short, while the lateral crura are long. The nasal tip widens because the lateral crura become more dominant in the tip area.
- The convex nature of the lateral crura and the distorted reclining angle of the lateral crura result in the tip appearing wide and round (**FIG 2**).

PATIENT HISTORY AND PHYSICAL FINDINGS

- Noses that are not in harmony with the face and have flawed internal proportions may disturb patients from an aesthetic viewpoint.
- Patients generally complain that their nasal tip is big and that they find the bridge disturbing.
- Inspection: A visual examination is most important; problems are clearly diagnosed with the help of photographs.
  - The nasal tip is wide.
  - The lobule is generally short.
  - The lateral crura are generally convex, long and wide.
  - The cephalic edge of the lateral crus is more anteriorly located than the caudal edge.
  - The dorsal septum and the nasal bones are hypertrophic.
  - Because the septum pushes the tip forward, the more than normally projecting nasal tip is likely to be pulled downward when the patient laughs.
- Palpation
  - Skin thickness directly influences the results. Strong cartilages and thin skin respond better to rhinoplasty surgery. By touching the nasal skin and examining the inside of the nasal tip with the help of a light source, we can gain valuable information about the soft tissue and cartilages.

IMAGING

- Front, base, top, lateral, and oblique photographs are standard procedure. A lateral photograph of the patient smiling gives clues about the dynamics of the nasal tip.

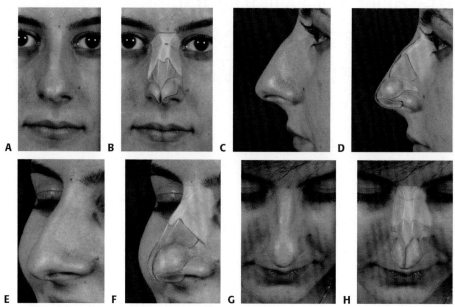

FIG 2 • A–H. The lobule is formed short, the lateral crura long. Because the lateral crura become more dominant in the tip area, the nasal tip widens. The lateral crura's convex nature and the distorted reclining angle of the lateral crura result in the tip appearing wide and round.

- An SLR camera of medium quality is sufficient. One can obtain a detailed and standard photographic archive with a 100- or 105-mm fixed macro lens.
- On close-up photographs, the nasal tip appears wider. In order to objectively depict the changes in the nasal tip, the camera's focal length has to remain the same.
- A black or blue background is preferable. A black background prevents a black shadow and looks better but may render the hair invisible. Blue is a color more appropriate for scientific purposes.
- Lighting changes the photographic results. The double softbox system is standard. To obtain standardized photographs, patient, the doctor and the lighting need to remain in the same location. It is advisable to draw a circle on the floor about 1 to 2 m in front of the background curtain.
- Lighting: To understand the lighting technique, one has to look at the eyes first. If the light reflection is not the same between the preoperative and postoperative photographs, it is difficult to make a comparison.
- Fish-eye effect: If the before photograph is taken with a fish-eye effect, the ears will not be visible. It is not possible to draw a meaningful comparison between two photographs with unequal focal distances.

SURGICAL MANAGEMENT

- Rhinoplasty surgery began in the form of closed reduction; however, a more controlled resection and reconstruction with an open rhinoplasty technique have become more popular.
- Closed surgery based on an intracartilaginous approach, where the surgeons could not see the tip cartilages, has quickly lost popularity. Because control is difficult to achieve, more inexperienced surgeons do not prefer this technique because it is difficult to achieve control.
- Because it is easy to learn and perform open rhinoplasty, this technique has gained great popularity in recent years.
- Although open rhinoplasty allows for more control, side effects such as rigidity and numbness are quite bothersome.

- In an effort to combine the control of open rhinoplasty techniques with the fast healing of the closed rhinoplasty, "open rhinoplasty with endonasal approach" has become an alternative approach. We named this philosophy as the "preservation rhinoplasty."

Preoperative Planning

- It is important to do the imaging work on a lateral photograph before the surgery.
- By doing the imaging work together with the patient, we can learn about the patient's expectations.

Approach

- Make a transfixion incision on one side (if the surgeon is left handed, on the left side; if right handed, on the right).
- Enter under the dorsal perichondrium from the septal angle and dissect as far as under the dorsal bone. In this area, the Daniel-Cakir blunt perichondrium elevator is particularly useful.
- Enter under the upper lateral perichondrium and dissect caudally as far as the scroll area (**FIG 3**).
- If there exists a caudal excess of the lateral crus, make an intracartilaginous incision in such a way that 2 to 3 mm of the caudal edge of the lateral crus is left in the skin. The cartilage left in the skin is called an auto-rim flap.[1]

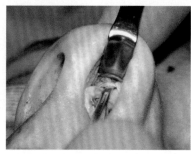

FIG 3 • Enter under the upper lateral perichondrium and dissect caudally as far as the scroll area.

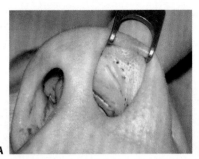
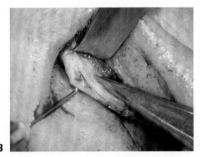
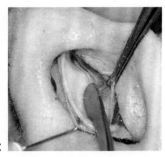

FIG 4 • A–C. Beginning from the turning point of the lateral crus, dissect the lower lateral cartilage by means of a subperichondrial dissection.

- Make an infracartilaginous incision to the dome and medial crus.
- Beginning from the turning point of the lateral crus, dissect the lower lateral cartilage by means of a subperichondrial dissection (**FIG 4**).
- Pulling the domes laterally with a hook, dissect the domes. Dissect the medial crura subperichondrially to the level of the footplates. In this area, the Daniel-Cakir sharp perichondrium elevator is particularly useful (**FIG 5**).
- Join the two dissections in the scroll region and expose the caudal edge of the bones.

- Enter under the periosteum by scratching the caudal edge of the bones with an elevator.
- Dissect the nasal and maxillary bones subperiosteally. In this area, the Daniel-Cakir periosteum elevator is particularly useful.
- Carefully join the subperiosteal dissection planes in the midline.
- Beginning from the upper lateral caudal edge, dissect the internal valve mucosa subperichondrially.

FIG 5 • A,B. Pull the domes laterally with a hook and dissect the domes. Dissect the medial crura subperichondrially until the footplate. In this area, the Daniel-Cakir sharp perichondrium elevator is particularly useful.

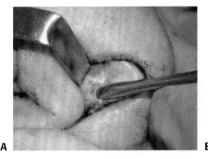
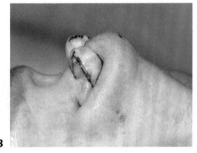

■ Dorsal Resection

- Resect the cartilage hump as a composite (**TECH FIG 1A,B**).
- Resect the exposed right and left nasal bone with bone scissors (**TECH FIG 1C,D**).
- If the radix is high, rasp the radix. Reduce the radix in a controlled way without causing the glabella to swell.
- File down any asymmetries of the bony surface to create a symmetrical appearance. A bone file, mastoid bur or rasp can be used for this purpose.
- Medialize the bone flaps with the help of lateral osteotomy, or lateral osteoectomy and median oblique and transverse osteotomies (**TECH FIG 1E,F**). Performing this procedure after tip surgery reduces swelling.

Tip Surgery

- Extract the domes from each nostril by dissecting the superficial musculoaponeurotic system (SMAS) from the deep SMAS.
- Determine the correct length of the lateral crus by stealing from the lateral crus.
- Shape the new domes with a cephalic dome suture[1] (**TECH FIG 2A,B**).

- Extract both domes through the nostril closer to you and let the assistant hold the dome farther away from you at the midline with the help of a hook.
- Join the domes by suturing the soft tissue between the domes. This suture will assist with equalizing the domes (**TECH FIG 2C,D**).
- Equalize the domes with a figure-of-8 suture.
- Place the strut graft between the medial and middle crura with sutures. Stabilize the tip of the strut cartilage graft with a U suture passing through the domes, stabilize the tip of the strut cartilage graft.
- Reconstruct the columellar break point, the lobule and the columella with a 6-0 PDS suture (**TECH FIG 2E**).
- Place the lower lateral cartilages in such a way that the superficial SMAS fits into the gap between the medial and middle crura.

Dorsal Reconstruction

- Shape the cartilage that has been resected as a composite and place it as a spreader graft (**TECH FIG 3A–D**).
- Repair the scroll ligaments (**TECH FIG 3E,F**).
- Close the mucosa with a 6-0 Monocryl.

For more detail, see the handbook on Aesthetic Septorhinoplasty.

TECHNIQUES

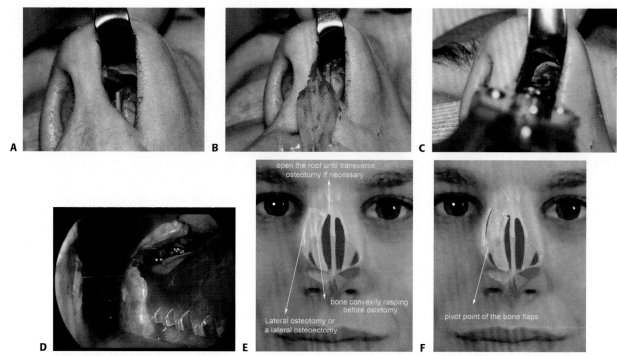

TECH FIG 1 • A,B. Resect the cartilage hump as a composite. **C,D.** Resect the exposed right and left nasal bone with bone scissors. **E,F.** Medialize the bone flaps with the help of lateral osteotomy, or lateral osteoectomy and median oblique and transverse osteotomies.

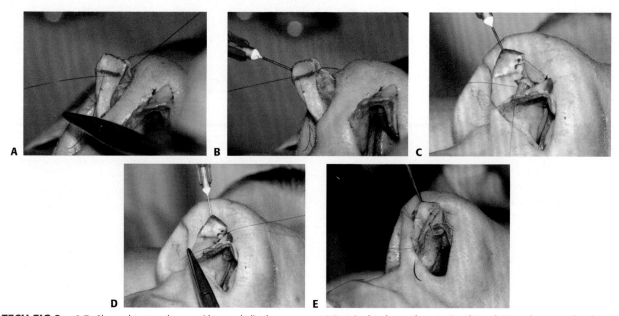

TECH FIG 2 • A,B. Shape the new domes with a cephalic dome suture. **C,D.** Join the domes by suturing the soft tissue between the domes. This suture will assist with equalizing the domes. **E.** Reconstruct the columellar break point, the lobule and the columella with a 6-0 PDS.

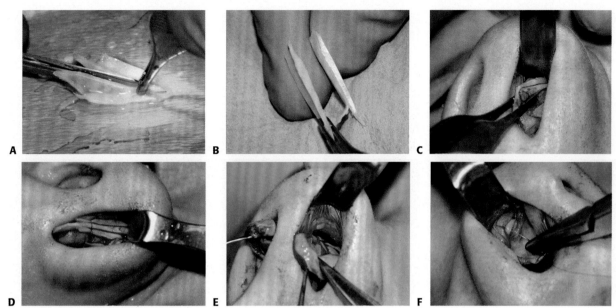

TECH FIG 3 • A–D. Shape the cartilage that has been resected as a composite and place it as a spreader graft. **E,F.** Repair the scroll ligaments.

PEARLS AND PITFALLS

Osteotomy contraindications	▪ When performing a wide dissection to the dorsum, an osteotomy with a lateral osteotome is contraindicated. The bones may collapse. If you perform an osteotomy, do so by entering from the cut on the skin or the rim incision with a 2-mm chisel.
Dissection	▪ Subperichondral dissection decreases the risk of damage and progressive thinning of the soft tissue, and it helps to protect the scroll ligament. It is easy to enter the subperichondral plane where the cartilage is thick. A good dissection is the best camouflage.
Pitanguy midline ligament	▪ A closed approach does not interfere with the Pitanguy ligament next to the columellar system. This is very beneficial to control the supratip skin.
Bruising, swelling	▪ Insert an intravenous tube splinted with a scalpel next to the nasal bone to decrease swelling.
Imaging	▪ We can plan rotation, projection, and resection with the help of the imaging work. Increasing the tip rotation and projection as well as filling the deep radix reduces the amount of dorsal resection. Imaging prevents us from over-resection.
Head lamp	▪ For closed surgery, a headlight is absolutely necessary. In order to be able to see the deepest areas of the dissection, surgeons should align the lamp with their own radix.

POSTOPERATIVE CARE

▪ Carefully tape the nose without squeezing the tip. If the tape pinches the nose tip caudally, the positioning of the tip cartilages can be damaged.

▪ Because thermoplastic plaster is water resistant, the patient may shower every day.

▪ Applying tape underneath the eyes decreases swelling and bruising.

▪ The patient can be discharged after 3 to 4 hours.

▪ In case of swelling, a cold compress can be applied. Cold compresses are not routinely used after wide dissection and inserting drains.

▪ The patient rests in bed with the head elevated.

▪ Paracetamol with codeine is sufficient for pain management.

▪ To treat bone edema, diclofenac potassium can be prescribed from day 5 to 10.

▪ After the preoperative prophylaxis, there is no need for antibiotics after preoperative prophylaxis.

▪ Saltwater irrigation can be done for 10 days.

▪ Internal silicone dolly splints can be removed after 2 to 4 days.

▪ After 10 days, the cast is removed. Generally, no more tape is used.

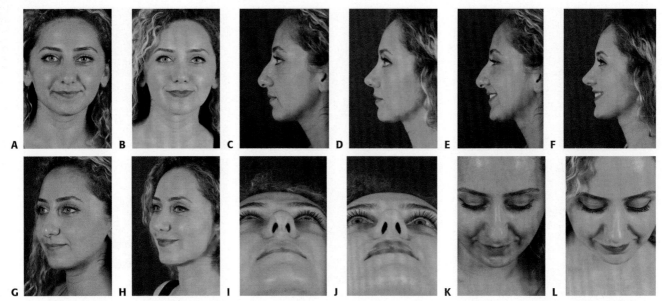

FIG 6 • A–L. Patient example. 1-year result.

OUTCOMES

- Over the past 10 years, we have performed approximately 2000 rhinoplasties.
- In 5% of the cases, a revision was necessary. As experience increases, the percentage of revisions decreases.
- Most revisions are performed due to rotation loss and dorsal residual hump and irregularities.
- For the first 3 years, we performed open rhinoplasty. During that time, we observed a more frequent occurrence of supratip deformity.
- Thereafter, we performed closed rhinoplasty for 7 years. Protecting the Pitanguy ligament increased control of the supratip skin.
- Over the past 4 years, we have been mobilizing the bone at the level of the medial canthus by performing a lateral osteoectomy rather than a lateral osteotomy. In this way, less of an infracture occurs at aperture. We receive fewer complaints concerning breathing problems.
- A case study with hump and bulbous tip (**FIG 6**).

COMPLICATIONS

- Irregularity of the dorsum
- Loss of rotation
- Loss of projection
- Tip asymmetry
- Bleeding
- Infection

REFERENCE

1. Cakır B, Oreroğlu AR, Daniel RK. Surface aesthetics in tip rhinoplasty: a step-by-step guide. *Aesthet Surg J*. 2014;34(6):941-955.

Indications and Technique for Treating the Narrow Midvault in Closed Rhinoplasty

Shruti C. Tannan, Jeffrey R. Claiborne, and Mark B. Constantian

DEFINITION

- A narrow middle vault can be defined anatomically or functionally.
- Anatomically, a narrow middle vault is defined as any part of the upper cartilaginous vault that is at least 25% narrower than the upper or lower nasal third.
- Functionally, a narrow middle vault is defined as inadequate internal nasal valve support.

ANATOMY

- The middle vault is composed of the paired upper lateral cartilages (ULCs) and the dorsal nasal septum.
- The ULCs extend superiorly beneath the paired nasal bones approximately 5 mm, in a region known as the keystone area.
- Laterally, the ULCs attach to the bony piriform aperture via the piriform ligament.
- Inferiorly, the ULCs are supported by their attachment to the lower lateral cartilages in a region called the scroll area.
- Aesthetically, the middle vault is the location of a smooth transition from the narrower nasal bones superiorly to the wider nasal base inferiorly.
- In the midline, the ULCs fuse with the septum to create a T in cross section, an intersection that creates an angle known as the internal nasal valve (**FIGS 1** and **2**).

- The internal nasal valve is bounded medially by the septum, laterally by the ULCs, and inferiorly by the inferior turbinate.
- The internal nasal valve is the narrowest portion of the nasal airway and therefore the site of highest airflow resistance.
- The width and stability of the middle vault, the critical area of the internal nasal valve, is determined by three factors:
  - Width of the nasal bony vault
  - Height and width of the middle vault roof
  - Soft tissue rigidity

PATHOGENESIS AND NATURAL HISTORY

- As air enters the region of the narrow internal nasal valve, airflow speed increases according to the Poiseuille law and the Venturi principle: when air goes through a narrow passage, it speeds up and increases the transmural pressure on the nasal sidewall, just as water running through a brook speeds up as it passes between a narrow channel. Additionally, the Bernoulli principle dictates that with increased flow speed, the intraluminal pressure decreases, which places the valve at risk for collapse from the lower pressure.

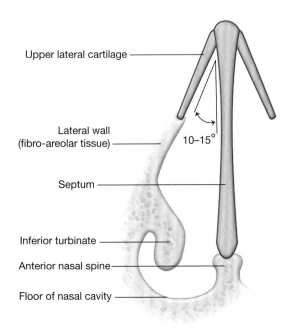

Upper lateral cartilage

Lateral wall
(fibro-areolar tissue)

10–15°

Septum

Inferior turbinate

Anterior nasal spine

Floor of nasal cavity

FIG 1 • Internal nasal valve.

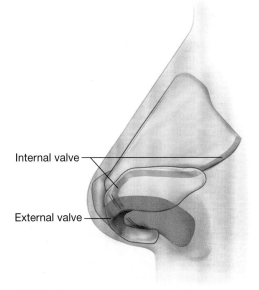

Internal valve

External valve

FIG 2 • Nasal valves.

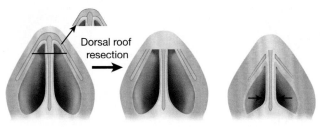

FIG 3 • Pathogenesis of iatrogenic middle vault collapse.

- Poiseuille law states that flow is proportional to the radius to the fourth power. Thus, seemingly diminutive changes in middle vault size have dramatic implications in nasal airflow.
- A decrease in middle vault size or weakening of the structural integrity of the nasal valve places the patient at risk for nasal airflow obstruction.
- Any resection of the middle vault roof greater than 2 mm during hump reduction destabilizes this most critical area, allowing the upper lateral cartilages to fall medially and produce a characteristic "inverted V" deformity and result in obstruction at the internal valves (**FIG 3**).
- Reducing the dorsum and creating an open middle vault and interval valvular incompetence will decrease the postoperative airway by 50%.
- The middle vault and internal nasal valve are at risk in three specific circumstances:
  - The midvault is congenitally narrow.
  - The nasal bones are short, therefore leaving a larger proportion of nasal sidewall supported by the ULCs (internal valves) and the lateral crura (external valves).
  - The surgeon reduces the dorsum by more than 2 mm, which in most patients will open the cartilaginous roof.
- The most common motivation for secondary rhinoplasty is an iatrogenic deformity from the previous surgery.[1]
- A narrow middle vault has been shown to be present preoperatively in 38% of primary and 87% of secondary rhinoplasty patients.[2]
- A study of 600 consecutive patients undergoing surgery for airway obstruction between 1991 and 2008 with a mean follow-up of 27 months found the following[2]:
  - Septal and valvular surgery corrected the airway obstruction in more than 95% of patients in a single operation, despite the fact that two-thirds of patients were secondary rhinoplasty patients with more severe deformities.
  - Septoplasty improved airflow ipsilateral to an obstruction but made no impact on total nasal airflow.
  - Internal valvular reconstruction with dorsal or spreader grafts doubled nasal airflow.
  - Dorsal and spreader grafts were equally effective at improving nasal airflow.
  - External valvular reconstruction doubled nasal airflow.
  - The greatest improvement in nasal airflow was observed after both internal and external valvular reconstruction (a fourfold improvement in airflow).
  - Septoplasty in addition to valvular surgery did not offer any clinical benefit compared with valvular surgery alone.
  - In patients with lateralized symptoms, the septum was deviated away from the obstructed side in 45% of cases, thus emphasizing the importance of valvular obstruction in creating airway symptoms.
  - Of the 384 secondary rhinoplasty patients, 94% had previously undergone adequate septoplasties but were still

symptomatically obstructed. Within this group, valvular reconstruction alone corrected the airway in 97% after one operative procedure.
- When primary and secondary rhinoplasty patients were stratified, the improvement in primary patients equaled or exceeded the improvement achieved in secondary rhinoplasty patients in six of the eight obstructed sites examined.
- Valvular obstruction was 4 times more common than pure septal obstruction in primary rhinoplasty patients and 12 times more common than pure septal obstruction in secondary rhinoplasty patients.
- When the entire 600-patient group was stratified, the greatest improvement was observed in those patients observed for more than 12 months, suggesting that the airway continues to enlarge as postoperative edema resolves.
- By measuring airflow during quiet and forced inspiration, sidewall stiffness could be quantified and increased following valvular reconstruction by dorsal, spreader, or alar wall grafts.
- Based on this study indicating that reconstruction of the internal nasal valve can double airflow, iatrogenic injury to the internal nasal valve can conversely reduce airflow by 50%, and this assumption has been corroborated by recent studies.[3]

PATIENT HISTORY AND PHYSICAL FINDINGS

- Four anatomic findings place patients at high risk for unfavorable results and should be identified preoperatively.[4]
  - Low radix or low dorsum
  - Inadequate tip projection
  - Narrow middle vault
  - Alar cartilage malposition
- Of these four, narrow middle vault and alar cartilage malposition (cephalic rotation of the lateral crus) impact the airway because they indicate preoperative threats to the internal and external nasal valves, respectively.
- The exam findings of an obstructing septum or turbinate do not often correlate well with patient symptoms.[2]
- Patients frequently breathe better on the apparent "obstructed" side, indicating that septal and turbinate obstruction do not explain the entire airway dysfunction.
  - Eighty percent of nasal septa in the population are deviated, yet only a small portion have clinical obstruction
- Patients with straight septa or prior successful septoplasty and turbinectomy frequently still have persistent symptoms of nasal obstruction.
- History
  - Organized approach to obtaining history: first inquire about the airway and subsequently discuss aesthetic concerns.
  - Many patients become accustomed to a poor nasal airflow and have forgotten how much better their airway used to be prior to trauma or other surgeries—thus, this part of the history requires that the physician guide the interview with direct questions.
  - It is important to inquire about a history of prior trauma because unhealed septal fracture lines may extend to the dorsal septal edge and therefore threaten dorsal strut stability.
  - Recent trauma (within 3 months) is an indication to postpone the rhinoplasty until any fractures have healed and until postoperative edema allows accurate judgment of the aesthetic contours.

- Ask about periodic or cyclic airway obstruction including which airway is worse, any nasal trauma history, seasonal allergies, clear rhinitis and suppurative sinusitis, snoring, epistaxis, sinus headache, frequent nose blowing, and what nonsurgical remedies the patient has tried to date.
- Often, secondary rhinoplasty patients with poor airways chronically self-medicate with steroid or vasoconstrictive sprays that must be identified and discontinued before surgery.
- Also important are the patient's work environment and a history of tobacco or alcohol consumption (either of which may cause nasal congestion) and cocaine use.
- Valve examination: Watch your patients breathe!
  - Sidewall collapse with inspiration is surprisingly common. If this occurs, it is important to determine the etiology (prior surgery, intrinsic weakness, cartilage malposition).
  - Perform a modified Cottle maneuver and compare airflow between sides. This maneuver is not specific, because even with septal deviation, traction on the sidewall will open the airway. Obstruction must be localized at the valves before valvular surgery is undertaken.
    - Support the collapsing area with a cotton-tipped applicator soaked in 1% pontocaine hydrochloride for the patient's comfort. Patients with valvular incompetence will notice an obvious and gratifying increase in airway size; thus, you can guarantee that valvular reconstruction will improve the airway similarly.
  - It is important to assess whether a high septal deviation exists because hump removal will unmask the curvature: in the middle of the operation, the nose can suddenly look newly asymmetrical. When a high septal deviation exists, the surgeon needs to be prepared to place unilateral or asymmetric spreader grafts. The correction is straightforward, but the surgeon must be attentive to new intraoperative deformities.
- Turbinates
  - Obstructing turbinates are relatively low in the hierarchy of causes of nasal obstruction.
  - Given their function to warm and humidify air, turbinate reductions should be planned conservatively.
  - Because the majority of turbinate hypertrophy is due to bony (not mucosal) overgrowth, most patients should be treated with turbinate crushing and outfracture.[5] If septal and valvular causes of airway obstruction have been corrected, the turbinates will not become enlarged again, unless the patient is atopic.

IMAGING

- Accurate photographs are imperative for consultation, formulation of an operative plan, and intraoperative guidance.
- Views should include full head and close-up frontal views, both oblique views (which often differ, particularly in patients with nasal asymmetry), both lateral views, and an inferior view.
- Photographs are best taken with a portrait focal length lens (90 to 105 mm) against a medium–dark background, lit so that symmetries and contours will be depicted accurately.
- Camera-mounted flash units are inferior to studio systems with umbrella lights or wall-mounted strobes to light the face evenly, provide backlighting, and illuminate the face and hair.

SURGICAL MANAGEMENT

- The great majority of functional nasal deformities can be corrected with only one of two operative strategies: spreader or dorsal grafts for internal valvular obstruction and alar wall grafts for external valvular obstruction. Each at least doubles airflow in most patients. Done correctly, these three procedures always work.
- For the patients presenting with nasal obstruction and/or a narrow middle vault, spreader grafts or dorsal grafts must be placed to support the lateral walls.
- Although some surgeons prefer autospreader grafts or spreader flaps where redundant ULC is turned in medially, their effectiveness at treating internal valve collapse has not shown promising results.[6,7]
- Other options for middle vault support include spreader flaps, tension suturing techniques,[8] and butterfly grafts.[7,9,10] Long-term functional outcome studies supporting these alternative techniques are lacking at this time, and current evidence indicates that tension sutures are ineffective. There is another theoretical problem with tension sutures: creating a barrel effect in the middle vault is not physiologic. The nasal airway needs variable resistance (which means a movable sidewall) during both inspiration (so that the alveoli can open) and exhalation (so that O_2 and CO_2 transfer can occur). The constant, widely open middle vault eliminates that necessary movement. Spreader grafts, however, have a solid foundation of literature supporting their long-term efficacy in both preventing and correcting middle vault collapse.[2]

Preoperative Planning

- Fallacies in planning: there are two common false assumptions that underlie the logic of reduction rhinoplasty that lead to unsatisfactory results.
- False assumption number one: *The nasal soft tissue cover has the infinite ability to contract to the shape of any underlying skeleton.*
- The nasal skin sleeve contracts according to its quality, thickness, and preoperative distribution, and not necessarily to the shape of the surgically reduced skeleton. The vectors of skin sleeve contraction are related to the volume and contour of the underlying skeleton, and the end result of reduction with a skin sleeve that cannot sufficiently contract to the reduced skeleton is the supratip deformity.
- False assumption number two: *Alterations in the nasal skeleton produce purely regional changes.*
- The classic application of this assumption is the common strategy in which the surgeon plans to resect all nasal dorsum anterior to a straight line drawn from the nasal radix to the point of the tip. Underlying this strategy is the assumption that dorsal reduction affects bridge height alone. Changes in the nasal skeleton are not independent, however, but rather have global effects outside their areas. Resection of the nasal bridge affects nasal width and length, apparent nasal base size, middle vault support, alar rim contour, and columellar position. Similarly, alar cartilage reduction can affect tip support and projection, nasal length, alar rim contour, and external valvular support. These structural interdependencies are not just regional. Recognizing this interplay is essential to effective preoperative planning, interpretation of intraoperative nasal appearance, postoperative success, and predictable correction of secondary deformities.

- One of the most important preoperative unknowns is the condition and quality of the cartilage graft material available. The appeal of alloplastic materials is their predictability on the day of surgery. However, the consistent longevity and intrinsic characteristics of autografts has not been duplicated with any alloplastic materials currently commercially available.
- The dorsum requires the straightest, smoothest graft—ideally septum, but autologous rib works as well.
- In planning graft placement, the surgeon should consider areas needing augmentation based on preoperative assessment as well as areas that may need grafts because of the surgical approach; for example, disequilibrium that the surgeon has created during reduction (ie, spreader grafts to support the internal valves after resection of the cartilaginous roof).
- The augmentation phase of any rhinoplasty re-establishes the preoperative nasal equilibrium and alters contours in ways that reduction alone cannot. The nose that is equilibrated at the conclusion of the procedure is less likely to change during healing and therefore gives the surgeon greater control over the result.

Positioning

- The operation is routinely performed under general anesthesia.
- The patient is placed supine, and the table is positioned in 10 to 15 degrees reverse Trendelenburg to minimize bleeding.
- The nose is blocked with 1% Carbocaine with epinephrine 1:100 000 (Carbocaine has a longer analgesic effect and intrinsic vasoconstrictive properties).

- Nasal vibrissae are shaved and the nose is thoroughly cleaned, inside and out, with povidone-iodine solution.
- Cotton packs soaked in 4% cocaine solution are placed in each airway.

Approach

- Endonasal rhinoplasty is an operation designed around changes in the skin surface—the underlying framework is adjusted only as much as is necessary to accomplish skin surface changes and functional airway changes.
- The endonasal rhinoplasty surgeon exposes only those anatomical parts that need correction and are directly related to changes that the patient wants. This principle creates the unique advantage of not subjecting any other nasal areas to possible iatrogenic deformities. *Primum non nocere* (first, do no harm)—if you expose areas unnecessarily, you put them at risk for postoperative problems.
- Skin sleeve movement, nasal balance changes, and the effects of reduction and augmentation all depend on an ability to see the undisturbed nasal surface accurately. This is what the patient sees and what matters.
- The nasal soft tissues create half the nasal shape: without being able to assess the skin surface accurately, the surgeon forfeits half of the information that is available to make the operation a success.
- Making changes through limited incisions and judging progress by feeling the surface simplifies some maneuvers and minimizes the need for graft fixation; crushed grafts can be used in ways that would be tedious or impossible with the open approach.

TECHNIQUES

■ Endonasal Access

- Unilateral or bilateral intercartilaginous incisions are preferred—the incision runs from the lateral end of the caudal reflection of the upper lateral cartilage around the septal angle. The surgeon making only functional corrections needs a single intercartilaginous incision that exposes the septal angle (**TECH FIG 1**).

- Joseph scissors and then a broad Cottle periosteal elevator are used to elevate the soft tissues off the bony and upper cartilaginous vaults if the surgeon plans a rhinoplasty; if not, the dorsum is not skeletonized.
- If no transfixion incision is necessary, the intercartilaginous incision stops at the junction of the anterior and middle thirds of the membranous septum; if the caudal septum requires shortening, the incision can be carried toward the anterior nasal spine.

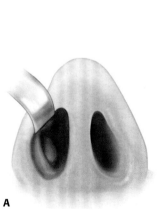 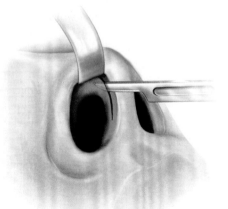 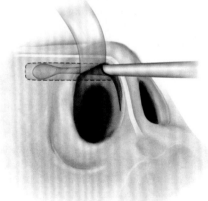

A   B   C

TECH FIG 1 • Endonasal access and creation of spreader graft tunnels. It is important to leave an adhesion between the mucoperichondrial edge and the anterior edge of the septum to prevent graft displacement.

■ Spreader Graft Tunnels

- When needed, spreader graft tunnels are performed before septoplasty. Spreader graft tunnels are facilitated by prior infiltration beneath the mucoperichondrium with local anesthetic.
- By identifying the septal angle, the surgeon can incise to cartilage beneath each mucoperichondrial flap and develop the tunnels with the sharp end of a Cottle perichondrial elevator (**TECH FIG 1**).

- Each tunnel must follow the dorsal septal edge and should extend beneath the caudal edge of the bony arch on each side, *leaving a narrow mucoperichondrial attachment along the anterior septal edge. This intact adhesion creates a pocket that will hold the spreader graft precisely; performed this way spreader grafts never rotate or displace. Done technically properly, they improve the airway reliably and virtually never require revision.*

■ Septoplasty

- For the septoplasty, the surgeon should perform the resection through a Killian incision, not from the dorsal edge, and leave 15 to 20 mm of intact, undissected cartilage along the nasal dorsum and 15 mm caudally to preserve stability and to facilitate spreader graft placement (**TECH FIG 2**).
- Do not perform a purely functional operation (septoplasty, crushing, and outfracture the inferior turbinates, spreader grafts, or alar wall grafts) through an open rhinoplasty approach because the risk of creating iatrogenic deformities is much too high and because it is unnecessary to take the tip apart to access the septum and internal valves. Spreader grafts are easily placed through an intercartilaginous incision; septoplasty is done through a Killian incision; and alar wall grafts are placed through short vestibular incisions to brace the anatomically unstable areas.
- Do not strip the mucoperichondrium from the dorsal or caudal struts, not only for stability but because such stripping has been experimentally shown to increase septal fibrosis and decrease chondrocytes in rabbits; we should assume that the same applies in humans.[11]
- If significant trauma has occurred, even in the distant past, the surgeon should enter the septum very cautiously and check for old fractures, as fractures through the anterior septal edge will destabilize the dorsal strut. It is preferable to avoid simultaneous septoplasty and bilateral osteotomies or to postpone osteotomy if the surgeon is not confident of septal support.
- In practice, the need for bilateral osteotomies in the severely traumatized nose is generally uncommon because

a unilateral osteotomy on the outfractured side achieves better symmetry than bilateral osteotomies.
- For septoplasty access, the initial mucoperichondrial Killian incision is made 15 mm above (cephalad to) the caudal septal edge; and using first the sharp and later the blunt end of a Freer elevator in one hand and a Frazier suction in the other, dissection proceeds under the mucoperichondrial flap onto the perpendicular plate of the ethmoid and over any posterior bony obstructions.
- Once the first flap has been developed, the sharp end of the elevator can score through the septal cartilage at the site of the opening incision; dissection then proceeds on the second side.
- Elevation of the perichondrium at the junction of septal cartilage and vomer is particularly difficult because the periosteal and perichondrial fibers are interlaced. The periosteal fibers are stronger, so mucosal tears are less likely if the surgeon begins dissection beneath the maxillary and vomerine mucoperiosteum and works cephalad.
- The first septal cut is made 15 to 20 mm below the dorsal septal edge with angled Knight septal scissors, which cut through septal cartilage and ethmoid; make sure that both blades are within the mucoperichondrial flaps before making the cut. A parallel cut is performed 8 to 10 mm inferiorly, and using Killian septal forceps, the first graft, now free on three sides, can be twisted so that the ethmoid fractures and allows removal in one piece. This maneuver often provides an initial graft 25 to 30 mm long containing the flattest, thickest, longest piece of septal cartilage, ideal for a dorsal graft.

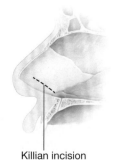 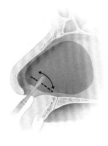 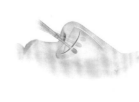 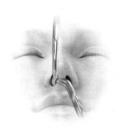 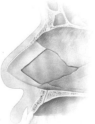

Killian incision

TECH FIG 2 • Septoplasty technique.

- Dissection continues posteriorly and caudally with the sharp end of a Cottle perichondrial elevator. The septal cartilage in the vomerine groove can often be dislodged by a bit of judicious wiggling with a narrow osteotome. With an osteotome and septal forceps, additional pieces of vomer or perpendicular plate of

the ethmoid can be removed if obstructing or if additional graft material is needed, always working under direct vision.
- In areas of severe deflection, tears in the mucoperichondrial flaps may be unavoidable, but the surgeon should nevertheless proceed cautiously and repair any tears.

■ Spreader Graft Placement

- Although septal cartilage provides the ideal spreader graft, strips of costal or conchal cartilage, ethmoid, or vomer may be used instead.
- Spreader grafts should provide confluence between the upper and lower nasal thirds, and they must span middle vault length from the bony arch almost to the septal angle.

- After spreader grafts are placed, caudal slippage can be avoided by a single 4-0 plain catgut transfixing suture placed at the septal angle.
- The width and contour of the middle vault should look and feel stable and symmetric once spreader grafts have been placed. In this regard, the closed approach provides significant advantages because the external surface configuration will guide the surgeon.

PEARLS AND PITFALLS

Pathogenesis	■ The middle vault and internal nasal valve are at risk in three circumstances: (1) when the midvault is congenitally narrow; (2) when the nasal bones are short, therefore creating a larger portion of the cartilaginous sidewall that is supported only by cartilage; (3) when the surgeon reduces the dorsum by more than 2 mm.
Planning	■ All key planning decisions can be made preoperatively from the nasal surface. Each anatomical point translates directly to a diagnosis and then to a surgical step: the entire rhinoplasty strategy can be set before surgery. ■ Reconstruct anatomically, never forgetting function and considering the patient's own aesthetic. ■ Reconstruction of internal valves doubles airflow in most patients.
Approach	■ The surgical outcome depends on the aesthetics and function of the nose, which are determined by both the soft tissue and structural support. ■ These contributions are easily assessed by the endonasal approach because the soft tissues, which determine 50% of the final result, are largely undisturbed.

POSTOPERATIVE CARE

- If septal or turbinate surgery has been performed, the nose is packed with petroleum gauze impregnated with bacitracin/mupirocin ointment.
- The packing should not overstuff the nose as it may dislodge the nasal bones or grafts.
- A no. 18 suction catheter is placed in the floor of each nasal airway to provide some airway patency and help equalize middle ear pressure.
- Oral antibiotics are prescribed for the first week while nasal packing is in place.
- A nasal splint is fashioned from layers of paper tape placed across the dorsum, tip, and cheeks, and then cloth tape is layered over it. Several layers of moistened 2-in. plaster are cut to fit and secured with another layer of cloth tape. The splint must be applied precisely but not too tightly to prevent nasal tip ischemia. Tip color should be checked frequently in the postoperative period, and the tip sling cut and nasal packs or splint removed as necessary.
- The nasal splint and any remaining packing are removed on postoperative day 6 to 7. By then, the nasal lining has healed, the nose is making mucus, and the packing slides out painlessly. Upon splint removal, the airway should instantly be excellent.

- If only septal and valvular surgery has been performed, swelling is minimal. If an entire rhinoplasty is performed, most patients are quite presentable at 7 days and may easily return to work in 10 days except in unusual circumstances. The nose will narrow after that for up to a year, but the dorsal line should be set.
- Patients should be seen as needed during the first 2 weeks to clean the nose of accumulated secretions, to ensure maintenance good alignment, and to educate the patient of expected changes over time. Patients must not exert themselves for at least 2 weeks following surgery to avoid hemorrhage and must slowly increase their activity after that to full athletic function at 6 weeks.

OUTCOMES (FIG 4)

- With good planning and technique, septal and valvular surgery can correct airway obstruction in up to 95%.[2]
  - That percentage reflects a combination of primary and secondary patients, some of whom required more than one surgery because of their preoperative deformities.
  - In primary patients, spreader grafts will uniformly increase airflow and, with experience, almost never require a second surgery.
- The airway will continue to improve throughout the first year, indicating that the airway enlarges as the edema resolves.[2]

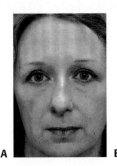 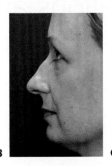 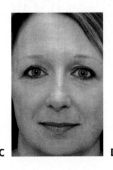 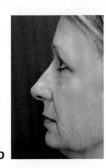

FIG 4 • Patient before (**A,B**) and after (**C,D**) septoplasty.

COMPLICATIONS

- Iatrogenic airway obstruction
  - More common than any complication and entirely preventable is iatrogenic decrease in the postoperative airway size. That cannot occur with proper preoperative septal, valvular, and turbinate diagnosis and treatment.
  - Most new postoperative obstructions are due to increased internal valvular incompetence or an incomplete septoplasty with residual obstructions posteriorly or along the floor. A new internal valvular incompetence will cut the preoperative airway by 50%.
  - Inadequate turbinate resection, columellar widening, and nostril stenosis are rare but do occur.
- Skeletal
  - Visibility of the caudal edge of the bony vault is often mischaracterized as inadequate reduction but is usually the result of middle vault collapse—the bony arch stands out relative to the depressed and over-resected middle vault.
  - New frontal asymmetry can occur when dorsal resection uncovers a high septal deviation. When recognized preoperatively or seen intraoperatively after dorsal resection, the surgeon can correct the deviation with asymmetrical spreader grafts and/or camouflage the deviation with a dorsal graft.
- Grafts
  - For those surgeons who augment often, graft imperfections are the most common reason for secondary revision.
  - Spreader grafts may be too wide or too narrow
- Septal perforation
  - Septal perforations can be minimized with careful dissection posteriorly and inferiorly where the perichondrium is densely adherent by repairing any mucosal tears and by placing silicone splints prior to nasal packing.
  - Even in the best of hands, the occasional small perforation will occur. Fortunately, many of these remain asymptomatic.
  - Smaller perforations may present as whistling, while larger ones as crusting, epistaxis, obstruction, or rhinitis.
  - Repair of perforations is difficult with a high recurrence rate. Repair involves debriding the exposed septal tissue and coverage with a local mucoperichondrial flap.
- Rhinitis and empty nose syndrome
  - Temporary rhinitis may occur for several weeks after an obstructed airway has been opened up.
  - An overaggressive turbinectomy can cause persistent rhinitis and is not easily correctible.
- Septal collapse
  - Loss of cartilaginous support has global ramifications for nasal support and airway because the intact septal partition is necessary for normal bridge contour, nasal length, base support, internal valvular competence, and upper lip carriage.

- Septal collapse can be avoided by identifying unhealed or unstable septal fractures before surgery and by leaving a minimum 15 mm width of undissected septal cartilage and mucoperichondrium along the dorsum to avoid jeopardizing septal support if unexpected, unhealed fracture lines are encountered.
- It is safer to access the septum through a Killian incision rather than through the dorsal edge. Leaving the mucoperichondrium undissected over the L-strut protects against collapse, prevents exposure of potentially weakened cartilage, and makes placement of spreader grafts easier.
- Infection
  - Fortunately, bacterial infection with rhinoplasty is quite rare but has become more common with the emergence and increasing prevalence of methicillin-resistant *Staphylococcus aureus* as a community-acquired pathogen. Patients should be routinely cultured for MRSA preoperatively and treated with mupirocin if necessary.
  - Using systemic antibiotics while nasal packing is in place may minimize the chance of maxillary sinusitis, although its necessity is unproven.

REFERENCES

1. Constantian MB. What motivates secondary rhinoplasty? A study of 150 consecutive patients. *Plast Reconstr Surg*. 2012;130:667.
2. Constantian MB, Clardy RB. The relative importance of septal and nasal valvular surgery in correcting airway obstruction in primary and secondary rhinoplasty. *Plast Reconstr Surg*. 1996;98:38.
3. Grymer LF. Reduction rhinoplasty and nasal patency: change in the cross-sectional area of the nose evaluated by acoustic rhinometry. *Laryngoscope*. 1995;105(4 pt 1):429-431.
4. Constantian MB. Four common anatomic variants that predispose to unfavorable rhinoplasty results: a study based on 150 consecutive secondary rhinoplasties. *Plast Reconstr Surg*. 2000;105:316.
5. Berger G, Hammel I, Berger R, et al. Histopathology of the inferior turbinate with compensatory hypertrophy in patients with deviated nasal septums. *Laryngoscope*. 2000;110:2100-2105.
6. Saedi B, Amali A, Gharavis V, et al. Spreader flaps do not change early functional outcomes in reduction rhinoplasty: a randomized control trial. *Am J Rhinol Allergy*. 2014;28(10):70-74.
7. Eren SB, Tugrul S, Ozucer B, et al. Autospreading spring flap technique for reconstruction of the middle vault. *Plast Reconstr Surg*. 2014;38(2):322-328.
8. Geissler PJ, Roostaeian J, Lee MR, et al. Role of upper lateral cartilage tension spanning suture in restoring the dorsal aesthetic lines in rhinoplasty. *Plast Reconstr Surg*. 2014;133(1):7e-11e.
9. Friedman O, Cook TA. Conchal cartilage butterfly graft in primary functional rhinoplasty. *Laryngoscope*. 2009;119(2):255-262.
10. Jalali MM. Comparison of effects of spreader grafts and flaring sutures on nasal airway resistance in rhinoplasty. *Eur Arch Otorhinolaryngol*. 2015;272(9):2299-2303.
11. Basaran K, Basat SO, Ozel A, et al. The effects of mucoperichondrial flap elevation on septal L-strut cartilage: a biomechanical and histologic analysis in a rabbit model. *Plast Reconstr Surg*. 2016;137(6):1784-1791.

54

CHAPTER

Indications and Techniques for Increasing and Decreasing Tip Projection in Closed Rhinoplasty

Barış Çakır and Mithat Akan

DEFINITION

- One of the reference points in the face is the vertical line intersecting the pupil, or "midpupillary line." The horizontal distance from the midpupillary line to the highest point of the tip is called the tip projection (TP).
- The horizontal distance from the midpupillary line to the apex of the nostril is called the nostril apex projection (NAP).
- The horizontal distance from the nostril apex to the tip's highest point is called the lobule projection (LP).
- The NAP together with the LP constitutes the TP (**FIG 1**).
- Examining the nose in this manner, element by element, will assist with the treatment.

ANATOMY

- The lower lateral cartilages consist of the footplate, the medial crus, the middle crus, the domes and the lateral crus.
- The lower lateral cartilages rest on the lip, the septum and the upper lateral cartilages.
- With its thickness of 2 to 4 mm, the Pitanguy midline ligament, which fills the space between the septal angle and the domes, ensures an elastic projection (**FIG 2A,B**).

PATHOGENESIS

- Tip projection = nostril apex projection + lobule projection
  - High NAP: Hypertrophic anterior and caudal septum, hypertrophic maxillary spine
  - High LP: Long medial and middle crus

- Low NAP: Hypoplastic maxilla, footplate sitting posteriorly, hypoplastic caudal septum, previous septoplasty surgery, aggressive resection of caudal septum
- Low LP: Short middle crus, short medial crus

PATIENT HISTORY AND PHYSICAL FINDINGS

- If the premaxillary support is weak, the nasolabial angle will be narrow, and when pulling up the lips, one can see that the maxillary mucosa is deep.
- Pressing on the nose tip will give us an idea about its support.
- In patients with posteriorly located maxilla it is difficult to obtain enough nasal projection. Patients who do not want a LeFort osteotomy may require a tongue in groove, an aggressive augmentation in premaxilla, or a long, strong columellar strut graft.

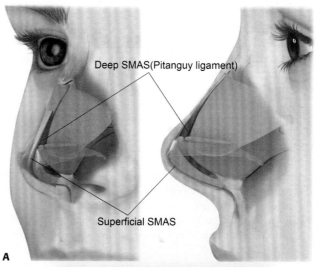

Deep SMAS(Pitanguy ligament)

Superficial SMAS

A

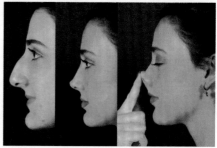

B

FIG 2 • **A,B.** With its thickness of 2 to 4 mm, the Pitanguy midline ligament, which fills the space between the septal angle and the domes, ensures an elastic projection.

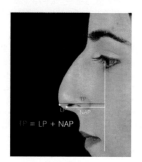

TP = LP + NAP

FIG 1 • Tip projection (*TP*), lobule projection (*LP*), nostril apex projection (*NAP*).

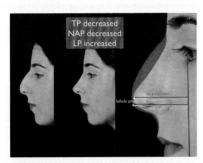

FIG 3 • One can easily plan changes to the TP, LP, and NAP by superimposing the newly planned nose over the old nose with a 50% contrast.

- It is noteworthy that in patients with high projection, the caudal and dorsal septa are hypertrophic.
- A hypertrophic septum can cause a hanging columella, tense lips and a wide footplate.
- Because the septum pushes the footplates more anterior than normal, the depressors are extremely tense. For this reason, the nasal tip may be more active when speaking.
- Skin thickness should be noted.

IMAGING

- Front, base, top, lateral, and oblique photographs are standard. A lateral smiling photograph can give clues about the dynamics of the nose tip.
- Imaging programs facilitate better analysis of the problems and planning of treatment.
- One can easily plan changes to the TP, LP, and NAP by superimposing the newly planned nose over the old nose with a 50% contrast (**FIG 3**).

SURGICAL MANAGEMENT

- The treatment needs to directly address the problem.

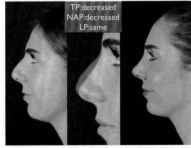

FIG 4 • Although a patient's LP may be normal, the high TP can be linked to a high NAP. In this case, LP did not change; TP decreased by decreasing NAP. Three months post-op photo is similar with the simulation.

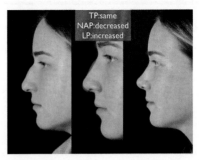

FIG 5 • A patient may have a normal TP, a high NAP, and a low LP. In order to protect the TP, one has to increase the LP in the same measure as one decreases the NAP.

Preoperative Planning

- It is important to observe how much the nasal tip contributes to the patient's facial expressions. One should observe the nose while the patient speaks. If the depressors are very active, this should be noted.
- Although a patient's LP may be normal, the high TP can be linked to a high NAP (**FIG 4**).
- A patient may have a normal TP, a high NAP and a low LP. In order to protect the TP, one has to increase the LP in the same measure as one decreases the NAP (**FIG 5**).
- A low TP may be linked to a low NAP as well as a low LP. Projection is the horizontal axis of the tip cartilage length. Rotation of the droopy tip also increases the projection (**FIG 6**).
- In thick-skinned noses, the projection needs to receive stronger support.

Approach

- A double-sided infracartilaginous incision and a single transfixion incision are sufficient.

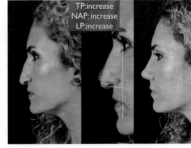

FIG 6 • A low TP may be linked to a low NAP as well as a low LP. Projection is the horizontal axis of the tip cartilage length. Rotation of the droopy tip also increases the projection.

■ Reducing the Nostril Apex Projection

- The surgical procedures outlined below all decrease the tip projection (TP). The techniques below can be applied in succession, until the desired projection is achieved.
- Dissect the caudal septum bilaterally in a subperichondrial plane (**TECH FIG 1A**).
- If this is not sufficient, resect the excess caudal septum. This procedure is recommended if the length of the nose needs to be shortened or if more rotation is needed. Only these two procedures are enough to resolve most of the excess TP (**TECH FIG 1B**).
- If this is not sufficient, dissect the caudal periosteum of the maxillary spine.
- If this is not sufficient, widen the dissection of the spine laterally.
- If this is not sufficient, resect the maxillary spine. This resection results in a dramatic deprojection (**TECH FIG 1C**).

- In those rare cases where the above procedures are insufficient, resect more bone from the maxillary spine and the surplus of periosteum an perichondrium at the septum maxillary spine junction.
- Even a deprojection of 3 to 5 mm greatly reduces the excursion of the depressor nasi muscle. Therefore, in patients with an active depressor muscle, an additional depressor resection may not be necessary if sufficient deprojection is performed.
- To decrease the NAP, shorten the lateral crura. If the lobule is short, we can not only extend the lobule but also shorten the lateral crus by performing a lateral crural steal.
- If the lobule is beautiful, a long lateral crus can be treated with a dissection and overlap in the region of the aperture.
- In patients in whom not only the projection is decreased but also the length shortened, there may exist an excess of mucosa in the membranous septum. Here, a conservative elliptical mucosal resection can be performed (**TECH FIG 1D**).

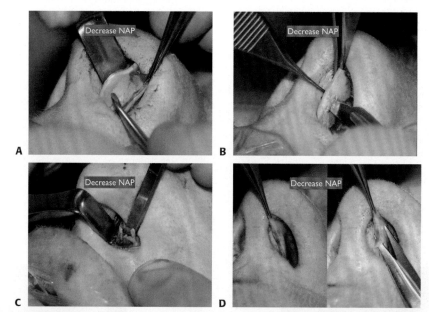

TECH FIG 1 • A. Dissect the caudal septum bilaterally in a subperichondrial plane. **B.** If this is not sufficient, resect the excess in the septum's caudal. **C.** Resection of the maxillary spine results in a dramatic deprojection. **D.** In patients where not only the projection is decreased but also the length shortened, an excess of mucosa may occur in the membranous septum. Here, a conservative elliptical mucosa resection can be performed.

■ Reducing Lobule Projection

- The most effective treatment for a long lobule is a medial crus overlap (**TECH FIG 2**).
- The most suitable location for this procedure is the break point of the columella.
- An oblique cut from the columella's break point toward the caudal-posterior direction increases the contact area.
- For an overlap, dissect the cartilage 2 to 3 mm from the mucosa.

- Tuck the medial crus underneath the middle crus, create an overlap of 2 to 3 mm, and suture it with a 6-0 PDS suture.
- Rarely is an overlap of 7 to 8 mm necessary. In this case, a resection of 2 to 4 mm can be combined with an overlap of 3 to 4 mm. In cases of long lateral crura shortened by lateral crural steal with high lobule projection (LP), an overlap of more than 4 to 5 mm may be necessary.
- A medial crus overlap is the most effective treatment for a hanging columella.

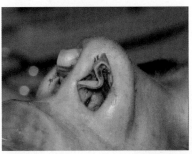 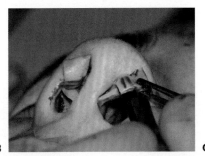 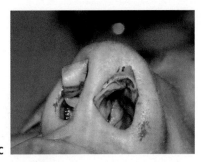

TECH FIG 2 • A–C. The most effective treatment for a long lobule is a medial crus overlap.

■ Increasing Lobule Projection

- The best technique for extending the lobule is a lateral crural steal (**TECH FIG 3A–F**). The LP increases at the same rate as the length of the lobular polygon.[1]
- A lateral crural steal will also increase rotation. Patients with a short lobule generally tend to need greater rotation.
- In closed rhinoplasty surgery where the Pitanguy and scroll ligaments are protected, only 5% to 10% of patients require a tip graft (**TECH FIG 3A**). Even though adequate rotation can be achieved by means of a steal, this may not be sufficient for adequate LP. In this case, tip grafts are preferable.
- If the ligaments are not protected, the cushioning underneath the domes disappears and the domes collapse into the septum. The Pitanguy ligament withdraws

underneath the supratip skin and fills up the supratip area. Depending on the increased height of the tip and supratip, the TP may appear insufficient. The need for a tip graft generally occurs due to a loss of projection of 3 to 4 mm, when the Pitanguy ligament has not been protected (**TECH FIG 3G–I**).
- If the lobule extends too much due to a lateral crural steal, this can be treated with a medial crus overlap.
- A lobule extended with the help of a steal should be supported by a strut graft.
- For an LP of 1 to 2 mm, minuscule free grafts to the tip are sufficient. After the mucosa has been closed, these grafts can be placed on and in between the dome cartilages.
- An LP of 2 to 3 mm necessitates tip grafts. An onlay graft in the shape of a boomerang facilitates the correct projection for tip highlights (**TECH FIG 3J**).

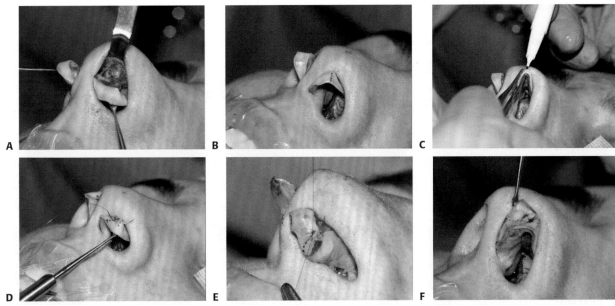

TECH FIG 3 • A–F. Lateral crural steal procedure.

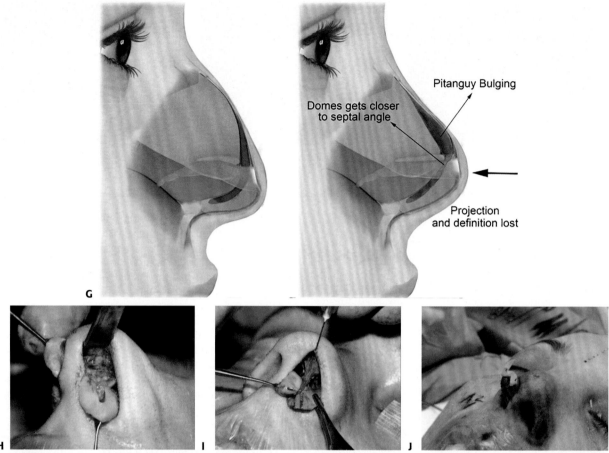

TECH FIG 3 (Continued) • **G–I.** If the ligaments are not protected, the cushioning underneath the domes disappears, and the domes collapse into the septum. The Pitanguy ligament withdraws underneath the supratip skin and fills up the supratip area. Depending on the increased height of the tip and supratip, the TP may appear insufficient. The need for a tip graft generally occurs due to a loss of projection of 3 to 4 mm, when the Pitanguy ligament has not been protected. **J.** An LP of 2 to 3 mm necessitates tip grafts. An onlay graft in the shape of a boomerang facilitates the correct projection for tip highlights.

■ Increasing Nostril Apex Projection

- If the footplates are wide, narrowing them with sutures will facilitate a TP of 1 to 2 mm (**TECH FIG 4A–G**).
- If the front of the maxilla is empty, perform a subperiosteal dissection to the front of the maxilla and fill it with cartilage pieces (**TECH FIG 4H,I**).
- In patients with a recurrent droopy tip, an aggressive augmentation in front of the maxilla is an effective technique.

- A long strut graft that extends to the maxilla and fixes the interdomal gap is the most effective technique for tip projection (**TECH FIG 4J–M**).
- Fixing the strut graft while the assistant pulls the dome cartilages anteriorly makes this technique easier.
- Increasing NAP also increases the rotation.

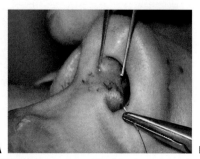
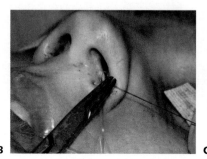
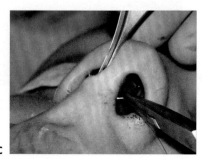

TECH FIG 4 • **A–G.** If the footplates are wide, narrowing them with sutures will facilitate a tip projection of 1 to 2 mm.

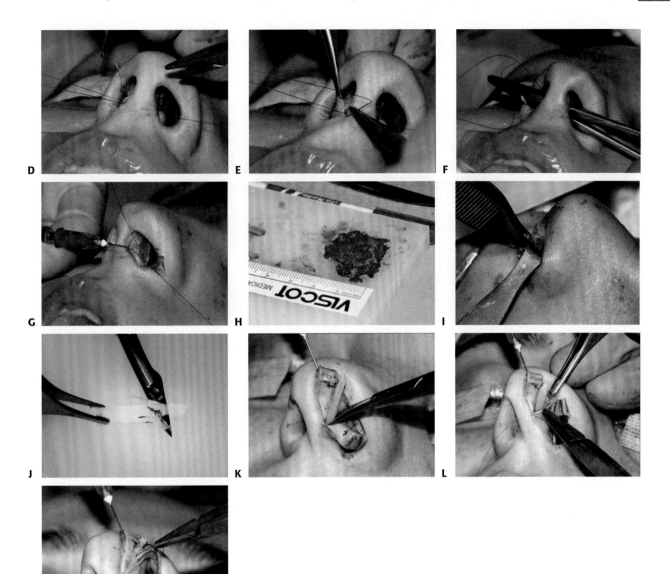

TECH FIG 4 (Continued) • **H,I.** If the front of the maxilla is empty, perform a subperiosteal dissection to the front of the maxilla and fill it with cartilage pieces. **J–M.** A long columellar strut graft that extends to the maxilla and fixes the interdomal gap is the most effective technique for tip projection.

PEARLS AND PITFALLS

Lateral crural steal	■ Every steal of 1 mm results in a rotation of about 6 to 8 degrees. The amount of the rotation obtained by means of a steal decreases logarithmically.
Lower lateral cartilage division	■ In big noses, it is generally necessary to cut the lower lateral cartilage at some point. The safest region for this cut is the middle crus.
Relationship between projection and rotation	■ Deprojection techniques will also reduce tip rotation. For this reason, it is necessary to equally shorten the lateral crus.
Tip projection analysis	■ Analyzing the TP in NAP and LP makes treatment more accurate.

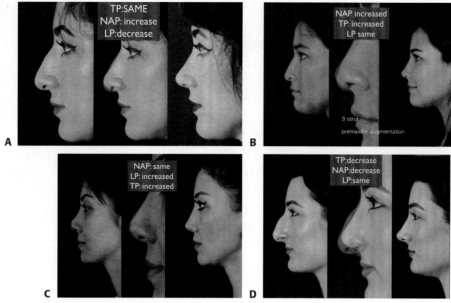

FIG 7 • **A–D.** Case examples.

POSTOPERATIVE CARE

- Carefully tape the nose without squeezing the tip. If the tape pinches the nose tip caudally, the positioning of the tip cartilages can be damaged.
- Because thermoplastic plaster is water resistant, the patient may shower every day.
- Applying tape underneath the eyes decreases swelling and bruising.
- The patient can be discharged after 3 to 4 hours.
- In case of swelling, a cold compress can be applied. Cold compresses are not routinely used after wide dissection and insertion of a drain.
- The patient rests in bed with the head elevated.
- Paracetamol with codeine is sufficient for pain management.
- Against bone edema, diclofenac potassium can be prescribed from day 5 to 10.
- After the preoperative prophylaxis, there is no need for antibiotics.
- Saltwater irrigation can be done for 10 days.

- Internal silicone dolly splints can be removed after 2 to 4 days.
- After 10 days, the cast is removed. Generally, no more tape is used.

OUTCOMES

- Sample preoperative photographs can be seen in **FIG 7**.

COMPLICATIONS

- Loss of rotation
- Loss of projection
- Tip asymmetry
- Bleeding
- Infection

REFERENCE

1. Cakır B, Oreroğlu AR, Daniel RK. Surface aesthetics in tip rhinoplasty: a step-by-step guide. *Aesthet Surg J.* 2014;34(6):941-955.

Techniques for Controlling Tip Rotation in Closed Rhinoplasty and Rhinoplasty Anesthesia

Barış Çakır and Mustafa Özgön

55

CHAPTER

DEFINITION

- A droopy nasal tip is one of the most frequently encountered indications for rhinoplasty.

ANATOMY

- The following anatomical features impact nasal tip rotation:
  - Maxilla
  - Columella
  - Lateral crus
  - Caudal septum
  - Upper lateral caudal
  - Pitanguy, scroll and interdomal ligaments
- All these anatomical structures have to be of the right dimension in order to ensure the desired nasal tip position (**FIG 1**).

PATHOGENESIS

- The most frequent problem causing a droopy nasal tip is the "tension nasal." Septum that extends too far caudally shapes the domes by bending the nasal tip cartilages from the middle crura.
- Septum pushes the footplates forward.
- Because the depressor and orbicularis muscles are under tension, an excessively droopy nasal occurs when laughing.
- Because the domes emerge from the middle crura, we encounter a long, wide and generally convex cartilage.
- Also, trauma or a resection of the caudal septum creates projection and loss of rotation.

NATURAL HISTORY

- The nasal tip has an elastic rotation and projection.
- The nasal tip contributes to minimal facial expressions. A nasal tip that remains stiff when speaking is one of the last remaining stigmata of rhinoplasty.
- It is important for the nasal tip to be mobile, so that the patient is able to comfortably lie face down and to kiss.
- Techniques such as septal extension graft and tongue in groove are proven solutions for rotation and projection; however, the nasal tip loses its softness.
- The nasal ligaments, and most importantly the Pitanguy ligament, ensure an elastic rotation and projection (**FIG 2**).

PATIENT HISTORY AND PHYSICAL FINDINGS

- The patient complains about a "droopy nasal tip."
- The nasolabial angle is narrow.
- The patient's skin type is of significance. Patients with thick skin and a nasal tip that droops excessively when laughing are more likely to experience loss of rotation.

IMAGING

- Front, base, top, lateral, and oblique photographs are standard. A lateral smiling photograph gives clues about the dynamics of the nasal tip. Taking a photograph of a beautiful nose, rotating it by 90 degrees, and looking at it in this way will facilitate the decision-making process concerning rotation during the surgery.

NONOPERATIVE MANAGEMENT

- Filler and Botox can be applied to the nasal base. This cannot substitute for rhinoplasty, however.

SURGICAL MANAGEMENT

- Suggested treatments for rotation control consist of different ways of attaching the medial crura to the septum.

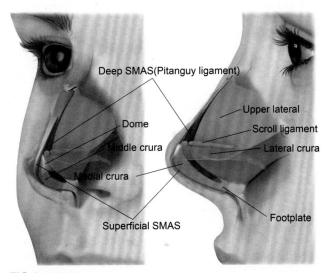

Deep SMAS(Pitanguy ligament)
Dome
Middle crura
Medial crura
Superficial SMAS
Upper lateral
Scroll ligament
Lateral crura
Footplate

FIG 1 • Anatomy.

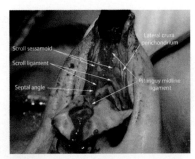

Scroll sessamoid
Scroll ligament
Septal angle
Lateral crura perichondrium
Pitanguy midline ligament

FIG 2 • Pitanguy and scroll anatomy.

- ■ The medial crura can be sutured to the septum named tongue-in-groove technique
    - ■ Permanent sutures can be applied from the medial crura to the septum named rotation control suture.
    - ■ The rotation can be stabilized with a septal extension graft.
- ■ However, these techniques may lead to a stiff nasal tip.
- ■ When deprojection is performed, the footplates, which are connected to the depressor muscles, change place posteriorly. This procedure decreases the muscle's excursion and weakens its function. For deprojection, it is generally sufficient to dissect the caudal septum in the subperichondrial plane.
- ■ For proper rotation, it is necessary to shorten the lateral crural cartilage, the upper lateral cartilage and caudal septum.
- ■ Shortening the lateral crus by means of the lateral crus steal technique increases lobule projection.
- ■ Without performing deprojection, a steal does not guarantee projection. The steal procedure re-establishes the projection lost due to deprojection.[1]
- ■ The basic effect of the lateral crus steal technique is an increase in rotation.
- ■ A strut graft is important to strengthen the support of the columella. In patients with weak columella support, 2 to 3 struts can be placed. Loss of projection causes loss of rotation.
- ■ In patients with an insufficient maxilla support, it is difficult to obtain rotation and projection. In these patients, the front of the maxilla should be filled with cartilage and bone (**FIG 3**).
- ■ In thick-skinned patients, it is necessary to select a strong and long cartilage as a strut graft and to use septocolumellar suture with 5-0 Prolene passing through the medial crus or the strut graft.

Positioning

- ■ The patient is positioned in the Trendelenburg position and lumbar flexion, with the neck in an extension of 20 to 30 degrees and parallel to the floor. In this position, intracranial blood pressure and surgical bleeding decrease. Keeping the head always parallel to the floor makes it less likely for errors to occur in rotation.
- ■ The patient is positioned on the back, with a pillow under the head, the arms on belly, and supported by a silicone cushion placed under their legs in such a way that their heels do not touch the operating table. The arms are secured by wrapping them with a sheet so that the chest is left either exposed or covered.
- ■ In the operating room, the anesthesia device is placed at a 45-degree angle next to the patient's head, to their right side. Thus, the surgeon can access the patient's head and check for symmetry (**FIG 4**). If the surgeon is right handed, the anesthesia device is placed to the left side.

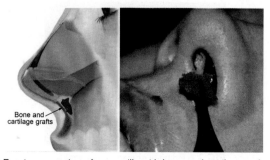

FIG 3 • Augmentation of premaxilla with bone and cartilage grafts.

Bone and cartilage grafts

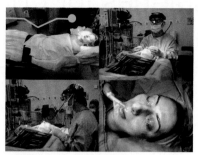

FIG 4 • Position of patient.

Anesthesia

- ■ Goal: Anesthesia aims to ensure the patient's safety and a bloodless surgical field during rhinoplasty and to prevent pain, nausea, and shivering, especially in the postoperative phase.
- ■ Application: On the day of the surgery, the patients, generally young adult outpatients whose anesthesia exam and workout (complete blood count, coagulation parameters, hepatitis markers, and ECG) have been completed 1 day earlier, are taken to the preop assessment room. The patient is monitored (ECG, SpO₂, NIBP), the tympanic temperature is measured, and the baseline values are recorded. An intravenous line is started, and 250 mL 0.9% isotonic NaCl with 1 g metamizole + 100 mg tramadol + 45.5 mg pheniramine maleate is administered.
- ■ A first-generation cephalosporin is used for surgical prophylaxis.
- ■ Pseudoephedrine nasal spray is used for septal mucosa vasoconstriction.
- ■ As premedication, an IV bolus of 1 mg midazolam + 10 mg metoclopramide + 50 mg ranitidine + 40 mg methylprednisolone is administered. Dexmedetomidine is administered with an infusion pump at a rate of 40 mcg/h.
- ■ Once these preparations are completed, the patient can be taken into the operating room and will be monitored again.
- ■ Infusions of propofol 50 mg/h and remifentanil 250 mcg/h are administered. Over the IV—after an infusion of 60 mg 2% lidocaine + 50 mcg fentanyl—5 mg rocuronium is given for the purpose of priming, and the timer is started. Following 150 mg of propofol, another 25 mg of rocuronium is administered. Fentanyl 50 mcg and another 50 mg of propofol are administered.
- ■ Once the eyelash reflex has disappeared, the eyes are covered with a line of polymyxin B eye cream and 1 cm of transparent tape. After 3 minutes, the patient is endotracheally intubated with a 7.0 spiral tube. The cuff is inflated with a cuff pressure of 25 cm H₂O, and during the operation, the cuff pressure is constantly measured, having been connected to a manometer with an 850 psi 120-cm extension, so that small adjustments can be made to keep it at 25 ± 5 cm H₂O.
- ■ The endotracheal tube is fixed at 21 to 23 cm to the right side (for left-handed surgeon) of the mouth, at a distance of 1 cm and such that the upper lip is not pulled askew, with 2 cm of Hypafix tape in the shape of an omega around the tube. Then the tube is connected to the anesthesia device in a semiclosed circuit with the help of an extension tube. In the volume control mode, breathing support is secured with 44% oxygen + 50% nitrous oxide and 6% desflurane at ET CO₂: 30 mm Hg (VT 8 to 10 mL/kg, f: 10 to 12/min, rate of fresh gas flow 2 L/min).

- The mouth and stomach are checked with a 16 G orange aspirator cannula. Then the surgery is started.
- Over 30 minutes, 1 g paracetamol is given.
- After the first hour, the dexmedetomidine infusion will be adjusted to 20 mcg/h, and in each half hour thereafter, the dose will be decreased by half, until it reaches zero after the 2nd hour.

Administering Local Anesthesia

- Local anesthesia is performed with 3-cc solution 1/80 000 (5 cc bupivacaine + 5 cc 2% lidocaine + 9 cc 0.9% NaCl + 1 cc 1/4 adrenaline) nasally, 2 cc 1/160 000 (2 cc 0.9% NaCl + 2 cc 1/80 000 lidocain-adrenaline solution. Jetokain®) solution for septal mucosa in 10 minutes. Generally, this should not lead to any significant lengthening of the QT interval or any other arrhythmia, and the increase in $ETCO_2$ should not exceed 10%. (Based on the adrenaline contained in the local anesthesia, the increase in $ETCO_2$ and the lengthening of the QT interval in the ECG are accepted as early warning signs to suspend the administration of local anesthesia, and normocapnia is ensured by increasing the minute volume on the ventilator.)
- Wait until the systolic blood pressure decreases below 90 mmHg for the local solution injection. If the local solution infiltration to nasal increases the blood pressure over 100 to 110 mm Hg, optimal adrenaline vasoconstriction cannot be achieved.
- During the surgery, generally, no further intervention is necessary. Rather than focusing on the same fixed numerical values in terms of the hemodynamic parameters for all patients during the surgical procedure, one should ensure the individual patient's regular pulse and blood pressure in such a way that they facilitate a surgical field without bleeding (**FIG 5**).

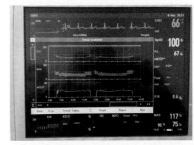

FIG 5 • Patient's parameters stabilization during the surgery.

- Based on the surgeon's feedback and the patient's hemodynamic parameters, the infusion dosages can be decreased in a controlled manner after the first hour.
- Toward the end of the surgery, while the silicone doyle splints are being placed, the nitrous oxide and desflurane are turned off. After a washout with 100% oxygen, 44% oxygen and 56% air are administered.
- Dexamethasone 8 mg and 4 mg ondansetron are administered intravenously.
- Upon completion of the surgery and before applying the bandages, the mouth and stomach are aspirated with an 18 G green aspirator cannula. Infusions of propofol are discontinued.
- While applying the bandages, the patient may sometimes open the eyes when coming into contact with cold water; if the patient can follow verbal directions, he or she can be extubated and given oxygen with a simple mask at 5 to 6 L/min. If the patient has not woken up at this stage, the team waits until the patient spontaneously does so, which generally occurs within 20 minutes. A conscious patient with sufficient spontaneous breathing is kept on the operating table for 5 more minutes and then transferred to the postoperative recovery room.

■ Securing an Elastic Rotation by Protecting the Pitanguy Ligament

- With the posterior transfixion incision, the perichondrium of the caudal septum is left attached to the Pitanguy ligament.
- Leaving 1 mm of cartilage from the caudal septum attached to the perichondrium makes it easier to suture it back.

- The surgeon delivers the caudal septum, then determines the excess caudal septum by forcing the tip rotation, and removes that excess (**TECH FIG 1A**).
- In the area of the membranous septum, the perichondrium and 1-mm cartilage flap that has been left attached to the Pitanguy ligament are fixed to the septum with 3 to 5 sutures with 5/0 PDS in the desired projection and rotation (**TECH FIG 1B**).

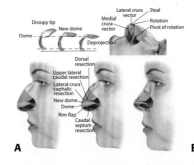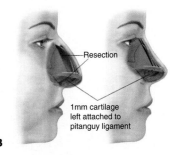

TECH FIG 1 • **A.** Resection for rotation. **B.** Resection of caudal septum and suturing caudal septal perichondrium and 1-mm cartilage flap to septum.

TECHNIQUES

T
E
C
H
N
I
Q
U
E
S

■ Shortening a Long Lateral Crus

- The surgeon delivers the tip cartilages and completes the surgery on the tip.
- The lateral crus must absolutely be shortened to the correct length.
- In patients with a short lobule and weak domes, the best technique to shorten the lateral crus is the lateral crus steal (**TECH FIG 2**).
- Cephalic resection also increases rotation but not as much as shortening the lateral crura.

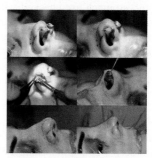

TECH FIG 2 • Lateral crura steal (because of long lobule after lateral crura steal, medial crura overlap performed).

■ Shortening a Long Upper Lateral

- After the desired tip position has been achieved, the caudal part of the upper lateral cartilages should be double-checked. Any kind of surplus should be resected (see **TECH FIGS 1A** and **3**).
- While repairing the scroll ligament, the surgeon can pass one suture through the upper lateral.

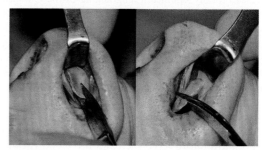

TECH FIG 3 • Caudal resection of upper lateral cartilage.

■ Projection is Important for the Nasal Tip Rotation

- The rigidity of the nasal tip needs to be double-checked. The nasal tip should be mobile but should still have adequate support when pressed with a finger. If support is not adequate, an additional strut should be placed.
- In secondary patients and patients with recurrent tip rotation and loss of projection, one should consider an augmentation in front of the maxilla.

PEARLS AND PITFALLS

Projection	■ Loss of projection causes loss of rotation. Therefore, the support for the tip should be double-checked at the end of the surgery.
Skin	■ Thick-skinned noses are more likely to experience loss of rotation. Projection should be well supported, and for that purpose, the surgeon may want to perform an over-rotation of 1 to 2 mm.
Loss of rotation	■ The most frequent reason for loss of rotation is a long lateral crus, a long upper lateral, and insufficient support of the nasal tip.
Impact of anesthesia	■ The patient is our main priority. ■ A harmonious collaboration between the anesthesia and surgical teams impacts the surgical outcome. ■ Nasal spray 20 min before surgery supply bloodless septal surgery. ■ We applied pre-emptive multimodal analgesia, multimodal nausea prophylaxis, combined H1 + H2 receptor blockage, and a balanced general anesthesia supported by nitrous oxide. (Noah pudding anesthesia*.) ■ We supported the premedication with an alpha 2 agonist (dexmedetomidine). ■ We used neither beta-blockers nor nitroglycerin. ■ We administered the local anesthesia-adrenaline solution in fractions and over a span of more than 10 min. Rather than waiting for suitable conditions to occur, the surgeon should create them. ■ We continuously monitored the pressure in the balloon of the intubation tube and kept it at a level that would not damage the trachea's mucosa. ■ At the end of the surgery, oral and pharyngeal suction as well as gastric emptying were performed when the patient was still under general anesthesia. ■ The patient was awakened at the position and the conditions that the anesthesia induction was started. ■ During the surgery, easy listening type of music was listened.

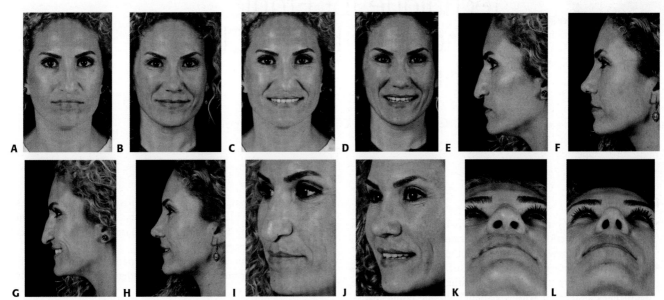

FIG 6 • A,B. A case example for rotation frontal view (3 months result). **C,D.** Smiling frontal view. **E,F.** Lateral view. **G,H.** Smiling lateral view. **I,J.** Oblique view. **K,L.** Base view.

POSTOPERATIVE CARE

- The patient is on bed rest for the first hour. After 1 hour, the patient may drink water. If the patient does not complain about nausea, he or she is allowed to eat a sandwich and drink fruit juice, followed by another hour of bed rest. If the patients have no further complaints, they may sit up and be mobilized. If their general condition is satisfactory, the intravenous line can be removed. The patient should be advised not to drink alcohol or operate a vehicle in the first 24 hours. Patients should be transferred by wheelchair to the vehicle taking them home.

OUTCOMES

- A case example for nasal tip rotation can be seen in **FIG 6**.

COMPLICATIONS

- Loss of rotation
- Over-rotation

REFERENCE

1. Cakır B, Oreroğlu AR, Daniel RK. Surface aesthetics in tip rhinoplasty: a step-by-step guide. *Aesthet Surg J*. 2014;34(6):941-955.

56 CHAPTER

Technique for Ethnic Rhinoplasty by the Closed Technique

Shruti C. Tannan, Clayton Crantford, and Mark B. Constantian

DEFINITION

- Closed rhinoplasty allows the surgeon to achieve the patient's aesthetic and functional goals as accurately as possible without introducing new deformities with the surgical approach.
- Ethnic rhinoplasty refers to surgery of the non–Northern European nose that respects the aesthetics and particular challenges associated with a patient's unique ethnic background. However, in practice, the distinction is somewhat artificial because each patient, regardless of his or her ethnic background, deserves a result that matches, as much as possible, the patient's aesthetic goals and that takes into account the degree of change (or preservation) of ethnic, familial, or personal characteristics that the patient desires.
- Specifically, some patients with distinctive familial, ethnic, or personal characteristics may wish to retain them, whereas others may want a type change. *It is critical that the surgeon be aware of these expectations to prevent patient dissatisfaction with the surgical result.*
- As with all preoperative discussions, a conversation with the patient about his or her goals and expected outcomes should be a critical part of every rhinoplasty, ethnic or not.
- The principles of forming and then performing the surgical plan do not differ; thus, ethnic rhinoplasty in many ways does not differ from any other rhinoplasty.
- The surgeon must consider the technique that allows him or her to deliver what the patient wants while also maintaining his or her personal identity.
- One of the most common motivations for secondary rhinoplasty is the loss of a familial, ethnic, or personal nasal characteristic.[1] For example, the surgeon may assume the dorsal hump is to be taken down, but the patient may prefer that the dorsal hump remain as a distinctive feature; this and all areas to be addressed during rhinoplasty should be discussed together preoperatively.
- A detailed discussion of specific aesthetic goals with the patient is imperative. The closed approach offers the surgeon the ability to see the result on the table; therefore, it is possible to set goals and deliver.
- Some patients intend to maintain some of the characteristics of their noses that are a part of their shared heritage, whereas others wish to alter them; it is up to the surgeon to initiate this discussion for a thorough understanding of the operative plan.

ANATOMY

- Although there is a large spectrum of variability in the so-called ethnic nose, there are common characteristics and features. It is important to recognize these findings in

advance so that a preoperative discussion is complete and so the operative plan addresses the concerns the patient wishes to alter while maintaining the characteristics the patient wishes to preserve.
- Four anatomic findings place all patients at high risk for unfavorable results and should be identified preoperatively.[2]
  - Low radix or low dorsum
    - Dorsal length and height, balanced against lower nasal size, determine the attractiveness of nasal proportion. A low radix or low dorsum begins caudal to the level of the upper lash margin with the patient's eyes in primary gaze.
    - When the radix begins low, nasal length is shorter and the nasal base size therefore appears larger. The surgeon must raise the dorsum segmentally or entirely to balance the patient's nasal base. In thicker-skinned patients, the strategy is particularly attractive because it requires less soft tissue contraction.
    - However, dorsal length must also be balanced against nasal base size. In patients with a very short nasal base (eg, some Asian noses), the radix should begin lower than the upper lash margin. Ethnicity and patient preference is one aspect; good nasal proportion is another.
  - Inadequate tip projection
    - Tip projection reflects cartilage strength, not skin volume, specifically the length of the alar cartilage middle crust. Adequate tip projection, in which the tip supports itself independent of dorsal height, is necessary for a straight profile line.
    - A tip with inadequate projection is any tip that does not project to the level of the anterior septal angle. Adequately projecting tips do not need increased support, whereas inadequately projecting tips do.
    - A patient may have a large nasal base but still have inadequate tip projection. An oversized, unbalanced lower nose does not mean that the patient has excessive tip projection.
    - Failure to recognize inadequate tip projection causes dorsal over-resection, supratip deformity, and deformity from soft tissue contraction.
  - Narrow middle vault
    - A narrow middle vault signals an internal valve that is already compromised.
    - The middle vault narrows following cartilaginous roof resection, so hump removal can inadvertently worsen the airway. Resection of even 2 mm of the cartilaginous roof during hump removal ablates the stabilizing confluence that braces the middle vault, which can now collapse toward the anterior septal edge, restricting airflow at the internal valves and producing a characteristic inverted "V deformity."

- Reconstruction of incompetent internal valves by either dorsal or spreader grafts doubles mean nasal airflow in most patients.[3]
- Alar cartilage malposition
  - Describes cephalically rotated lateral crura whose long axes run toward the medial canthi instead of toward the lateral canthi.
  - The abnormal cephalic position of the lateral crura places them at special risk if an intercartilaginous incision is made at its normal intranasal position. This will transect the entire rotated lateral crus instead of splitting the intended cephalic portion.
  - The majority of malpositioned lateral crura do not provide adequate external valvular support, leading to external valvular incompetence in addition to boxy or ball tips.
  - Adequate treatment of cephalic rotation of the lateral crura requires resection and replacement of these structures, relocation of the lateral crura to support the external valves, or supporting the areas of external valvular collapse with autogenous grafts.
  - Correction of external valvular incompetence doubles mean nasal airflow in most patients.[4]

PATIENT HISTORY AND PHYSICAL FINDINGS

- Patient history
  - Airway and aesthetic concerns
  - History of prior nasal trauma
  - Airway obstruction
- Internal nasal exam
  - Valves
  - Septum
  - Turbinates
- External nasal exam
  - Cartilage size and substance
  - Bony vault length
  - Nasal sidewall stiffness
  - Soft tissue thickness/distribution
    - Soft tissue *thickness* determines the degree of reduction possible and the character of augmenting or stabilizing grafts. Soft tissue *distribution* determines ultimate nasal size and proportion.
  - Nasal shape overall: width, length, bridge contour, tip shape, nostril size, columella and upper lip position, and any asymmetries.

IMAGING

- Software imaging systems exist that allow improved communication between surgeon and patient, although it represents a simulated, not guaranteed result. Imaging is only useful if the surgeon can simulate those structural and contour changes that the patient's anatomy and biological principles will permit.

SURGICAL MANAGEMENT

- The objectives of ethnic rhinoplasty are in keeping with the goals of as any other rhinoplasty: to achieve the patient's aesthetic and functional goals as accurately as possible without introducing new deformities.
- The closed approach to ethnic rhinoplasty offers many advantages.
- Closed rhinoplasty requires less dissection, always allowing the surgeon an undisturbed view of the nasal surface, which determines 50% of the final outcome.

- Closed rhinoplasty allows the surgeon the ability to control tip contours more accurately because there is less intraoperative soft tissue manipulation and the dorsal and tip skin never leave their preoperative positions.
- Tip grafts are easier to place in precise pockets in closed rhinoplasty because they do not have to be sutured into place. Multiple grafts of different thickness and substance can be placed to create particular aesthetic goals because the surgeon controls the soft tissue pocket. These techniques are not possible through the open approach.
- Columellar struts are never needed because the medial crura are not routinely disrupted from the adherent columellar skin and tip projection is not routinely lost through the closed approach access.
- Fewer variables are introduced by the surgical approach, and this reduces postoperative problems and greatly decreases the chance of new iatrogenic deformities.
- Closed rhinoplasty avoids problems that are almost unique to open rhinoplasty: columellar widening or notching, significant alar rim, and alar cartilage distortions.
- There are no contraindications to the closed approach to rhinoplasty, as this approach allows the surgeon to minimize morbidity in even the most difficult of cases.

Preoperative Planning

- The preoperative exam consisting of an internal and external nasal exam is critical.
- Specific attention should be paid to the valves, septum, turbinates, and basic nasal aesthetics.
- Always identify the four anatomical variants first so that their treatment can be included in the surgical plan.
- Preoperative photographs are imperative.
- Setting goals with the patient and discussing potential complications and revisions are vital.
- Three soft tissue parameters are used to form the authors' rhinoplasty plan: skin thickness, skin distribution, and tip lobular contour.[5]
- Virtually all primary and secondary nasal deformities can be solved by one of two surgical strategies that follow the necessary reduction maneuvers: (1) radix, spreader, and tip grafts or (2) dorsal grafts and tip grafts plus or minus (3) alar wall grafts.
  - This means that the surgeon need master only four graft types (because radix/dorsal grafts are the same graft in different lengths) to solve most nasal problems.
  - Maxillary augmentation for retrusion, lateral wall grafts for asymmetries, composite grafts for alar retraction, and other procedures are relative details.
  - The primary aesthetic and airway problems can be corrected using only the four graft types mentioned, using the two strategies outlined. This gives the surgeon much less to master.

Positioning

- The patient is placed supine with the arms and legs padded and the knees slightly flexed; the operating table is 10 to 15 degrees reverse Trendelenburg position to minimize bleeding.

Approach

- Closed rhinoplasty
- Rhinoplasty offers the possibility of individualizing a result as much as or more than any other aesthetic procedure, and the closed approach is often the key to doing so.

- The techniques for performing the closed approach to ethnic rhinoplasty are the same as any closed rhinoplasty.

- The key is addressing the patient's desires and goals without creating incongruity with a patient's heritage or an awkward, "operated" appearance.

■ Skeletonization

- Endonasal access via unilateral or bilateral intercartilaginous incisions is preferred.

- For details on closed rhinoplasty exposure, see Chapter 53, Indications and Technique for Treating the Narrow Middle Vault in Closed Rhinoplasty.

■ Dorsal Resection

- Bony vault reduction is performed under direct vision using a sharp rasp, judging the result by assessing surface contours.
- Next, resection of the dorsal border of the septum is accomplished with a no. 11 blade from which the tip has been broken to avoid lacerating the contralateral dorsal skin (**TECH FIG 1**).
- The dorsum should feel and appear perfectly smooth through the skin surface after dorsal resection.
  - Watch for a depressed discontinuity in the mid-dorsum; this is a "mid-dorsal notch" and signifies dorsal over-resection beyond the limits of soft tissue contraction.
  - Treatment is placement of a thin dorsal graft under the notch, not more skeletal resection.[6]

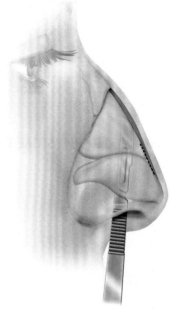

TECH FIG 1 • Resection of the dorsal border of the septum is accomplished under direct vision with a no. 11 blade from which the tip has been broken to avoid lacerating the contralateral dorsal skin.

■ Nasal Spine–Caudal Septum

- Through a transfixion incision, the caudal septum and nasal spine can be accessed and resected as necessary to change the relationship of the columella to nostril rim, nasal length, subnasale contour, and upper lip carriage (**TECH FIG 2**).

- If the nasolabial angle and upper lip relationships are satisfactory, no transfixion incision and no caudal septal or nasal spine modifications are necessary.
- Be cautious about over-resection; 1 or 2 mm makes the difference between normal columellar position and retraction.

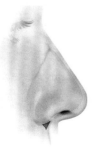
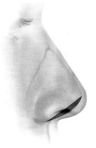
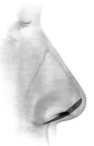
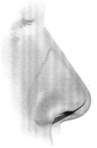

A Nasal spine reduction only

B Caudal septal reduction without shortening

C Caudal septal reduction with shortening

D Caudal septal reduction with lengthening

TECH FIG 2 • The specific maneuvers for the nasal spine and caudal septum depend on the need.

■ Alar Cartilage Resection

- Orthotopic or nondeforming cephalically rotated (mal-positioned) lateral crural cartilages are modified retrograde through the intercartilaginous incisions; rarely, more than 2 to 3 mm is removed, leaving lateral crura of 8 to 10 mm in width.
- The domes can be narrowed by vertical wedge resections performed at the lateral genu.
- Distorted or severely convex "boxy" or "ball" tips that must be significantly modified are dissected free from their vestibular and overlying skin and (1) resected and replaced after trimming to create the flattest segment, (2)

resected and replaced by septal or ear cartilage grafts, or (3) delivered as a medially based flap and rotated into the alar rim, with care to ensure that distortion or notching at the soft triangle or lateral genua does not occur.
  - Most "boxy" or "ball" tips are also malpositioned, so that a functional problem accompanies the aesthetic deformity and should be corrected simultaneously.[7]
- Freeing of the lateral crura, dome resection, or division of the alar cartilage arch reduces tip projection: thus, tip grafts are necessary to reconstruct the lobule.
- In order to avoid vestibular stenosis and iatrogenic airway obstruction, nasal lining should never be resected.

■ Upper Lateral Cartilages and Shortening the Nose

- A single hook is used to draw the caudal edge of the upper lateral cartilage downward, exposing the caudal edge for submucosal resection with Joseph scissors.
- The posterior edges of the upper lateral cartilages should be left to abut the lateral crura; mucosa should never be resected.
- A variety of interventions shorten the nose. In descending order of their effect, they are dorsal resection, caudal septal resection, resection of the cephalic edges of the alar cartilages lateral crura, and resection of the anterocaudal ends of the upper lateral cartilages (**TECH FIG 3**).
  - This final step is unnecessary unless substantial nasal shortening is required.

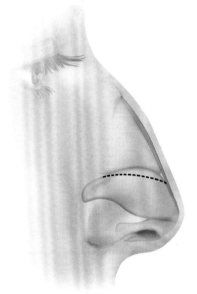

TECH FIG 3 • The cephalic portion of the lateral crus is resected.

■ Septoplasty and Spreader Graft Tunnels

- Spreader graft tunnels should be performed prior to septoplasty.

- For details on septoplasty and spreader grafts, see Chapter 63, Indications and Technique for Treating the Narrow Middle Vault in Closed Rhinoplasty.

■ Turbinectomy

- Turbinate crushing and outfracture suffice in most patients.
- If resection is necessary, for example, in severely atopic patients, biopsy forceps are used to trim the anterior

edge sufficient to obtain 3 mm of clearance to the septum or nasal floor.
- Be conservative, as over-resection and its resulting physiologic disturbances are not correctable.

■ Graft Placement and Wound Closure

- Spreader grafts are sized to the dimensions of the tunnel and the length of the upper lateral cartilages. They may be adjusted in width or configuration to provide symmetry.
- The skin of the nasal dorsum and radix is thinnest, and slight imperfections/asymmetries may be easily noticed. Dorsal and radix grafts must fit the configuration of the defect and suit the soft tissue cover. These grafts should

feel and look perfectly on the operating room table beneath the soft tissue envelope.
- Important principles of tip grafting include the following: graft length should be suited to its purpose and graft substance/contour must match the soft tissue cover.
- Multiple softened grafts work well for patients who still have their alar cartilages and only need improved definition.

- For the patient with an undefined and unsupported tip, solid cartilage or bone graft is placed to establish projection and define the angle of rotation. By itself, a single tip graft looks too artificial and pointed. Accordingly, softened cartilage grafts are placed anterior to the defining graft to re-create a normal lobule.

- As grafts are placed (in that order), 5-0 plain catgut sutures close each access incision so that graft position will be easier to maintain.

Osteotomy

- A single lateral osteotomy with a guarded osteotome, which begins intranasally, low at the pyriform aperture, and ends higher toward the nasal root, is sufficient to narrow the upper nasal third.
  - If the bony vault is low and broad and will be augmented, the nasal bones are short, or if the upper nasal third is already sufficiently narrow, osteotomy is not necessary (**TECH FIG 4**).
- Gentle digital pressure is used to greenstick fracture the remaining cephalic attachment and will reform the bony pyramid.

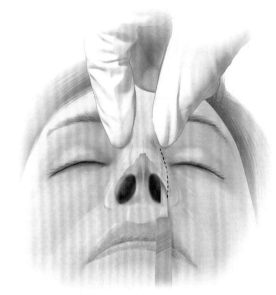

TECH FIG 4 • Intranasal osteotomies are performed with a guarded, curved 4-mm osteotome beginning at the base of the piriform and advancing toward the medial canthus.

Alar Wedge Resection

- When necessary, an external incision is made slightly outside the alar crease in order to not destroy this important landmark.
  - Remember that the alar wall has two surfaces, external and vestibular, and that they can be treated independently. In other words, the alar lobule can be narrowed without reducing nostril size, or both alar lobule and nostril can be reduced.
- It is important to retain a small medial flap as the surgeon incises the nasal floor to provide a smooth closure line and avoid notching. 6-0 nylon is used for closure and sutures are removed at 5 days.

PEARLS AND PITFALLS

Ethnic rhinoplasty	• Ethnic rhinoplasty does not differ from any other type of rhinoplasty from a technical standpoint: treatment of a low dorsum and large nasal base under a thick soft tissue cover is the same whether the patient's ethnic background is Slavic or African American.
	• It is imperative that the surgeon and patient communicate about the particular aspects of the appearance of the nose he or she wishes to preserve and which ones he or she would like to address surgically.
	• Knowledge of common characteristics of each ethnic group provides a starting basis for the preoperative discussion, but it is the patient's specific nasal contour and aesthetic goals that should dominate. Individuals are too unique to make sweeping generalizations about the characteristics of any ethnic groups.
Approach	• Closed rhinoplasty does not mean blind rhinoplasty. Rather, the mental exercise that distinguishes endonasal rhinoplasty from open rhinoplasty is precisely the same thought process that distinguishes liposuction from abdominoplasty.
	• The surgeon accepts limited access and makes intraoperative judgments based on the appearance and "feel" of the surface because doing so gives the surgeon more control and precision and therefore benefits the patient.
	• The more difficult the deformity and the more difficult the case, the stronger the argument can be made for limiting access, limiting incisions, and minimizing morbidity by minimal disruption of the nose.

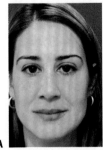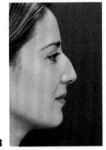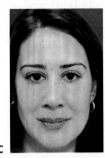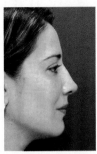

A   **B**   **C**   **D**

FIG 1 • A young woman of Greek ancestry for whom it was critically important to maintain ethnic identity, which she defined as preserving her dorsal convexity. The surgical procedure involved dorsal reduction, spreader grafts to maintain valvular competence following resection of the cartilaginous roof, tip grafts to increase projection, and deliberate maintenance of dorsal height. **A,B.** Preoperative views. **C,D.** Two-year postoperative views.

POSTOPERATIVE CARE

- Nasal packs are placed in all patients who undergo septoplasty or have had grafts placed. Nasal packs, tape, and plaster splints immobilize the reconstruction for 1 week, until the grafts and modified skeleton are stable and packing can be removed without pain or bleeding.
- See each patient frequently in the early postoperative period and for at least the first postoperative year, documenting postoperative changes.

OUTCOMES

- With a thorough informed discussion preoperatively, the surgeon can achieve functional and aesthetically pleasing results that are in keeping with a patient's expectations about maintaining his or her ethnic identity (**FIG 1**).
- Because only four graft types need to be mastered, with experience, the need for revisions should not be common.

COMPLICATIONS

- Skeletal problems
- Soft tissue problems
- Graft problems
- Asymmetry
- Using the surgical planning and techniques described, the following complications virtually never occur.
  - Iatrogenic airway obstruction
  - Intraoperative and postoperative hemorrhage
  - Septal perforation
  - Rhinitis
  - Circulatory problems
  - Infection
  - Septal collapse

- Red nose
- Racial incongruity
- Treatment of more common complications is straightforward. Because the underlying anatomy has not been disturbed, and no sutures or struts have been placed, not much can go wrong.
  - Dorsal grafts can move out of position but can be easily adjusted in a small secondary procedure.
  - Spreader grafts virtually never require revision and can be expected to double nasal airflow in most patients.
  - Alar wall grafts occasionally bow or are under corrected or overcorrected but still double airflow if external valvular incompetence existed preoperatively.
  - Tip grafts can be placed insufficiently, or in excess, or heal asymmetrically.
  - In any of these occasions, local adjustments through limited incisions are corrective.

REFERENCES

1. Constantian MB. What motivates secondary rhinoplasty? A study of 150 consecutive patients. *Plast Reconstr Surg.* 2012;130:667.
2. Constantian MB. Four common anatomic variants that predispose to unfavorable rhinoplasty results: a study based on 150 consecutive secondary rhinoplasties. *Plast Reconstr Surg.* 2000;105:316.
3. Constantian MD, Clardy RB. The relative importance of septal and nasal valvular surgery in correcting airway obstruction in primary and secondary rhinoplasty. *Plast Reconstr Surg.* 1996;98:38-54.
4. Constantian MB. Functional effects of alar cartilage malposition. *Ann Plast Surg.* 1993;30:487.
5. Constantian MB. Experience with a three-point method for planning rhinoplasty. *Ann Plast Surg.* 1993;30:1.
6. Constantian MB. The mid-dorsal notch: an intraoperative guide to overresection in secondary rhinoplasty. *Plast Reconstr Surg.* 1993;91:477.
7. Constantian MB. The boxy nasal tip, the ball tip, and alar cartilage malposition: variations on a theme, a study in 200 consecutive primary and secondary rhinoplasty patients. *Plast Reconstr Surg.* 2005;116:268.

57

CHAPTER

Indications and Technique for Open Rhinoplasty in Patients With Dorsal Hump and Wide Tip

Charles H. Thorne and Sammy Sinno

DEFINITION

- *Dorsal hump* refers to excess height in the upper third of the nose. When examining a patient in the lateral view, ideally the nose should be in line with a line drawn from the radix to the tip (or slightly behind this line in females); any excess projection anterior to this line is a dorsal hump.
- *Wide tip* refers to a variety of configurations of the lower lateral cartilages that create the appearance of bulbous and poorly defined nasal tip.

ANATOMY

- The anatomy of the dorsal hump is usually both cartilaginous and bony. The nasal bones and the dorsal septum can both or independently be excessive. Any of these situations can contribute to a dorsal hump.
- A wide tip is primarily related to positioning and orientation of the lower lateral cartilages. Dr. Rohrich and colleagues categorized three types of boxy tip relating to a wide intercrural angle, a wide domal arch, or both.[1] Wide or bulbous tips can also result from bifidity of the nasal tip, excess or convex lateral crura, or lower lateral cartilage malposition.

PATIENT HISTORY AND PHYSICAL FINDINGS

- Dorsal hump and wide nasal tip are the two most commonly encountered patient complaints regarding their nose.
- On palpation of the dorsum, a dorsal hump can be bony or cartilaginous, or in some instances both.

- Palpation of the tip cartilages is important to give information regarding integrity, positioning, and recoil of the lower lateral cartilages.

IMAGING

- Although CT imaging can be useful in nasal surgery for airway abnormalities, routine scans are not obtained for patients presenting for correction of dorsal hump and wide nasal tips.

SURGICAL MANAGEMENT

- A clear surgical plan should be outlined prior to any rhinoplasty procedure.

Preoperative Planning

- The patient is counseled extensively in preoperative discussion regarding surgical outcomes and recovery. Photographs are taken and will be used intraoperatively. Currently, we do not use 3D imaging software.

Positioning

- The patient is in the supine position with the head slightly extended.

Approach

- The open approach is used for full visualization of deformities in the dorsum and tip.

TECHNIQUES

■ Correction of the Dorsal Hump

- An inverted V or upright V incision is used to open the nose along with bilateral infracartilaginous incisions (**TECH FIG 1A**).
- Using converse tip scissors, the nasal skin and soft tissues are dissected immediately on the surface of the nasal cartilages from caudal to cranial (**TECH FIG 1B**). A Joseph periosteal elevator is used to elevate the periosteum off the nasal bones in the midline (**TECH FIG 1C**).
- Once full exposure is achieved, a no. 15 blade is used to separate the upper lateral cartilages from the septum (**TECH FIG 1D**). An assessment is then made regarding the anatomical features that contribute most to the dorsal hump.

- Separation of the upper lateral cartilages from the septum:
  - If primarily cartilaginous, the dorsal septum is scored with a no. 11 blade and then excised with Swedish or Foman scissors.
  - If the hump is primarily bony, a bone rasp is used to bring down the dorsum (**TECH FIG 1E**).
- The nasal skin must be redraped and constantly reassessed by lateral visualization and palpation to determine adequacy of reduction.
- The dorsum is then restored by either suturing the upper lateral cartilages back together with 5-0 PDS sutures or spreader grafts placed and secured between the upper lateral cartilages and septum.

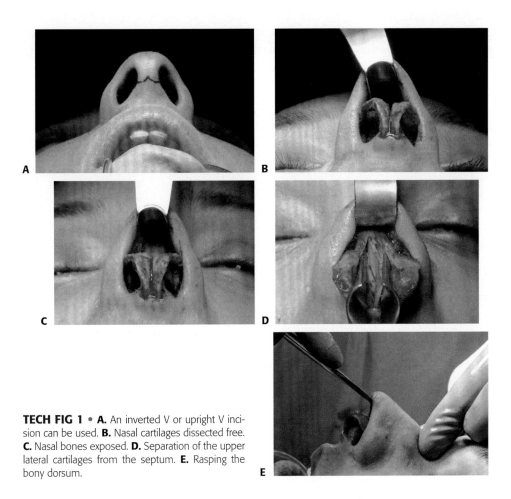

TECH FIG 1 • A. An inverted V or upright V incision can be used. **B.** Nasal cartilages dissected free. **C.** Nasal bones exposed. **D.** Separation of the upper lateral cartilages from the septum. **E.** Rasping the bony dorsum.

■ Correction of the Wide Tip

- Correction of the wide tip has several components. A cephalic trim is often performed first by marking, scoring, and then excising the cephalic aspect of the lateral crura, making sure to leave an adequate width of residual lateral crura (at least 5mm) (**TECH FIG 2A**).

- Tip sutures can also be powerful in correcting a wide tip; these are placed with 6-0 PDS:
  - Intradomal sutures can also be used to refine the tip and correctly orient malpositioned lower lateral cartilages into the correct plane (**TECH FIG 2B–D**).
  - Interdomal sutures, placed from one dome to the other and tied, also can have a drastic impact on refining the tip.

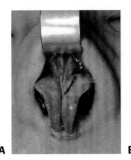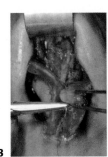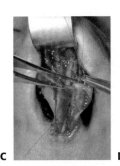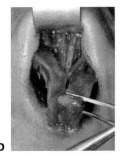

TECH FIG 2 • A. Marking of the cephalic aspect of the lateral crura to be excised. **B–D.** Intradomal suture placement.

PEARLS AND PITFALLS

Exposure	■ It is critical to expose the nasal architecture in a subperichondrial and subperiosteal plane to avoid excess bleeding and leave maximal soft tissue covering of framework modifications.
Dorsal reduction	■ Reduce the dorsum in an incremental fashion to avoid over-resection. ■ Avoid over-resection of the upper lateral cartilages. ■ If the patient has had a prior septoplasty, exercise caution in reducing the hump as an 8- to 10-mm L strut is necessary.
Osteotomies	■ Perform the infracture as low as possible to avoid a step-off deformity.
Wide tip	■ Use a graduated approach toward refining tip aesthetics: cephalic trim, then intradomal sutures, and then interdomal suture.

POSTOPERATIVE CARE

- The nose is taped, and an Aquaplast splint is applied.
- The tape, splint, and sutures are removed in 5 days.
- Patients are encouraged to sleep on their backs with head elevated for 2 weeks following surgery.
- All patients are encouraged to gently clean their nostrils with cotton swabs and a mixture of water and peroxide.

OUTCOMES

- Typically, correction of dorsal humps and wide tips yield very high patient satisfaction in rhinoplasty procedures.

COMPLICATIONS

- Undercorrection can occur and patients must be counseled extensively preoperatively.

REFERENCE

1. Rohrich RJ, Adams WP Jr. The boxy nasal tip: classification and management based on alar cartilage suturing techniques. *Plast Reconstr Surg.* 2001;107(7):1849-1863.

Treating the Narrow Midvault

Eric J. Culbertson and Jason Roostaeian

DEFINITION

- The brow-tip dorsal aesthetic lines on frontal view are paired gentle curvilinear lines starting at the medial brow curving medially along the nasal bridge before transitioning laterally to the tip. This line can be disrupted by bony irregularities of the upper third of the nose, middle vault contour deformities in the middle third, and deviations of the tip or asymmetry of the lower lateral cartilages in the lower third. Restoration of this and other nasal aesthetic contours is key to achieving an optimal result following rhinoplasty (**FIG 1A**).[1]
- Narrowing of the midvault can cause both aesthetic deformity, commonly appearing as an "inverted V," and functional airway obstruction due to narrowing of the internal nasal valve (**FIG 1B**).[2]

ANATOMY

- The middle vault is composed of the paired upper lateral cartilages, overlying soft tissue and skin, and underlying attached mucosa. Superiorly, the keystone area (also referred to as the K area) is the junction of the upper lateral cartilages with the nasal bones. Inferiorly in the scroll area, the upper and lower lateral cartilages are connected by loose areolar and fibrous attachments (**FIG 2**).
- The internal nasal valve is defined by the caudal border of the upper lateral cartilage, the septum, the head of the inferior turbinate, and the piriform aperture. Nasal airway resistance accounts for more than 50% of total airway resistance during nasal breathing, and the internal nasal valve has the smallest cross-sectional area of the nasal airway. The normal angle between the septum and upper lateral cartilage is 10 to 15 degrees (**FIG 3A**). An angle below this range can contribute to nasal obstruction (**FIG 3B**).[3]

PATHOGENESIS

- Midvault narrowing is a common sequela of rhinoplasty, particularly following dorsal hump reduction. Reduction of the cartilaginous component frequently disrupts the relation and attachments of the septum with the upper lateral cartilages, which form a single entity. Cartilage resection can result in an open roof deformity and allow collapse of the upper lateral cartilages, narrowing the internal valve angle and resulting in an inverted-V deformity and nasal obstruction. Often, this may not become apparent for months or years after surgery.
- Patients at particular risk are those with short nasal bones, thin skin, weak cartilages, or a combination thereof.[2]
- Scar contracture from tumor resection or trauma involving the lower portion of the nose may distort the internal nasal valve.
- Facial paralysis may cause internal and external valve collapse through ptosis of the lateral nasal soft tissues and loss of muscle tone that normally prevents valve collapse, particularly on inspiration.
- Weakening of the attachments between the upper and lower lateral cartilages with age may lead to senile tip ptosis that can also cause internal valve narrowing.

PATIENT HISTORY AND PHYSICAL FINDINGS

- A detailed nasal history should be obtained, in particular to include a history of symptoms related to nasal obstruction, nasal allergies, prior nasal trauma, and nasal surgeries. Any patient aesthetic concerns and goals should be elicited and clearly defined.[3,4]
- A complete external and internal nasal examination should be conducted in all patients.
- Evaluate symmetry of the upper lateral cartilages. An inverted-V deformity may be present as a result of collapse of the upper lateral cartilages.

Normal

Inverted–V

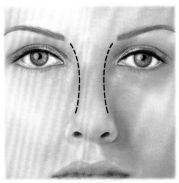
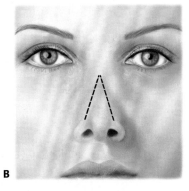

FIG 1 • Normal brow-tip aesthetics form paired curvilinear lines from the medial brow to the tip (**A**). Midvault narrowing can disrupt these lines and distort the aesthetics of the nose, with a visible inverted-V deformity (**B**).

A   B

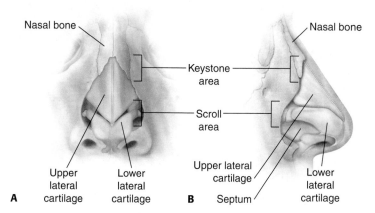

FIG 2 • A,B. Normal nasal anatomy.

- Perform a Cottle maneuver, where the cheek immediately adjacent to the nasal sidewall is displaced laterally to assess for improvement in nasal airway obstruction with widening of the internal nasal valves. Gentle internal elevation of the upper lateral cartilages using a cotton-tipped applicator will also improve breathing in patients with midvault narrowing. Patency of the internal nasal valve during inspiration should also be assessed.
- A nasal speculum is used to evaluate the septum for deformities and the inferior turbinates for hypertrophy.
- Standardized photographs including frontal, lateral oblique, and basal views should be obtained in all patients.

IMAGING

- Imaging is seldom required for diagnosis or treatment; however, supplemental testing can be performed to assess airway dynamics. Rhinomanometry measures pressure and flow during inspiration and expiration and provides a measure of airflow resistance and nasal patency. Acoustic rhinometry analyzes reflected sound waves directed through the nostrils and can be used to measure cross-sectional area and nasal volume to quantify nasal obstruction.[5]

SURGICAL MANAGEMENT

- The primary objective is to correct any functional airway obstruction caused by narrowing of the internal nasal valve.

- Aesthetic concerns and goals for treatment discussed with the patient may also be addressed, particularly to restore symmetric and pleasing dorsal aesthetic lines.
- The use of spreader grafts to reconstruct the roof of the middle nasal vault and open the internal nasal valve was first described by Jack Sheen, originally through an endonasal approach.[2] Either an open or endonasal approach may be used for spreader graft placement. The use of the upper lateral cartilages as autospreader grafts or flaps, reducing the need to harvest cartilage grafts, was subsequently described.

Preoperative Planning

- In planning the operative approach, it is important to carefully review the preoperative photos and establish clear goals of treatment with the patient. Consideration of previous operations, extent of previous nasal trauma, and involved structures and available septal and other potential cartilage grafts (ear, rib) should be taken into account. The patient should be informed of the possible need to harvest cartilage from these other donor sites such as the ear or rib.

Positioning

- The patient is positioned supine on the operating table with arms tucked at the side.
- An oral right angle endotracheal tube is used for intubation, and should extend inferiorly in the midline away from the nose, and secured without distorting the upper lip and nose.
- Nasal hairs may be trimmed, if desired.

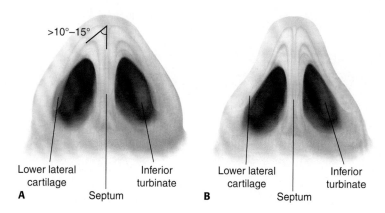

FIG 3 • Normal middle nasal vault anatomy is demonstrated. The normal angle between the septum and upper lateral cartilages is 10 to 15 degrees **(A)**. A more acute angle may narrow the midvault and cause obstruction of the internal nasal valve **(B)**.

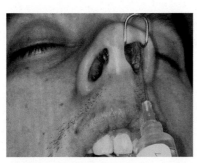

FIG 4 • Local anesthetic is injected into the nasal sidewalls, columella, and inside the nostril along the lower lateral cartilages.

- Local anesthetic consisting of 1% lidocaine with 1:100 000 epinephrine is infiltrated into the nasal sidewalls and columella and inside the nostril along the lower lateral cartilages (**FIG 4**).

- Oxymetazoline or 4% cocaine-soaked pledgets are placed in each nostril.
- A throat pack is placed to prevent gastric accumulation of blood.
- The face is prepped with dilute Betadine.
- A sterile head wrap is placed followed by surgical drapes.

Approach

- The open or closed (endonasal) approach to rhinoplasty may be used to correct the narrow midvault, depending on the technique used, extent of prior surgery or trauma, and other treatment goals.
- Spreader graft placement, using either cartilage or auto-spreader flaps, corrects the lack of dorsal support and helps restore a normal dorsal profile. If additional cartilage is needed, this may be harvested from the rib or ear.

■ Open Spreader Graft Placement

- After prepping and draping, the nasal pledgets are removed.
- A gull wing or stair-step incision is marked on the columella at the narrowest point, approximately at the midpoint, and extending along the side of the columella just into the nostril.
- This is incised with a no. 15 blade just through the dermis.
- Infracartilaginous incisions are made laterally on each side (**TECH FIG 1A**).
- The columella and alar incisions are connected.
- Fine curved iris or converse scissors are used to complete the columellar incision, with care taken to avoid injury to the medial crura.
- The nasal tip is elevated from the lower lateral cartilages with scissors, and dissection continued over the upper lateral cartilages up to the bony dorsum (**TECH FIG 1B**).
- The upper lateral cartilages are separated from the septum at the anterior septal angle using fine iris scissors or a no. 15 blade, and the mucoperichondrium on either side of the septum is incised onto the septal cartilage (**TECH FIG 1C**).
- Mucoperichondrial flaps are raised on either side of the septum using a Cottle elevator (**TECH FIG 1D**).
- The more proximal portion of the upper lateral cartilages is then separated from the septum after complete release of the mucoperichondrium using a no. 15 blade

to upstroke from distal to proximal. A converse retractor should be used to protect the nasal skin.
- Adequate septal cartilage is removed for spreader and any other needed grafts as well as to correct any significant septal deviation, preserving 1 to 1.5 mm dorsal and caudal septal struts (**TECH FIG 1E**).
- Spreader grafts are designed, typically measuring 1 to 3 mm in thickness, 3 to 5 mm in width, and 15 to 30 mm in length, depending on the patient's anatomy and degree of correction needed (**TECH FIG 1F–H**).
- The spreader grafts are placed on each side of the septum, just below the level of the upper lateral cartilages, extending from above the bony-cartilaginous junction beneath the nasal bone to the caudal end of the upper lateral cartilages (**TECH FIG 1I**).
- The spreader grafts are secured in place with 2 to 3 interrupted 5-0 PDS sutures passing through the spreader graft on one side, the septum, and then the other graft (**TECH FIG 1J**).
- The upper lateral cartilages are then reapproximated to the septum at the midline over the spreader grafts using 2 to 3 interrupted 5-0 PDS sutures.
- Mattress sutures of 4-0 plain gut are placed through the mucoperichondrial flaps to close the dead space where septal cartilage was harvested.
- The nose is thoroughly irrigated, hemostasis is achieved, and the nasal skin is redraped.

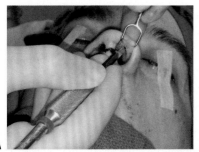
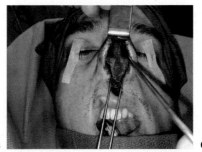
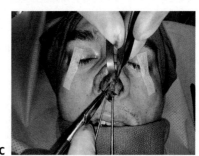

TECH FIG 1 • **A.** The columella incision is made, followed by infracartilaginous incisions laterally on each side. The columella and alar incisions are then connected. **B.** The nasal tip is elevated from the lower lateral cartilages and dissection continued over the upper lateral cartilages up to the bony dorsum. **C.** The upper lateral cartilages are separated from the septum, and the mucoperichondrium on either side of the septum is incised onto the septal cartilage.

T E C H N I Q U E S

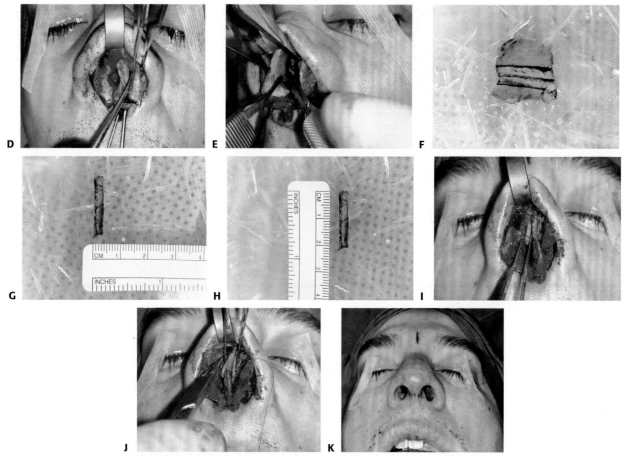

TECH FIG 1 (Continued) • **D.** Mucoperichondrial flaps are raised on either side of the septum. **E.** Septal cartilage is harvested with preservation of 1 to 1.5 mm dorsal and caudal septal struts. Spreader graft are designed **(F)**, typically measuring 1 to 3 mm in thickness, 3 to 5 mm in width **(G)**, and 15 to 30 mm in length **(H)**. **I.** The spreader grafts are placed on each side of the septum, just below the level of the upper lateral cartilages. **J.** The spreader grafts are secured in place with interrupted sutures passing through the spreader graft on one side, the septum, and then the other graft. **K.** The columellar skin is reapproximated with interrupted 6-0 Prolene, and the infracartilaginous incisions are closed with interrupted 5-0 chromic.

- The columellar skin is reapproximated with interrupted 6-0 Prolene, and the infracartilaginous incisions are closed with interrupted 5-0 chromic (**TECH FIG 1K**).
- Internal nasal splints are placed in each nostril and sutured through the septum with a single 3-0 Prolene mattress suture.

- Tape strips are applied to the nasal dorsum to limit postoperative swelling.
- The throat pack is removed prior to extubation. A nasogastric tube may be used to suction gastric contents to remove accumulated blood.
- A mustache gauze dressing is applied across the upper lip to absorb any nasal drainage.

■ Endonasal Spreader Graft Placement

- The patient is positioned and prepared as previously described.
- The nasal pledgets are removed after prepping and draping.
- A Killian incision, approximately 1 to 1.5 cm cranially from the caudal septal border, or a hemitransfixion incision at the caudal septal border is performed through the mucoperichondrium using a no. 15 blade (**TECH FIG 2A**).
- Submucoperichondrial dissection is performed using a Cottle elevator, preserving the attachments to the septum

dorsally for approximately 1 cm for later spreader graft pocket creation (**TECH FIG 2B**).
- The septum is incised vertically with a no. 15 blade or Freer knife with care to preserve the contralateral mucoperichondrium.
- Submucoperichondrial dissection is performed on the contralateral side, again preserving attachments dorsally (**TECH FIG 2C**).
- The septal cartilage can now be harvested using a no. 15 blade or Freer knife, preserving an L strut of at least 1 cm dorsally and caudally.

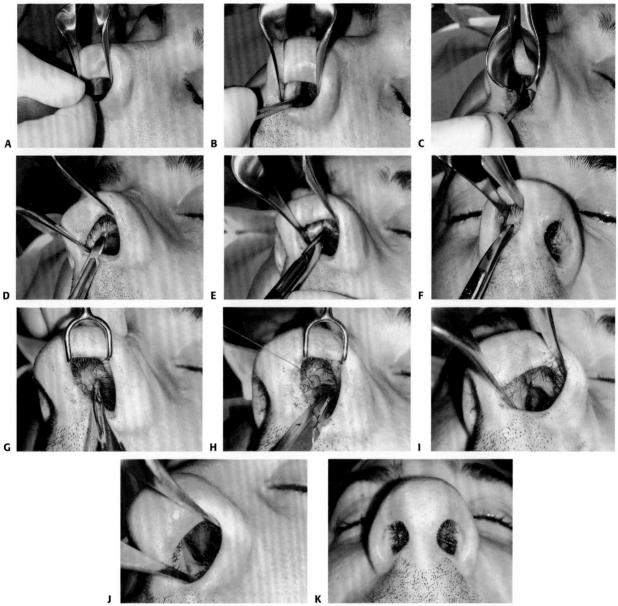

TECH FIG 2 • A. A Killian incision is made approximately 1 to 1.5 cm cranially from the caudal septal border through the mucoperichondrium. **B.** Submucoperichondrial dissection is performed, preserving the attachments to the septum dorsally for approximately 1 cm for later spreader graft pocket creation. **C.** Submucoperichondrial dissection is performed on the contralateral side, again preserving attachments dorsally for later spreader graft placement. **D.** The mucosa at the internal nasal valve is incised, and a submucoperichondrial pocket is developed on each side between the septum and upper lateral cartilages. **E.** An approximately 5-mm-wide pocket for spreader graft placement is developed along the dorsal septum beneath the upper lateral cartilages to the level of the nasal bones. **F.** This is repeated on the other side. **G.** The spreader grafts are inserted into each pocket, and the caudal aspects are secured to the septum in a horizontal mattress fashion **(H)**. **I.** The mucosa is closed over the spreader grafts. **J.** Mattress sutures are placed through the mucoperichondrial flaps to close the dead space where septal cartilage was harvested. **K.** Internal nasal splints are placed in each nostril and sutured through the septum.

- Spreader grafts are shaped from the harvested cartilage, one or two depending on whether unilateral or bilateral placement is desired.
- Spreader grafts typically measure 1 to 3 mm in thickness, 3 to 5 mm in width, and 15 to 30 mm in length, depending on the patient's anatomy and degree of correction needed.
- The mucosa at the internal nasal valve is incised with a no. 15 blade, and a submucoperichondrial pocket is developed on each side between the septum and upper lateral cartilages (**TECH FIG 2D**).

- Mucoperichondrial attachments to the septum between this plane and the previous septal dissection are left intact for support along the floor of the pocket.
- An approximately 3 to 5 mm wide pocket for spreader graft placement is developed along the dorsal septum beneath the upper lateral cartilages to the level of the nasal bones using fine iris scissors. This is then repeated on the other side (**TECH FIG 2E,F**).
- The spreader grafts are inserted into each pocket, and the caudal aspects are secured to the septum with a 4-0 chromic suture in a horizontal mattress fashion (**TECH FIG 2G,H**).

- The mucosa is closed over the grafts using 5-0 chromic suture (**TECH FIG 2I**).
- Mattress sutures of 4-0 plain gut are placed through the mucoperichondrial flaps to close the dead space where septal cartilage was harvested (**TECH FIG 2J**).
- Internal nasal splints are placed in each nostril and sutured through the septum with a single 3-0 Prolene mattress suture (**TECH FIG 2K**).

- The throat pack is removed prior to extubation. If necessary, a nasogastric tube may be used to suction gastric contents to remove accumulated blood.
- A moustache gauze dressing may be applied across the upper lip to absorb any nasal drainage.

■ Autospreader Flaps

- Positioning and prepping proceed as previously described.
- The open approach is used to elevate the skin of the nasal tip and dorsum and expose the upper and lower lateral cartilages and dorsal septum.
- The upper lateral cartilages are separated from the septum using a no. 15 blade, and the mucoperichondrium on either side of the septum is incised onto the septal cartilage.
- Mucoperichondrial flaps are raised on either side of the septum using a Cottle elevator.
- 5-0 PDS sutures are placed caudal to the upper edge of the upper lateral cartilages, thereby infolding the superior edge of the upper lateral cartilages, serving a spreader-type function (**TECH FIG 3**).
- The nose is thoroughly irrigated, hemostasis is achieved, and the nasal skin is redraped.
- The columellar skin is reapproximated with interrupted 6-0 Prolene, and the infracartilaginous incisions are closed with interrupted 5-0 chromic.
- Tape strips are applied to the nasal dorsum to limit postoperative swelling.
- The throat pack is removed prior to extubation. A nasogastric tube may be used to suction gastric contents to remove accumulated blood.
- A mustache gauze dressing is applied across the upper lip to absorb any nasal drainage.

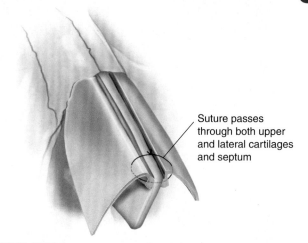

Suture passes through both upper and lateral cartilages and septum

TECH FIG 3 • Sutures are placed through the upper lateral cartilages caudal to their upper edges, thus infolding the superior edges against the septum and serving an autospreader flap function.

PEARLS AND PITFALLS

Preoperative	■ A thorough discussion of the planned goals and risks should be conducted with the patient to ensure appropriate expectations are met.
Technique	■ The open technique provides greater control of spreader graft placement and facilitates other alterations to the nasal structure, particularly tip refinement. ■ The endonasal technique is especially useful in patients with long, thin noses that are straight. ■ To minimize widening of the nasal dorsum and potential palpability, place the spreader grafts just below the level of the upper lateral cartilages. ■ Autospreader grafts may not be adequate to straighten the deviated dorsum, and spreader grafts are preferred.
Postoperative	■ Have the patient avoid sleeping on a side as it will worsen edema to one side and increase concern for deviation.
Prevention	■ Spreader grafts may be beneficial prophylactically following dorsal hump reduction, particularly in patients with a high bony-cartilaginous junction or weak upper lateral cartilages, in which closure of the open roof with nasal bone infracturing alone may be inadequate. ■ Preservation of the upper lateral cartilages during dorsal hump reduction and reapproximation along the dorsal septum with tension spanning sutures will frequently restore the midvault without the need for spreader grafts.[6]

POSTOPERATIVE CARE

- Surgery is performed on an outpatient basis.
- Usual postrhinoplasty precautions are followed.
- Keep the intranasal mucosa moist with frequent application of ointment and saline nasal spray.
- Any internal and/or external nasal splints are removed at 1 week.
- Prolonged edema may occur and in some cases can take up to 1 year to fully resolve.

OUTCOMES

- The goals of functional and aesthetic improvement can be accomplished with any of the described techniques.[7,8] Optimal outcomes will be attained using the technique with which the surgeon is most comfortable and able to achieve consistent results.

COMPLICATIONS

- Spreader grafts may widen the nasal midvault and/or tip, which may or may not be desired. This is more likely with autospreader flaps.
- Other possible short-term and long-term complications include infection, hematoma, nasal asymmetry, septal perforation, worsening of nasal obstruction, scarring, nasal bleeding/crusting, empty nose syndrome, and prolonged edema that may last up to 1 year.

REFERENCES

1. Rohrich RJ, Muzaffar AR, Janis JE. Component dorsal hump reduction: the importance of maintaining dorsal aesthetic lines in rhinoplasty. *Plast Reconstr Surg.* 2004;114(5 suppl):1298-1308.
2. Sheen JH. Spreader graft: a method of reconstructing the roof of the middle nasal vault following rhinoplasty. *Plast Reconstr Surg.* 1984;73(2 suppl):230-239.
3. Howard BK, Rohrich RJ. Understanding the nasal airway: principles and practice. *Plast Reconstr Surg.* 2002;109(3 suppl):1128-1146; quiz 1145-1126.
4. Rohrich RJ, Ahmad J. A practical approach to rhinoplasty. *Plast Reconstr Surg.* 2016;137(4 suppl):725e-746e.
5. Aziz T, Biron VL, Ansari K, Flores-Mir C. Measurement tools for the diagnosis of nasal septal deviation: a systematic review. *J Otolaryngol Head Neck Surg.* 2014;43:11.
6. Roostaeian J, Unger JG, Lee MR, et al. Reconstitution of the nasal dorsum following component dorsal reduction in primary rhinoplasty. *Plast Reconstr Surg.* 2014;133(3 suppl):509-518.
7. Hassanpour SE, Heidari A, Moosavizadeh SM, et al. Comparison of aesthetic and functional outcomes of spreader graft and autospreader flap in rhinoplasty. *World J Plast Surg.* 2016;5(2 suppl):133-138.
8. Erickson B, Hurowitz R, Jeffery C, et al. Acoustic rhinometry and video endoscopic scoring to evaluate postoperative outcomes in endonasal spreader graft surgery with septoplasty and turbinoplasty for nasal valve collapse. *J Otolaryngol Head Neck Surg.* 2016;45:2.

59 CHAPTER

Indications and Technique for Increasing and Decreasing Tip Projection in Open Rhinoplasty

David A. Sieber and C. Spencer Cochran

DEFINITION

- Proper tip projection can be determined through multiple methods.
  - The authors' preferred method is to have a tip projection that is equal to the length of the upper lip as measured from the white roll to the base of the columella. This line should equal the distance from the base of the columella to the tip-defining point. This method assumes that the upper lip is of normal length and may not be applicable in all patients (**FIG 1A**).
  - Another method places a line from the alar crease to the tip-defining points (lines A to B). A perpendicular line is then drawn from the upper lip through lines A to B. Ideal tip projection is when A, 50% to 60% of AB (**FIG 1B**).
  - Goode method: a triangle is formed from a line drawn from the nasion through the alar crease (A). The other sides are composed of a line from the nasion to the tip-defining point (B) and another line from the alar crease to the tip-defining point (C). An ideal tip has a B:C ratio of 0.55 to 0.6 (**FIG 1C**).

ANATOMY

- Tip projection is dependent on numerous interrelated nasal structures:
  - Length and strength of lateral crura
  - Length and strength of medial crura
  - Septal angle
  - Fibrous attachments from the feet of the medial crura to the caudal septum
  - Attachments between the upper lateral and lower lateral cartilages at the scroll area
  - Interdomal ligaments connecting the cephalic margins of the domes
  - Nasal skin and soft tissue envelope (this is the limiting factor in tip projection)

PATHOGENESIS

- Overprojection of the tip may be the result of one or many abnormalities in nasal anatomy such as a prominent septal angle or excessively long and/or strong medial or lateral crura.[1]
- Likewise, underdevelopment or underprojection of the nasal tip may be due to a weak septal angle or short and weak medial or lateral crura.[2]
- More commonly, underprojection is the result of a poorly planned primary rhinoplasty in which proper support either through the use of a columellar strut or tip suturing was not employed, resulting in loss of tip support as the soft tissue envelope contracts.[3,4]

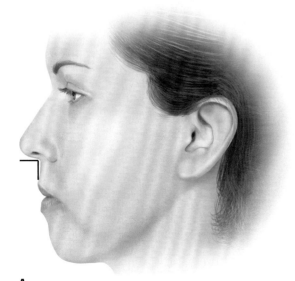

A

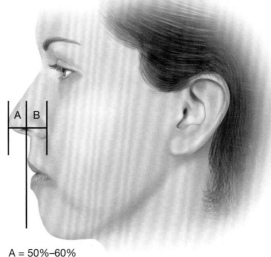

A = 50%–60%
B   of AB

FIG 1 • A–C. Common methods for determining proper tip projection.

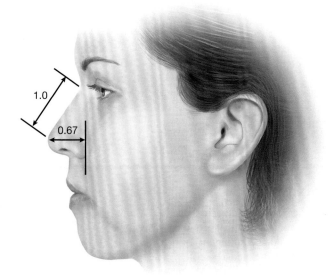

FIG 1 (Continued)   **C**

- The tripod method for understanding tip projection is both relevant and important to comprehend (**FIG 2**). As each leg of the tripod is modified to re-establish proper tip projection, there is a resulting effect on tip rotation.
- Proper support of each leg of the tripod is critical in maintaining tip projection over time through the use of:
  - Columellar strut graft: forms foundation of the tip, maintains projection, and prevents distortion
  - Extended alar contour grafts
  - Dorsal spreader grafts

PATIENT HISTORY AND PHYSICAL FINDINGS

- Patients presenting for primary rhinoplasty will complain of a nose that "sticks out too far" or will state that they do not like the appearance of their nose on profile view.

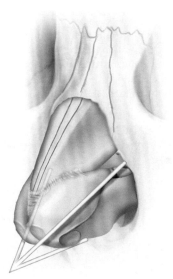

FIG 2 • Tip support is dependent on three independent structures much like the legs of a tripod. The paired lateral crura and the columella/medial crura form the three legs of support.

- Secondary rhinoplasty patients may complain of a "short" nose, stating that their nose has become smaller over time.
- Confirmation of nasal over- or underprojection should be confirmed using the aforementioned methods.

IMAGING

- Imaging may be performed using Vectra (Canfield, Parsippany, NJ) or standard photographs and should be employed to establish preoperative anatomy as well as to help determine surgical goals with the patient.

NONOPERATIVE MANAGEMENT

- Although soft tissue fillers such as hyaluronic acid are used by some surgeons as a nonsurgical option to change nasal contour, we do not advocate the use of fillers in the tip to increase tip projection; the risk of vascular occlusion or embolization that can result in injury to the remaining nasal vascular network may lead to irreversible skin loss.

SURGICAL MANAGEMENT

- Surgical management of tip projection should follow an organized and incremental approach including the following:
  - Determine the cause of tip over- or underprojection.
  - Incrementally address each of the aforementioned factors.
  - Reset the desired tip projection based on preoperative planning and intraoperative results.
  - Re-establish proper support in each leg of the tripod.

Preoperative Planning

- Preoperative imaging should be reviewed with the patient to ensure that the patient has realistic goals for surgery and that the desired surgical result can be achieved.

Positioning

- Patient is placed in the flat supine position.
- General anesthesia and endotracheal intubation are preferred for this procedure.
- Approximately 5 cc of 1% lidocaine with 1:100 000 epinephrine is injected into the planned columellar and marginal incisions.
- The nose is packed with oxymetazoline-soaked gauze to assist with hemostasis.
- The patient is then prepped and draped in a sterile fashion.

Approach

- Any change in tip projection should be performed through an open approach for maximal control of tip positioning and support.
- Tip projection is typically a result of a combination of factors and therefore requires a stepwise approach for correction.
- After each aforementioned factor is addressed, tip projection should be reassessed by redraping the soft tissue envelope.

■ Opening the Nose

- A transcolumellar incision is made as an inverted V or chevron shape across the narrowest portion of the columella and extends around the columellar roll to terminate on the midportion of the medial crura.
- The soft tissue envelope is elevated from the tip and nasal dorsum to expose the osteocartilaginous framework.

- The soft tissue envelope should be widely undermined from the lateral crura toward the piriform aperture. The destabilization of the nasal tip that occurs when the soft tissue envelope is elevated in the open approach establishes a modest amount of deprojection.
- Any additional dorsal refinement is then preformed at this time prior to tip modification.

■ Separation of Lower Lateral Cartilages

- Divide the ligamentous attachments between the lateral crura and the upper lateral cartilages. Also divide the suspensory ligaments traversing the septal angle connecting the cephalic margins of the domes.
- After the suspensory ligament has been divided, patients with a prominent septal angle may require judicious trimming of the lower portion of the cartilaginous dorsal septum. This can help prevent a "polly beak" deformity resulting from excess dorsal septum in the supratip area.
- If additional deprojection is required, the fibroelastic attachments between the feet of the medial crura and the caudal septum should be released.

- This is accomplished by dividing the lower lateral cartilages in the midline to elevate mucoperichondrial flaps on either side of the caudal septum beginning at the septal angle and extending to the nasal spine area.
- These maneuvers will cause a deprojection of approximately 2 to 3 mm.
- When all other factors have been addressed and the desired decrease in tip projection still has not been achieved, the length and strength of the medial and/or lateral crura must be altered.

■ Isolation of Lower Lateral Cartilages

- Approximately 1.5 cc of 1% lidocaine with epinephrine is infiltrated into each dome, lateral, and medial crura to hydrodissect the vestibular mucosa off of the underside of the lower lateral cartilages.
- If indicated, a cephalic trim is then performed using a no. 15 blade to remove the cephalic excess from the lateral crura, making sure to leave at least 6 mm of cartilage in place.
- Using angled converse scissors, a spreading motion is used to separate the vestibular mucosa from the cartilage.
- Care must be taken not to tear the mucosa when developing the correct plane of dissection.
- Both the cephalic and caudal borders of the lower lateral cartilages must be completely free from mucosal attachments.
- The nasal mucosa needs to be freed from the lateral third of the lower lateral crura down to the lower third of the medial crura. The medial and lateral portions need to

maintain some attachments to the mucosa so as to not avulse the cartilage completely.
- Once these maneuvers have been performed, the lower lateral cartilages should be present as a single, continuous ribbon of cartilage (**TECH FIG 1**).

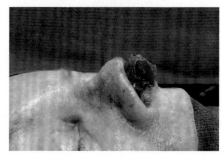

TECH FIG 1 • Appearance of lower lateral cartilages with vestibular mucosa dissected off of cartilage. Lower lateral cartilage should be present as a single continuous "ribbon" of cartilage.

Determination of Tip Projection

- This ribbon of lower lateral cartilage may then be reformed into the appropriate segments composed of the lateral, middle, and medial crura.
- The first step is to determine where the new dome should be located.
- The location of the new dome will determine three inter-related factors:
  - Nasal length
  - Tip rotation
  - Tip projection
- As the dome is moved from a more medial (caudal) to a lateral (cephalic) position on the lower lateral cartilage, there will be a resultant decrease in nasal length and projection with an increase in tip rotation (**TECH FIG 2**).
- The caveat is that because you are creating a new dome, increasing tip rotation, and causing tip deprojection, there will be an excess of cartilage in the new medial crura.

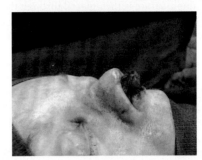

TECH FIG 2 • Location of new domes has been established, causing deprojection and rotation of the tip. Excess cartilage is now present in the area of the medial crura.

- Using these same concepts, additional tip projection can be created through formation of a new dome in a more medial (caudal) position along the lateral crura. This will in turn result in a decrease in tip rotation and an increase in nasal length.

Resupporting the Tip

- It is the senior author's (CSC) preferred technique to routinely use a columellar strut for all rhinoplasties.
- Using angled converse scissors, a pocket is created in the midline within the soft tissue caudal to the edge of the septum. Some soft tissue needs to be left between the columellar strut and septum to prevent "clicking" of the cartilage postoperatively (**TECH FIG 3A**).
- The length of the columellar strut helps to determine tip projection, and the angle at which the soft tissue pocket is created helps to determine final tip rotation (**TECH FIG 3B**).

- A horizontal mattress using 5-0 PDS is made to secure the medial crura to the columellar strut. This suture knot should be tied between the medial crura and the columellar strut so as to prevent a palpable knot from forming postoperatively.
- Once the appropriate location for the dome has been determined, a simple 5-0 PDS is passed through the new dome and into the columellar strut. The position of this suture into the caudal vs cephalic portion of the dome will also determine the degree of dome divergence. Typically, the suture is placed in the cephalic third of the dome.
- An identical suture is placed on the contralateral side.

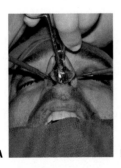
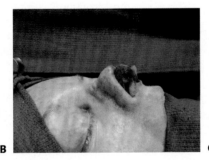
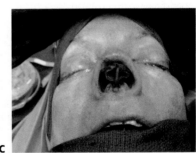
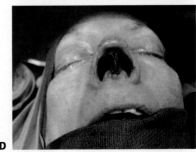

A B C D

TECH FIG 3 • **A.** A precise pocket is created for the columellar strut which will act to re-establish and support the new nasal tip location. **B.** The orientation and height of the columellar strut help to determine tip rotation and projection. **C.** Appearance of the lower lateral cartilages once the new domes have been secured to the columellar strut. With tip deprojection and cephalic rotation, excess lower lateral cartilage is forced into the medial crura as depicted here. **D.** Excess cartilage has been excised and is secured to the columellar strut. Cut edges of cartilage should be placed within the soft triangle so as to not create visible ridges postoperatively.

T
E
C
H
N
I
Q
U
E
S

- A third simple suture is then placed through the cephalic portion of one dome, then through the cephalic portion of the columellar strut, and through the contralateral dome.
- At this point, the excess cartilage that has been forced into the medial crura must be assessed (**TECH FIG 3C**).
- A small amount of cartilaginous excess in the medial crura with a minimal convexity may be plicated to the columellar strut using a 5-0 PDS as a horizontal mattress.
- If too much excess cartilage exists in the medial crura so that it creates a visible convexity not correctable with a suture, then this excess will need to be excised.
- The segment of medial crural cartilage should be cut in a way so that the cut edges of the cartilage lie within the

soft triangle. This can either be in an end-to-end fashion or with the proximal segment overlapping on top of the distal segment. Leaving the ends of the cartilage too far posteriorly will create a visible ridge on the columella postoperatively.
- Two to three horizontal mattress sutures are then used to tie down the cephalic, caudal, distal, and proximal edges of the cartilage to the columellar strut (**TECH FIG 3D**). Failure to do so will again result in a visible ridge.
- These techniques help incremental manipulation of tip projection, which when properly supported, should provide the patient with a lasting result.
- The soft tissue is then redraped, and the vestibular and columellar incisions are closed.

PEARLS AND PITFALLS

Pitfall	- Skin thickness is often the limiting factor in the amount of possible tip deprojection because the skin must be able shrink around the osteocartilaginous framework for the nose to have sufficient tip definition.
Pitfall	- Changing the length of the lateral crura or medial crura can have the potential to affect rotation.
Pitfall	- The surgeon should be cognizant of the possibility of alar base flaring and be prepared to correct the flaring with an alar base resection.
Pearl	- Multiple factors contribute to tip projection. Incrementally eliminating these factors will allow the surgeon to decrease tip projection in a controlled manner.
Pearl	- When the ligamentous attachments and fibroelastic attachments are eliminated, the main support to the tip comes from the length and strength of the lower lateral crura, especially in an open rhinoplasty where the support from the skin has been eliminated.

POSTOPERATIVE CARE

- Steri-Strips are applied to the dorsum with one in the infratip region to support the new tip position.
- A Denver Splint is placed onto the dorsum.
- The Denver Splint and Steri-Strips are removed 7 days postoperatively.

OUTCOMES

- **FIGS 3** and **4** demonstrate representative examples of successful tip modification using the described techniques.

COMPLICATIONS

- Because of the destructive nature of tip refinement, the most common complication requiring reoperation is a distortion or twisting of the nasal tip due to abnormal scarring. This is typically resolved by releasing the soft tissue envelope and the cartilaginous interfaces causing the distortion. The tip must then be resupported as described.
- The strength of the lateral crura needs to be evaluated intraoperatively. If they are weak and are not resupported,

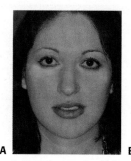 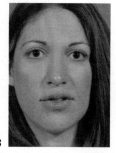 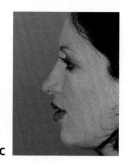 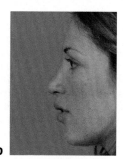

A   B   C   D

FIG 3 • **A,B.** Frontal view of a 27-year-old female pre- and 1-year postoperative from open primary rhinoplasty with tip deprojection. **C,D.** Lateral view of a 27-year-old female pre- and 1-year postoperative from open primary rhinoplasty with tip deprojection.

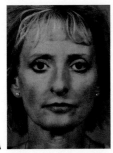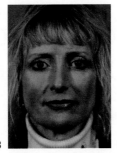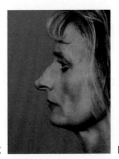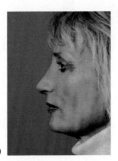

FIG 4 • A,B. Frontal view of a 48-year-old female pre- and 1-year postoperative from primary open rhinoplasty with tip deprojection. **C,D.** Lateral view of a 48-year-old female pre- and 1-year postoperative from primary open rhinoplasty with tip deprojection.

then external nasal valve collapse may occur postoperative. Support is best maintained through the use of a lateral crural strut graft or extended alar contour graft.

■ After deprojection of the tip, the patient may have excess flaring of the alar bases. This needs to be evaluated preoperatively with the patient as there may be a need for an alar base resection to restore proportional nasal aesthetics.

REFERENCES

1. Johnson CM Jr, Godin MS. The tension nose: open structure rhinoplasty approach. *Plast Reconstr Surg.* 1995;95:43.
2. Petroff MA, McCollough EG, Hom D, Anderson JR. Nasal tip projection: quantitative changes following rhinoplasty. *Arch Otolaryngol Head Neck Surg.* 1995;117:783.
3. Rich JS, Friedman WH, Pearlman SJ. The effects of lower lateral cartilage excision on nasal tip projection. *Arch Otolaryngol Head Neck Surg.* 1991;117:56.
4. Tardy ME Jr, Walter MA, Patt BS. The overprojecting nose: anatomic component analysis and repair. *Facial Plast Surg.* 1993;9:306.

60
CHAPTER

Techniques for Controlling Tip Rotation in Open Rhinoplasty

Nicolas Tabbal and Geo N. Tabbal

DEFINITION

- Nasal tip rotation can be assessed in various ways, but the nasolabial angle is the preferred measurement. It is defined as the angle formed by the intersection of a line between the most anterior and posterior points of the nostril and a line perpendicular to the horizontal facial plane (**FIG 1**). Tip rotation determines nasal length; increasing tip rotation (larger angle) shortens the nose, and decreasing tip rotation (smaller angle) lengthens the nose.
- A nasolabial angle of 95 to 110 degrees in women and 90 to 95 degrees in men is frequently cited as ideal, but a variety of cultural, ethnic, and other influences are taken into consideration.
- Increasing tip rotation entails cephalad rotation of the tip, thereby increasing the nasolabial angle and shortening the nose by decreasing the distance between the radix and the tip-defining points.
- Decreasing tip rotation results in a decreased nasolabial angle and lengthening of the nose as the distance between the radix and the tip-defining points increases.

ANATOMY

- Tip position results from the interplay between cutaneous attachments to the cartilaginous framework, fibrous attachments between the upper and lower cartilages, abutment of

the lower lateral cartilages (LLCs) against the piriform aperture, prominence of the caudal septum, location and attachment of the medial crura and the caudal septum, length of the upper lateral cartilages, and location of the anterior septal angle.

PATIENT HISTORY AND PHYSICAL FINDINGS

- Physical inspection of the external nasal features and an intranasal evaluation using a speculum and light source are necessary to construct a treatment plan.
  - Ballottement of the nasal tip provides information about tip support.
  - Assessment of skin thickness helps determine the degree of cartilage modification required to achieve the desired result.
- Standard medical photography should include standard rhinoplasty views such as the frontal, lateral (ie, profile), basal, and oblique views.
- Many patients present with complaints of tip descent on animation, suggesting that the action of the depressor septi nasi is causative for this dynamic rotation of the nasal tip (**FIG 2**). Recent studies contradict this mechanism and suggest that the tip does not move significantly on smiling, but rather the alar bases are pulled cephalad, creating the appearance of a plunging tip.

IMAGING

- Standard 2D medical photography is necessary for accurate preoperative analysis, intraoperative decision-making, and assessing postoperative outcomes. In addition, the surgeon may choose to use an imaging system to aid in communicating desired postoperative outcomes.

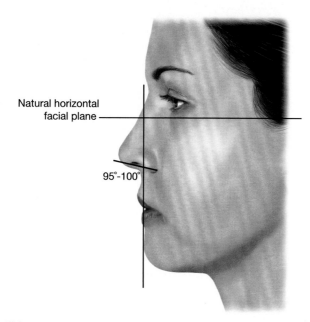

Natural horizontal facial plane

95°-100°

FIG 1 • Analyzing tip rotation by measuring the nasolabial angle.

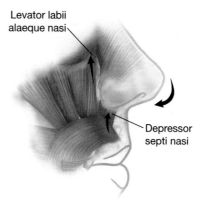

Levator labii alaeque nasi

Depressor septi nasi

FIG 2 • The depressor septi nasi muscle draws the tip down with animation.

SURGICAL MANAGEMENT

- The first step in any surgical procedure, and particularly in rhinoplasty, is an accurate diagnosis.
- Patients' expectations and surgeons' views on surgical limitations must be effectively communicated. No patient will get the exact nose that he or she wants.

Preoperative Planning

- Prior to infiltration with local anesthetic, a more thorough intranasal examination is performed to confirm that the preoperative plan is accurate and feasible.

Positioning

- The patient is placed supine on the operating table with the vertex of the scalp located just beyond the end of the bed.
- After intranasal intubation or placement of a laryngeal mask airway, the eyelids are taped shut with tape placed sufficiently far laterally to not interfere with the procedure.

- A throat pack is inserted.
- Oxymetazoline-soaked pledgets may be placed in each nare with the aid of a nasal speculum and a headlight for accurate placement. There is no role for cocaine in rhinoplasty.
- The nasal framework is infiltrated with local anesthetic that includes epinephrine.

Approach

- The debate over the open vs closed approach continues. Any technique for tip rotation is more easily and, by most surgeons, more accurately performed using the open approach. The exposure is better, and the ability to fix the tip in the desired position and to keep it there is also better.
- The closed approach is reasonable when the tip rotation will not be altered significantly, but, even then, one must be willing to convert to an open approach if the desired tip rotation/projection cannot be achieved.

■ Skin Undermining

- The attachments between the tip cartilages and the skin restrict the rotation of the nasal tip and are effectively released when initial exposure is obtained whether the approach is open or closed.

■ Division of the Scroll Area

- Release of the fibrous, or sometimes cartilaginous, attachments between the lateral crura and the upper lateral cartilages is necessary to rotate the tip and is achieved by performing a cephalic trim. If no cephalic trim is performed, then an intercartilaginous incision or division of

the scroll area is necessary. In cases when significant tip rotation is performed, an intercartilaginous incision may be necessary in addition to the cephalic trim to maximally liberate the lateral crura. Similarly, division of the attachments between the medial crura and the caudal septum is necessary for significant tip rotation (**TECH FIG 1A**).

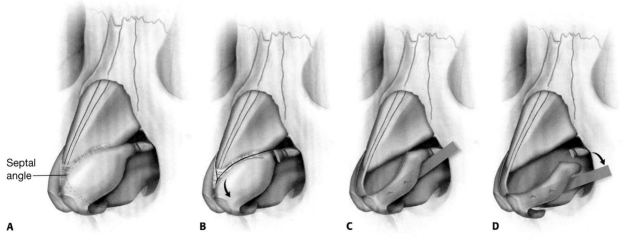

Septal angle

A **B** **C** **D**

TECH FIG 1 • A. The attachments between the upper lateral cartilages and lateral crura and between the medial crura and septum must be divided to allow adequate tip rotation. **B.** Release of the lateral crura from the accessory cartilages. **C,D.** Lateral crural strut grafts are then needed to prevent loss of tip support and potential alar rim collapse.

T E C H N I Q U E S

- In tip over-rotation, the lateral crura can be divided at their junction with the accessory cartilages (**TECH FIG 1B**). Reinforcement is usually necessary by placement of lateral crural strut grafts that both lengthen and stabilize the counter-rotated tip structures, preventing the loss of tip support and potential alar rim collapse (**TECH FIG 1C,D**).

- When increasing tip rotation, this abutment of the lateral crura to the piriform aperture may also require division, but, in these cases, suturing the overlapping edges of the divided lateral crura can frequently be performed to decrease the likelihood of alar collapse.

■ Lateral Crural Strut Grafts

- Both upward and downward rotation of the nasal tip can be augmented with the use of lateral crural strut grafts. These grafts help reposition the nasal tip and provide increased strength to the lateral crura. The pocket for each graft is designed to orient the tip as desired (**TECH FIG 2**).

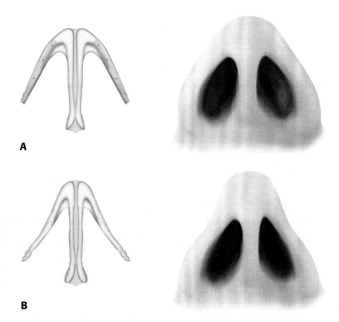

A

B

TECH FIG 2 • Placement of lateral crural strut grafts not only strengthens the lateral crura but also can be used to differentially increase or decrease tip rotation depending on orientation and pocket placement.

■ Septal Resection

- Typical cases where cephalad rotation of the tip is desired will require resection of the anterior septum and septal angle, whereas derotation or lengthening of the nose requires resection of the posterior aspect of the caudal septum (**TECH FIG 3**). In truth, both these maneuvers promise more than they deliver, and modern-day approaches, particularly to lengthening the nose, necessitate extended spreader grafts or caudal septal extension grafts.[1]

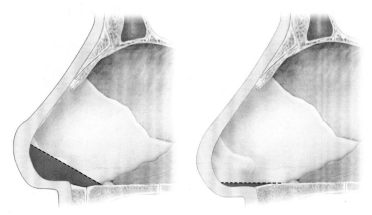

TECH FIG 3 • Anterior resection of the caudal septum causes tip rotation, while inferior resection causes counter-rotation.

Suture Techniques

- Various suspension suture techniques have been described to aid in nasal tip rotation, although the power of these methods to change tip rotation remains limited. However, a secondary and equally desirable effect is the ability of suture techniques to provide support to the weakened tip complex.
- Placement of medial crural septal sutures or medial crural columellar strut sutures can be utilized to either deproject or counter-rotate the tip. When placed more anteriorly along the caudal septum, they will act to upwardly rotate the tip and increase tip projection (**TECH FIG 4A,B**).
- Tip rotation sutures push the tip in a cephalad rotation while retracting the columella and refining tip shape.
- Horizontal mattress sutures placed between the domes of the middle crura, referred to commonly as transdomal sutures, will slightly counter-rotate the tip as the middle crura are shortened slightly (**TECH FIG 4C**).
- Degloving of the caudal septum with sutures used to affix the cephalic borders of the medial crus to the septum will also result in cephalic rotation of the tip and shortening of the nose.

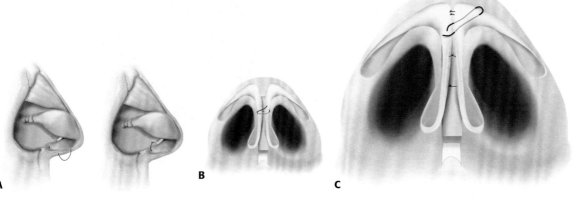

TECH FIG 4 • A. The medial crural septal suture. **B.** Medial crural columellar strut suture. **C.** Transdomal sutures slightly counter-rotate the tip.

Columellar Struts

- Routine use of columellar strut grafts is an effective mean to control tip rotation and projection:[2]
  - The strut is harvested from a straight and strong portion of autologous cartilage (usually arising from the septum).
  - Skin hooks are used to gently retract the medial crura anteriorly and establish the appropriate amount of tip projection such that a subcutaneous pocket for the graft can be developed from between the medial crura by extending from the tip of the medial crura to the just above the level of the nasal spine.
  - A 25-gauge needle is used to temporarily stabilize this configuration while it is sewn into place (**TECH FIG 5**).

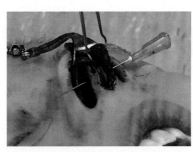

TECH FIG 5 • The skin hooks are used to displace the medial crura anteriorly, and then a 25-gauge needle allows the surgeon to secure placement of the columellar strut and effect the desired rotation and projection of the tip.

Tongue-and-Groove Technique

- The single most powerful method to rotate the tip is direct suturing of the medial crura to the caudal septum (**TECH FIG 6**).[3] This is a maneuver that is ideally used in the long nose requiring cephalic rotation and shortening and is probably underutilized.

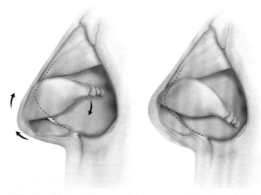

TECH FIG 6 • The tongue-and-groove technique repositions the medial crura onto the septum and thereby allows control of tip rotation.

■ Cartilage Grafts

- Placement of cartilage grafts affixed to the septum can rotate or counter-rotate the nasal tip depending on their shape, length, and positioning. First described by Byrd et al., all three varieties of septal extension grafts rely on a stable caudal septum and differ only in their site of anchorage to the septum:

- Placed as paired spreader grafts, the first type is placed at the junction of the upper lateral cartilages and the septum.
- Also placed as a pair, the second variety consists of two batten grafts that extend diagonally over the caudal and dorsal end of the septum's L strut.
- The third type is a direct extension graft that is affixed to the anterior septal angle with figure-of-8 sutures (**TECH FIG 7**).

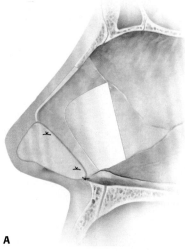
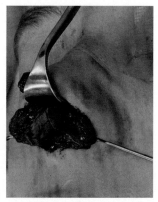

A   **B**

TECH FIG 7 • A,B. Septal extension grafts can be used to rotate or counter-rotate the tip depending on their shape, length, and positioning.

PEARLS AND PITFALLS

Patient communication	■ Paramount to successful rhinoplasty outcomes is effective and clear communication between the patient and the surgeon. This begins with understanding the goals of the patient during the consultation at which time the surgeon helps establish reasonable expectations.
Nasal analysis	■ Precise and accurate nasal analysis must be performed for accurate diagnosis of the deformity.
Surgical technique	■ Once the etiology for the nasal deformity has been understood given the anatomical findings, one can choose a corrective surgical plan that minimizes unwanted sequelae. ■ The options for tip rotation or counter-rotation include skin undermining, division of the scroll area, septal resection, tongue-and-groove technique, cartilage grafts, and suture techniques.

POSTOPERATIVE CARE

- At the conclusion of the procedure, the nose is painted with Mastisol and carefully taped. The tape is itself painted with Mastisol and a splint is applied. The splint is removed on approximately the 5th postoperative day. If an open approach has been used, the columellar sutures are removed as well. Longer periods of taping probably do not add to the stability of the result and are to be avoided. Injection of Kenalog into the nasal tip may increase the rate that the swelling resolves but is unpredictable and can thin the skin. If injected, Kenalog should be injected with extreme conservatism.

OUTCOMES

- Techniques to rotate the tip are much more easily performed and are much more reliable than techniques to derotate or lengthen the nose, and patients should be counseled accordingly.

COMPLICATIONS

- Iatrogenic loss of tip support with concomitant loss of tip projection is a known and feared complication that should be minimized whenever possible. It is preferred to use incremental and reversible methods of tip rotation prior to or instead of destructive, irreversible modifications to the tip-supporting elements. Re-establishment of tip support should be employed whenever possible.

REFERENCES

1. Byrd HS, Burt JD, Andochick S, et al. Septal extension grafts: a method of controlling tip projection shape. *Plast Reconstr Surg.* 1997;100:999.
2. Rohrich RJ, Kurkjian TJ, Hoxworth RE, et al. The effect of the columellar strut graft on nasal tip position in primary rhinoplasty. *Plast Reconstr Surg.* 2012;130:926.
3. Guyuron BG, Varghai A. Lengthening the nose with a tongue and groove technique. *Plast Reconstr Surg.* 2003;111:4.

Technique for Ethnic Rhinoplasty Using the Open Approach

Dean M. Toriumi and Jeffrey T. Steitz

DEFINITION

- The ethnic nose is very diverse and can encompass many different nasal contours and anatomic variations. It is outside the scope of this chapter to cover all of these anatomic variations. For this chapter, I will cover the Black and Asian nose and how I use the open approach to perform structural grafting to augment the nose.
- When I use the term "ethnic" in this chapter, I will be referring to primarily Black and Asian patients. These techniques may also prove to be effective in the thick-skinned "Mestizo" nose. This is with the understanding that there are many other forms of ethnic noses that have significantly different anatomy but will not be emphasized in this chapter.
- Many ethnic patients have an underprojected nose with a wide alar base and poorly defined nasal tip. These patients also tend to have thicker skin. They can have a low wide dorsum lacking definition on frontal view. Some ethnic patients may have a dorsal hump with a low radix. All of these different configurations require different management.
- In general, most Black and Asian patients require augmenting their nose to stretch the thick skin envelope to create improved contour. This requires cartilage grafting to push out and stretch the thick skin envelope making the lateral view larger to enhance the appearance of the frontal view.

ANATOMY

- The anatomy of the Black and Asian nose can vary significantly from patient to patient. Most ethnic patients will tend to have thicker sebaceous skin that is much thicker in the lower half of the nose. They tend to have weak lower lateral cartilages that can make controlling and preserving tip projection very difficult.
- Ethnic patients tend to have a short weak nasal septum that lacks caudal projection leaving a deficiency in tip support. For this reason, adding structural support is critical to providing a good aesthetic and functional outcome.
- Ethnic patients may demonstrate a reversal of the normal "gull in flight" appearance of the transition from alar margin to infratip lobule (**FIG 1**).[1] Many of these patients will demonstrate a reversal of normal with retraction of the columella in relation to the hanging alar lobule (**FIG 2**). Correction of the retracted columella requires a large caudal septal extension graft that can push the columella and infratip lobule inferiorly to create a more normal "gull in flight" appearance to the alar lobular transition to the infratip lobular projection.[2] This graft will act to move the columella/infratip lobule or central compartment inferiorly to create a more favorable relationship between the ala and infratip lobule.
- Ethnic patients also tend to have a wide alar base that creates a discrepancy between the width of the upper third of the nose and the width of the lower third of the nose. It is preferable to avoid overnarrowing the upper third of the nose with aggressive lateral osteotomies to create narrowing and then accentuate the imbalance between the upper third and lower third widths.

PATIENT HISTORY AND PHYSICAL FINDINGS

- The patient should be examined to assess nasal tip support and caudal projection of the septum.
- Intranasal examination should be performed using a nasal speculum, appropriate lighting, and preferably examination

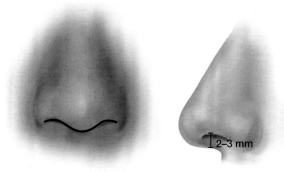

FIG 1 • The normal relationship between the infratip lobule and ala demonstrates a "gull in flight" appearance on the frontal view. This translates to a 2- to 3-mm columellar show on the lateral view.

2–3 mm

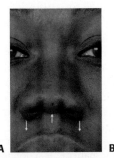
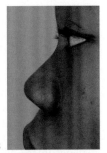

A   B

FIG 2 • A Black patient with retracted columella and hanging ala to create the opposite of the normal "gull in flight" orientation between the infratip lobule and ala. **A.** Frontal view showing the ala projecting inferiorly to greater extent than the columella/infratip lobule. **B.** Lateral view showing hidden columella.

with an endoscope. Assess the nasal septum and status of the inferior turbinates. Watch the patient breathe in to determine if there is any lateral wall weakness, which is rare in Black and Asian patients.

- Discuss with the patient what the primary goal of the surgery should be. Determine their primary deformities they would like corrected.

- The deficiency in nasal tip support and reversal of the normal "gull in flight" orientation of the ala and columella must be pointed out to the patient.

- Preoperative computer imaging is critical in the ethnic patient and should be used in most patients. This will enhance your ability as the surgeon to determine what the patient's goals are and to point out specific concepts to the patient. This will help ensure your aesthetic goals align with those of the patient.

- The linkage between lack of structural support and the large thick skin envelope must be pointed out to the patient as well.

- One of the key concepts in ethnic rhinoplasty (Black and Asian) is to realize that it is usually necessary to augment the lateral view via dorsal augmentation, place a caudal septal extension graft and possibly a shield-type tip graft to stretch the thick skin, and create a narrowing effect on the lateral view. By stretching the skin on the nose, particularly in the nasal tip area, definition can be increased and narrowing can be achieved. This can be very difficult for both the surgeon and patient to understand, but thick-skinned patients rarely look better when the nose is reduced unless the skin is able to contract. Typically, the thicker skin of the lower third of the nose will not contract significantly, potentially leaving a polly beak deformity, a wider scarred nasal tip, and an underprojected tip complex.

- Expanding and augmenting the lateral view can also improve the lateral view by lifting the upper nasal dorsum to match the projection of the prominent thicker supratip skin by creating a straighter profile (**FIG 3**).

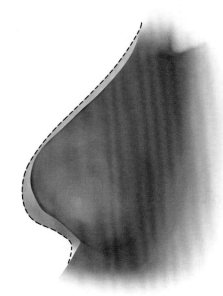

FIG 3 • By augmenting the lateral view, the upper nasal dorsum can frequently be elevated to the level of the prominent supratip skin creating a straighter dorsal line.

SURGICAL MANAGEMENT

- It is preferable to perform these surgeries under general anesthesia. With the patient intubated, the airway is protected from blood contacting the vocal cords and potentially causing laryngospasm. A protected airway is particularly important if any work is planned on the nasal septum or turbinates.

- Local anesthetic agent (1% lidocaine with 1:100 000 epinephrine) is injected into the nose to provide hemostasis. Injections are made along the septum, along the marginal incisions, over the nasal dorsum and middle vault, and in the nasal tip area. At least 10 minutes should pass before the procedure is initiated to allow the full vasoconstrictive effect to set in.

■ Harvesting Cartilage for Grafting

- Auricular cartilage can be harvested but is not ideal for grafting. The auricular cartilage is softer and weaker than costal cartilage and usually not adequate for augmentation cases. If auricular cartilage is harvested, the posterior approach is preferred to minimize the chance of ear deformity or change in position.

- In most ethnic patients, a larger amount of cartilage is needed for grafting. Costal cartilage is preferable and can be harvested from a smaller 11-mm incision[3] (**TECH FIG 1A**). It is recommended to use a larger incision when less experienced because safety is most important when harvesting costal cartilage.

- The 6th or 7th ribs are ideal for cartilage grafting material in the ethnic patient. If a longer dorsal graft is needed, it is preferable to use the seventh rib as it is straighter and longer. The 6th rib tends to have a genu that will shorten the straight segment that could be used for dorsal augmentation. If both dorsal augmentation

and premaxillary augmentation need be performed, two costal cartilage grafts may be harvested.

- Costal perichondrium should be harvested as well, because this material can be used for camouflage and to aid in fixation of the dorsal graft to the underlying dorsal nasal bone. In these cases, the costal perichondrium is

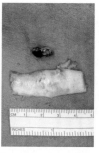

TECH FIG 1 • A 4.5-cm segment of costal cartilage harvested through an 11-mm incision.

placed as an interpositional graft that is sutured to the undersurface of the dorsal graft. The nasal dorsum is rasped or perforated with a 3-mm straight osteotome, and then the dorsal graft with perichondrium is placed over the nasal dorsum. The perichondrium will rigidly fix the dorsal graft to the underlying nasal dorsum.

Open Approach

- An inverted-V incision is made at the level of the midcolumella (**TECH FIG 2A**). The position of the incision can be varied depending on the goals of the surgery. In most ethnic patients, the goal is to increase nasal tip projection.
- The columellar incision is connected to bilateral marginal incisions made along the caudal margin of the lateral crura.

- The columellar flap is elevated off of the medial crura. Care is taken to avoid damaging the columellar flap.
- During flap elevation, dissection can be performed just below the subdermal plexus leaving the fibrofatty tissue of the nasal tip and supratip on the cartilages to then be excised (**TECH FIG 2B,C**).

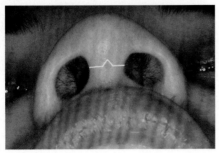 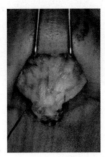 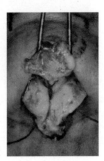

TECH FIG 2 • A. Position of the inverted-V midcolumellar incision marked out in *yellow*. **B.** A Black patient with thick skin after flap elevated leaving fibrofatty tissue on the lower lateral cartilages. **C.** After fibrofatty tissue dissected from cartilages.

Exposing the Nasal Septum

- Dissection is performed between the medial crura to access the caudal septum. Typically, the caudal septum is further cranial than in most Caucasian patients (**TECH FIG 3**). After identifying the caudal septum, mucoperichondrial flaps are elevated.
- Septal deviations can be corrected, and septal cartilage can be harvested for grafting purposes. Most ethnic patients have small harvestable segments of cartilage that are available.

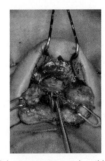

TECH FIG 3 • Caudal septum exposed and bilateral mucoperichondrial flaps elevated. Note how far cranial the caudal septum is set back.

Managing the Nasal Dorsum

- In most ethnic patients, the nasal dorsum needs augmentation. Major dorsal augmentation with costal cartilage will be covered in another chapter.
- Many ethnic patients will require radix augmentation to elevate a deep radix. When placing a radix graft, smaller grafts can be fixated using a transcutaneous suture (**TECH FIG 4A–C**).
- If a modest degree of dorsal augmentation is required, septal cartilage can be used. It is helpful to camouflage

the lateral margins of the dorsal graft with soft tissue (costal perichondrium, temporalis fascia, etc.) (**TECH FIG 4D,E**).
- Larger dorsal grafts will be fixated to the nasal dorsum by suturing costal perichondrium to the undersurface of the dorsal graft (**TECH FIG 4F**).[3,4] The dorsal graft is then placed on the nasal dorsum after perforating the nasal bones with a 3-mm straight osteotome. The perichondrium ossifies, resulting in rigid fixation of the dorsal graft to the nasal dorsum. This method of fixation is covered in Chapter 76.

TECHNIQUES

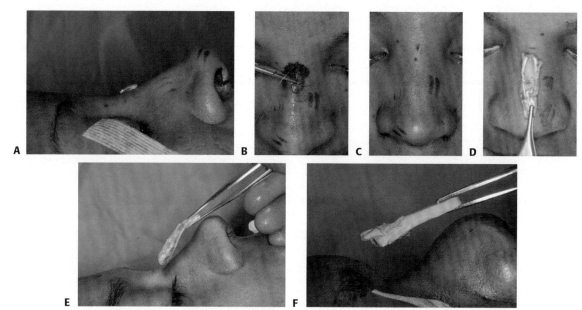

TECH FIG 4 • **A.** Soft cartilage radix graft over radix area. **B.** A 6-0 Monocryl suture placed transcutaneously to fix radix graft into position. **C.** Transcutaneous fixation suture in place over radix area. **D.** For lesser degrees of dorsal augmentation, septal cartilage can be used. Septal cartilage dorsal graft with costal perichondrium sutured to the lateral margins to camouflage the graft. **E.** Lateral view showing the perichondrium draped over the edges of the dorsal graft. **F.** For major dorsal augmentation, costal perichondrium is sutured to the undersurface of the dorsal graft and placed on top of the nasal bones after they have been perforated with a 3-mm straight osteotome. The perichondrium will act to ossify the dorsal graft and fixate it to the bridge.

■ Middle Nasal Vault

- Most ethnic patients do not require dorsal hump reduction. In this case, there is no need to open the middle nasal vault unless deviated. The spreader grafts can be placed into submucoperichondrial pockets to stabilize the dorsal septum and extended caudally to stabilize the caudal septal extension graft.
- Submucoperichondrial tunnels are dissected using a narrow Cottle elevator. The elevator is advanced superiorly in a submucoperichondrial plane up to the nasal bones (**TECH FIG 5**).
- After the tunnels are created, spreader grafts are fashioned and placed into the submucoperichondrial tunnels. The spreader grafts should fit rather snugly into the pockets. The grafts are left to extend beyond the caudal septum to stabilize the caudal septal extension graft.
- The spreader grafts are fixated using a single 5-0 PDS suture that traverses the spreader grafts and septum.

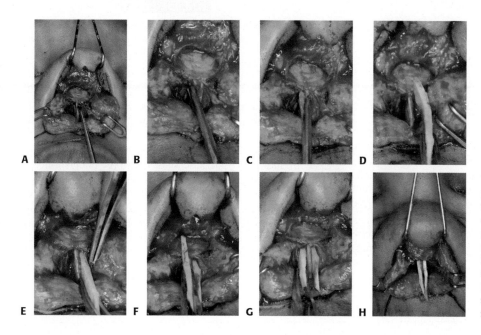

TECH FIG 5 • Spreader grafts placed into submucoperichondrial tunnels. **A.** Cottle elevator used to create the tunnels. **B.** Making the right tunnel. **C.** Making the left tunnel. **D.** Left spreader graft ready to be inserted into the tunnel. **E.** Left spreader graft being positioned. **F.** Right spreader graft. **G.** Both spreader grafts in place. **H.** Bilateral spreader grafts in place.

■ Stabilizing the Nasal Base

- The nasal base is stabilized using a caudal septal extension graft. Typically, the extension graft is slightly wider along the anterior margin (**TECH FIG 6A–D**). The extension graft is stabilized anteriorly using the extended spreader grafts and inferiorly using thin slivers of cartilage placed across the caudal septum and the extension graft.[5,6] The grafts are sutured in place with 5-0 PDS sutures.

- After the extension graft is stabilized, the medial crura are fixed to the septal extension graft using a 4-0 plain on an SC-1 needle. It is helpful to pull the medial crura and columella anteriorly to open the nasolabial angle and increase projection (**TECH FIG 6E–G**). This suture is followed up with a 5-0 PDS suture that is placed between the medial crura catching the caudal septum as well.

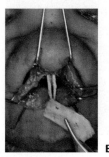
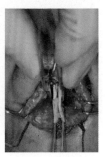
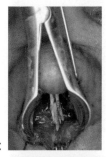
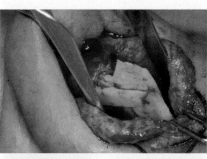
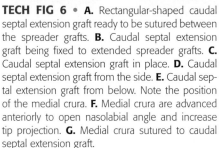
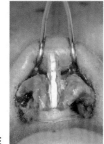
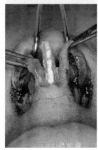
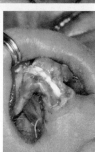

TECH FIG 6 • A. Rectangular-shaped caudal septal extension graft ready to be sutured between the spreader grafts. **B.** Caudal septal extension graft being fixed to extended spreader grafts. **C.** Caudal septal extension graft in place. **D.** Caudal septal extension graft from the side. **E.** Caudal septal extension graft from below. Note the position of the medial crura. **F.** Medial crura are advanced anteriorly to open nasolabial angle and increase tip projection. **G.** Medial crura sutured to caudal septal extension graft.

■ Managing the Nasal Tip

- Nasal tip contour and definition are controlled by what is done at the tip lobule. In most ethnic patients, a tip graft is placed over the domes to provide additional tip projection and tip definition.[7] There is rarely any need to reduce the lateral crura as the tip grafting is what achieves the change in lobular contour. Furthermore, the lateral crura tend to be very weak, and any reduction can result in weakening of the tip structure.

- An onlay-type tip graft can be sutured horizontally over the domes (**TECH FIG 7A,B**). These tip grafts are typically softer cartilage and are sutured over the domes using two 6-0 Monocryl sutures.

- In most patients with thicker skin, a shield-type tip graft is used. In these cases, if the shield-type tip graft extends more than 2 mm but less than 3 mm above the existing domes, a buttress graft is used to stabilize the posterior surface of the graft to prevent it from rotating cephalically (**TECH FIG 7C–E**).[9] This graft prevents over-rotation of the nasal tip lobule.

- If shield-type tip graft projects more than 3 mm above the domes, lateral crural grafts are used to stabilize the shield-type tip graft. These grafts are angled at 45 degrees off of the midline and sutured to the posterior surface of the shield graft to stabilize it and prevent it from rotating cephalically (**TECH FIG 7F–H**). Lateral crural grafts are different from lateral crural strut grafts that are placed under the lateral crura between lateral crus and the underlying vestibular skin. Lateral crural grafts are placed on top of the lateral crura and are used to stabilize the shield-type tip graft.[3,7]

Alar Rim Grafts

- In some patients after placing the shield-type tip graft and stabilizing it with a buttress graft or bilateral lateral crural grafts, additional camouflage is needed to prevent visibility. In such cases, alar rim grafts can be placed. Alar rim grafts are usually sutured to the lateral margin of the shield-type tip graft with a 6-0 Monocryl suture (**TECH FIG 8A–F**). Then, the alar rim graft is placed into pockets along the marginal incision. The alar rim graft is placed into the pockets by suturing a guide suture to the end of the alar rim graft. Then, the alar rim graft is advanced using the guide suture

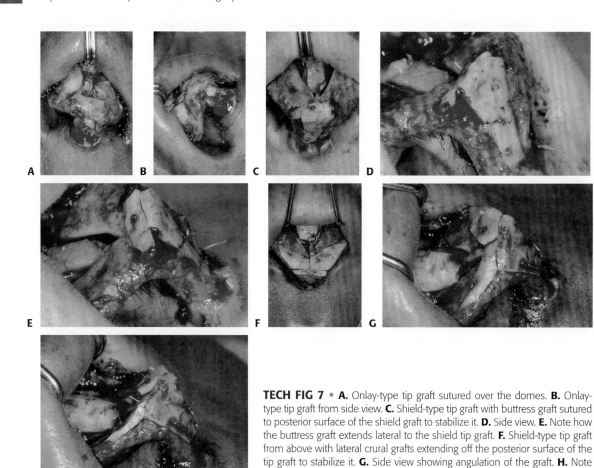

TECH FIG 7 • A. Onlay-type tip graft sutured over the domes. **B.** Onlay-type tip graft from side view. **C.** Shield-type tip graft with buttress graft sutured to posterior surface of the shield graft to stabilize it. **D.** Side view. **E.** Note how the buttress graft extends lateral to the shield tip graft. **F.** Shield-type tip graft from above with lateral crural grafts extending off the posterior surface of the tip graft to stabilize it. **G.** Side view showing angulation of the graft. **H.** Note the shield shape of the tip graft.

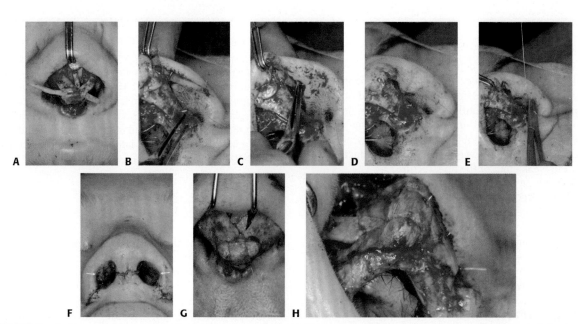

TECH FIG 8 • A. Alar rim grafts sutured to the lateral margins of the shield-type tip graft. **B.** Guide suture sutured to the end of alar rim graft. **C.** Alar rim graft placed into pockets along marginal incision. **D.** Guide suture pulled taught to pull alar rim graft into the depth of the pocket. **E.** Tying guide suture over the vestibular skin. **F.** Basal view at the end of the operation with *yellow arrows* pointing to knots tied over vestibular skin. **G.** Costal perichondrium sutured over leading edge of the shield-type tip graft for camouflage. **H.** Lateral view showing perichondrium over tip graft.

into the depth of the pocket, and the suture is sutured over the mucosa with a loop and left until the cast is removed. This helps to prevent the alar rim graft from becoming displaced.

- If additional camouflage is needed, soft tissue (scar tissue, fascia, or costal perichondrium) can be sutured over the domes using a 6-0 Monocryl suture (**TECH FIG 8G,H**).

■ Managing the Alar Base

- If necessary, alar base reduction can be performed to decrease the size of the nostrils and to narrow the nasal base. In most ethnic patients, a lateral alar base reduction can be used to decrease alar flare (**TECH FIG 9A–C**).

In patients with larger nostrils, a combination of internal and external alar base reduction is performed (**TECH FIG 9D–K**). This type of resection involves extending the excision into the nostril and onto the nostril sill. The design of the excision depends on the size of the nostril and the amount of lateral alar flare.

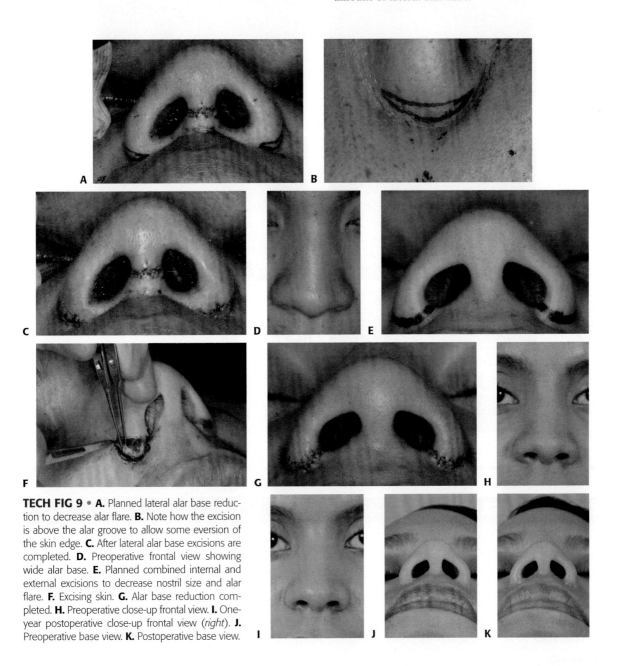

TECH FIG 9 • A. Planned lateral alar base reduction to decrease alar flare. **B.** Note how the excision is above the alar groove to allow some eversion of the skin edge. **C.** After lateral alar base excisions are completed. **D.** Preoperative frontal view showing wide alar base. **E.** Planned combined internal and external excisions to decrease nostril size and alar flare. **F.** Excising skin. **G.** Alar base reduction completed. **H.** Preoperative close-up frontal view. **I.** One-year postoperative close-up frontal view (*right*). **J.** Preoperative base view. **K.** Postoperative base view.

- After making the skin excision, a subcutaneous 6-0 Monocryl suture is placed to help with approximation of the nostrils. The skin edges are approximated using 7-0 nylon vertical mattress sutures with some interspersed 6-0 fast-absorbing gut sutures.

Nasal Base Bunching

- In some ethnic patients, excision alone is not adequate to narrow the base of the nose. In these cases, a nasal base bunching suture can be used to further narrow the base of the nose (**TECH FIG 10A**). A 3-0 Mersilene suture is passed from one alar base excision site to the other and cinched down to narrow the nasal base (**TECH FIG 10B–E**). It is helpful to place some fibrous tissue around the suture as it is passed through the skin to act a "stop" to prevent the suture from tearing through the tissues.

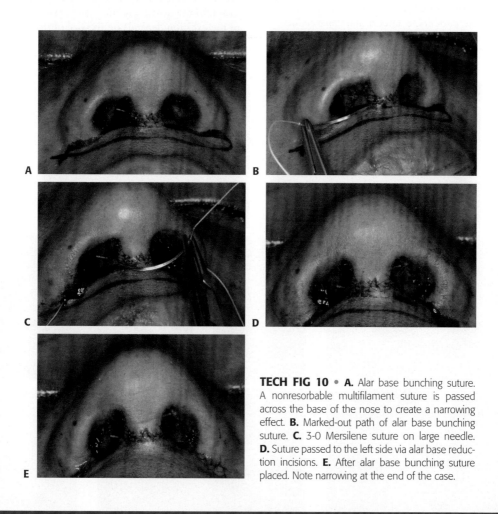

TECH FIG 10 • A. Alar base bunching suture. A nonresorbable multifilament suture is passed across the base of the nose to create a narrowing effect. **B.** Marked-out path of alar base bunching suture. **C.** 3-0 Mersilene suture on large needle. **D.** Suture passed to the left side via alar base reduction incisions. **E.** After alar base bunching suture placed. Note narrowing at the end of the case.

PEARLS AND PITFALLS

Approach	■ Avoid making columellar incision too high or too low. Keep incision away from the soft tissue triangle.
Grafting material	■ Harvest adequate cartilage for grafting to avoid suboptimal outcomes.
Nasal dorsum	■ Avoid excessively narrowing the nasal bones and potentially creating imbalance between upper and lower third of the nose.
Approach to managing the ethnic nose	■ Avoid reducing the Black or Asian nose as most of these patients require expansion of the skin envelope using cartilage grafts and stabilization of the nasal base.
Stabilizing nasal base	■ Make sure the nasal base is adequately stabilized. In most cases, a columellar strut may be inadequate.
Managing nasal tip	■ If a shield-type tip graft is placed, make sure it is adequately stabilized using a buttress graft, lateral crural grafts, or alar rim grafts.
Managing the alar base	■ When performing alar base reduction, avoid excessive excision.

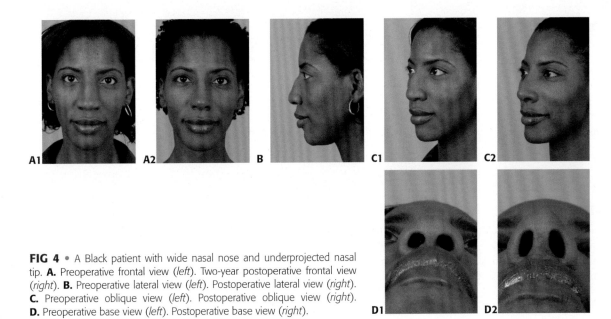

FIG 4 • A Black patient with wide nasal nose and underprojected nasal tip. **A.** Preoperative frontal view (*left*). Two-year postoperative frontal view (*right*). **B.** Preoperative lateral view (*left*). Postoperative lateral view (*right*). **C.** Preoperative oblique view (*left*). Postoperative oblique view (*right*). **D.** Preoperative base view (*left*). Postoperative base view (*right*).

POSTOPERATIVE CARE

- No nasal packing is used in the rhinoplasty patients. A running quilting 4-0 plain gut suture is used to approximate the septal flaps.
- Cast is removed on the 7th postoperative day.
- Patients should avoid salty foods postoperatively to minimize edema.
- Kenalog (10 mg/mL) can be injected deep into the tissues of the nasal tip to decrease edema and help to prevent scarring. These injections can be started at 1 month postoperatively and repeated every 3 months.

OUTCOMES

- Improved nasal tip definition and stronger profile can be expected after augmenting the nose using structural grafting (**FIG 4**).

COMPLICATIONS

- Infection is rare but can occur when extensive cartilage grafting is performed.
- Potential complications include asymmetries, deviation, and irregularities.

- If costal cartilage is used, warping of the cartilage can occur.
- Postoperative polly beak deformity can occur if there is a loss on tip projection or if there is prolonged supratip edema.
- Postoperative loss of nasal tip projection can be seen if the nasal base is not adequately stabilized.
- Potential visibility of the shield-type tip graft over time.

REFERENCES

1. Gunter JP, Rohrich RJ, Friedman RM. Classification and correction of alar-columellar discrepancies in rhinoplasty. *Plast Reconstr Surg.* 1996;97(3):643-648.
2. Toriumi DM. Caudal septal extension graft for correction of the retracted columella. *Oper Tech Otolaryngol Head Neck Surg.* 1995;6(4): 311-318.
3. Toriumi DM, Pero CD. Asian rhinoplasty. *Clin Plast Surg.* 2010;37(2): 335-352.
4. Toriumi DM. Discussion: use of autologous costal cartilage in Asian rhinoplasty. *Plast Reconstr Surg.* 2012;130(6):1349-1350.
5. Bahman Guyuron MD, Amin Varghai BS. Lengthening the nose with a tongue-and-groove technique. *Plast Reconstr Surg.* 2003;111(4): 1533-1539.
6. Toriumi DM. Structure approach in rhinoplasty. *Facial Plast Surg Clin North Am.* 2002;10(1):1-22.
7. Toriumi DM. New concepts in nasal tip contouring. *Arch Facial Plast Surg.* 2006;8:156-185.

62 CHAPTER

Technique for Treating the Crooked Nose

Ali Totonchi, Navid Pourtaheri, and Bahman Guyuron

DEFINITION

- A crooked nose is a nose with a portion of its midline structures deviating away from the facial midline along any extent of its cranial to caudal or anterior to posterior dimension.

ANATOMY

- The crooked nose involves deviation or asymmetry of one or more structural components of the nose, including nasal bones, upper lateral cartilages, lower lateral cartilages, septum, and nasal spine.

PATHOGENESIS

- The crooked nose may be a result of trauma, collapse or cicatrix after surgery, cocaine abuse, infection, mass effect from tumor, congenital defects, or improper development.
- The crooked nose can affect nasal airway patency and sinus drainage in causing sinus or migraine headaches.

PATIENT HISTORY AND PHYSICAL FINDINGS

- A complete patient history, including prior nasal and facial reconstructive or aesthetic procedures, should be reviewed.
- It is essential to collect a history of nasal trauma, airway complaints, allergies, sinus symptoms, and headaches.
  - A crooked nose can be associated with sinus infections, sinus headaches and migraines, or nasal airway obstruction. Assessing for these factors and postoperatively tracking these symptoms aid in gauging the benefits of surgery beyond its aesthetic outcome.
  - Unilateral nasal airway obstruction that is persistent or obstructive symptoms during quiet and deep inspiration is a reliable indicator of mechanical airway compromise, such as an enlarged turbinate, septal or nasal deviation, or incompetent internal or external nasal valve that should be addressed during surgery. Cyclical nose obstruction is a physiological or occasionally pathological change that may not improve with surgery.
- It is crucial to obtain a history of medications that can lead to bleeding (ie, aspirin and NSAIDs) and behaviors that may affect wound healing (ie, smoking, poor diet, steroid use). Discussion of these deleterious factors and their potential impact on postoperative outcomes with the patient may improve patient compliance.
  - Patient expectations should be assessed and managed, and the patient's role in facilitating a successful outcome should be emphasized.

- Physical examination should include facial analysis to assess for overall symmetry, canting of the occlusal plane, alignment of the nose with the rest of the face, and chin position in relation to the upper and the lower incisor midlines, lips, and upper face midline.
  - The nasal midline should be at the intercanthal midline rather than the intereyebrow midline, because patients often pluck their eyebrows differentially to align the midline of the deviated nose with the altered eyebrow.
  - Nasal analysis should assess each structural component and their degree of deviation. This should include observation of asymmetric nasal bones, a deviated caudal dorsum (septum and upper lateral cartilages), or a deviated nasal base (septum and lower lateral cartilages).
  - Midvault deviation always involves anterior septal deviation and is commonly associated with mid- and posterior septal deviation.
  - By tilting the patient's head up for an examination of the basilar view, one can assess the deviation or asymmetry of the columella, tip, footplates, nostrils, and alar bases. An overhead view may detect the external nasal deviation more clearly. The most powerful view for observation of nose deviation is a full-smile frontal view.
- Palpation to assess the three-dimensional frame of the nose could prove helpful:
  - One can palpate the nasal bones, upper lateral, and lower lateral cartilages, as well as the membranous septum, tip support, the caudal cartilaginous septum, and the anterior nasal spine. The latter is done by placing this structure between the dominant index finger and the thumb and confirming the midline positioning of this structure precisely.
  - Percussion over the frontal, ethmoid, and maxillary sinuses can elicit tenderness. This may be indicative of inflammation of the underlying sinuses.
- To assess nasal valve competence or airway patency, one can occlude the patient's nostril one side at a time and ask the patient to inhale normally and then deeply.
  - During the modified Cottle test, the examinee asks the patient to breathe quietly while supporting the nostril open at the level of the external and then internal nasal valve with a cotton-tip applicator or the speculum. If breathing is improved, this represents a positive test and indicates internal and/or external nasal valve incompetence.
- An internal nasal exam using a speculum can detect septal deviation, enlarged turbinates, synechiae, perforation, spurs, and contact between the turbinates and the septum:
  - Septal deformities observed may include septal tilt, C- or S-shaped deviation in the anteroposterior or cephalocaudal dimensions, or localized deviation with septal spurs.

When there is a septal tilt, usually there is no curve to the septum, and the caudal septum is dislocated to one side of the vomer bone. This is the most common class of septal deviation, followed by C-shaped anteroposterior septal deviation.

- Crusting, purulence, ulceration, or presence of polyps should also be noted.
- It is important to observe and document the color and size of the turbinates—pale boggy turbinate mucosa may indicate allergic rhinitis, whereas erythematous mucosa may indicate infection or inflammatory rhinitis.
- Analysis of the turbinates may reveal hypertrophy that typically occurs on the side ipsilateral to the external deviation or a paradoxical curl, which can misdirect the air and increase turbulence of airflow through the nose.
- Analysis of the nasal valves and internal nose should be repeated before and after vasoconstriction of the nasal mucosa using 0.25% phenylephrine or 1% ephedrine sulfate delivered via an aerosolized misting system or topically with cottonoid pledgets:
  - Posterior rhinoscopy is often helpful in patients with nasal airway obstructive symptoms.
  - Visualization of the posterior nasal airway is best achieved using a 0- or 30-degree nasal endoscope.

IMAGING

- Life-sized photographic and cephalometric analysis should be performed to confirm the findings of the physical examination and allow for measurements used to plan for surgical correction, particularly on patients who are expecting aesthetic improvement.
- Computed tomographic (CT) imaging of the nose and perinasal sinuses is not obtained routinely but can provide valuable information in the following cases (**FIG 1**):
  - Patients with frequent sinus headaches, sinus infections, or migraine headaches
  - Patients for whom the extent of deviated structures are not clear after physical examination
  - Imaging provides clear visualization of the nasal bones, septum, turbinates, or a mass that may have contributed to the nasal deviation.
  - The CT may reveal many conditions such as septal deviation, large posterior spur sinusitis, concha bullosa, septal bullosa, Haller cell, and contact points.

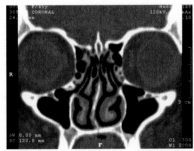

FIG 1 • Coronal CT image illustrating a deviated nasal septum and asymmetric turbinates. (Reprinted from Guyuron B. Correcting deviated noses, septoplasty, and turbinectomy. In: *Rhinoplasty*. Philadelphia, PA: Elsevier; 2012:306, with permission from Elsevier.)

SURGICAL MANAGEMENT

- The crooked nose usually presents with multiple deviated substructures, and successful surgical correction requires complete elimination of deviation from all substructures.
- Surgical techniques for correction of the crooked nose will be discussed for each substructure of the nose that may be involved.

Preoperative Planning

- Analysis of life-sized photographs and measurements of the deviation from the midline for each component of the nose can be valuable in correcting the deviation and discussing the surgical plan with the patient preoperatively. "Morphed" or simulated preoperative photos demonstrating the intended surgical changes can help the patient understand the surgical goals and manage the patient's expectations prior to obtaining final written consent for the procedure. It is crucial to clearly indicate to the patient that there cannot be any guarantee that the simulated or intended results may not be achieved.
- If there is a need for cartilage grafts, the first choice is septal cartilage as long as there is enough cartilage present. It is important to discuss with the patient the potential need for cartilage from a second site such as a conchal or costal graft if the septal cartilage is too deformed, absent, or insufficient to correct the nasal deformities planned.

Positioning

- The patient is placed in supine position with the arms tucked by their sides.
- After induction of general anesthesia, the airway is secured with dental floss or dental wire to the first premolar.
- The table is turned 90 degrees away from anesthesia to optimize access to the face and nose.
- The internal nasal hairs are trimmed with a pair of curved iris scissors, and the internal nose is cleansed with cotton swabs.
- The entire face is prepped with Betadine solution. After 1 to 2 minutes, the Betadine is wiped away with sterile saline solution.
- A split drape is placed sterilely around the face to expose the forehead up to the hairline and down to the chin.
  - This exposure allows for continual assessment of the nasal midline with respect to the facial midline and the effect of surgery on the upper lip position.

Approach

- An open approach is the authors' preferred method for correcting significant deviation or if other concomitant rhinoplasty maneuvers are planned.
- Deviation of the upper nasal third or bony vault involves the nasal bones and will require osteotomies for correction.
- Deviation of the midvault involves the septum and in most cases the upper lateral cartilages, which have to be separated from the septum and differentially trimmed after septoplasty and completion of nasal bone osteotomies. Other techniques, such as spreader grafts and/or septal rotational sutures, may be indicated.
- Deviation of the lower nasal third or nasal base involves the lower lateral cartilages, and successful correction may require elongation of the short side, shortening of the long side, reshaping, and/or the use of cartilage grafts.

■ Administration of Local Anesthesia

- It is important to achieve long-lasting and profound local anesthesia and vasoconstriction using the double-injection method:
  - Initial injection includes approximately 10 cc of 1% Xylocaine with 1:200 000 epinephrine solution.
  - If a turbinectomy is indicated, inject the turbinates using a 25-gauge spinal needle.
  - Cottonoid gauze saturated in oxymetazoline hydrochloride or phenylephrine solution is inserted deep in the nose as far cephalically and posteriorly as possible to produce vasoconstriction of the lining of areas that are difficult to reach with injection.
  - The injection should be performed with precision and in an organized manner, starting from the radix into soft tissues along the lateral and medial surface of the nasal bones profusely, along the medial surface of the nasal bones, followed by injection along the nasal base and columella, the dorsal septum on either side of the nasal roof, and the lining on either side of the vomer as far posteriorly as possible.
  - After a few minutes, the injection is repeated in the same order of initial injection using approximately 10 cc of 0.5% ropivacaine with 1:100 000 epinephrine.
  - This double-injection method starting with 1:200 000 solution reduces systemic uptake of the higher epinephrine concentration in the second injection that may otherwise cause hypertension, tachycardia, or arrhythmia. Ropivacaine in the second injection is longer lasting, which minimizes discomfort and the need for analgesics in the early postoperative period. Additionally, the initial injection by virtue of vasoconstriction renders the effects of the second injection more intense and produces protracted anesthesia.

■ Nasal Bone Correction

Unilateral Nasal Bone Correction

- Unilateral nasal bone deviation not affecting the internal nasal valve patency can be corrected with an onlay graft:
  - Septal cartilage (provides the most predictable outcome), conchal cartilage (gently crushed as a single or double layer), diced cartilage, soft tissue such as dermis, fascia graft, or fat injection may be used for this purpose.
  - An intercartilaginous incision is made to expose the target nasal bone.
    - A limited pocket is created by elevation of the periosteum using a Joseph periosteal elevator.
  - The graft is positioned in the subperiosteal plane and molded into place.
  - The incision is loosely approximated to allow for drainage.
- If the nasal bone shift is associated with medial transposition of the upper lateral cartilages, this may compromise ipsilateral internal valve function and requires correction by unilateral out-fracture.
  - A small vestibular incision at the pyriform aperture is made, and the periosteum is elevated using a Joseph periosteal elevator.
  - A low-to-low osteotomy and out-fracture of the nasal bone can be used to reposition the bone.
  - A spreader graft may be placed to avoid return of the nasal bone to its previous position as follows:
    - Make a 3-mm-long incision in the mucoperichondrium immediately caudal to the junction of the upper lateral cartilage and the septum as anteriorly as possible.
    - A septal elevator is used to create a pocket only large enough to accommodate the spreader graft between the septum and the upper lateral cartilage. The dissection is extended under the nasal bone.
    - A piece of folded Surgicel saturated in bacitracin ointment is placed between the nasal bone and septum and is left in position until it dissolves while the patient is maintained on oral antibiotics.

Bilateral Nasal Bone Deviation

- Bilateral nasal bone deviation is corrected with bilateral osteotomies and repositioning of the deviated nasal bones:
  - An onlay graft may be placed instead of osteotomy for mild deviation with no midvault deviation or compromise of internal nasal valve function.
  - If the nasal bone deviation also involves midvault deviation, a septoplasty is also needed, along with separation of the upper lateral cartilages from the septum.
  - The bilateral independent controlled osteotomy technique begins with medial osteotomy of the nasal bones (**TECH FIG 1**):
    - A 4- or 6-mm osteotome is placed medial to the nasal bones and is driven cephalically with gentle tapping of a mallet.
    - A wedge of bone is resected medially, unilaterally, or bilaterally, to reposition the nasal bones if the bones are too widely spaced from the septum.
  - Percutaneous anteroposterior vertical osteotomy of the nasal bones is performed next:
    - It is important to palpate the cephaloanterior border of the nasal bones to identify their point of divergence from the midline. This is where the osteotomy will begin.
    - A 2-mm osteotome is passed through the skin and muscle at this point, and osteotomy is performed through this small incision by sliding the osteotomy over the bone to avoid injury to the angular artery.
    - The osteotomy is advanced in the subperiosteal plane to make several interrupted puncture osteotomies in a linear fashion from anterior to posterior.

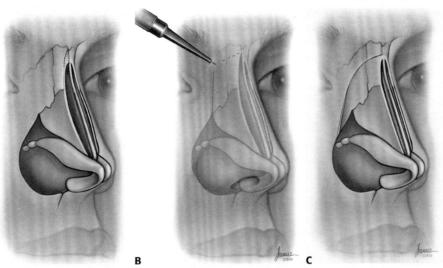

TECH FIG 1 • Nasal bone osteotomies. **A.** Medial wedge osteotomy is carried out using a 4- to 6-mm osteotome. **B.** Vertical osteotomy performed anterior to posterior percutaneously using a 2-mm osteotome. **C.** Low-to-low osteotomy is performed at the nose-face junction using a guarded osteotome to complete the nasal bone osteotomies. (Reprinted from Guyuron B. Correcting deviated noses, septoplasty, and turbinectomy. In: *Rhinoplasty*. Philadelphia, PA: Elsevier; 2012:117-119, with permission from Elsevier.)

- Finally, perform a low-to-low lateral osteotomy:
  - A no. 15 blade is used to make an incision in the vestibular lining close to the piriformis aperture.
  - A Joseph periosteal elevator is used to elevate the periosteum in a protected manner (it provides a barrier to reduce diffusion of blood that may otherwise cause periorbital ecchymosis).

- A guarded osteotome is placed at the nasofacial junction. A low-to-low osteotomy is completed to avoid a step deformity with gentle tapping of a mallet.
- The osteotomies are repeated on the contralateral side.
- Reposition the nasal bones with direct pressure.

■ Septoplasty

- Correction of the deviated septum can be accomplished using an open approach or closed technique through a left-sided L-shaped (Killian) incision.
- Open approach
  - After separation of the upper lateral cartilages from the septum, the mucoperichondrium on the left side of the septum is elevated, starting from the caudal septal angle. A small incision in the mucoperichondrium anteriorly may be needed to facilitate opening into the correct subperichondrial plane.
  - Once in the correct plane, the glistening cartilage will be in view. The blunt end of a periosteal elevator is used to raise a mucoperichondrial flap.
  - Continue dissection posteriorly, cephalically, and caudally until the junction of the quadrangle cartilage and the vomer bone is reached. It is often easier and safer to start the dissection from the posterocaudal septum anteriorly to facilitate dissection of the firm anterocaudal fibrous attachments.
- Closed approach:
  - An L-shaped (Killian) incision is used on the left mucoperichondrium (for the right-handed surgeon) to enter the subperichondrial plane and to elevate the mucoperichondrium on the left side.
- From this point on, the septoplasty technique is the same, regardless of whether an open approach or closed Killian incision was used.
- Using the sharp end of the septal elevator, one can continue an L incision through the quadrangular

cartilage, leaving an L strut at least 20 mm wide anteriorly and 10 mm wide caudally:
  - This L strut helps maintain long-term dorsal and columellar support, particularly if the operative plan includes repositioning of the nasal bones or manipulation of the upper lateral cartilages.
- Beyond the L strut, only the deviated portion of the septum that cannot be straightened with scoring needs to be resected. If more cartilage is needed to serve as a graft in other parts of the nose, then the remainder may be harvested. In other words, only the deviated portion of the posterocaudal septum is removed.
- The mucoperichondrium is elevated posterior and cephalad to the L incision only. Gentle separation of the caudal portion of the septal cartilage from the maxillary crest of the vomer bone is performed using the sharp end of the septal elevator.
- The sharp end of the septal elevator is also used to separate the cartilage from the perpendicular plate of the ethmoid bone.
- Once the septal cartilage is freed, it is removed using cartilage forceps (Adson-Brown).
- Correction of bony septal deviation and spurs
  - Septal deviation and spurs are often corrected by posterocaudal resection of the septal cartilage. Spurs, if present, are usually at the junction of the vomer bone, quadrangle cartilage, and perpendicular plate of the ethmoid bone.
  - If the maxillary crest or any portion of the vomer bone is deviated or if there is a bony spur on one side of the septum, it is important to remove this portion of bone using a rongeur.

- It is imperative to dissect the mucoperichondrium and the periosteum on the concave side of the septum first to prevent a tear in the mucoperichondrium. If a tear occurs, it can be addressed after septoplasty is complete (see below).
- Deviation or protrusion of the anterior nasal spine (ANS)
  - By palpating the ANS with the thumb and index finger of the dominant hand, the position of and size of the ANS is assessed. If the ANS is deviated or protruding, it can be reduced. If it is deviated, it can be repositioned with a greenstick fracture using a 2-mm osteotome.
- When the posterocaudal portion of the remaining septal cartilage is dislodged to one side of the maxillary crest, it is paramount to correct this septal tilt (see below).
- The caudal septum is affixed to the ANS spine using a figure-of-8 5-0 PDS suture placed from the septal cartilage to the periosteum of the ANS.
- The deviated portion of the vomer bone and the perpendicular plate are removed as thoroughly as possible to completely eliminate any internal septal deviation posteriorly.
- The remaining portion of the septoplasty technique depends upon the type of septal deviation observed.
- Correction of septal tilt (**TECH FIG 2**):
  - Disengaging the dislodged caudal and posterior portion of the retained L strut from the vomerine groove and ANS is accomplished using a periosteal elevator.
  - Removal of the overlapping redundant caudal portion of the septal cartilage with a no. 15 blade scalpel provides a "swinging-door"-type free movement of the cartilage.
  - Repositioning and fixation of the septum at midline to the periosteum of the anterior nasal spine are performed by placing a 5-0 PDS figure-of-8 suture.

- Prior to repositioning the septum, it is important to ensure that the ANS is in the midline or correct its position as discussed earlier.
- Correction of C- or S-shaped septal deviation
  - The posterocephalic portion of the septum is resected as described above.
  - Using a 2-mm osteotome, the ANS is greenstick fractured to reposition it in the midline as needed.
  - The perpendicular plate of the ethmoid and remaining portion of the quadrangular cartilage beyond the L strut is may be partially resected only if needed to correct deviation in the anterior and cephalic third of the septum.
  - Typically, removal of the posterior and caudal portion of the cartilage and creation of a swinging-door-type movement will release enough tension from the cartilage to eliminate the curvature.
  - If still deviated, one can score the L-shaped frame on its concave surface using a scalpel.
  - Specific differences in septal cartilage scoring based on the type of C- or S-shaped deviation are as follows:
    - Anteroposterior C-shaped deviation—the cartilage is scored in a cephalocaudal direction on the concave surface of the septal cartilage.
    - Cephalocaudal C-shaped deviation—the cartilage is scored in an anteroposterior direction on the concave surface of the septal cartilage.
    - Anteroposterior S-shaped deviation—the cartilage is scored in a cephalocaudal direction on both surfaces.
    - Cephalocaudal S-shaped deviation—the cartilage is scored in an anteroposterior direction on both surfaces.
  - Because the final outcome of scoring is not predictable, it is mandatory to place bilateral extramucosal stents (Simple Stent, Supramed) which are fixed into position using a through-and-through suture (**TECH FIG 3**). This will mold the septal cartilage while it is healing to further remove the deviation.

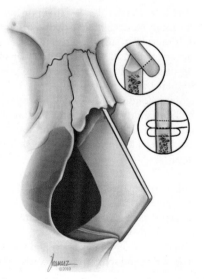

TECH FIG 2 • Septal tilt correction. The overlapping and displaced caudal portion of the deviated septal L strut is resected, moved into position at midline, and sutured into place. Deviated nasal spine correction may be needed prior to medializing the septum. (Reprinted from Guyuron B. Correcting deviated noses, septoplasty, and turbinectomy. In: *Rhinoplasty*. Philadelphia, PA: Elsevier; 2012:316.)

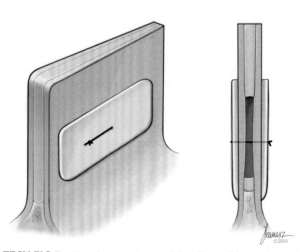

TECH FIG 3 • Septal stents. To control the effects of the scoring and eliminate dead space, simple stents are applied on both sides and sutured in position. (Reprinted from Guyuron B. Correcting deviated noses, septoplasty, and turbinectomy. In: *Rhinoplasty*. Philadelphia, PA: Elsevier; 2012:322.)

- Correction of mucoperichondrial perforation
  - Inadvertent tears in the mucoperichondrium if unilateral or bilateral without apposing perforations may be managed with nasal stents (Doyle or Simple) to prevent synechiae.
  - A bilateral tear with apposing perforations should be corrected by replacing a straight piece of septal cartilage, perpendicular plate of the ethmoid bone, or a PDS synthetic plate between the mucoperichondrial flaps, spanning the full width of the perforation.
- Correction of the deviated caudal dorsum
  - Despite a thorough septoplasty, if the caudal portion of the dorsal L-shaped strut remains deviated to one side along the caudal third of the anterior septum, one has to place spreader grafts and possibly a septal rotation suture as follows.
  - The spreader grafts are cut to size from the harvested septal cartilage or secondary donor site such as rib cartilage and are sutured along the dorsum of the septum after septal scoring using 5.0 PDS horizontal mattress sutures (**TECH FIG 4**).
  - After placement of the spreader grafts, a septal rotation suture is placed (**TECH FIG 5**). On the side that the anterior septum needs to be shifted toward, a 5-0 PDS suture is passed through the caudal portion of the upper lateral cartilage and then through the spreader grafts and the septum and further caudal through the upper lateral cartilage on the side where the septum needs to be shifted away. The suture is then returned through the upper lateral cartilage, spreader grafts, septum, and upper lateral in mattress fashion.
  - As the suture is tied, the composite layers, including the spreader grafts and the septum, are pulled toward the somewhat fixed upper lateral cartilage on the side where the suture was placed more cephalically.

- The suture is tied incrementally until the septum becomes perfectly aligned with a line bisecting the intercanthal line and the upper incisor midline (as long as these structures are positioned centrally).
  - A second suture may be required to avoid bowing of the upper lateral cartilage on the side toward the septum that is being rotated.
- Turbinate reduction:
  - Repositioning the septum requires reduction of the turbinates for optimal correction of the septal position and to prevent nasal airway obstruction after correction of the deviated septum.
  - Partial turbinectomy is more versatile and predictable than submucous resection, because it addresses both the hypertrophic mucosa and the underlying bone while leaving a normal-sized turbinate behind, which leads to less morbidity and greater success than complete turbinectomy.
  - Excising medial aspects of the turbinate evenly across the full length of the turbinate using a pair of turbinate scissors will produce a reliable outcome. Submucous resection with a microdebrider (XPS blade) combined with out-fracture of the turbinate is another reasonable option.
  - One can out-fracture the middle turbinate or partially or completely remove the middle turbinate if there is hindered sinus drainage or other indications, such as migraine headaches.
  - Concha bullosa can be treated by removal of the medial wall or on rare occasions, resection of most of the turbinate.
- Use of septal stents
  - After completion of septoplasty, a Doyle stent or a Simple Stent is placed on either side of the septum and fixed in position using a through-and-through 4-0 polypropylene suture (see **TECH FIG 3**).

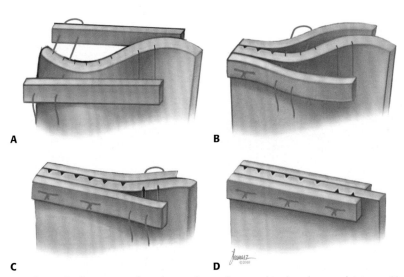

TECH FIG 4 • A–D. Spreader graft placement. Bilateral spreader grafts are placed and sutured into position along the dorsal septum to correct septal curvature after septal scoring. (Reprinted from Guyuron B. Correcting deviated noses, septoplasty, and turbinectomy. In: *Rhinoplasty*. Philadelphia, PA: Elsevier; 2012:322, with permission from Elsevier.)

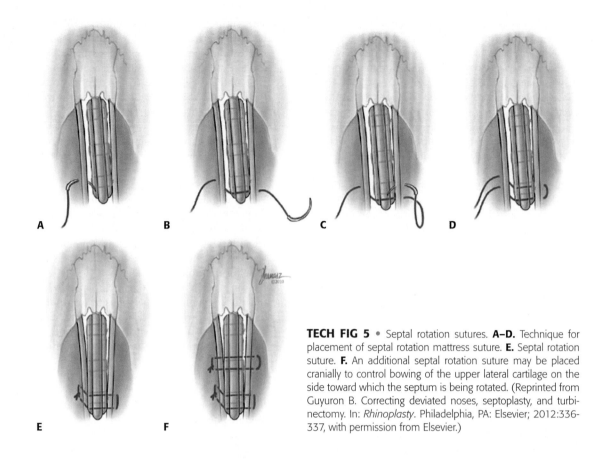

TECH FIG 5 • Septal rotation sutures. **A–D.** Technique for placement of septal rotation mattress suture. **E.** Septal rotation suture. **F.** An additional septal rotation suture may be placed cranially to control bowing of the upper lateral cartilage on the side toward which the septum is being rotated. (Reprinted from Guyuron B. Correcting deviated noses, septoplasty, and turbinectomy. In: *Rhinoplasty*. Philadelphia, PA: Elsevier; 2012:336-337, with permission from Elsevier.)

■ Upper Lateral Cartilage Correction

- For a deviated midvault dorsum, an open approach is preferred.
- It is important to separate the upper lateral cartilages from the septum and assess for symmetry after the septum is pushed to midline and nasal bones have been repositioned (**TECH FIG 6**).

- Repositioning of the septum may require differential trimming of the upper lateral cartilages using a Joseph scalpel and then sutured along the septum with spreader grafts (see **TECH FIG 4**) if indicated using 5.0 PDS horizontal mattress sutures or a septal rotation suture (see **TECH FIG 5**) as discussed in the sections above.

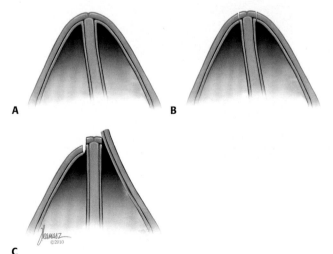

TECH FIG 6 • Importance of differential trim of the upper lateral cartilages after septoplasty and nasal bone repositioning. **A.** Deviated septum and upper lateral cartilages. **B,C.** Trimmed upper lateral cartilages prior to nasal bone osteotomies and septal repositioning may result in residual excess or shortage of the upper lateral cartilages on either side. (Reprinted from Guyuron B. Correcting deviated noses, septoplasty, and turbinectomy. In: *Rhinoplasty*. Philadelphia, PA: Elsevier; 2012:314, with permission from Elsevier.)

■ Lower Lateral Cartilage Correction

- The lower lateral cartilages may be accessed for correction using an open rhinoplasty approach.
- If the caudal septum is displaced, straighten it prior to adjusting the length of the lower lateral cartilages.
- The tripod concept is used to determine the appropriate length that each side of the lower lateral cartilages must be matched in order to correct the deviation and nasal projection. For example, a nasal base that is deviated to the left will require lengthening of the lateral crus of the left lower lateral cartilage or shortening of the lateral crus of the right lower lateral cartilage, depending on what the appropriate tip projection would be. In the underprojected nose, the lateral crus on the side the base is deviated toward is lengthened, whereas in the overprojected nose, the lateral crus on the side the base is deviated away from is shortened.

- If correction requires shortening of the lower lateral cartilage on one side, one can mobilize the lower lateral cartilage, transect and overlap it laterally and if necessary medially, and then repair it preferably after placement of a Gunter lateral crus strut with 5.0 PDS sutures (**TECH FIG 7**).
- If correction requires lengthening of the lower lateral cartilage on one side, the lateral crus is dissected, transected, and elongated, and the cut ends are secured to a Gunter lateral strut using 5.0 PDS sutures (**TECH FIG 8**). A lateral crus strut, if used, should be placed bilaterally for symmetry.
- After correction, the lower lateral cartilages are secured to a columellar strut graft to provide long-term stability.
- A perfect alignment of the nasal domes and the midline of the dorsum is checked repeatedly.

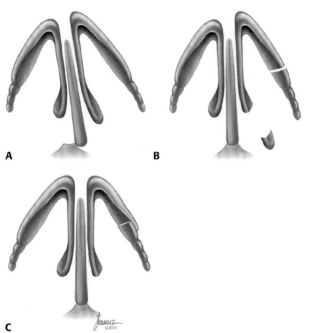

TECH FIG 7 • Lower lateral cartilage trim after septal tilt correction. **A,B.** Lower lateral cartilage exposed and mobilized after septal tilt correction, a portion of the medial crus portion is resected or overlapped as needed. **C.** Lateral crus is overlapped depending on the orientation of the lower lateral cartilage and taking into consideration the tripod concept. (Reprinted from Guyuron B. Correcting deviated noses, septoplasty, and turbinectomy. In: *Rhinoplasty*. Philadelphia, PA: Elsevier; 2012:341, with permission from Elsevier.)

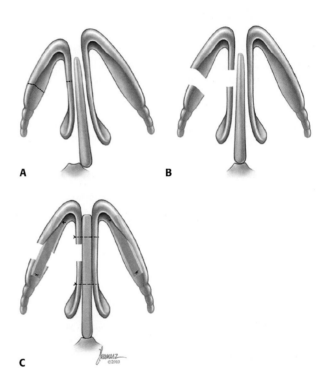

TECH FIG 8 • Lower lateral cartilage extension after septal tilt correction. **A,B.** Mobilization of the lower lateral cartilage and anterior advancement after septal tilt correction. **C.** Segments fixed in position with a columella and lateral crus strut. (Reprinted from Guyuron B. Correcting deviated noses, septoplasty, and turbinectomy. In: *Rhinoplasty*. Philadelphia, PA: Elsevier; 2012:342, with permission from Elsevier.)

PEARLS AND PITFALLS

Preoperative examination	■ Careful preoperative analysis of the face, nasal framework, and internal structures allows for thorough correction, including important observation of eyebrow alteration. A full-smile frontal view will best elucidate nasal deviation. ■ Failure to do so may result in residual deviation.
Mucoperichondrial tears	■ It is important to identify any mucoperichondrial tears before repair of the incisions. ■ Bilateral apposing tears can result in a persistent septal perforation if not addressed.
Turbinate reduction	■ Turbinates must be conservatively reduced intraoperatively before or after the septoplasty. ■ Failure to reduce the turbinates on the side toward which the septum was corrected may result in relapse of the septal deviation.
Trim the upper lateral cartilages last	■ Trimming these structures prior to repositioning the septum and nasal bones may result in upper lateral cartilage excess on one side and shortage on the opposite side.
Protect the periosteum during lateral osteotomy	■ The periosteum provides a barrier to limit diffusion of blood into the periorbital tissues. ■ If disrupted, this can result in significant periorbital ecchymosis.

POSTOPERATIVE CARE

- Stents:
  - If a septoplasty was performed, at the end of the procedure, Doyle stents are placed on either side of the septum and fixed to the membranous septum using a through-and-through mattress 4-0 polypropylene suture. Doyle stents allow further stabilization of the septum and eliminate dead space. These stents are removed after 3 to 8 days, depending on the condition and the amount of dissection or manipulation of the septum.
  - Extramucosal internal stents (Simple Stents) that are placed for septal scoring or stents placed for bilateral apposing perforations of septal mucoperichondrium should be removed after 2 to 3 weeks.
  - The patient is kept on oral antibiotics throughout the period that any internal stents are in position to prevent toxic shock syndrome. An oral first-generation cephalosporin is preferable.
- Dressing:
  - Place Steri-Strips transversely across the nasal dorsum and sidewall touching down onto the midface on either side as well as one vertically along either sidewall connecting beneath the tip to help maintain the new shape of the nose and facilitate collapse of the dead space.
- Splint:
  - If nasal bone osteotomy was performed, a dorsal nasal splint (aluminum and thermoplastic) is applied over the Steri-Strips.
  - The dorsal splint is removed after 7 to 8 days and after Doyle stent removal to prevent nasal bone shift.

- A Medrol dose-pack may be prescribed postoperatively to minimize swelling and bruising from osteotomies. Corticosteroids are to be avoided in patients with active acne or a propensity for severe acne.
  - The patient should avoid wearing glasses for 5 weeks after nasal bone osteotomy.
- The patient can bathe on postoperative day 1 but is instructed to not get the nasal dressings wet.
- Patients are prevented from strenuous activity for 3 weeks to avoid intranasal bleeding.

OUTCOMES

- Although the goal is correction of all of the nasal deviation in a single surgery, secondary procedures may become necessary to achieve optimal results even for the most skilled surgeon.
- It is important to discuss this possibility with patients who undergo rhinoplasty for any reason, especially those with a significantly crooked nose.

COMPLICATIONS

- Hematoma
- Persistent epistaxis
- Infection
- Graft loss
- Dorsal nasal collapse—from L-strut fracture or collapse
- Synechiae—can be avoided by use of Doyle stents
- Empty nose syndrome—from over-resection of the inferior turbinate

Technique for Treating the Long Nose

Michael R. Lee and Rod J. Rohrich

63
CHAPTER

DEFINITION

- *Long nose* is a term used to describe a nose that extends beyond the ideal nasal length. Multiple subsites may be responsible for creating a long nose and will be discussed.
- *Nasal length* is measured from the root of the nose to the most projected part of the nasal tip. Ideally, nasal length should measure 0.67 of the midfacial height (eyebrow to subnasale).
- *Nasal projection* is measured from the alar groove to the most projected part of the nasal tip. Ideally, nasal projection should measure 0.67 of the ideal nasal length.[1]
- *Nasal rotation* is determined by using the nasolabial angle. On lateral view, a line is drawn bisecting the long axis of the nostril, whereas a second vertical line is drawn through the anterior most aspect of the upper lip. The angle created should fall between 90 and 110 degrees in women and between 90 and 95 degrees in men. A more obtuse angle is associated with over-rotation of the tip, whereas a more acute angle is associated with a decreased tip rotation. The latter is often seen with the long nose.

ANATOMY

- Increased nasal length may result from multiple anatomic subsites including the radix and nasal bones, dorsal and caudal nasal septum, and/or excess paired nasal cartilages. These structures may be solely responsible for the long nose, but more often it is a combination of subsites (**FIG 1**).
- The nasal skin and musculature envelop the underlying bone and cartilage. Soft tissue attachments work to keep proper relationships between nasal bone and cartilage. These attachments provide support for the nasal tip.
- Nasal tip support structures can be divided into major and minor. Major tip support structures include the fibrous attachments between the upper and lower lateral cartilages (scroll ligament), lateral crura and pyriform aperture, medial crura and caudal septum, and the interdomal tip ligament. Minor tip support structures include fibrous attachments of alar cartilage to the cartilaginous dorsum, alar cartilage attachments to overlying skin, and the membranous septum.[1]

PATHOGENESIS

- A long nose may occur as the result of congenital development, traumatic injury, iatrogenic injury, and/or aging.[2,3] Congenital overgrowth may lead to volume excess.

Traumatic injury may displace or activate growth of bone or cartilage. Iatrogenic injury may create a long nose when tip support is not properly established. Aging results in loss of tip projection and midface volume loss, both of which contribute to a long nose.
- The illusion of a long nose may occur in patients with subnasale malposition, periapical hypoplasia, short midface, or inadequate chin projection.
- A true increase in nasal length may occur with a high radix, excess volume of the upper lateral cartilages, lower lateral cartilages, nasal septum, and/or loss of tip projection.

PATIENT HISTORY AND PHYSICAL FINDINGS

- Aesthetically, patients may feel their nose is simply too large for their face. As the focal point of the face, a long nose often disrupts nasofacial balance.
- Patients may point out a large hump caused by excess bony or cartilaginous dorsum. They may complain of a prominent or hanging columella that results from excess of the caudal septum. Patients may also report a drooping tip from inadequate support.

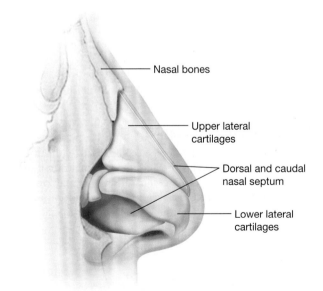

FIG 1 • Illustration depicting the nasal substructure. Increased nasal length may result from multiple anatomic subsites including the radix and nasal bones, dorsal and caudal nasal septum, and/or excess paired nasal cartilages.

Labels: Nasal bones; Upper lateral cartilages; Dorsal and caudal nasal septum; Lower lateral cartilages

- Examination begins with assessment of facial widths and vertical heights. This is important as the overall surgical goal is to create improved balance between the face and nose. If the facial proportions grossly deviate from aesthetic ideals, this is taken into consideration when creating the operative plan.
- The nose is evaluated in all classic rhinoplasty views with attention focused on areas responsible for creating a long nose. The patient is examined in repose, animation, and respiration as the nose is a dynamic structure.
- Anterior inspection is useful to determine symmetry and straightness, both of which contribute to the dorsal aesthetic lines (DALs). A large dorsal hump may distort the DALs.
  - Tip definition and position are also noted.
- Lateral and oblique views are useful in the long nose. Evaluation begins with critique of the radix or nasal root. A high radix may be responsible for creating a long nose, whereas a low radix may give the nose an overprojected appearance. Next, the dorsum is inspected for the presence of a convexity (hump) or irregularities. Overgrowth of the upper lateral cartilages and/or dorsal septum is typically responsible for dorsal convexity. Distally, overgrowth of the caudal septum can downwardly displace the lower lateral cartilages. Overgrowth of the lower lateral cartilages can further contribute to caudal tip position. Caudal septal excess may also distort the alar-columellar relationship and create excess columella show.
- Basal view analysis provides additional information in the long nose patient. Excess lower lateral cartilage volume may create domal fullness and disrupt the ideal columellar:tip ratio of 2:1. The basal aesthetic lines (BALs)[4] are studied as they may be distorted by excess lower lateral cartilage volume and malposition of the medial crura.

IMAGING

- 3D imaging is extremely helpful in the long nose and improves communication between the surgeon and patient. Modern-day imaging software can readily display the anticipated changes of hump reduction, increased nasal rotation, and decreased nasal projection.
- Imaging can also be useful to illustrate to patients the difference chin surgery or midface volume restoration can make in overall nasofacial harmony.

SURGICAL MANAGEMENT

- Surgical management is best accomplished with an open surgical approach. This provides direct visualization of the radix, upper lateral cartilages, nasal septum, and lower lateral cartilages. Direct visualization and inspection of these structures optimize the ability to correctly diagnose and treat the problem(s).[5]

Preoperative Planning

- A comprehensive consultation is required as with all patients seeking rhinoplasty. Communication is an essential component of a successful outcome. This communication allows the patients to voice their desired changes and the surgeon to determine if expectations are obtainable. Furthermore, patients may not want all aspects of their long nose addressed, and each anticipated change should be discussed. The result of this discussion helps establish an ideal operative plan.

Positioning

- Once in the operating room, the patient is intubated and positioned on the table. The most cephalic portion of the head extends just beyond the table (**FIG 2**). The patient's head may be elevated 15 degrees to minimize venous pooling in the operative field. A throat pack is gently placed and removed at the end of the surgery. Local anesthetic with epinephrine is injected into the planned incision sites.

Approach

- Overall treatment of the long nose involves reduction of oversized nasal structures and establishment of adequate tip support. With the nasal skin envelope elevated, nasal bone and cartilages are easily inspected. Direct visualization and palpation help to determine cartilage size and integrity.
- The relationships between these structures are also studied. Excess dorsal septum may be associated with excess or normal upper lateral cartilage volume. Excess upper lateral cartilages may caudally displace excess or normal-sized lower lateral cartilages. Excess caudal septum may also caudally displace excess or normal-sized lower lateral cartilages. The open surgical approach allows an exact inspection of each structure to determine the appropriate surgical technique(s) to be implemented.

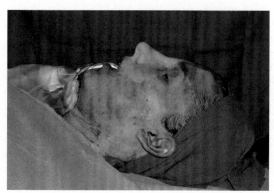

FIG 2 • Photograph depicting proper positioning of patient undergoing rhinoplasty.

Component Dorsal Hump Reduction

- The component dorsal hump reduction[6] may be used to address multiple causes of a long nose. Such causes include a high radix, dorsal septum excess, and/or upper lateral cartilage excess.
- Dissection continues to the anterior septal angle.
  - Once identified, bilateral mucosal flaps are elevated to expose the cartilaginous septum.
  - The elevator is used to dissect away the mucosa from the medial portion of the upper lateral cartilages (**TECH FIG 1A**).

- This move facilitates separation of the upper laterals from dorsal septum while minimizing mucosal trauma. Next, the upper lateral cartilages are separated from the dorsal septum with scalpel or scissors.
- Subsequently, short-angle scissors are used to remove excess of the cartilaginous dorsal septum.
- The rasp can be used to lower a high radix and smooth out any bony humps that exists. If excess upper lateral cartilage volume is present, it is trimmed with scissors.
- Reconstitution of the dorsum is completed with upper lateral crura tension spanning sutures[7] (**TECH FIG 1B**).

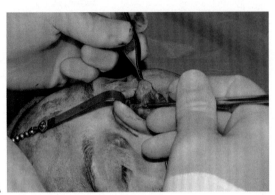 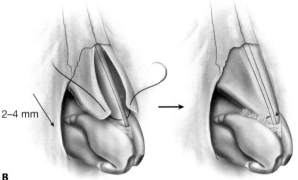

2–4 mm

A   **B**

TECH FIG 1 • **A.** Component dorsal hump reduction. Mucosa is freed from the medial upper lateral cartilages and nasal septum to minimize trauma during separation of these structures. **B.** Upper lateral cartilage tension spanning suture. Suture is used to advance the upper lateral cartilages anteriorly and fixate them to nasal septum. This reconstructs the middle vault and smoothens the dorsum.

Caudal Septal Reduction

- The caudal septum is easily exposed with further dissection of the septal mucosal flaps (**TECH FIG 2A**).

- Once exposed, scissors are used to excise the excess caudal septum.
- Often in the long nose, an angulated excision is performed for increased tip rotation (**TECH FIG 2B**).

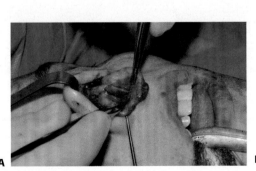 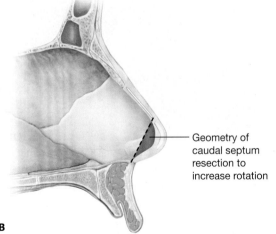

Geometry of caudal septum resection to increase rotation

A   **B**

TECH FIG 2 • **A.** Caudal septal exposure provided with open approach rhinoplasty. **B.** Geometry of the caudal septal resection is designed to increase rotation of the nasal tip.

■ Excess Lower Lateral Cartilages

- Excess volume of lower lateral cartilages can be improved with a cephalic trim (**TECH FIG 3A**).

- This disrupts the scroll ligament (major tip support) and permits upward rotation of the nasal tip often needed in the long nose (**TECH FIG 3B**).

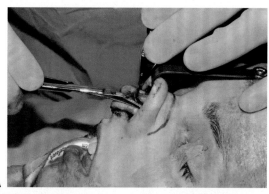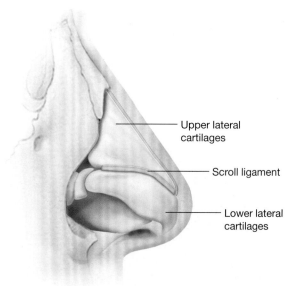

Upper lateral cartilages

Scroll ligament

Lower lateral cartilages

TECH FIG 3 • A. Cephalic trim to reduce lower lateral cartilage volume and increase tip rotation. **B.** Disruption of the scroll ligament is often required to allow cephalic rotation of the lower lateral cartilages.

■ Optimizing Tip Support

- Once the dorsum is established at the appropriate level, ideal tip position is determined and secured. This is most commonly accomplished with the use of a columella strut and tip sutures (**TECH FIG 4A**).

- Alar contour grafts may also be used to provide additional support to the lower third (**TECH FIG 4B**).

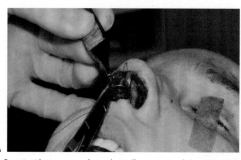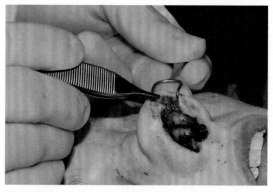

TECH FIG 4 • A. Placement of a columellar strut and tip sutures for stabilization. **B.** Alar contour graft placement just above the alar rim.

■ Adjuvant Procedures

- Subnasal retraction from periapical hypoplasia typically requires fat grafting or application of filler to augment. Chin augmentation and genioplasty are typically used to improve a weak chin.

POSTOPERATIVE CARE

▪ Nasal dressing is placed at the end of the surgery. Taping is done to support and minimize swelling of the nasal tip. A nasal splint is also applied. Tape and splint are discontinued at postoperative day 7 when the transcolumellar incision sutures are removed. Patients are started on saline intranasal spray and topical antibacterial ointment for the incision. Once the incision is healed, scar care is initiated and continued for 6 to 12 months.

OUTCOMES

▪ Reduction rhinoplasty to treat the long nose is an overall reliable operation. The aesthetic result may be limited by a thick overlying soft tissue envelope. Patients with thick skin should be made aware of this prior to surgery. Failure to thoroughly recognize all instigating factors may result in a less than desirable result.

COMPLICATIONS

▪ Cartilage reduction must stop short of creating a secondary deformity. Disruption of the upper lateral cartilage soft tissue connection with the nasal bones and/or dorsal septum can result in middle vault collapse. Overzealous resection of the lateral crura and failure to establish proper tip support can lead to lower nose collapse and/or problems with the nasal ala. Any number of these untoward outcomes can create aesthetic and functional problems.

REFERENCES

1. Lee MR, Geissler P, Cochran S, et al. Decreasing nasal tip projection in rhinoplasty. *Plast Reconstr Surg.* 2014;134:41e.
2. Rohrich RJ, Hollier LH, Janis J, Kim J. Rhinoplasty with advancing age. *Plast Reconstr Surg.* 2004;114:1936.
3. Lee MR, Malafa M, Roostaeian J, et al. Soft tissue composition of the columella and potential relevance in rhinoplasty. *Plast Reconstr Surg.* 2014;134:621.
4. Lee MR, Tabbal G, Kurkjian J, et al. Classifying columellar deformities in rhinoplasty. *Plast Reconstr Surg.* 2014;133:464e.
5. Rohrich RJ, Lee MR. External approach for secondary rhinoplasty—advances over the last twenty-five years. *Plast Reconstr Surg.* 2013;131:404.
6. Rohrich RJ, Muzaffar AR, Janis J. Component dorsal hump reduction: the importance of maintaining dorsal aesthetic lines in rhinoplasty. *Plast Reconstr Surg.* 2004;114:1298.
7. Roostaeian J, Unger JG, Lee MR, et al. Reconstruction of the nasal dorsum following component dorsal reduction in primary rhinoplasty. *Plast Reconstr Surg.* 2014;133:509.

64
CHAPTER

Technique for Treating the Short Nose

Nicholas Lahar and Jason Roostaeian

DEFINITION

The short nose is defined as a perceived excess upward tilt of the nasal tip that results in a foreshortened appearance. Common defining features include a decreased distance from nasofrontal angle to tip defining point, an over-rotated tip, and an increased nasolabial angle. Other commonly associated features can include decreased dorsal nasal length, increased nostril show, cephalic over-rotation of tip, low/deep radix, and long upper lip.[1] The perceived deficits of the nose must be evaluated with respect to the other facial features, but there are generally accepted measurements of facial harmony (see below).

ANATOMY

- The structural nose is composed of the paired nasal bones, upper lateral cartilages, and lower lateral cartilages. The midline septum also offers significant support for dorsal height and projection.

PATHOGENESIS

- Tip projection is highly dependent on support of the lower lateral cartilages. In cases of poor lower lateral cartilage support, tip support becomes more dependent on septal cartilage. Other supporting structures include intercartilaginous ligament between the upper and lower lateral cartilages, lateral crural complex extending from the piriform rim, interdomal ligaments, and medial crural attachments to the septum.
- Deformities are typically acquired or congenital.
- Acquired causes: iatrogenic, trauma, chemical (eg, cocaine), autoimmune disorders, and infections
- Scar contracture from tumor resection or trauma involving the lower portion of the nose may distort and retract the nasal tip.

PATIENT HISTORY AND PHYSICAL FINDINGS

- A detailed nasal history should be obtained, in particular to include a history of symptoms related to nasal obstruction, nasal allergies, prior nasal trauma, and nasal surgeries. Any patient aesthetic concerns and goals should be elicited and clearly defined.[2]
- A complete external and internal nasal examination should be conducted in all patients.
- Facial harmony is evaluated with particular attention to the relationships of the facial thirds on the profile view, nasofrontal angle, tip defining point, nasal length, nasolabial angle, and nostril show.

- Via palpation and examination, identify typical findings such as lack of nasal cartilage, weakened or fractured osseous/cartilaginous support, scar tissue, and contracture of soft tissue.
- Evaluate the nose with respect to the other facial features to assess facial harmony.
- There are generally accepted measurements for nasal length and nasolabial angle that can be used to assess the appearance.
  - Nasal length is typically about two-thirds the height of the midface (supraorbitale to subnasale).[1]
  - Ideal nasal length: nasal length/nasal projection ratio of 5:3.[1]
- Ideal nasolabial angle:
  - Caucasian women: 95 to 105 degrees
  - Caucasian men: 90 to 95 degrees[1]
- The columella protrudes 3 to 4 mm below the alar rim. The ideal ala-columella relationship creates a symmetrical oval outline on profile view bisected by a line connecting the most anterior to most posterior portion of the nostril.
- Assess the nasal alae and soft tissues aesthetically and for skin quality.
- A nasal speculum is used to evaluate the septum and the inferior turbinates for abnormalities.
- Standardized photographs including frontal, lateral oblique, and basal views should be obtained in all patients.
- Assess septal cartilage and other potential donor sites (ear and/or rib), particularly if the patient has had nasal surgery previously.
- Priority should be given to strong, straight pieces of cartilage for dorsal and columellar strut grafts.

IMAGING

- No specific imaging is required if attention is being paid specifically to a shortened nose.
- A nasal x-ray can be helpful in cases of prior trauma or asymmetric nasal bones.
- Computed tomography (CT) imaging can help evaluate nasal bones, septal deviation, turbinate pathology, and the sinuses when the history warrants further investigation.

SURGICAL MANAGEMENT

- The primary objective in correction of the short nose is to increase overall radix to tip length. This often requires a concomitant increase in tip projection while reducing tip rotation and the nasolabial angle.[2]

- Adjunctive procedures, eg, functional modifications, should also be determined and made part of the operative plan accordingly.

Preoperative Planning

- Risks, benefits, and expectations must be discussed with the patient prior to surgery.
- Consideration of the soft tissue envelope and its overall compliance, previous operations, extent of previous nasal trauma, and involved structures and available septal and other potential cartilage grafts (ear, rib) should be taken into account. The patient should be informed of the possible need to harvest cartilage from these other donor sites such as the ear or rib. In cases of severe soft tissue contracture, preoperative discussion to set expectations accordingly and/or attempts to increase compliance via mechanical means such as frequent downward massaging should be considered.
- Principles of nasal lengthening
  - Precise assessment of length deficiency
  - Accurate identification of deficient tissues
  - Adequate release of soft tissue envelope
  - Pertinent modification of skin, mucosa, and/or skeletal deformities to restore length
  - Maintaining patency of the nasal airway

Positioning

- The patient is positioned supine with arms tucked. The head is placed at the very end of the bed.
- An oral right angle endotracheal tube is used for intubation, and should extend inferiorly in the midline away from the nose, and secured without distorting the upper lip and nose.
- Nasal hairs may be trimmed, if desired.
- Oxymetazoline or 4% cocaine-soaked pledgets are placed in each nostril.
- Local anesthetic consisting of 1% lidocaine with 1:100 000 epinephrine is infiltrated into the nasal sidewalls, into the columella, and inside the nostril along the lower lateral cartilages.
- A throat pack is placed to prevent gastric accumulation of blood.
- The face is prepped with dilute Betadine.
- A sterile head wrap is placed followed by surgical drapes.

Approach

- An endonasal approach is indicated for simple refinements of the nasal tip. Otherwise, an open approach is preferred particularly when there is poor support for the nasal tip or when more complex nasal tip adjustments are necessary.

▪ Shield-Tip Graft

- Indication: Mild shortening attributed to a deficient infratip lobule or columella
- Concept: Cartilage graft is placed at the tip of the lower lateral cartilages to increase the length or manipulate contour.

- A gull wing or stair-step transcolumellar incision is made at the narrowest point of the columella (**TECH FIG 1A**).
- An incision is made in the nostril margin at the caudal margin of the lower lateral cartilages and extends to the transcolumellar incision medially (**TECH FIG 1B**).

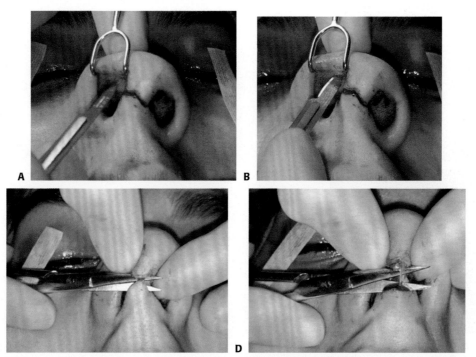

TECH FIG 1 • A. A transcolumellar incision is made with care to avoid injuring the medial crus. **B.** An infracartilaginous incision is made at the lower margin of the lower lateral cartilages. **C,D.** The transcolumellar incision is completed.

- Fine curved iris or Converse scissors are used to complete the columellar incision, with care taken to avoid injury to the medial crura (**TECH FIG 1C,D**).
- A nasal skin flap is elevated from the columellar incision and lower lateral cartilages using sharp double hooks for traction.
- If the relationships of the lower lateral cartilages are to be preserved, a Killian incision is performed approximately 1 to 1.5 cm cranially from the caudal septal border through the mucoperichondrium using a no. 15 blade.
- Submucoperichondrial dissection is performed using a Cottle elevator.
- The septal cartilage can now be harvested using a no. 15 blade or swivel knife, preserving an L strut of at least 1 cm dorsally and caudally.
- The shield tip graft is shaped from the harvested cartilage.
- The graft is laid in the desired location to augment tip projection and/or nasal length. It is secured in place with

6-0 polyglactin (Vicryl) suture. Graft position is adjusted to augment lengthening vs projection depending on the needs of the patient.
- Other preoperatively planned functional and aesthetic adjustments are made as needed.
- The nasal skin flap is laid back down and secured with 5-0 chromic sutures intranasally and 6-0 polypropylene in the columella.
- Tape strips are applied to the nasal dorsum to limit postoperative swelling and to help shape and refine the tip.
- The throat pack is removed prior to extubation. A nasogastric tube may be used to suction gastric contents to remove accumulated blood.
- A mustache gauze dressing is applied across the upper lip to absorb any nasal drainage.
- An ice pack may be used on the midface to minimize swelling.

■ Septal Extension Graft

- Indicated for moderate length deficiency.
- Allows for a relatively stable construct and control of the length deficiency.
- A gull wing or stair step incision is made at the narrowest point of the columella.
- An infracartilaginous incision is made in the nostril margin at the caudal margin of the lower lateral cartilages and extends to the transcolumellar incision medially.
- Fine curved iris or Converse scissors are used to complete the columellar incision, with care taken to avoid injury to the medial crura.

- A nasal skin flap is elevated from the columellar incision using sharp iris or Converse tip scissors. Care is taken to keep the perichondrium on the lower lateral cartilages (**TECH FIG 2A**).
- Intercartilaginous ligament attachments are divided sharply, allowing the lower lateral cartilages to splay and to expose the septum (**TECH FIG 2B**).
- The lower lateral cartilages are splayed open with sharp hooks, and an incision is made on the dorsal septum.
- Submucoperichondrial dissection of the septum is performed bilaterally using a Cottle elevator.

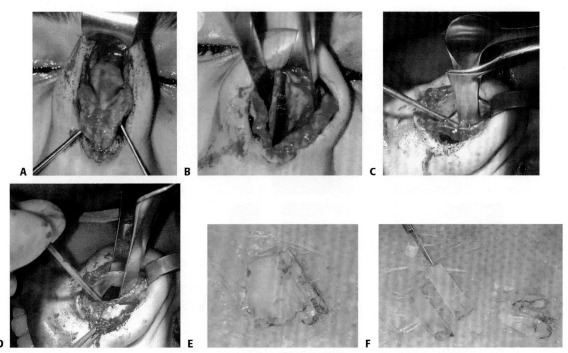

TECH FIG 2 • A. The nasal soft tissues are elevated in the subperichondrial plan, revealing the lower lateral cartilages, the upper lateral cartilages, and nasal dorsum. **B.** After separating the lower lateral cartilages via the intercartilaginous ligament, the mucoperichondrium is elevated off the nasal septum, revealing the entire cartilaginous septum. **C,D.** A 1-cm dorsal L strut is preserved while harvesting septal cartilage for various grafts. **E,F.** The septal cartilage is carefully crafted to create septal extension grafts, spreader grafts, or tip grafts.

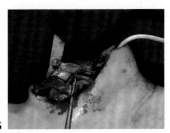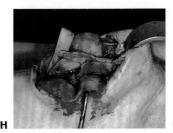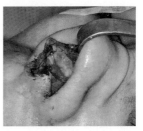

TECH FIG 2 (Continued) • **G,H.** The crafted extension grafts are secured to the caudal septal cartilage. **I.** The lower lateral cartilages are secured to the extension graft.

- The septum is incised anteroposteriorly with a no. 15 blade with care to preserve a 1-cm dorsal and caudal strut for nasal support (**TECH FIG 2C,D**).
- The septal extension graft is shaped from the harvested cartilage (**TECH FIG 2E,F**).
- Often two small septal grafts are needed if the septal extension graft need to be placed midline; otherwise, inherent bend in septal cartilage graft and L strut can be used to place graft on right or left side of septum to ensure the tip is in the midline.
- The septal extension graft is secured to the anterior septal angle/caudal septum with multiple 5-0 PDS sutures (**TECH FIG 2G,H**).
- The domes of the lower lateral cartilages are advanced and secured to the septal extension graft as needed to increase tip projection (**TECH FIG 2I**).
- Once structural lengthening has occurred, it must be verified that soft tissues can cover the new length. Wide

undermining of the dorsal and lateral nasal soft tissues may be necessary to sufficiently advance the skin flap.
- Mattress sutures of 4-0 plain gut are placed through the mucoperichondrial flaps to close the dead space where septal cartilage was harvested.
- The columellar skin is reapproximated with interrupted 6-0 Prolene, and the infracartilaginous incisions are closed with interrupted 5-0 chromic sutures.
- Internal nasal splints are placed in each nostril and sutured through the septum with a single 3-0 Prolene mattress suture.
- The throat pack is removed prior to extubation. If necessary, a nasogastric tube may be used to suction gastric contents to remove accumulated blood.
- A mustache gauze dressing may be applied across the upper lip to absorb any nasal drainage.
- An ice pack may be used on the midface to minimize swelling.

■ Tongue-and-Groove Technique

- Indication: Moderate to severe nasal length deficiency[5–8]
- This technique allows for more stable construct and control of the length deficiency.
- A gull wing or stair-step incision is made at the narrowest point of the columella.
- An infracartilaginous incision is made in the nostril margin at the caudal margin of the lower lateral cartilages and extends to the transcolumellar incision medially.
- Fine curved iris or Converse scissors are used to complete the columellar incision, with care taken to avoid injury to the medial crura.
- A nasal skin flap is elevated from the columellar incision using sharp iris or Converse tip scissors.
- Intercartilaginous ligament attachments are divided sharply, allowing the lower lateral cartilages to splay, exposing the septum.
- The lower lateral cartilages are splayed open with sharp hooks, and an incision is made through the perichondrium on the dorsal septum.
- Submucoperichondrial dissection of the septum is performed bilaterally using a Cottle elevator.
- The septum is incised anteroposteriorly with a no. 15 blade with care to preserve at least 1-cm dorsal and caudal strut for nasal support.
- The cartilage is wedged off the bony septum and removed from the operative field.

- The dorsal septal extension grafts and columellar strut grafts are shaped from the harvested cartilage.
- Two septal grafts are cut to length in proportion to deficiency. For instance, if the nose is deficient by 3 mm, the graft will extend beyond the septum by 3 mm.
- These septal grafts will be placed along the dorsal septum with the deficiency extending beyond the margins of the septum, projecting anteriocaudally (**TECH FIG 3**).
- The width of the septal grafts is dependent on the dorsal septum width. The septal grafts can be thinned appropriately to make the total desired dorsal width. Nasal bone osteotomies may be required to narrow the nasal dorsum depending on the needs of the patient.
- The dorsal grafts are secured to the dorsal septum bilaterally with 5-0 PDS or Vicryl sutures.

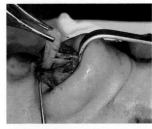

TECH FIG 3 • A columellar strut is secured between two extended spreader grafts to create a stable construct for lengthening the nose.

- A columellar strut is then prepared from the septal cartilage.
  - The width of the strut will be the width of the medial crus plus the desired additional length (the deficiency).
- The columellar strut is placed between the bilateral spreader grafts, interdigitating. The strut is secured to both the caudal septum and the extended spreader grafts into a position that helps to lengthen the nose and increase projection.
- The medial crura are advanced anteriorly and caudally on the columellar strut as needed to increase tip projection. This medial crura are sewn and secured to the columellar strut using 5-0 PDS or Vicryl suture.
- Lower lateral cartilage tip refinements (eg, interdomal, transdomal, etc.) can be made at this time.
- Once structural lengthening has occurred, it must be verified that soft tissues and lateral tissues can cover the new length. Wide undermining of the dorsal and lateral nasal

soft tissues may be necessary to sufficiently advance the skin flap.
- Mattress sutures of 4-0 plain gut are placed through the septal mucoperichondrial flaps to close the dead space where septal cartilage was harvested.
- The columellar skin is reapproximated with interrupted 6-0 Prolene, and the infracartilaginous incisions are closed with interrupted 5-0 chromic sutures.
- Internal nasal splints are placed in each nostril and sutured through the septum with a single 3-0 Prolene mattress suture.
- The throat pack is removed prior to extubation. If necessary, a nasogastric tube may be used to suction gastric contents to remove accumulated blood.
- A mustache gauze dressing may be applied across the upper lip to absorb any nasal drainage.
- An ice pack may be used on the midface to minimize swelling.

PEARLS AND PITFALLS

Preoperative	- A thorough discussion of the planned goals and risks should be conducted with the patient to ensure appropriate expectations are met.
Technique	- Wide undermining of the nasal skin is required to redrape the skin over the cartilaginous framework. - Columellar strut grafts or septal extension grafts should not extend past domes/tip defining points. - When there is insufficient septal strut cartilage, consider septal extension graft given the minimal cartilage requirements. Lower lateral cartilages can be strengthened with lateral crural strut grafts or alar rim grafts if nasal lengthening causes excess alar retraction. - Be mindful of overwidening the nose with spreader grafts that are too wide and high along the dorsal strut.
Postoperative	- Have the patient avoid sleeping on a side as it will worsen edema to one side and increase concern for deviation.

POSTOPERATIVE CARE

- Surgery is usually performed on an outpatient basis.
- Usual postrhinoplasty precautions are followed.
- Keep the intranasal mucosa moist with frequent application of ointment and saline nasal spray.
- Any internal and/or external nasal splints are removed at 1 week.
- Prolonged edema may occur and in some cases can take up to 1 year to fully resolve.

OUTCOMES

- The goals of functional and aesthetic improvement can be accomplished with any of the described techniques.[3,4] Optimal outcomes will be attained using the technique with which the surgeon is most comfortable and able to achieve consistent results.

COMPLICATIONS

- Possible short-term and long-term complications include infection, hematoma, nasal asymmetry, septal perforation,

worsening of nasal obstruction, scarring, nasal bleeding/crusting, cartilage exposure, and prolonged edema that may last up to 1 year.

REFERENCES

1. Gunter JP, Rohrich RJ. Lengthening the aesthetically short nose. *Plast Reconstr Surg.* 1989;83(5):793-800.
2. Katira K, Guyuron B. Contemporary techniques for effective nasal lengthening. *Facial Plast Surg Clin North Am.* 2015;23:81-91.
3. Howard BK, Rohrich RJ. Understanding the nasal airway: principles and practice. *Plast Reconstr Surg.* 2002;109(3):1128-1146.
4. Rohrich RJ, Ahmad J. A practical approach to rhinoplasty. *Plast Reconstr Surg.* 2016;137(4):725e-746e.
5. Guyuron B, Varghai A. Lengthening the nose with a tongue-and-groove technique. *Plast Reconstr Surg.* 2003;111(4):1533-1539.
6. Gruber RP. Lengthening the short nose. *Plast Reconstr Surg.* 1993;91(7):1252-1258.
7. Çakır B, Öreroğlu AR, Daniel RK. Surface aesthetics in tip rhinoplasty: a step-by-step guide. *Aesthet Surg J.* 2014;34(6):941-955.
8. Erickson B, Hurowitz R, Jeffery C, et al. Acoustic rhinometry and video endoscopic scoring to evaluate postoperative outcomes in endonasal spreader graft surgery with septoplasty and turbinoplasty for nasal valve collapse. *J Otolaryngol Head Neck Surg.* 2016;45:2.

Technique for Dorsal Augmentation Using Costal Cartilage Graft

Dean M. Toriumi

DEFINITION

- Low nasal dorsum is when the bridge of the nose demonstrates inadequate height/projection.
- A low dorsum can appear wide and flat on frontal view with inadequate lateral wall shadowing.
- Asian patients tend to have inadequate dorsal height and frequently are in need of dorsal augmentation.
- Inadequate dorsal height may be directly related to excessive nasal tip projection. The relationship between dorsal height and tip projection frequently requires creating balance between these two parameters.

ANATOMY

- The anatomy of the low dorsum can vary from patient to patient.
- In the Asian patient, the nasal dorsum can be low and wide (**FIG 1**).
- Asian patients tend to have a low radix (low nasal starting point) as well.
- Asian patients tend to have very small and thin septal cartilage that provides insufficient stock for dorsal augmentation.
- Some patients have a congenitally low dorsum.
- Patients that suffered from trauma can present with a low dorsum or saddle nose deformity.
- Most patients with a saddle nose deformity have a deficiency in the middle nasal vault usually with a normal bony nasal vault. Many of these patients may actually have a dorsal convexity above the saddled area.

PATIENT HISTORY AND PHYSICAL FINDINGS

- Any evidence of previous trauma or surgery should be elicited in the history.
- Any prior placement of alloplastic implants should be elicited in the history.
- Physical exam should reveal any septal deviations or fractures.
- Asian patients who have a low dorsum also tend to have an underprojected nasal tip.
- All patients should be queried as to any previous injectable fillers placed into their nose.

SURGICAL MANAGEMENT

Anesthesia

- It is preferable to perform these surgeries under general anesthesia. With the patient intubated, the airway is protected from blood contacting the vocal cords and potentially causing laryngospasm. A protected airway is particularly important if any work is planned on the nasal septum or turbinates.
- Local anesthetic agent (1% lidocaine with 1:100 000 epinephrine) is injected into the nose to provide hemostasis. Injections are made along the septum, along the marginal incisions, over the nasal dorsum and middle vault, and in the nasal tip area. At least 10 minutes should pass before the procedure is initiated to allow the full vasoconstrictive effect to set in.

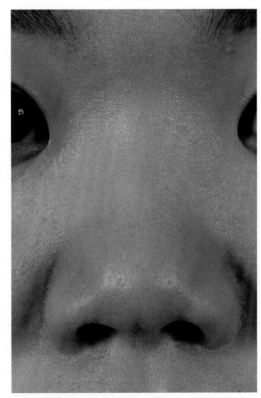

FIG 1 • Asian patient with low dorsum showing lack of lateral wall shadowing and flat appearance to nasal dorsum.

Harvesting Costal Cartilage for Dorsal Augmentation

- Costal cartilage can be harvested from relatively small incisions with low morbidity. Costal cartilage of adequate length and width can be harvested through an 11-mm chest incision.[1,2]
  - When less experienced, a larger incision should be used to safely harvest the costal cartilage.
  - Consider using a 3-cm incision until you are comfortable with the chest wall anatomy and have significant experience harvesting costal cartilage.
- Avoid cutting the muscle layer.
  - It is preferred to separate the muscle fibers bluntly.
  - This allows the muscle layer to be tightly resutured at the end of the operation to provide good support to the area.
- Costal perichondrium should be harvested from the surface of the rib. Costal perichondrium can be used for camouflage or as a soft tissue graft.
- The best rib to harvest for dorsal augmentation is typically the 7th rib. The 7th rib is longer and straighter and provides the best cartilage stock for major dorsal augmentation[3,4] (**TECH FIG 1A,B**).

- The 5th rib is curved and not appropriate for large dorsal augmentations.
- The 6th rib is relatively straight but has a genu that could shorten the straight segment that can be used for the dorsal graft.
- The 7th rib is also more superficial than the 6th rib, so it is easier to harvest through a smaller incision.
- The 7th rib cartilage is sharply dissected away from the 6th and 8th ribs using a Freer elevator and lifted off of the underlying perichondrium.
  - Typically, a 3.5- to 4.5-cm segment of costal cartilage should be harvested.
- Perform a Valsalva maneuver after the rib is harvested to see if there is a tear in the pleura.
  - If so, a red rubber catheter can be placed during closure, and then the chest can be expanded and the catheter removed after the closure is completed.
- The 7th rib tends to lie below the level of the diaphragm and therefore lessens the likelihood of a pneumothorax. As you move medially on the 7th rib, it may move above the diaphragm.

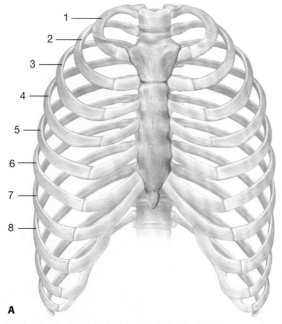
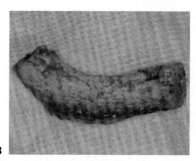

TECH FIG 1 • **A.** Chest wall showing rib anatomy. The 7th rib is longer and straighter than the 5th and 6th ribs. The 6th rib has a genu where the rib passes below the breast. **B.** Harvested rib.

Preparing and Affixing the Dorsal Graft

- The harvested costal cartilage should be initially carved into three separate segments (**TECH FIG 2A**), which are then assessed for the most ideal curvature.
  - If a very thick dorsal graft is needed, the rib should be carved differently by taking thinner peripheral segments to provide a thicker dorsal graft (**TECH FIG 2B**). In this case, the middle segment is typically used for the dorsal graft.

- If the central core of the costal cartilage has a soft (pearlike) texture, this increases the likelihood of warping of the cartilage. In this case, it is preferable to use the outer core of the rib for the dorsal graft.
  - If this cartilage must be used, it is recommended to laminate the cartilage by suturing two thinner layers of cartilage together to create one dorsal graft. The lamination acts to decrease the likelihood of warping.

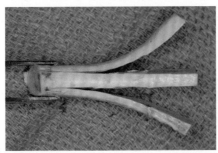
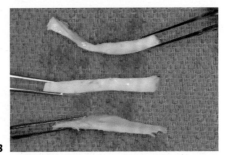

TECH FIG 2 • A. Younger patient with the rib being carved into three separate segments. Note the bending of the cartilage. **B.** For larger dorsal grafts, the central segment of the rib can be made thicker to allow for a thicker dorsal graft.

- The dorsal graft should be carved into a canoe shape that is narrower at both ends (**TECH FIG 3A**).
  - It should be carved to provide appropriate dorsal height. Care should be taken to avoid making it too narrow. It is carved so it is curved anterior to posterior (**TECH FIG 3B**).
  - The graft is fashioned so the concave surface is facing inferior or toward the nasal dorsum. This is critical to prevent the upward bending of the cartilage graft creating a prominent radix and supratip.
- The dorsal graft is carved slightly wider than what would be considered ideal, as contracture over time will tend to make the dorsum look narrower.
  - If costal perichondrium is sutured to the sidewalls of the dorsal graft, it will look a bit wider, and this should be accounted for when carving the graft. Perichondrium that is so sutured acts to camouflage the graft and prevent visibility of its lateral margins (**TECH FIG 4A,B**).
  - The perichondrium should overlap the junction between the lateral margins of the dorsal graft and the nasal dorsum (**TECH FIG 4C**).
  - If the perichondrium is placed at the junction between dorsal graft and nasal dorsum, the perichondrium will form bone and create an osseous bridge between the dorsal graft and nasal dorsum.
- A strip of costal perichondrium is sutured to the undersurface of the superior aspect of the dorsal graft, where it would sit on top of the nasal bones (**TECH FIGS 4C** and **5**).
  - The perichondrium is sutured to the undersurface of the upper portion of the dorsal graft with a running 5-0 PDS suture. Care is taken to make sure the costal

perichondrium is oriented so the surface that was initially against the cartilage is oriented so it is facing the bone.
  - Costal perichondrium is at the bone/cartilage interface and will ossify, creating a bony union between the dorsal graft and nasal dorsum. This ossification and rigid fixation occur within the 1st month after surgery.
- The nasal dorsum is rasped with a narrow rasp, or multiple perforations are made in the bony nasal vault at the interface with the dorsal graft. Using a narrow rasp decreases the likelihood that the dorsal pocket will be enlarged (**TECH FIG 6**).
  - Multiple perforations are made in the bone using a 2-mm straight osteotome. At least 8 to 10 perforations are made in the bone to expose cancellous bone and allow more rapid ossification of the dorsal graft with perichondrium interface to the underlying bony dorsum.
  - This ossification typically occurs within the first month after surgery. Once the ossification is complete, the dorsal graft becomes immobile and cannot be moved or shifted. This rigid fixation acts to prevent bending or warping of the dorsal graft.
- For the dorsal graft with costal perichondrium interface to ossify and fix to the nasal dorsum, there must be a tight subperiosteal space that will force the dorsal graft against the bone.
  - Thus, at the beginning of the operation, the surgeon should use a Joseph periosteal elevator to raise the periosteum off the bone, leaving a relatively narrow tunnel. This will ensure a tight fit when the dorsal graft is inserted into the subperiosteal space.

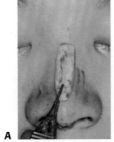
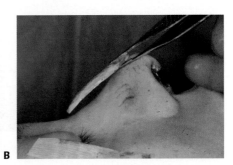

TECH FIG 3 • Shape of dorsal graft. **A.** Dorsal graft is typically canoe shaped tapering inferiorly. **B.** The dorsal graft is curved with the concave surface facing the nasal dorsum.

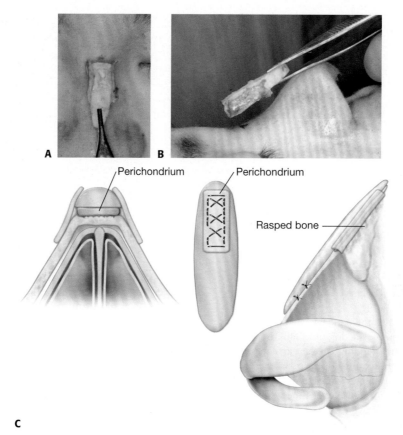

TECH FIG 4 • Dorsal graft with perichondrium. **A.** Dorsal graft with perichondrium sutured to the sides of the graft. **B.** Lateral view of the dorsal graft with perichondrium. **C.** Dorsal graft with perichondrium sutured to the undersurface of the dorsal graft and placed into a tight subperiosteal pocket to force the dorsal graft against the bone. Perichondrium is also placed along the sides of the dorsal graft.

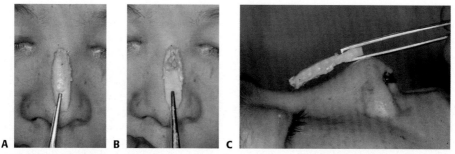

TECH FIG 5 • Dorsal graft with perichondrium. **A.** Dorsal graft over the dorsum. **B.** Perichondrium sutured to the undersurface of the dorsal graft. **C.** Dorsal graft with concave surface facing the bony dorsum.

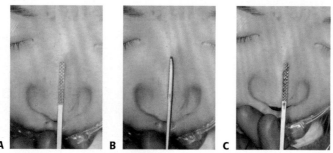

TECH FIG 6 • Rasping the nasal dorsum. **A.** Narrow rasp to roughen the nasal dorsum. **B.** Side view of the low-profile rasp. **C.** After rasping bone dust on the rasp.

■ Use of a Transosseous Suture or K-Wire

- If a tight subperiosteal space is not possible as a result of removal of a previous implant or deformity, a transosseous suture can be used to fix the dorsal graft with interpositional costal perichondrium to the bony nasal vault (**TECH FIG 7**).
  - In this case, small stab incisions are made along the side of the dorsum, and holes are created across the nasal dorsum approximately 4 to 5 mm below the leading edge of the dorsum just below the level of the medial canthus (**TECH FIG 8**). This is done using multiple 16-gauge needles. Care must be taken to make sure the holes are directly opposite each other at the same level across the bridge of the nose.
  - The transdorsal path should be above the level of the intranasal mucosa. This can be ensured by dissecting the intranasal mucosa to make room for passage of the 16-gauge needle (see **TECH FIG 7**).
    - Protect the eye when drilling the hole to avoid ocular damage.
- Once the transdorsal hole is created, a 4-0 PDS suture can be passed through the needle and passed back through the dorsum. The suture is then passed back through the same skin incision and over the top of the upper part of the dorsal graft. Then, the suture is passed back through the opposite skin incision and tied tightly to force the upper segment of the dorsal graft with intervening costal perichondrium tightly against the bony nasal dorsum.
  - This tight contact between costal cartilage dorsal graft, costal perichondrium, and underlying perforated bone allows rigid fixation of the dorsal graft to the bony dorsum.

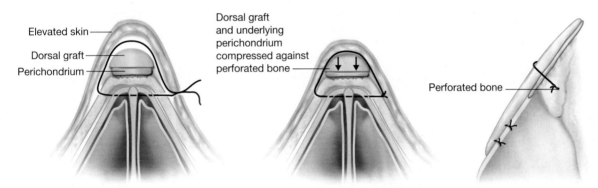

TECH FIG 7 • Transosseous hole drilled across the dorsum above the mucosa. The suture is passed across the dorsum and then over the top of the dorsal graft to hold it snugly against the bony dorsum.

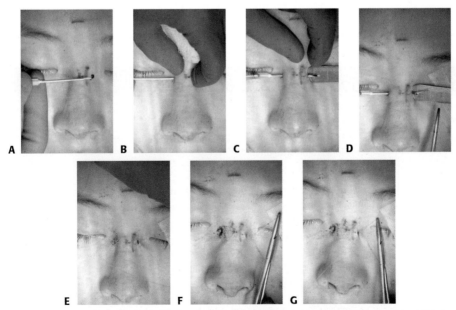

TECH FIG 8 • Transosseous suture placement to hold dorsal graft in position. **A.** A 16-gauge needle used to drill hole across the dorsum. **B.** Needle is used to drill a hole across the dorsum through small stab incisions on the side of the dorsum. **C.** Needle passed across the dorsum protecting the opposite eye. **D.** A 4-0 PDS suture needle is placed into the core of the 16-gauge needle to pass back across the dorsum. **E.** Suture passed across the dorsum. **F.** Suture passed back through stab incision and over the top of the dorsal graft and through the opposite incision. **G.** Tying down suture to force dorsal graft with interpositional costal perichondrium against the perforated bony dorsum.

T
E
C
H
N
I
Q
U
E
S

- In some cases, in which a large dorsal pocket is created and a transosseous suture is not possible (very low dorsum), a 0.45 threaded Kirschner wire can be passed through a small upper dorsal skin incision, through the upper dorsal graft, and into the bony dorsum (**TECH FIG 9**). The K-wire should pass only 3 to 4 mm into the underlying bony dorsum.
  - It is left in place until the 7th postoperative day and then gently backed out in the office using a hemostat

or needle holder. The small stab incision will close in a couple of days, leaving a small scar on the nasal dorsum.

- In most patients, the dorsal graft with costal perichondrium interface is ossified into position by the 21st day postoperative. At 1 month, the dorsal graft is difficult to move.

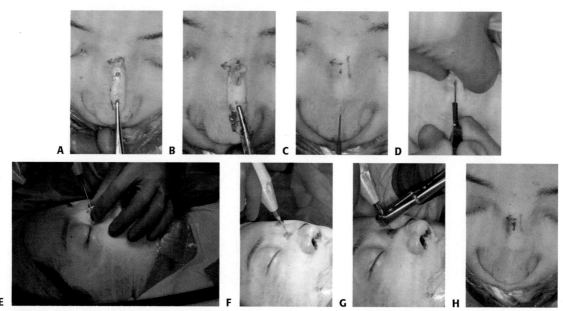

TECH FIG 9 • Use of a Kirschner wire to fix the dorsal graft. **A.** Canoe-shaped dorsal graft over the nasal dorsum. **B.** Costal perichondrium sutured to the undersurface of the upper aspect of the dorsal graft. **C.** Dorsal graft in position and placement of 0.45 threaded Kirschner wire planned. **D.** Making a small stab incision over the dorsal graft. **E.** Drilling the threaded Kirschner wire through the dorsal graft and then 4 mm into the underlying bony dorsum. **F.** Drilling Kirschner wire into position. **G.** Cutting the Kirschner wire with a wire cutter. **H.** Kirschner wire in place.

PEARLS AND PITFALLS

Choosing the grafting material for dorsal augmentation	▪ Auricular cartilage is insufficient. Costal cartilage provides larger cartilage stock and allows for carving of larger dorsal grafts.
Harvesting costal cartilage	▪ Chose the proper rib to insure adequate cartilage. For most larger dorsal grafts, the 7th rib is ideal as it is longer and straighter.
Harvesting costal perichondrium	▪ Harvest costal perichondrium from the surface of the rib.
Managing warping of costal cartilage grafts	▪ Observe for curvature as the dorsal graft is carved. Splint cartilage grafts to prevent further bending. Lamination is very effective.
Fixation of dorsal grafts	▪ Suture costal perichondrium to undersurface of the dorsal graft and place on top of bony dorsum after perforated with 2-mm osteotome.
Dorsal graft pocket	▪ Make a tight narrow subperiosteal dorsal pocket to force dorsal graft with interpositional costal perichondrium tightly to the perforated bone.
Contour dorsal graft	▪ Dorsal graft should be canoe shaped and should be oriented with the concave surface facing the perforated bone.
Other modes of fixation of dorsal graft	▪ If tight subperiosteal pocket is not possible, consider transosseous suture fixation.

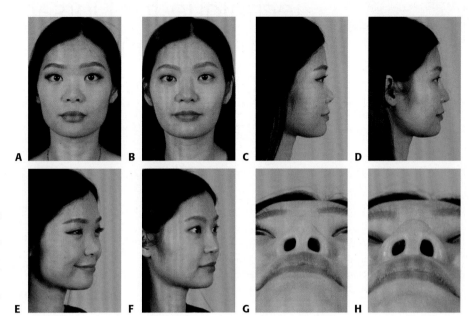

FIG 2 • Asian patient who underwent dorsal augmentation using costal cartilage. **A.** Preoperative frontal view. **B.** Postoperative frontal view. **C.** Preoperative lateral view. **D.** Postoperative lateral view. **E.** Preoperative oblique view. **F.** Postoperative oblique view. **G.** Preoperative base view. **H.** Postoperative base view.

POSTOPERATIVE CARE

- No nasal packing is used in the rhinoplasty patients. A running quilting 4-0 plain gut suture is used to approximate the septal flaps.
- Cast is removed on the 7th postoperative day.
- Patients should avoid salty foods postoperatively to minimize edema.

OUTCOMES

- Most patients that undergo dorsal augmentation using costal cartilage with dorsal graft fixation using the costal perichondrium interface do well over time. The incidence of warping is relatively low, and the nasal dorsum looks very natural (**FIG 2**).

COMPLICATIONS

- Infection is rare but occurs when extensive cartilage grafting is performed.

- Warping or displacement of the dorsal graft is possible but can be minimized if preventive measures are taken.
- Pneumothorax is a potential problem with harvesting of costal cartilage.
- Resorption of the dorsal graft is rare.
- Aesthetic problems such as undercorrection or overcorrection are possible if appropriate sizing is not accomplished.
- Potential visibility of the dorsal graft is possible as the dorsal nasal skin contracts or thins.

REFERENCES

1. Toriumi DM, Pero CD. Asian rhinoplasty. *Clin Plast Surg.* 2010; 37(2):335-352.
2. Toriumi DM. Discussion: use of autologous costal cartilage in Asian rhinoplasty. *Plast Reconstr Surg.* 2012;130(6):1349-1350.
3. Toriumi DM. Caudal septal extension graft for correction of the retracted columella. *Op Tech Otol Head Neck Surg.* 1995;6(4):311-318.
4. Toriumi DM, Swartout B. Asian rhinoplasty. *Facial Plast Surg Clin North Am.* 2007;15(3):293-307.

66
CHAPTER

Technique for Dorsal Augmentation Using Alloplastic Material

Man-Koon Suh and Nguyen Phan Tu Dung

DEFINITION

- A low nasal dorsum is one of the main characteristics of Asian noses. Dorsal augmentation is one of the most frequently performed procedures in Asian rhinoplasty.
- There is a distinctive difference in preferences of materials used for dorsal augmentation between surgeons from Asia and other countries.
  - Autogenous tissues preferred by Western surgeons provide better safety but have several disadvantages:
    - Less satisfaction aesthetically
    - Scars on the donor site
    - Decreased height or irregularity of the nasal dorsum due to tissue resorption
    - More complex surgical procedure compared with implants
  - Thus, use of an implant is still preferred for dorsal augmentation in Asia.
- Owing to the thick and fibrotic soft tissue envelope of Asian noses, as opposed to that of Westerners' noses, implant visibility or an operated looking appearance after dorsal augmentation with implant is considerably less likely. The appropriate surgical technique complemented by a high-quality implant surely minimizes the frequency of adverse effects.[1-3]

ANATOMY

- The structure of an Asian nose is shown in **FIG 1**.
- Use of an implant is limited to dorsal augmentation. Tip projection should be carried out by various tip-plasty techniques including suture techniques and cartilage grafting.

It is safe to use an implant only from the radix to the supratip area (**FIG 2**).
- Application of an implant extending to the tip area should be avoided, since it may cause thinning and redness of the tip skin or a rupture of the tip skin with implant exposure.

PATIENT HISTORY AND PHYSICAL FINDINGS

- The following must be checked during the preoperative evaluation:
  - Presence of facial asymmetry
  - Presence of nasal axis deviation
  - Presence and underlying causes of tip and nostril asymmetry
  - Dorsal skin characteristics, including the texture, color, and any skin problems such as visible veins or telangiectasias
- The surgeon must decide the following during the preoperative consultation:
  - How high the nasal dorsum should be raised
  - Whether the profile should be straight or curved
  - The type of prosthesis to be used for dorsal augmentation
  - The type of cartilage to be used for tip projection

SURGICAL MANAGEMENT

- Dorsal augmentation material for Asians is chosen from either autogenous tissues or implants.
- In cases in which the dorsal skin is too thin, autogenous tissues are recommended.
  - Dermofat graft or diced cartilage wrapped with the temporal fascia is preferred.

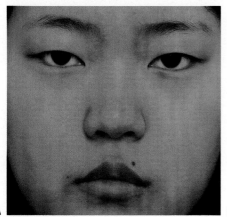
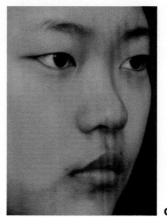
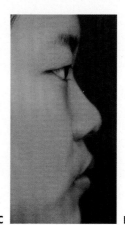
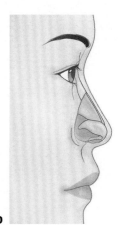

FIG 1 • A–D. Asian nose with a low and short nasal dorsum. Nasal bone is flat and low, and alar cartilage is small and weak as well. (**D.** Copyright Man Koon Suh, MD.)

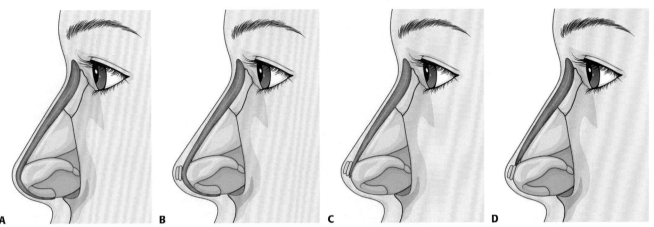

FIG 2 • Four types of dorsal and tip augmentation strategies in Asian noses. **A.** L-shaped implant only for dorsal and tip augmentation. **B.** L-shaped implant combined with cartilage graft on the tip of the implant. **C.** Long I-shaped implant combined with cartilage graft on the tip of the implant. **D.** Short I-shaped implant with cartilage graft on the alar cartilage. This is the most recommended technique for the Asian rhinoplasty. (Copyright Man Koon Suh, MD.)

- A rib cartilage block used for dorsal augmentation for a patient with thin skin may result in a visible contour of the rib cartilage graft, increasing the possibility for revision surgery.
- The implant can be relatively safe and bring aesthetically beautiful results for Asians when the skin is not thin.

Preoperative Planning

Implant Selection

- Each material has advantages and disadvantages. Silicone and e-PTFE (expanded polytetrafluoroethylene) are used most commonly for dorsal augmentation, but other products are available, such as Medpor.
  - Characteristics of silicone implants
    - There is no change in the implant height as time progresses.
    - Capsular formation.
    - The frequency of calcification on the surface of the implant is higher than that of an e-PTFE implant over a long period.
  - Characteristics of e-PTFE implants
    - Micropores are present within implant, allowing tissue ingrowth. As a result, there is less implant mobility and no capsular formation.
    - Calcification occurs less in e-PTFE implants than in silicone implants.
    - Delayed spontaneous hematoma also occurs less in e-PTFE implants.
    - The height of an e-PTFE implant decreases to about 5% to 20%.[4] Accordingly, the height predictability decreases, and tissue ingrowth makes it difficult to remove an e-PTFE implant as opposed to a silicone implant.
- The answer to which type of implant is better between silicone and e-PTFE implant depends largely on the experience and preference of the surgeon. Silicone implants are generally used because there is no morphologic change over time and height predictability is excellent. Nevertheless, an e-PTFE implant may be considered for the following cases:
  - A contracted nose due to capsular contracture
  - Wide dorsum due to hypertrophied capsule

  - Weak periosteum (cases with fragile periosteum are prone to implant mobility; e-PTFE implants have higher adherence to the nasal bones or adjacent tissues, so that implants are less mobile)
  - Calcification on the surface of a silicone implant
  - Foreign body reaction to silicone
  - Late spontaneous hematoma inside the capsule of a silicone implant
- Thin dorsal skin is not an indication for an e-PTFE implant.
  - An e-PTFE implant inserted into a patient's nose with thin dorsal skin may force the thin skin to adhere closely to the implant without capsular formation. Thus, the implant edges may be more conspicuous.
- There are I-shaped (boat shape) and L-shaped silicone implants (**FIG 3**).
  - An I shape is mainly used for dorsal augmentation, whereas an L shape is used to simultaneously raise both the dorsum and the tip.
  - An L shape is not recommended because it has a risk of the nasal tip becoming too hard, tip skin thinning, and implant exposure through the nasal tip skin.

Implant Design

- The patient is asked to look straight ahead, and the starting and end points of an implant are marked on the nose (**FIG 4A,B**).
  - The starting point of an implant would coincide with the double eyelid line for Westerners. However, it looks natural to have the implant starting point coincide with the eyelash line for Asians.

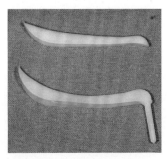

FIG 3 • I- and L-shaped silicone implants.

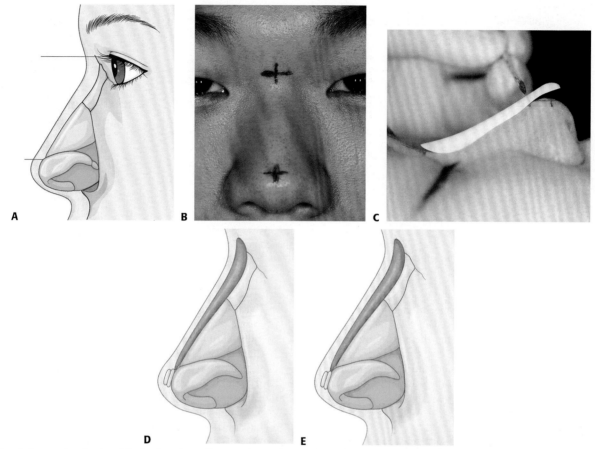

FIG 4 • A. Start and end point of the implant. **B.** Markings. **C.** The implant tip should be shortened and adjusted to fit to its ending point, which is 3 to 5 mm above the tip defining point. The dorsal line should be slightly curved and have a higher nasal tip and supratip break in women **(D)** but be straight in men **(E).** (**A,D,E.** Copyright Man Koon Suh, MD.)

- The starting point of an implant would be somewhat higher for patients with a protruding forehead. The more protruding the forehead, the higher the position of the implant starting point. The flatter the forehead of a patient, the lower the implant starting point.
- The distal end of an implant should not extend to the nasal tip but to the area just above the nasal tip. Hence, the length of an implant would be approximately 35 to 45 mm.
  - No part of an implant should enter into the nasal tip under any circumstance, and the nasal tip must be projected with cartilage graft (**FIG 4C**).
- Raising the radix area high like that of the Westerner creates a fierce-looking face for Asians. It is pertinent for Asians to have the line extending from the forehead to the radix to be natural.

- The nasal tip of a female should be slightly higher than the dorsal line so as to form the natural supratip break. Accordingly, the nasal tip should also be projected by a cartilage graft. The side view line from dorsum to the nasal tip should be a straight line in males (**FIG 4D,E**).

Approach

- Dorsal augmentation can be done through an intranasal or an open approach.
- An open approach is needed in cases requiring tip plasty, whereas the intranasal approach is adequate for dorsal augmentation using a simple implant. In these cases, an inframarginal incision is recommended.

■ Implant Carving

- The operator must be equipped with implants of various shapes and heights provided by the manufacturer (**TECH FIG 1A**).
- Until recently, an e-PTFE block was carved into nasal implant shape (**TECH FIG 1B**). Now, however, ready-made products that are precarved in various shapes facilitate ease of carving (**TECH FIG 1C**). The carving process for an e-PTFE prosthesis is similar to that for a silicone implant.

Carving Process

- The operator selects the most appropriate implant in consideration of nasal profile and the desired nasal shape of a patient.
- The proximal beginning part of the implant is placed on the starting point marked on the nose, and then distal ending point of the implant is marked (**TECH FIG 2A,B**).

- The marked distal end of the implant is cut, and then the thick distal end is thinly carved (**TECH FIG 2C,D**).
- The bottom of the implant is carved and trimmed to the curvature of the dorsum (**TECH FIG 2E,F**).
- With respect to carving of an implant, various techniques exist depending on the surgeon. However, it is convenient to use a no. 11 scalpel blade for a novice surgeon. A number of blades must be prepared so that a slightly dull blade can be replaced with a new one.

Carving Precautions

- Implants are available with a variety of width profiles, ranging from 8 to 12 mm. While the most common implant width for Asians is 10 mm, the width is individually determined depending on the width of the nasal bone.
- With respect to the hardness of the silicone implant, the soft type has advantages of better adherence to the nasal bone and less mobility as opposed to the hard type.

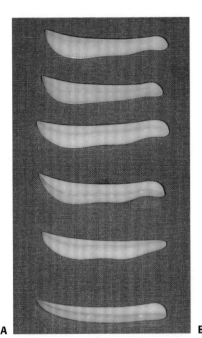
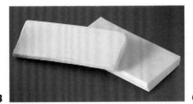
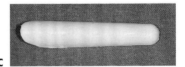

TECH FIG 1 • **A.** Various silicone implant shapes. **B.** e-PTFE implant block that would be carved into shape. **C.** Preshaped e-PTFE implant.

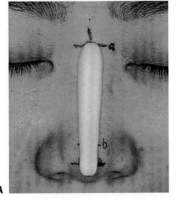
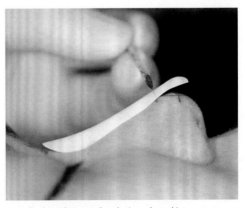

TECH FIG 2 • Silicone implant carving. **A,B.** Placing the company-supplied implant on the designed marking.

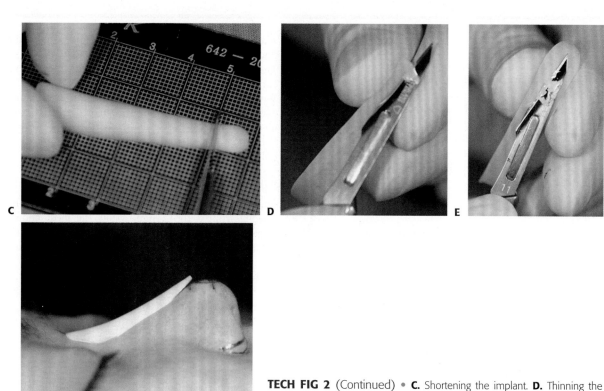
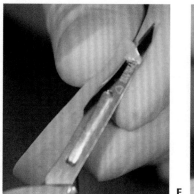
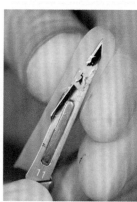
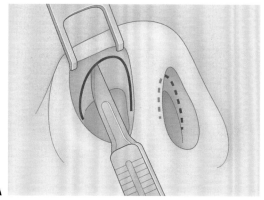

TECH FIG 2 (Continued) • **C.** Shortening the implant. **D.** Thinning the thickness of the tip. **E.** Carving the implant body according to the patient's dorsal irregularity. **F.** Final shape after carving.

- The shape of the bottom side of an implant should be curved or concave, so that the surface adheres to the nasal skeleton. Thus, implant mobility is less likely to occur.
- The end of an implant should be carved very thin.

- A thick terminal end of an implant may lead to capsular contracture, which can occasionally cause skin indentation.
- The author avoids both hatching and making holes in silicone implants.

■ Incision

- The endonasal approach would be sufficient for cases desiring a simple augmentation of the dorsum and tip. In such a case, an infracartilaginous incisional approach is recommended (**TECH FIG 3A**).
- An incision begins initially along the inferior margin of the medial crus, at 2 to 3 mm inward from the columella border of the midpoint of the columella (**TECH FIG 3B**).

- Once the incision is made to the dome area, it changes direction and moves laterally along the inferior border of the medial crus (**TECH FIG 3C**).
- The inferior margin of the lateral crus can be visualized by turning over the alar rim inside out.
- The incision lies deep medial to the alar rim (**TECH FIG 3D**). Incisions made along the lines of the alar rim must not be performed because they cause a nostril deformity.

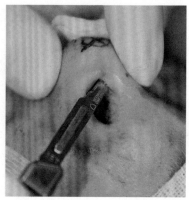

TECH FIG 3 • **A–D.** Inframarginal incision. (Copyright Man Koon Suh, MD.)

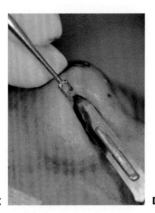 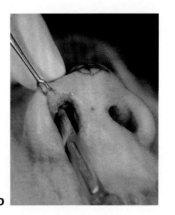

TECH FIG 3 (Continued) **C** **D**

- In cases requiring an additional operation, such as tip plasty, open rhinoplasty incisions are used.
- Implant deviation occurs in the process of making a pocket for an implant. When an operation creates a pocket by making incisions in the right side, a pocket in the radix may easily deviate toward the left side. Therefore, it is safe to create a symmetrical pocket by making incisions bilaterally.

■ Dissection for the Pocket

- A space for inserting an implant is referred to as a pocket. A dissection to form a straight and symmetrical pocket is the most significant part of dorsal augmentation.
- The dissection plane is supraperichondrial and subperiosteal, which means that dissections are performed above the perichondrium in the lower lateral and upper lateral cartilages and under the periosteum in the nasal bone area.
  - Metzenbaum scissors are used for the dissections over the lower and upper lateral cartilages while making sure a maximum amount of the soft tissues is included in the skin envelope.
- Implants should be inserted into the subperiosteal pocket to prevent mobility and shifting of the implant and to reduce visibility of the implant through the skin.
  - A Joseph knife is used to cut the periosteum transversely about 1 mm above the inferior margin of the nasal bone. Then, a Joseph elevator is used to lift the periosteum.

- At that time, lifting the periosteum a little bit at a time, step by step, can avoid periosteal damages, rather than lifting a large portion of the periosteum all at once. Once the operator is acquainted with this procedure, he or she may proceed by using only a Joseph elevator without the knife.
- Dissection and pocket formation mentioned above are performed through the opposite side incision to form a symmetric pocket (**TECH FIG 4**).
- Some surgeons prefer that the implant pocket be exactly the same size as the implant, but this author recommends a slightly larger pocket size.
  - Theoretically, fitting snugly and precisely to the width of a pocket prevents shifting of an implant. In reality, there is no assurance of having accurate identical left and right dimensions of a pocket. Thus, having a pocket width slightly wider than that of the implant allows room for prompt manual correction of implant shifting externally in the event of a development of implant deviation later on.

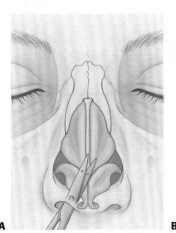 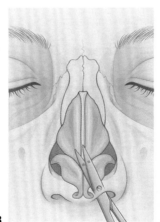 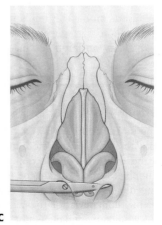

A **B** **C**

TECH FIG 4 • A–C. Dissection around the nasal tip and over the upper lateral cartilage.

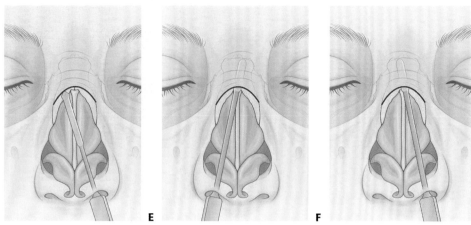

TECH FIG 4 (Continued) • **D–F.** Periosteal elevation. (Copyright Man Koon Suh, MD.)

- The time it takes for an implant in a pocket to be fixed by capsular formation is 10 to 14 days after surgery. A deviated implant may be properly positioned by moving it by hand during the time.
- In cases in which the nasal dorsum is not straight or uniform (eg, the nasal dorsum is skewed to one side of the nose), an inserted implant may easily be deviated if the gradient difference of the slope of the nasal dorsum has not been properly compensated by carving the implant properly before inserting it.

Pretreatment of e-PTFE Implant

- Unlike a silicone implant, an e-PTFE implant has internal pores of 25 to 40 µm in size. The size of bacterium is smaller than that of the pore. Bacteria may enter through these pores and reside within an e-PTFE implant, whereas a macrophage is larger than the pore, which makes it impossible to enter and combat these bacteria through the pores within an e-PTFE implant. Accordingly, a pretreatment is required for infection prevention.
- For the prevention of infection, a thorough aseptic technique and removal of the powders in the gloves are necessary.
- A liquid mixture of povidone-iodine and antibiotics is used for implant washing. Simply soaking an e-PTFE implant within a bowl of antibiotic does not allow infiltration of an antiseptic solution within the pores. Thus, the antiseptic solution should be forced to flow through these pores by using negative pressure.
- The author inserts an e-PTFE implant within a syringe and draws into the syringe a 10-cc antiseptic solution, for which an antibiotic is reconstituted with a

povidone-iodine solution. Then, in an attempt to fill these pores with the antiseptic solution, negative pressure is applied by pulling the syringe plunger (along with the piston in the syringe) (**TECH FIG 5**).

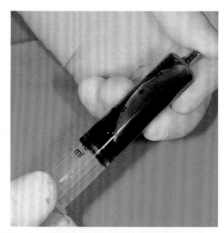

TECH FIG 5 • Pretreatment of the e-PTFE using the negative pressure.

Implant Insertion

- Washing the inner pocket with a povidone-iodine solution mixed with an antibiotic before implant insertion is helpful for the prevention of infection.
- When the implant is inserted into the pocket through an incisional opening, make sure it is positioned in the center of the pocket without deviation to one side (**TECH FIG 6A**).
- Insertion of a silicone implant is not that difficult, but an operator needs to take precautions for insertion of e-PTFE implant.

- If a soft type e-PTFE implant is being used, the implant may be pressed or wrinkled or may produce a dead space during insertion, which can increase the possibility of infection. An e-PTFE implant should not be pushed to be inserted. Rather, it is pulled into place with thread (**TECH FIG 6B**). This technique also facilitates proper positioning of the implant in the midline.
- There is no need to fix the distal end of an implant. A prospect of implant shifting may require suturing of the distal implant to the septal angle or alar cartilage (**TECH FIG 6C**).

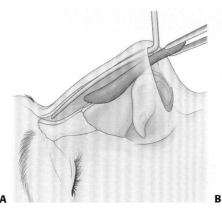
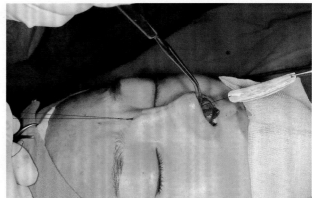
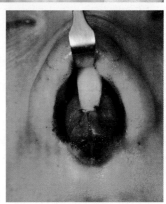

TECH FIG 6 • **A.** Silicone implant insertion. **B.** Pullout technique for the e-PTFE insertion. **C.** Fixation of the silicone implant tip to the alar cartilage. (**A.** Copyright Man Koon Suh, MD.)

■ Management of Supratip Area

- Theoretically, female patients should have a break point in the supratip area, so that there is a slight curvature, from the dorsum to the nasal tip.
- A formation of a natural-looking supratip break requires two elements:
  - Adequate tip projection
  - Prevention of supratip bulging
- The thickness of the terminal end of a prosthesis should be thinly carved for the prevention of supratip bulging.
- Supratip bulging may occur in cases where a tip projection is inadequate, thick supratip soft tissues that existed before surgery have not been corrected, or the distal end of an implant is thick. Thus, these issues need to be solved.
- A supratip groove occurs due to a height discrepancy at the area where the thinly carved distal end of an implant meets the cartilage onlay graft of the tip (**TECH FIG 7A**).
  - The groove is largely inconspicuous in cases with thick skin. Nevertheless, the existence of a groove should be verified by palpating it by hand before wound closure.
- If the surgeon is concerned with an unsightly groove on the nose, it can be resolved by using dermis or cartilage graft in the area (**TECH FIG 7B–E**). A graft should be placed between the skin envelop and the distal end of an implant.

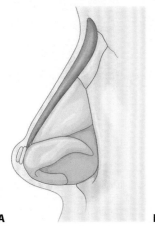
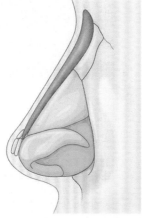
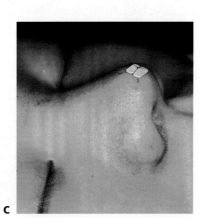

TECH FIG 7 • **A.** Visible groove between the implant tip and grafted cartilage on the tip. **B.** Cartilage or dermis graft is placed at the visible groove between the implant tip and cartilage onlay graft. **C.** Groove on the supratip area.

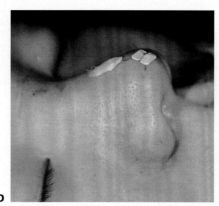
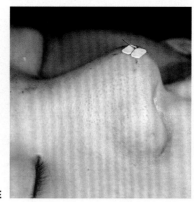

TECH FIG 7 (Continued) • **D.** Cartilage graft on the groove. **E.** Groove disappears after the cartilage graft. (**A,B.** Copyright Man Koon Suh, MD.)

■ Implant Wrapped With Temporal Fascia or Allograft Dermis

- If an implant is needed in patients with thin dorsal skin, covering it with temporal fascia or allograft dermis can reduce the issue of an implant visibility.
- The temporal fascia does not leave visible scar in the donor area, while donor harvesting is easy. Both superficial and deep temporal fascia may be used, but this author uses the latter.
- Temporal fascia may be easily harvested under local anesthesia and is performed from the area between the temporal crest and the superior root of the ear helix (**TECH FIG 8A**).
- An incision of a 3 cm in length is made, 1 cm anterior and 3 cm superior to the superior root of the helix.

The surgeon should take precaution not to injure the superficial temporal vessels.
- The glittering and lustrous deep temporal fascia can be seen after retracting the superficial temporal fascia. This fascia is appropriately incised and carefully removed from the temporal muscle (**TECH FIG 8B**) and the wound is closed (**TECH FIG 8C**).
- An implant is carved to coincide with the curvature of the nasal dorsum. Then, all sides of the implant, except for the bottom, are covered with the harvested temporal fascia.
  - After the fascia is trimmed along the margin of the implant, the fascia is fixed to the implant by using an absorbable suture material (**TECH FIG 8D**).
- An identical effect may be obtained from allograft acellular dermis used in place of a fascia.

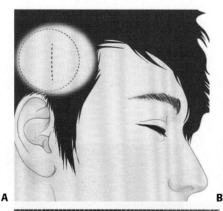
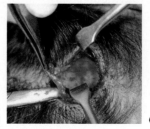
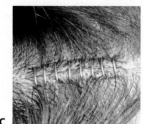
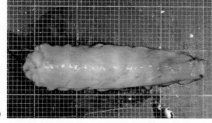

TECH FIG 8 • A. Donor site for the harvest of temporal fascia. **B.** Harvest of the deep temporal fascia. **C.** The temporal wound is closed with glue and staples. **D.** Silicone implant covered with temporal fascia. (**A.** Copyright Man Koon Suh, MD.)

■ Completion

- An absorbable suture material is used to repair the intranasal wound.
- Joseph dressing is done using paper tape (**TECH FIG 9A**). The paper tape is applied starting from the radix and proceeding caudally.

- This author applies compression by implementing an AquaSplint as well as a Joseph dressing. They both serve to minimize postoperative swelling (**TECH FIG 9B,C**).

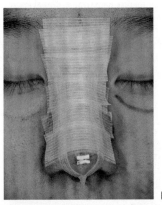 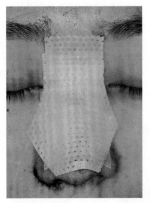 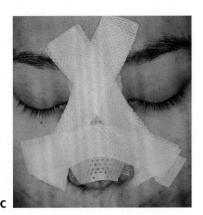

TECH FIG 9 • **A.** Joseph dressing. **B,C.** AquaSplint.

■ Correction of Implant Deviation

- In the event that prosthetic deviation is detected after 2 to 3 weeks of surgery, making it difficult to manipulate manually, a surgical revision is made as follows.
- Deviated silicone implant
  - A small inframarginal incision is made on the contralateral side of implant deviation.
  - Unilateral capsulotomy is performed along the lateral margin of the posterior capsule by using a D knife or a pair of scissors (**TECH FIG 10**).
  - A small additional pocket is made for movement of an implant in the area slightly lateral to the capsulotomy site.
  - After moving the implant manually, the implant is fixed by using a paper tape and AquaSplint.
- Deviated e-PTFE implant
  - After incisions are made in the inner nose, an elevator is used to separate the implant from the upper lateral cartilage and nasal bone.
  - The implant is moved to its proper position.

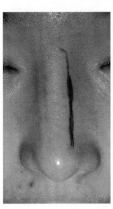

TECH FIG 10 • Design for the unilateral capsulotomy.

PEARLS AND PITFALLS

Good candidate for an implant	■ Low-profile nasal dorsum with thick dorsal skin
Implant position	■ Eyelash: right above the nasal tip ■ Pocket: subperiosteal, supraperichondral plane ■ Pocket size: slightly larger than the width of an implant
Patients with thin skin	■ Autograft using patient's own dermis or diced cartilage, rather than an implant, is recommended. ■ Implant wrapped up with the fascia or dermis is recommended for patients who must have an implant. ■ There is no truth in the opinion that e-PTFE implants used in patients with thin skin would show less visibility through the skin. ■ In patients with thin skin, both sides of the edge of the implant are sometimes more visible rather for a non–capsule-forming e-PTFE implant.

PEARLS AND PITFALLS (Continued)

How to manage the supratip area	■ In an attempt to prevent supratip bulging, it is important to thinly carve the implant tip and provide sufficient tip projection. ■ Additional cartilage or dermis graft may be necessary in some cases for the sunken groove between the implant tip and cartilage onlay graft.
Carving the silicone implant	■ Some surgeons make multiple partial-thickness cuts on the bottom of an implant to improve accurate contact and adherence to the nasal bone in the nasofrontal area (**FIG 5A**). This can cause an uneven thickness of the posterior capsule and late spontaneous hematoma, however, as well as a higher probability of infection secondary to increased surface area of an implant, so this practice should be avoided as much as possible. ■ Occasionally, several holes are drilled into an implant to prevent implant mobility (**FIG 5B**). This should also be avoided since it can cause dorsal skin dimpling, secondary to capsular contracture formed within the hole, or can lead to late spontaneous hematoma following tearing of the thread-shape capsule in the hole.

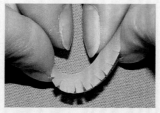 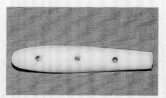

FIG 5 • **A.** Hatching on the undersurface of the silicone implant is not recommended. **B.** Making several holes in the implant is not also recommended.

POSTOPERATIVE CARE

■ An AquaSplint and paper dressing are removed 4 to 5 days after surgery.
■ Implant deviation should be frequently verified up to 2 weeks after surgery.
■ Detected implant deviation may be corrected by manual manipulation of the implant within 2 weeks after surgery.

COMPLICATIONS

■ Immediate complications
  ▪ Implant deviation

  ▪ Hematoma
  ▪ Infection
■ Delayed complications
  ▪ Thinned dorsal skin with visible implant contour (**FIG 6A**)
  ▪ Redness of the dorsal skin
  ▪ Capsular contracture resulting in upturned nasal tip or visible implant contour on both sides (**FIG 6B**)
  ▪ Delayed spontaneous hematoma (**FIG 6C**)
  ▪ Calcification on the surface of the implant or on the inner surface of capsule
  ▪ Implant extrusion through the tip skin or vestibular mucosa (**FIG 6D–I**)

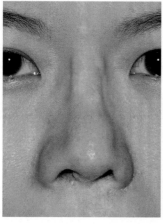 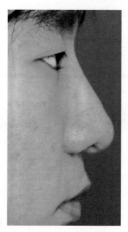 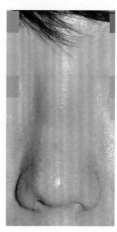

FIG 6 • **A.** Rib cartilage contour is visible through the thinned skin, and there is dorsal irregularity because of the focal partial resorption of the graft. **B.** Capsular contracture at the thick implant tip results in a supratip groove. **C.** Delayed spontaneous hematoma developed 3 years after dorsal augmentation with a silicone implant that had been hatched. Complications of L-shaped or long nasal implant include nasal tip skin thinning (**D,E**), contracted nose with redness of the tip skin (**F,G**), and exposure of the implant through the tip skin (**H,I**).

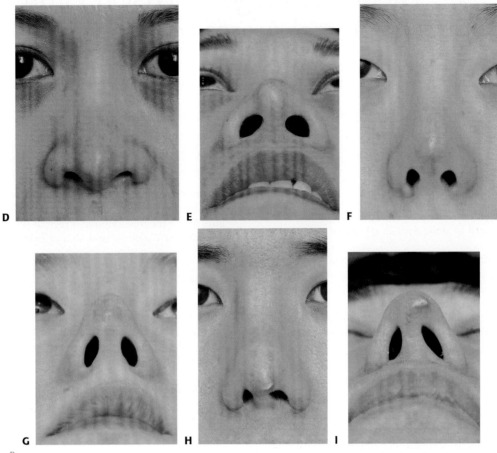

FIG 6 (Continued)

REFERENCES

1. Tham C, Lai YL, Weng CJ, Chen YR. Silicone augmentation rhinoplasty in an oriental population. *Ann Plast Surg.* 2005;54:1-5.
2. Deva AK, Merten S, Chang L. Silicone in nasal augmentation rhinoplasty: a decade of clinical experience. *Plast Reconstr Surg.* 1998;102:1230-1237.
3. Godin MS, Walderman SR, Johnson CM. Nasal augmentation using Gore-Tex: a 10-year experience. *Arch Facial Plast Surg.* 1999;1:118-121.
4. Jung YG, Kim HY, Dhong HJ, et al. Ultrasonographic monitoring of implant thickness after augmentation rhinoplasty with expanded polytetrafluoroethylene. *Am J Rhinol Allergy.* 2009;23:105-110.

67
CHAPTER

Diced Cartilage in Fascia Graft for Dorsal Augmentation in Rhinoplasty

Aaron M. Kosins and Rollin K. Daniel

DEFINITION

- Dorsal augmentation refers to augmentation of the nasal dorsum, which can be done with alloplastic or autogenous materials.
- Dorsal augmentation with a diced cartilage in fascia graft refers to augmentation of the nasal dorsum using autogenous tissues—the patient's cartilage from the nasal septum, ear, and/or rib that is diced into small pieces and wrapped in deep temporal fascia. The methods outlined herein include refinements to the techniques initially proposed by Daniel and Calvert.[1-3]

ANATOMY

- The normal or "ideal" dorsum exhibits a smooth transition from the nasal radix to the nasal tip. In a male, this relationship is classically identified as a smooth line, whereas in a Caucasian female, the ideal dorsum lies 2 mm behind this line. Patients with deficiency of the nasal dorsum (low dorsum) lie behind this line.
- In non-Caucasian patients, the ideal dorsum may be different, and patient preferences must be identified.

PATHOGENESIS

- Dorsal deficiency can be congenital, genetic, traumatic, or a consequence of previous surgery. Some patients are born with a low dorsum, and many ethnicities have a naturally occurring low dorsum (eg, Asian ancestry).
- Trauma to the nose can cause septal collapse resulting in a low dorsum or "saddle deformity."
- Previous over-resection of the nasal dorsum and aggressive septal surgery are the most common reasons for dorsal deficiency after rhinoplasty.

PATIENT HISTORY AND PHYSICAL FINDINGS

- In cases where no prior surgery has been performed, the diagnosis is clear and based on physical examination. The patient is viewed on profile, and the ideal radix and tip are visualized. The dorsum is designed to fit these ideals.
- If previous surgery has been performed, the rhinoplasty surgeon should be aware of the causes of a dorsal deficiency. Along with physical examination, photographs should always be taken and, again, the ideal radix and tip overlaid

on the profile photograph. A complete internal speculum examination should be done to assess the presence and integrity of the nasal septum. Previous operative reports are desirable in diagnosis and should help guide the surgical plan.

IMAGING

- CT scans are rarely indicated except in the presence of severe trauma or asymmetric developmental deviation of the nose (ADDN). CT scans are useful to assess the nasal bones, nasal septum, heights of the maxillae, and the presence of concha bullosa.

DIFFERENTIAL DIAGNOSIS

- Differentiate the causes of dorsal height deficiency with physical examination, speculum assessment, and previous operative reports.

NONOPERATIVE MANAGEMENT

- Theoretically hyaluronic acid fillers can be used as a temporary solution; however, the authors do not advocate this type of treatment. Results are marginal at best, and injections require a high level of accuracy and experience. Follow-up (repeat) treatments must be done at least twice per year.

SURGICAL MANAGEMENT

- The authors perform diced cartilage in fascia as the mainstay for dorsal augmentation whenever dorsal deficiency exists. Timing is dependent on patient age (patients should be older than 14 years old) and timing of previous operations. We advocate waiting *at least* 1 year from any prior nasal surgeries to perform secondary surgery.

Preoperative Planning

- Discuss again risks, benefits, and expectations with patient at both the preoperative visit and on the day of surgery. Risks include bleeding, infection, septal perforation, dorsal asymmetry, prolonged swelling of the graft (6 weeks), and cosmetic deformity. Harvest of the deep temporal fascia involves a temporal incision, and risks include alopecia and poor scarring. Finally, if auricular or rib cartilage must be taken, then these risks must be discussed as well.

Positioning

- The patient is positioned supine, and the hair, head, and neck are prepped and draped in sterile fashion.

Approach

- The temporal incision is planned. A line is drawn up from the most anterior point of the tragus into the temporal hair. A V-shaped incision is drawn so that the superficial temporal artery is avoided (**FIG 1**).

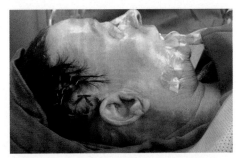

FIG 1 • A temporal V-shaped incision is used for access to the deep temporal fascia.

■ Deep Temporal Fascia Harvest

- The V-shaped incision is carefully planned and infiltrated subdermally with 5 cc of 1% lidocaine with epinephrine.
- The incision is made clearly through the dermis, and careful cauterization is used to avoid trauma to the hair follicles.
- Dissection is carried down to the superficial temporal fascia, which is identified and divided.
- Scissors are used to spread the loose areolar layer until the glistening white deep temporal fascia (superficial leaflet) is identified (**TECH FIG 1**).
- Retractors are used to expose the operative site, and a 4 × 3 cm graft is taken using a 15-blade scalpel. Care is taken to avoid trauma to the temporalis muscle below. A distinct vessel is always present below the fascia at the 4 or 5 o'clock position.
- The superficial temporal fascia is reapproximated as well as the skin with staples.

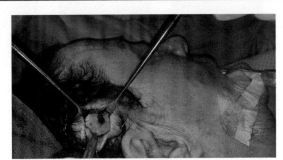

TECH FIG 1 • After incision through the skin, the superficial temporal fascia is divided, and scissor dissection is carried out to the glistening layer of the deep temporal fascia.

■ Diced Cartilage in Fascia Graft

- The fascia graft is measured in length to approximate the dorsal augmentation and 20 mm wide. The fascia is folded over on itself to fasten a 10-mm wide fascial sleeve. This is sewed on one side with a running 4-0 chromic suture. Two 4-0 plain gut sutures on straight needles are placed in the proximal portion so that the graft may be guided up to the radix.
- Cartilage from any donor site is prepared and diced into fine, less than 1 mm cubes with 10-blade scalpels or dermatome blades.
- The diced cartilage is placed in a tuberculin syringe for injection into the fascial sleeve. It is important that the cartilage is finely diced so that the cartilage is injected with minimal resistance. Excess fluid is removed before injection.

- Diced cartilage is injected into the fascial sleeve into the distal end. Once injected, it is molded on the back table to the predetermined height.
- Using the 4-0 plain gut sutures, the graft is guided into position up to the nasal radix and secured distally with a 4-0 plain gut suture. If cartilage needs to be removed, it can be done from the distal free end. Molding is then done on the table.
- After all incisions are closed, a Denver splint is placed for 6 to 7 days. The graft can be molded postoperatively for up to 2 weeks. At times, a percutaneous stitch is placed after graft insertion to prevent mobility.
- See **FIG 2** for a patient example.

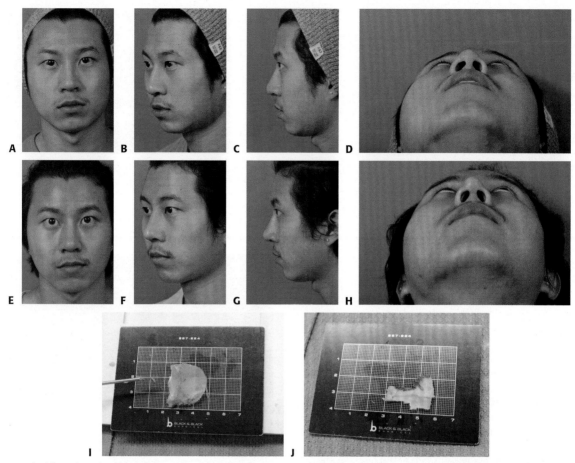

FIG 2 • Frontal, oblique, lateral, and basal views of a patient **(A–D)** preoperatively and 13 months postoperatively **(E–H)**. The patient requested dorsal augmentation and required a diced cartilage in fascia graft for dorsal augmentation. 0.6 cc of diced cartilage was placed inside the fascial sleeve. **I.** A large piece of septum and perpendicular plate of ethmoid bone were harvested using Piezo instrumentation. After making the cuts in the cartilage with a 15-blade scalpel, a Piezo saw was used under direct vision to cut the bony ethmoid. **J.** Tip projection was achieved by creating a septocolumellar "tomahawk" graft that was placed on the right side of the caudal septum for increased length and projection as well as derotation. 15 cc of fat grafting was also done to the forehead.

PEARLS AND PITFALLS

Do not overfill the graft. The designer dorsum is created to size.	■ Grafts made too high will maintain height postoperatively.
Tapering grafts is very difficult to do. Create a flat platform, and place a uniform graft.	■ Trying to change the thickness of the graft from proximal to distal does not work well and results in dorsal irregularities.
Avoid excessive molding on the table.	
Make the fascial sleeve wider than you think.	
Create a narrow tunnel to place the graft.	■ Excessive dissection allows for graft migration. If it moves, hyaluronidase can be used to help mobilize it versus revision rhinoplasty.

POSTOPERATIVE CARE

■ Typically, the nose stays swollen for 3 weeks after open rhinoplasty, but the full remodeling process takes 1 year. When a diced cartilage in fascia graft is used, this swelling persists for 6 to 8 weeks.

■ Once the Denver splint is removed, taping is done at night for 3 weeks to help with swelling.
■ No glasses are to be worn for 6 weeks.
■ Patients must be told not to mold his/her graft or massage it.

COMPLICATIONS

- Infection occurs in less than 1% of patients and is treated with doxycycline 100 mg twice daily for 1 week. Any infection that appears to be getting worse warrants an infectious disease consultation.
- Displacement of the graft. Hyaluronidase can be attempted to mobilize the graft, but operative intervention is often warranted.
- Undercorrection
- Overcorrection
- Palpable, diced cartilage can occur if the cubes are not made as small as possible.

REFERENCES

1. Daniel RK, Calvert JW. Diced cartilage grafts in rhinoplasty. *Plast Reconstr Surg.* 2004;113(7):2156-2171.
2. Daniel RK. Diced cartilage grafts in rhinoplasty surgery. *Plast Reconstr Surg.* 2008;112(6):1883-1891.
3. Daniel RK, Sajadian A. Secondary rhinoplasty: management of the overresected dorsum. *Facial Plast Surg.* 2012;28(4):417-426.

CHAPTER 68

Indication and Technique for Diced Cartilage and Fascia Grafting in Rhinoplasty

Ashkan Ghavami

DEFINITION

- Augmentation of the nasal bridge and radix has historically been a highly debated topic in rhinoplasty.
- Techniques include alloplastic materials such as silicone implants, Gore-Tex, and PTFE. Although these techniques continue to be popular worldwide, particularly in Asian countries, there has been a paradigm shift toward autogenous sources. Preferred cartilage grafts include septal, costal, and conchal cartilage. Each of these in isolation is fraught with problems in stability of shape and long-term contour.
- Erol's description of the "Turkish Delight," which is diced cartilage wrapped in Surgicel, provided a simple, less complicated option for dorsal augmentation.[1] Not long after, Daniel[2,3] described wrapping with autogenous temporal fascia (DCFG: diced cartilage fascia graft) as an alternative; this has become many surgeons' primary technique today. It should be noted that temporoparietal grafting to the nose in isolation was described long ago by Guerrerosantos in 1985.[4]
- The author's preferred material is conchal cartilage, but costal cartilage and/or septal remnants can be used.
- Fascial wrapping and/or overlay of the cartilage construct allows for incorporation of the graft and smooth contour in surgical outcomes. Contour irregularities from warping with other autogenous techniques have been a long-standing problem that is avoided with DCFG when properly executed.
- This technique can be particularly useful in secondary rhinoplasty.[2]

ANATOMY

- Anatomical landmarks and technical execution of harvesting the cartilage grafts to be diced/crushed are imperative to avoid injury or deformation of donor sites at the expense of obtaining cartilage source.
- Standard techniques for harvest of rib, septal, and conchal elements can be used based on the surgeon's personal preference.
- For conchal grafts, a postauricular approach is performed. Rib graft typically is taken from the sixth or seventh rib, and it is important to not harvest calcified portions that are difficult to dice and/or morselize sufficiently. The inframammary crease is used in both men and women.
- Temporal, mastoid, and rectus fascia can all be used.
- Goals are based on the desired contour and degree of augmentation/camouflaging required. This begins at the radix and proceeds caudally to the supratip and anterior septal angle region.

- Blending with the osteotomy lines and the ascending process of the maxilla as it transitions to the nasal bones is important to create a smooth nasal sidewall contour and soft contour shadow/highlight.
- "Spot" augmentation with DCFG can be done in radix alone or to fill specific contour irregularities (particularly in secondary revision cases).

PATIENT HISTORY AND PHYSICAL FINDINGS

- Particularly in the modern era of social media and a "selfie-obsessed" culture, it is absolutely critical to communicate the magnitude of augmentation desired by the patient while setting realistic expectations.
- Accounting for the somewhat unpredictable long-term absorption rates is also important to communicate with the patient.
- The author believes that the trade-off of minor to moderate long-term absorbability of DCFG for complications associated with traditional augmentation techniques (warping, extrusion, unnatural dorsal contour lines, need for removal, and replacement/reconstruction) is highly acceptable in favor of DCFG.
- After the standard workup for rhinoplasty with imaging and planning, desired dorsal contour is obtained during the consultation. Attention is given to the width and height of desired dorsal augmentation. If specific camouflaging or contour correction is planned, then these regions should be pointed out to the patient with the end points described or shown via imaging, drawings, or demonstration with saline (in-office).

IMAGING

- Three-dimensional imaging software as well as 2D imaging or drawings are helpful in communicating the amount of dorsal height and narrowing/widening with patients.
- The author currently prefers to demonstrate with description and reference to other surgical case examples during consultation. Hand drawings on printed out photographs are helpful, and only when necessary during repeat consultation(s) or during the preoperative office visit is 3D imaging utilized.
- X-rays or CT scans are not necessary unless there is history of recent or remote trauma or if concomitant nasal airway correction or sinus surgery is planned.
- When costal cartilage is used, assessment of possible excess calcification of the ribs should be done. This can include needle testing in the exam room using minimal local anesthesia and/or CT scan evaluation when truly necessary.

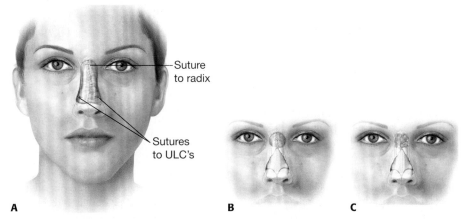

FIG 1 • **A.** Anteroposterior view of proper DCFG positioning on dorsum. **B.** Variation: radix-only DCFG. **C.** Variation: radix-only DCG. No fascia necessary due to thick nasal skin.

NONOPERATIVE MANAGEMENT

- There is no substitution for DCFG that is nonoperative and long term that is justified in the author's opinion. However, as an adjunct to planning and only when a patient is not ready for surgery for a year or more, temporary injectable fillers can be a useful tool and "buys time." Hyaluronic acid gel fillers are preferred, and any other filler material is not recommended.
- A major limitation of nonsurgical filler augmentation is that dorsal aesthetic lines in the anteroposterior view are difficult to optimize because narrowing of the nasal pyramid is not being simultaneously performed.
- The one region that may warrant dorsal augmentation with temporary fillers instead of DCFG is in the radix when all other aspects of the nasal shape are accepted by the patient. Consultation should include surgical options and informed consent of the temporary nature of injectable fillers for the radix or for minor contour correction.
- One of the best indications for injectable (nonoperative) dorsal augmentation is for minor/subtle contour correction of dorsal and other irregularities (primary and secondary rhinoplasty). Small molecule, highly cross-linked hyaluronic acid gel is best and must be injected with respect of vascular dermal capacitance.

SURGICAL MANAGEMENT

Preoperative Planning

- Planning DCFG augmentation in rhinoplasty involves many of the methods listed above:

- Detailed consultation with the patient with regard to the desired goals in dorsal augmentation is paramount. This includes dorsal height, dorsal aesthetic contour width, and supratip/other tip transition points to the dorsum.
- Imaging as discussed above can aid in this process.
- Saline solution can be injected in the office to show an approximate effect of dorsal augmentation on profile view if the surgeon and patient agree that this step is necessary to finalize the decision-making process.
- Standard rhinoplasty preoperative planning is performed including attention to internal and external valve sufficiency, airway assessment, Cottle maneuver, nasal endoscopy (when indicated), and evaluation of cartilage donor sites.
  - Note: augmentation of the dorsal height and/or narrowing of the bony pyramid and midvault can worsen airway functional issues. Dorsal height augmentation can mask these issues visually, while untreating the underlying insufficiency and patency of the airway. Dorsal width changes with DCFG must be reconciled with the need for spreader graft/flap techniques.
- DCFG is not a substitute for proper osteotomies and correction of sidewall irregularities and asymmetries. The platform for the DCFG construct must be stable, symmetric, and structurally sound prior to using DCGF for augmentation and/or contouring.
- Marking of the topographical dimensions can be done both on the patient in the holding area on day of surgery and on photographs.
- **FIGS 1** and **2** demonstrate typical positioning of the DCFG construct.

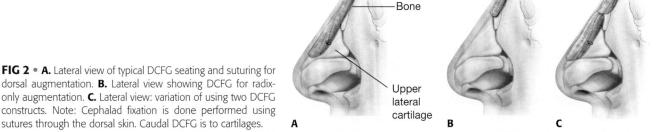

FIG 2 • **A.** Lateral view of typical DCFG seating and suturing for dorsal augmentation. **B.** Lateral view showing DCFG for radix-only augmentation. **C.** Lateral view: variation of using two DCFG constructs. Note: Cephalad fixation is done performed using sutures through the dorsal skin. Caudal DCFG is to cartilages.

- Donor sites:
  - Ear: The preferred sleeping side is avoided, and the contralateral ear is used when possible. Concomitant correction of prominent ears allows for more graft material, and discussion with the patient is indicated. If the patient has a small conchal area, then the larger concha is used, or bilateral conchal graft is planned.
  - Rib: The inframammary crease is marked in both men and women, and the rib is accessed through the smallest incision the surgeon is comfortable with. This is typically the sixth or seventh rib. Incision placement should be shown to the patient preoperatively.
  - Fascia: The temporal, mastoid, or rectal fasciae are all options. When using costal graft, the author prefers rectus fascia because it is thick and in the same donor site. When this would be too thick and not indicated for a particular nasal envelope, temporal fascia is then harvested. When using ear cartilage, mastoid fascia is taken. If mastoid fascia is not large enough and true wrapping is required, then ipsilateral temporal fascia is obtained through a pre-hairline approach.

Positioning

- Standard head positioning for rhinoplasty is used with the patient in the supine position and the head of bed in reverse-Trendelenburg, as well as head elevation, approximating a 30 to 45 degree angle.
- Bilateral conchal cartilage grafts are typically consented for and prepped, so access must be available with draping.
- If rib graft is to be used, this harvest site is prepped and accessible during the rhinoplasty.

Approach

- The donor cartilage that is planned for harvest will determine the approach taken to obtain it.
- Incisions should be designed to be as small as possible and as inconspicuous as possible.
  - Ear: retroauricular sulcus
  - Rib: inframammary crease
  - Septal: preferred septal approach (open vs Killian or transfixion incision)
  - Fascia: mastoid (posterior sulcus), temporal (posterior hairline), and rectus abdominis (inframammary crease)

■ Cartilage Harvest (TECH FIG 1)

EAR

- Prior to infiltration with local anesthesia, 7 mm of conchal height is marked on the conchal surface anteriorly in multiple points using a caliper.
- After infiltration, prepping, and draping, a posterior sulcus incision is made. Cautery guided and sharp scissor dissection is performed to expose the conchal donor in its entirety subperichondrially.
- Two 25-gauge needles are then passed through the anterior marked points to penetrate posteriorly. A line is marked connecting the two on the posterior surface of the conchal cartilage. This avoids the sometimes messy tattooing with methylene blue dye.
- If mastoid fascia is to be used, then posterior exposure of the fascia is accomplished by undermining in a posterosuperior direction to acquire both the periosteum and mastoid fascia. Mastoid fascia often requires thinning and can be placed as an onlay without wrapping. Care is taken to not injure and transect posterior nerves. Meticulous hemostasis is necessary.

- Conchal harvest is then completed by excising all conchal cartilage posterior to a line from needle to needle. This line should be curvilinear to avoid deforming the superior crura. The graft and fascia are placed in saline.
- Any rents in the skin should be repaired.
- A layered closure should be performed, and Xeroform/antibiotic ointment bolster is secured with a silk or nylon suture. This should be molded to compress the conchal space.

RIB

- The inframammary crease is marked at approximately 4 cm. Surgeons should not hesitate to make this incision as big as they need based on experience and comfort. Visualization is necessary for preventing complications.
- An incision is made and dissection carried down to the perichondrium of the rib. The rib is palpated and needle prick examination performed to assess for softness and suitability. The fascial and rectus abdominis fibers are vertically spread bluntly to expose the rib. If rectus fascia is to be used, see below for details regarding harvest.
- A midline incision is made through the perichondrium parallel to the orientation of the costal cartilage. Gentle elevation is performed to preserve a perichondrial sleeve around the removed rib segment that is later closed along with fascia and muscle forming a functionally rigid construct and prevents postoperative pain from any sensation of instability during deep respiration.
- Using direct visualization and staying subperichondrial, the posterior aspect of the rib is freed from the perichondrium with a blunt elevator. Curved endoscopic brow elevators and Cottle elevators are an excellent combination for this technique.

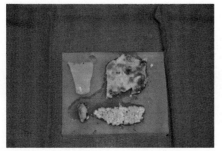

TECH FIG 1 • Components of DCFG: septal cartilage, cephalic trim cartilage, deep temporal fascia (4 × 6 cm), and diced conchal cartilage.

- Once the rib is removed using a 10 blade, it is placed in saline. If strut grafts and other grafts are needed, it is allowed to sit for at least 10 minutes after symmetrical carving; the remaining cartilage will be used to dice/crush.
- Long-acting local anesthetic is infiltrated into the deep subcutaneous tissues and in the rib dead space. The author prefers to place an angiocath in this space, followed by reinjection and removal of the angiocath prior to extubation. Some surgeons prefer a pain pump, which I have found to be unnecessary. The site is then closed in a layered fashion with absorbable sutures, from deep to skin: perichondrium, rectus fascia (if fascia is harvested, then closure is still possible, or spanning sutures can be used, and remaining muscle fibers and fascia can be approximated), Scarpa fascia, deep dermal, and subcuticular closure.
- Commonly, if the rib is used for DCFG, the costal cartilage is needed for other elements such as strut grafts, spreader grafts, etc. Rib cartilage simply for DCFG is sufficient without obtaining the conchal cartilage. However, there are circumstances when rib cartilage and ear are both required for different purposes particularly in very deficient dorsum or in complex revision rhinoplasty.

■ Dicing of Cartilage

- The cartilage to be diced or crushed is placed on a silicone block. A 10 or 11 blade is used to dice the pieces as small as possible so that they can pass through a "slip tip" (non-Luer locking) tuberculin syringe. Alternatively, sterilized razor blade can also be used. The size of the pieces is determined by the augmentative goals, the rigidity/memory of the cartilage donor, and the thickness of the dorsal skin envelope (**TECH FIG 2**).
  - For radix augmentation in thicker-skinned patients, finely diced cartilage can be used without fascial onlay or wrapping. Excessive crushing is not necessary and may increase absorption. However, fascial onlay or wrapping will help reduce the chance of untoward cartilage edge visibility long term and can also have a subtle augmentative benefit too, depending on the thickness of the fascia (rectus or mastoid vs temporal).

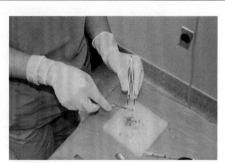

TECH FIG 2 ● Dicing of cartilage graft.

- If finer pieces are needed, a handheld (Ruben) morselizer is very useful and preferred over the classic morselizer which requires a mallet and is less refined in giving the exact degree of softening or morselizing of diced pieces. Once again, excessive morselization is not indicated.

■ Temporal Fascia Harvest

- If ear cartilage is harvested, the ipsilateral temporal region is approached.
- A 3-cm incision is made several centimeters posterior to the temporal hairline. If the hair is thin, the incision is placed further posteriorly (**TECH FIG 3**).
- Respect of hair follicles and the anterior beveled approach is used to limit injury and transection of hair roots.
- If proper preinfiltration of local anesthetic with epinephrine is used, then cautery can be minimized, which also aids in prevention of iatrogenic alopecia.
- After the incision is made, the subgaleal, supratemporal bloodless plane is entered. Blunt undermining superficial to the white fibers of the deep temporal fascia is visualized and exposure from the temporal crest cephalad from the supraorbital ridge toward the sentinel vein, and 3 to 5 cm posterior to the incision point is performed.
- Marking pen can be used to delineate the rectangular piece for harvest. Typically a 5 × 7 cm piece can be obtained. Using an 11 or 15 blade, the temporal fascia is scored, muscle is exposed along the marked lines, and then fascia is grasped and pulled off the muscle with the aid of angled scissors.

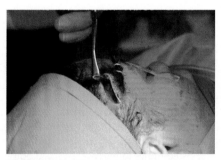

TECH FIG 3 ● Temporal fascial harvest.

- Inadvertent muscle fibers and any fatty tissue carried over should be trimmed off the fascia.
- Occasionally vessels deep to the fascia are injured, especially in the inferoposterior region and temporal crest caudally. These should be cauterized precisely without inadvertent heat injury of the fascial harvest.
- The incision is closed after irrigation of the pocket and confirmation of hemostasis. Three-point layered closure helps close the dead space. Staples or a running small caliber quick absorbing suture of the skin layer can be used. A drain is rarely used, but if it is, a round 7-French drain to bulb suction is preferred. No compressive wraps are necessary.

■ Fascial Wrapping

- There are two methods for wrapping:
  - Syringe method (**TECH FIG 4**):
    - Diced/crushed pieces are placed into a non–Luer-Lok ("slip tip") 1 cc tuberculin syringe. The plunger is used to squeeze pieces into a confluent mass within the syringe without gaps or air. The syringe is placed on top of the fascia, and the fascia is needle-fixed at two corners to the silicone block.
    - A running absorbable suture is used from proximal to distal and needles removed for circumferential closure of the fascial sleeve around the syringe.

The contents are injected into the sleeve, and final suture is placed to close the proximal open end of the sleeve. This suture can be cut with needle attached for placement and securing to the radix skin.
  - Onlay technique:
    - No syringe is required, and the diced cartilage is placed onto the fascia directly in the middle (similar to how a burrito is made), and the fascia is then wrapped around it and sutured in similar fashion as above. This technique is best for when the DCFG does not need to be as rigid and is best for lesser degree of augmentation, radix augmentation, and/or contour/camouflage grafting purposes.

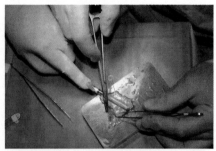

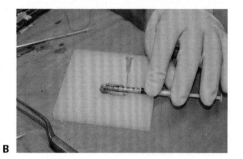

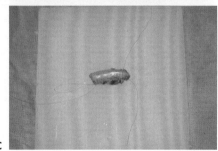

TECH FIG 4 ● **A.** Syringe fascial sleeve wrapping. **B.** Syringe and sleeve near complete. Cartilage will now be pushed into fascial tubular sleeve and final sutures placed at open end to close the DCFG construct. It is important to not leave openings so that diced cartilage cannot extrude and create irregular contours. **C.** DCFG construct completed. Sutures left long on either end to allow for immediate fixation.

■ Placement of DCFG

- DCFG can be placed through an open or "closed" endonasal approach. A closed approach requires passing through an infra or intra-cartilaginous access incision.
- The needle that is left attached to the DCFG construct is used to pass through the radix region at the cephalad end point of the desired augmentative footprint. This is done after osteotomies to narrow the nasal bony vault (if indicated). The DCFG is slid into a pocket that was previously undermined from the tip complex to the takeoff of the frontal bone in the nasofrontal angle/radix region. The needle is brought through the skin and grasped, and after the DCFG is positioned, it is tied to the skin and to itself as a loop. This can be removed upon splint removal on day 6 or 7 (**TECH FIG 5**).
- The lateral dimensions of the DCFG tunnel should not be overly released and undermined because this can result in inadvertent excessive blunting of the lateral dorsal aesthetic contour lines. In addition, if more height is needed, a tighter "wrap" of the DCFG and narrower tunnel will aid in driving the volumizing effect of the DCFG dorsally rather than laterally.

- If only radix augmentation is indicated, then the DCFG will be shorter, but skin securing with suture is still recommended.
- It is imperative that the caudal aspect of the DCFG is secured with at least two sutures to the anterior septal angle region. Typically the upper lateral cartilage and septum are great anchor points.
- The DCFG should be massaged in place to desired contour, width, and height.
- Note: After the remaining sequence of the primary or revision rhinoplasty is complete, it is important to create a balance between the dorsal augmentation and tip height as well as supratip transition. The caudal aspect of the fascial (DCFG) can extend to the lower lateral cartilages and/or domes depending on the desired aesthetic goals in this region.
- Splinting should take into account precise molding effects of the splint on the height and width of the DCFG. The author prefers an elastic splint (Aquaplast), but any splinting choice is acceptable as long as excessive narrowing is not created. Lastly, it is important to not have any irregularity or deviation in the splinting process because this may alter the shape and centralization of the DCFG.

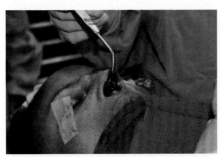 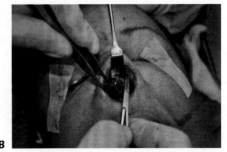

TECH FIG 5 • **A.** Passing DCFG with 5-0 chromic suture to secure at radix skin and **B.** two sutures placed to caudal upper lateral cartilage (approximately 7 o'clock and 5 o'clock positions).

■ Combined Techniques

- Case no. 1 demonstrates the benefits of combining DCFG with traditional costal cartilage dorsal augmentation (see **FIG 3**).
- It is important to secure the cephalad portion of the costal graft to the nasal bones and to adhere to classic carving and shaping principles. This avoids lateral migration and cantilevering of the costal graft.
- The DCFG is sutured on top of the rib graft. Skin securing as described above is also necessary, as is passing the threaded K-wire through the DCFG and costal graft chimera construct. The wire is trimmed at skin level and removed during splint removal (**TECH FIG 6**).
- This combination gives a large degree of augmentation and utilizes the benefits of lateral contour and camouflage.

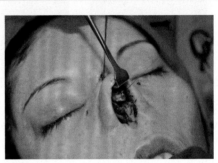

TECH FIG 6 • Variation of rib graft to the dorsum (wired to radix bone) and DCFG on top for warping prevention, contour blending, and further augmentation. K-wire has already been placed through the DCFG and Rib graft. Caudal suture left long and will be on two sutures to secure DCFG to the upper lateral cartilages. A third suture can also be placed if necessary so that the DCFG can drape and contour properly over the caudal dorsal structures. Patient is Case 1.

PEARLS AND PITFALLS

Obtaining proper dorsal height	■ Preoperative photographs and/or 3D imaging ■ Thorough discussion with the patient preoperatively on setting realistic goals with dorsal height ■ Saline test if necessary
Optimizing DCFG dimensions	■ Tighter wrapping and maximal filling provide more rigid and larger construct ■ Avoid overdissection of lateral dorsal tunnel dissection ■ Larger pieces can be used in thicker skin envelopes
Fixation	■ Cephalic DCFG suturing at radix skin ■ Three-point caudal fixation (one central and two lateral)
Early contour irregularity	■ Can be molded up to 3 wk in office ■ If necessary, no earlier than 9 mo, minor dorsal ridges if present or spicules can be rasped under local anesthesia in office
Radix-only augmentation	■ May not require fascia, but pieces should be small enough for camouflage

POSTOPERATIVE CARE

- Postoperatively, the DCFG has the great advantage of being malleable and able to be further shaped/molded for 3 weeks.
- If deviations or irregularities are seen, they can be softened and improved with gentle steady yet firm pressure much like clay. Occasionally local anesthesia may be required for patient comfort.

- The splint is removed at day 6 or 7.
- Retaping is preferred to help with edema and is a routine technique of the author in all primary and secondary rhinoplasties. The patient is instructed on how to tape and is encouraged to tape as shown nightly for 7 to 21 days, depending on the amount of edema present at splint removal.

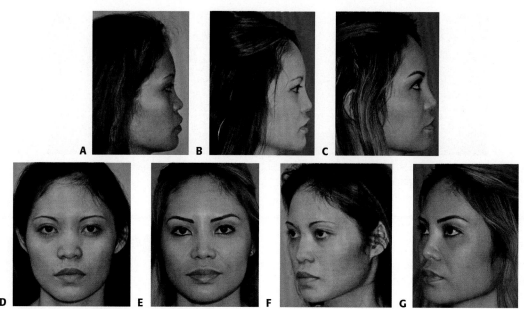

FIG 3 • Case 1: primary Asian rhinoplasty. Rib graft augmentation of the dorsum with overlying DCFG. Note: DCFG and rib graft are both K-wire fixed to the radix bone. Wire removed at 7 days with splint. **A.** Lateral view shows preop, 1.5 years postoperatively **(B)**, and 5 years postoperatively **(C)**. Notice the integrity of dorsal volume. Rib graft was relatively small in height. **D.** AP view. **E.** 5-year result. **F.** Oblique view. **G.** 5-year result.

- The DCFG effects and solidification occur at approximately week 3 and continue to be complete by 3 months where its effects can be seen.
- In the author's experience, desired outcomes can be assessed accurately as with most rhinoplasty aesthetic endpoints at 1 year postoperatively.
- Much like all rhinoplasty outcomes, aesthetic results will still continue to evolve even past a year, and patients should be informed about the process.

OUTCOMES

- Patient satisfaction is high and is likely dependent on thorough preoperative assessment, and proper informed consent of dorsal dimension end goals.
- Realistic expectations are important in the preoperative discussion and planning. It should be stressed to the patient that absorption and dorsal height long term have been shown to be acceptable and revision rates are low.
- Discussion of alternative techniques and their limitations should also be done preoperatively.
- Typical dorsal aesthetic contour lines and height are shown a year or more in these case examples (**FIG 3**).

COMPLICATIONS

- In general, the adverse events that can occur from the DCFG technique are rare and when present can be addressed via closed surgical approach.
- Loss of unacceptable DCFG volume has not been in issue in the author's practice and, if present to a small degree, has not driven any patient to seek revision.

- Excess dorsal height can be present and is addressed through a closed approach with sharp trimming or rasping. If other revisions are indicated and opening of the nose is indicated, then direct excision of regions of the DCFG can be accomplished.
- Irregular contour is managed by simple rasping via a closed approach.
- DCFG contour can appear edematous and irregular for a few months, and patience from both surgeon and patient is required. Once the subtle height and width dimensions plateau and no longer change after a few months, discussion of any undesirable contours and/or dimensions can proceed, and possible revision is planned.
- Infection is rare and has not been experienced by the author but should be addressed early with oral antibiotics, irrigation (if indicated), and removal if necessary. There are no reports of DCFG removal for infection. However, meticulous sterility of grafted cartilage during acquisition and creation of the DCFG construct is important.
- "Redness" of the skin overlying the DCFG has been witnessed by the author and has typically subsided without intervention.

REFERENCES

1. Erol OO. The Turkish delight: a pliable graft for rhinoplasty. *Plast Reconstr Surg.* 2000;105:2229-2241.
2. Daniel RK. Rhinoplasty: septal saddle nose deformity and composite reconstruction. *Plast Reconstr Surg.* 2007;119: 1029-1043.
3. Daniel RK, Calvert JC. Diced cartilage in rhinoplasty surgery. *Plast Reconstr Surg.* 2004;113:2156-2171.
4. Guerrerosantos J Temporoparietal free fascial grafts to the nose. *Plast Reconstr Surg.* 1985;76:328-329.

Technique for Surgical Management of the Depressor Septi Nasi Muscle

Michael R. Lee, Sammy Sinno, and Rod J. Rohrich

DEFINITION

- *Depressor septi nasi* (DSN) *muscle* is a paired structure occasionally responsible for deformity of the nasal tip and/or columella.[1]
- *Animation deformity* of the nasal tip and/or columella may result from action of the DSN. Such deformities typically include drooping of the nasal tip and/or columella on animation.
- *Basal aesthetic lines* (BALs) are created by the lateral borders of the columella. Excess soft tissue of the columella which includes the DSN muscle may cause distortion of the BALs.[2]
- *Medial crura footplate approximation* is a described multistep process designed to improve symmetry and architecture of the medial nasal base, thereby improving the BALs.[3]

ANATOMY

- Variations of DSN anatomy have been reported in the literature, particularly with ethnicity.[4]
- Muscular fibers of the DSN may originate from the maxillary periosteum and/or orbicularis oris muscle. Fibers may be diminutive in some patients.
- Muscle fibers of the DSN course through the columella and insert on the medial crura and nasal septum.
- Columella composition includes cartilage (caudal nasal septum and medial crura) and soft tissue (muscle fibers, fibroblast, collagen fibers, elastin fibers, adipocytes, and neurovascular structures).[5] Muscle fibers traversing the columella are from the DSN and orbicularis oris muscle.
- The caudal septum is firmly seated on the maxillary crest and does not move with contraction of the DSN. Flanking the caudal septum is the medial crura. These more mobile medial crura may descend with contraction of the DSN.

PATIENT HISTORY AND PHYSICAL FINDINGS

- Patients may report (1) tip descent on animation, (2) short upper lip on animation, (3) transverse crease in the mid-philtral area, (4) infratip/columellar decent on animation, and (5) columellar fullness and nostril deformity on basal view.
- Exam includes inspection of the nose in all classic rhinoplasty views. Inspection is initially performed in repose and then again with animation. Animation includes smiling and speaking.
- Frontal view is used to evaluate tip position both in repose and with animation. The tip is inspected to determine if descent is occurring or if the misconception of tip descent is occurring. Tip position in relation to the ala and cheek during animation helps to differentiate between the two deformities. The tip is inspected both in isolation and in comparison to the nasal ala and cheek mound. It is important to determine if the tip is truly descending or if elevation of the ala/cheek mound with subnasale repositioning are responsible for the deformity. The latter is an illusion of tip descent.[6] The infratip lobule is also studied to identity fullness and/or asymmetry.[7] Inspection of the upper lip for shortening and/or a transverse crease is also done.

- The lateral view is studied in repose and animation to study tip position, infratip architecture, and the alar-columellar relationship. Inspection of the nasal ala and check mound in relation to tip position is studied on animation. This lateral view allows a more focused inspection on the tip alone with animation. The alar-columella relationship is also assessed to identify the presence of alar retraction or a hanging columella. Fibers of the DSN attach to the mobile medial crura, and animation may distort the columella on animation.

- Basal view evaluation focuses on identifying and classifying columellar deformity. Four types of deformity exist all based on the underlying anatomy.[2] Excess or malpositioned cartilage and/or soft tissue can create a deformity in this area and distort the BALs.[2] Comprehensive evaluation of the nasal base and in particular the medial nasal base (columella) is important when treating the DSN.

IMAGING

- Imaging is typically not utilized for diagnosis of animation deformities.
- 3D imaging is used to discuss existing static deformities and illustrate anticipated surgical results. Many patients with the aforementioned complaints will receive increased tip rotation and placement of a columella strut to stabilize the nasal tip. These potential changes can be illustrated using an imaging system.
- Changes in alar-columellar relationships are also illustrated using the imaging system.

SURGICAL MANAGEMENT

- Proper diagnosis is essential for effective surgical treatment. Treatment of the DSN can be perceived as a static problem, dynamic problem, or both.[2,4]
- Excess muscle volume can disrupt aesthetic ideals of the medial nasal base creating a static lateralization of the BALs. Surgical management focuses on reduction of the DSN and adjacent soft tissue.
- Treatment of dynamic problems is deformity specific. Tip descent is managed with disruption of the DSN and stabilization. Illusion of tip descent is treated with increased rotation and stabilization. A shortened upper lip and/or transverse crease is addressed with treatment of the muscle and mucosal rearrangement.[1]

Preoperative Planning

- A focused discussion is undertaken with the patient to determine concerns. Patients should be educated in regard to limitations of deformity correction. Although all maneuvers are executed to maximize the aesthetic and functional outcome, the face and nose are dynamic, and perfection is rarely achievable.
- Examination of the nose under anesthesia is performed prior to local injection and prepping of the patient. Both visual and tactile examinations of the tip and columella are completed. Palpation of the tip helps to determine support and cartilage integrity. Gentle manipulation of the columella from side to side can help determine caudal septal position and soft tissue volume. The BALs are also inspected (**FIG 1**).

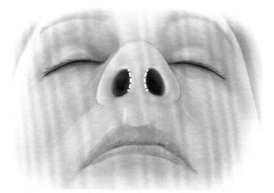

FIG 1 • Illustration of ideal basal aesthetic lines (BALs; *dashed lines*). The BALs should be smooth and exhibit a slight convexity, harmoniously transitioning the upper lip to the nasal tip. Excess soft tissue or cartilage malposition can disrupt this nasal harmony.

Positioning

- Once in the operating room, the patient is intubated and positioned on the table. The most cephalic portion of the head extends just beyond the table. The stretcher may be placed head up to 15 degrees to minimize venous pooling in the operative field. A throat pack is gently placed and removed at surgery end. Local anesthetic with epinephrine is injected into the planned incision sites (**FIG 2**).

Approach

- Though treatment of the DSN can be accomplished through intranasal incisions, the authors prefer an open surgical approach. The transcolumellar incision allows direct visualization and access to the tip and columella tissue. When the operative plan includes lengthening the upper lip and or treating a transverse crease, a transoral incision is also used. Techniques are dependent on the problem being treated as outlined below.

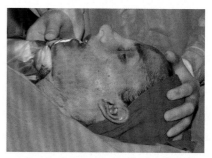

FIG 2 • Photographic example of patient position and exam under anesthesia.

T E C H N I Q U E S

■ Tip Descent

- A transcolumellar incision is made and connected to bilateral infracartilaginous incisions. As the nasal envelope is elevated, soft tissue is detached from the underlying cartilage of the lower lateral cartilages (**TECH FIG 1**). Muscle fibers are directly resected to release any attachment to the medial or domal crura.[5] The tip is well supported with columella strut and tip suturing. Collectively, these maneuvers stabilize the tip and correct the animation deformity. Patients with short upper lip or philtral crease may undergo treatment with transoral incision. When a transoral incision is used, the muscle may be transposed and sutured together with a 4-0 chromic. Alar contour grafts are also commonly used to provide additional support to the ala.

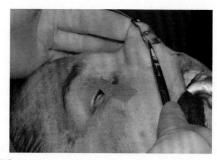

TECH FIG 1 • Demonstration of the transcolumellar incision with direct exposure of the medial crura cartilage.

■ Tip Descent Illusion

- An open surgical approach is performed as described above. Surgical maneuvers to increase tip rotation are

often needed in these patients. Release of the scroll ligament and possible cephalic trim is used with placement of a columella strut to reposition and strengthen the nasal tip (**TECH FIG 2A,B**).

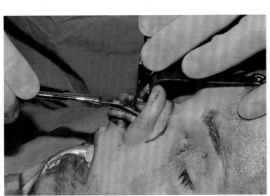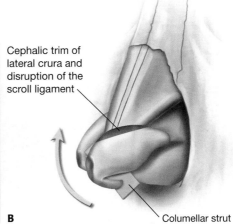

Cephalic trim of lateral crura and disruption of the scroll ligament

Columellar strut

TECH FIG 2 • **A.** Photograph showing release of the scroll ligament. Release of the scroll ligament allows for upward rotation of the nasal tip. **B.** Illustration of nasal tip mechanics. With disruption of the scroll ligament (in isolation or with cephalic trim), the nasal tip can be rotated upward and stabilized with a columellar strut.

■ Short Upper Lip/Transverse Crease

■ A 1-cm horizontal incision is made in the upper labial sulcus centered on the frenulum (**TECH FIG 3A**). Incision is made with pinpoint electrocautery, and dissection is continued until the DSN is identified. The DSN is released near the point of origin (either orbicularis or periosteum). The fibers are then transposed and sutured[1] together with 4-0 chromic (**TECH FIG 3B**).

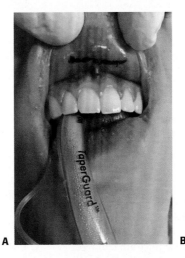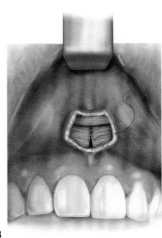

TECH FIG 3 • **A.** Transoral horizontal incision centered on the frenulum. This incision allows access to the DSN and orbicularis fibers. **B.** Illustration of release of the depressor septi nasi muscle and suture fixation.

■ Animation Deformity of the Columella

■ An open surgical approach is performed as described above. The DSN fibers (both superficial to and between the medial crura are resected away from the medial crura (**TECH FIG 4**). It is important to resect at least 2 to 3 mm so that the muscle does not scar back together. If posterior columella animation deformity is present, then any fibers inserting on the footplates are also removed. A columella strut is often placed to fortify tip position and stabilize the columella.

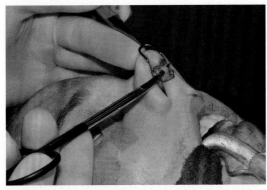

TECH FIG 4 • Photograph illustrating soft tissue that includes DSN fibers traversing the columella. At least 2 to 3 mm of muscle resection is needed to avoid recurrent animation deformity.

■ Columellar Base Deformity

- Excess DSN volume requires resection to recreate the ideal medial nostril and BALs. Through an open approach, this tissue is easily reduced as needed. If footplate flare is abnormal, then a MCFA[3] is also performed (**TECH FIG 5**). This may displace excess soft tissue inferiorly subsequently distorting the alar-columellar relationship. Resection of excess soft tissue avoids this complication.

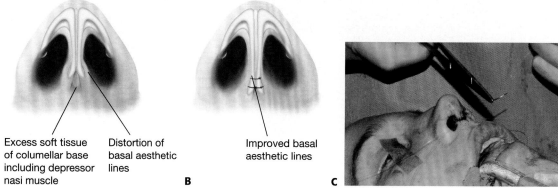

Excess soft tissue of columellar base including depressor nasi muscle   Distortion of basal aesthetic lines   Improved basal aesthetic lines

A   **B**   **C**

TECH FIG 5 • **A.** Premature flare of the medial crura footplates causes distortion of the basal aesthetic lines. **B.** Any excess soft tissue should be resected to prevent inferior displacement during the medial crura footplate approximation. **C.** A combination of gut and PDS sutures is used to approximate the tissue.

PEARLS AND PITFALLS

Patient communication	■ Of utmost importance is communication between the patient and surgeon. An understanding of patient goals is essential for successful rhinoplasty.
Proper diagnosis	■ Proper diagnosis provides the basis for operative planning. This requires a comprehensive evaluation of the face and nose during repose and animation.
Knowledge of relevant anatomy	■ An understanding of the anatomy responsible for existing deformities is crucial. Anatomically based classification systems are particularly useful.
Technique	■ Once the problem has been identified and diagnosed, surgical correction is planned. Understanding the problem is fundamental to correction as all DSN deformities are not treated the same.

POSTOPERATIVE CARE

- Nasal dressing is placed at surgery end. Taping is done to support and minimize swelling of the nasal tip. A nasal splint is also applied. Tape and splint are discontinued at postoperative day 7 when the transcolumellar incision sutures are removed. Patients are started on saline intranasal spray and topical antibacterial ointment for the incision. Once the incision is healed, scar care is initiated and continued for 6 to 12 months.

OUTCOMES

- Resolution of tip deformity with DSN treatment has been well documented in the existing literature.[4] Outcomes regarding nasal base aesthetics are limited. Composite outcomes reported included increased nasolabial angle, lengthened upper lip, improvement of lip crease, narrowed wide nasal base, and improvement in perceived tip descent/animation deformity.

COMPLICATIONS

- Described complications of DSN treatment are uncommon but include transient central upper lip paresthesia and upper lip asymmetry.[4] These typically resolve in 2 to 3 months.[1,4]

One might also expect recurrence of deformity if the muscle is not adequately treated.

REFERENCES

1. Rohrich RJ, Huynh B, Muzaffar AR, et al. Importance of the depressor septi nasi muscle in rhinoplasty: anatomic study and clinical application. *Plast Reconstr Surg.* 2000;105:375-383.
2. Lee MR, Tabbal G, Kurkjian J, et al. Classifying columellar deformities in rhinoplasty. *Plast Reconstr Surg.* 2014;133:464e-470e.
3. Geissler P, Lee MR, Unger J, et al. Reshaping the Medial Nostril and Columellar Base: Five-Step Medial Crural Footplate Approximation. *Plast Reconstr Surg.* 2013;132:553-557.
4. Sinno S, Chang JB, Chaudhry A, et al. Anatomy and management of the depressor septi nasi muscle: a systematic review. *Plast Reconstr Surg.* 2014;134:134-135.
5. Lee MR, Malafa M, Roostaeian J, et al. Soft tissue composition of the columella and potential relevance in rhinoplasty. *Plast Reconstr Surg.* 2014;134:621-625.
6. Kosins AM, Lambros V, Daniel R. The plunging tip: analysis and surgical treatment. *Aesthet Surg J.* 2015;35:367-377.
7. Rohrich RJ, Liu RJ. Defining the infratip lobule in rhinoplasty: anatomy, pathogenesis of abnormalities, and correction using an algorithmic approach. *Plast Reconstr Surg.* 2012;130:1148-1158.

Alar Contour Grafts

Jacob G. Unger and Rod J. Rohrich

DEFINITION

- The alar contour graft (ACG) is a cartilaginous strut utilized in rhinoplasty to strengthen and reinforce the alar rim placed along the alar margin[1] (**FIG 1**).
- ACG is synonymous with alar rim graft.
- Alar retraction is excessive elevation of the alar rim as evidenced from an AP or lateral view with >2 mm of elevation from the long axis of the nostril.[2]
- Alar collapse is a malformation of the rim on basal view that can occur when the lower lateral cartilage (LLC) is congenitally cephalically oriented, resulting in a loss of support along the anterior portion of the alar rim with a subsequent concavity. This deformity may be static, dynamic, or both.
- Alar notching is defined as a sharp angle within the ovular lateral contour. This can extend cephalically and sometimes be referred to as a "parenthesis deformity" or "ball tip."[3,4]

ANATOMY

- ACGs are intimately related to the aesthetics of the alar rim. The ideal alar rim is defined on lateral view by a smooth contour with a slight arch, peaking vertically between the level of the tip defining points and the columellar-lobular angle. Further, the height of the alae should be no higher than 2 mm above or 2 mm below the long axis of the nostril.
- The alar rim is largely composed of thick, lower nasal skin superficially and mucosa internally.
- The lateral crus of the LLC normally runs parallel to the alar rim. The LLC may be cephalically oriented, which predisposes to alar deformity. The orientation of the LLC helps

determine the shape of the ala anteriorly in the area of the soft triangle.
- The posterior half of the alar rim encompasses the alar lobule and is composed entirely of fibrofatty tissue and thick skin.[1,2]

PATIENT HISTORY AND PHYSICAL FINDINGS

- Visual inspection and manual palpation of the nose will indicate if any alar rim deformities are present in the preoperative state. Standard rhinoplasty imaging should be undertaken with AP, lateral, basal, and ¾ views of the nose. Visualization of the lateral crura of the LLC through the skin envelope can help diagnose a more vertical orientation, which may portend a higher risk of future alar deformities.
- Forced inspiration through the nares will uncover any dynamic external nasal valve collapse or evidence of alar collapse.

IMAGING

- No imaging is necessary or indicated to prepare for alar rim deformity correction with ACG.
- Three-dimensional imaging may be useful as a preoperative planning and patient communication tool. Caution is advised not to "lower" the alar position with a computer program if one does not feel that this is a consistently reproducible surgical outcome in his or her hands. However, this imaging may help educate patients how reinforcement of alar retraction or collapse with ACG may be very useful, as well as indicating changes in alar-columellar relationships.

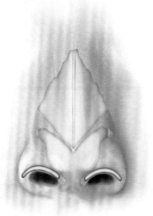
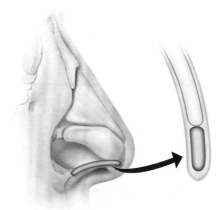

FIG 1 • Alar contour grafts.

SURGICAL MANAGEMENT

- It is crucial that the correct diagnosis is made to ensure the most accurate surgical treatment. Most crucially, if the patient has had severe mucosal loss and shortening due to previous surgery, this must be disseminated to the patient. This is a much more difficult problem to correct and may require mucosal grafts or other interventions beyond placing ACGs.
- In a virgin nose, alar retraction, notching, and collapse, both static and dynamic, can be treated with operative placement of ACGs. It is important to note the position of the LLCs as well. If they are cephalically oriented, some inferior repositioning may be indicated as well using lateral crural strut grafts or other techniques.

PREOPERATIVE PLANNING

- A discussion regarding the patients' concerns of lower nasal shape and alar position should be undertaken. The patient must understand that although this maneuver has a powerful impact on alar position and deformity correction, there is a definite possibility of only partial correction or asymmetry.
- Examination under anesthesia is performed prior to local injection and intranasal oxymetazoline-soaked pledget placement. This examination will help ensure that there is no internal mucosal shortage or scarring that can add to any alar deformity.

Positioning

- The patient is intubated and positioned on the table supine. The most cephalic portion of the head extends just beyond the table. One may choose to place the patient slightly asymmetrically on the table with the head and body closer to the edge of the bed to the surgeon's dominant hand side. If needed or desired, one may utilize a "head-up" position to 15 degrees to minimize venous pooling in the operative field.

Approach

- Although placement of ACG can be accomplished through medial or lateral approach, the authors prefer an open, medial approach. The transcolumellar, infracartilaginous incisions allow direct visualization and access to the desired location of the grafts. A laterally based approach through a radial incision within the base of the lobule on the mucosal side can be utilized but has the added difficulty of challenging angles of dissection and placement, as well as confirmation of the depth of placement.

T E C H N I Q U E S

■ Open, Medial Placement (Preferred Technique)

- A stair-step transcolumellar incision with bilateral infracartilaginous incisions is used to open the soft tissue envelope.
- The placement of the ACGs is performed at the end of the procedure, immediately prior to closing, because these grafts are delicate and can tend to become misplaced or fracture during soft tissue envelope manipulation.
- First choice cartilage is septal cartilage because it can be harvested within the primary surgical field, but an ear or rib cartilage graft may be used if septum is unavailable. A double hook is utilized to place traction on the soft triangle/columellar region to create tension for accurate dissection.
- The ACG pocket is carefully dissected between the vestibular and nasal skin below the infracartilaginous incision by using long, sharp Stevens scissors.
- The pocket should be carried down into the alar lobule and ideally to the level of the alar base.

- This dissection will secure the pocket for graft placement.
- Once the grafts are placed into their pockets, the nasal skin is redraped for closure.
- Any excess cartilage extruding medially from the pocket is resected[1,2] (**TECH FIG 1**; Video 1).

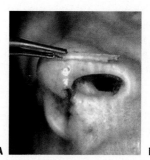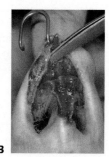

TECH FIG 1 ● **A.** Planned location for placement of ACG. **B.** Dissection of pocket for ACG placement.

■ Lateral Placement—Open Approach

- This technique helps placing the ACG via a radial incision within the alar base/alar lobule.
- A no. 15 blade is used to create a 0.5-cm incision in the base mucosa.
- Use a double hook to extend the alar rim laterally and create tension for dissection of a pocket.

- Carefully place Stevens scissors into the incision and spread, aiming toward the soft triangle until the tips are visible within the space at the edge of the infracartilaginous incision at the level of the soft triangle.
- Place the grafts from lateral to medial and excise the excess cartilage at the lateral margin of the incision.

■ Closed Approach

- This is a blind technique that requires extensive experience in rhinoplasty prior to attempt and has high risk for misplacement or asymmetric placement.
- Once the domes of the LLC have been delivered and there is a medial pocket rostral to the soft triangle, careful dissection with Stevens or Converse scissors is used to create a pocket along the alar margin between the mucosal and skin envelope.

- This requires bimanual palpation and constant checking to ensure accurate pocket dissection.
- Ensure dissection laterally to the same position bilaterally with palpation of scissor tips at the same position on each side.
- Place the grafts in the same manner and excise the excess medially.

PEARLS AND PITFALLS

Asymmetry	■ It is important to note that although alar contour grafts are not large (measuring on average 2 to 3 mm in width and 1.5 cm in length), they must be of equivalent size, strength, and design. If the grafts are not nearly identical in both dimension and strength, these powerful grafts can cause tip deviation toward the weak side or asymmetric alar contour upon healing.
Avoid nasal skin buttonhole	■ Use curved Stevens scissors with tips pointing toward the mucosal side at all times. This provides an anatomic dissection and ensures that if a rent is created in the soft tissue envelope, it is on the more forgiving mucosal side.
Difficulty of placement	■ Cut the leading edge of the graft on an angle of 30 to 45 degrees for an atraumatic advancement of the graft into the pocket. Undue force on the graft upon placement can result in fracture of this delicate graft.

POSTOPERATIVE CARE

- Nasal dressing is placed at surgery end.
  - Bacitracin-soaked 1 × 1 cm surgical squares are used to support the soft triangle where no suture is placed to avoid a teardrop nostril apex.
  - Taping is done to support and minimize swelling of the nasal tip.
  - A Denver nasal splint is also applied. Doyle splints are also commonly applied after septoplasty.
- Tape and splints are removed at postoperative day 7 when the transcolumellar incision sutures are removed.
  - Patients are started on saline intranasal spray and topical antibacterial ointment for the incision.
- Patients are encouraged to keep head of bed elevated while sleeping for the first 2 weeks to improve edema.
- No nose blowing for 2 weeks postoperatively
- Exercise is reintroduced on a graduated scale, beginning with light exercise at 2 weeks, heavy exercise (ie, jogging) at 4 weeks, and heavy lifting allowed and inverted maneuvers (ie, yoga head stands, etc.) at 6 weeks.

OUTCOMES

- Outcomes are well documented in the literature showing improvement in alar position, external nasal valve function, as well as prevention of postoperative alar complications such as collapse, notching, and retraction.[2,5,6]

COMPLICATIONS

- Complications related to ACG are minimal. It is a low-risk maneuver used to improve alar aesthetics and prevent complications. One must be cautious to avoid placing asymmetric grafts because this could influence tip position and cause asymmetry of tip position.

REFERENCES

1. Rohrich RJ, Raniere J Jr, Ha RY. The alar contour graft: correction and prevention of alar rim deformities in rhinoplasty. *Plast Reconstr Surg.* 2002;109(7):2495-2505.
2. Unger JG et al. Alar contour grafts in rhinoplasty: a safe and reproducible way to refine alar contour aesthetics. *Plast Reconstr Surg.* 2016;137(1):52-61.
3. Constantian MB. The boxy nasal tip, the ball tip, and alar cartilage malposition: variations on a theme—a study in 200 consecutive primary and secondary rhinoplasty patients. *Plast Reconstr Surg.* 2005;116(1):268-281.
4. Toriumi DM. New concepts in nasal tip contouring. *Arch Facial Plast Surg.* 2006;8(3):156-185.
5. Guyuron B. Alar rim deformities. *Plast Reconstr Surg.* 2001;107(3):856-863.
6. Guyuron B, Bigdeli Y, and Sajjadian A, Dynamics of the alar rim graft. *Plast Reconstr Surg.* 2015;135(4):981-986.

71
CHAPTER

Techniques for Treating Nasal Airway Obstruction

Michael R. Lee

DEFINITION

- Nasal airway obstruction (NAO) is a clinical diagnosis established through a focused history and physical examination. All patients undergoing rhinoplasty should be assessed for NAO.
- The external nasal valve is located at the nostril. Nasal ala forms the lateral aspect of the valve, whereas the columella makes up the medial portion. Collectively, these structures with the soft triangle create the external valve.
- The internal nasal valve is formed by the junction of the caudal portion of the upper lateral cartilage with the dorsal nasal septum.
- Nasal septum is the anatomic structure that divides the nasal cavity. Made of bone and cartilage, the septum provides support for the nasal dorsum and tip.
- Inferior turbinates are paired bones that extend medial into that nasal cavity from the lateral nasal wall. Turbinates regulate nasal airflow characteristics and provide mucociliary clearance.

ANATOMY

- NAO typically occurs at one of four areas:
  - External nasal valves
  - Internal nasal valves
  - Nasal septum
  - Inferior turbinates
- Understanding the anatomy of these structures is fundamental to treating NAO in rhinoplasty.
- The external nasal valve relies on structural support of the lower lateral cartilages and adjacent soft tissue.
  - Lateral support is provided by fibrofatty tissue of the nasal ala and structural integrity of the lateral crura.
  - Medial support is provided by the caudal septum, medial crura, and soft tissue of the columella.[1]
  - The term basal aesthetic lines (BALs) is used to describe this lateral border of the columella. BALs should exhibit a smooth slightly concave slope with no protrusion into the nostril (**FIG 1A**).
- Each upper lateral cartilage is supported cephalically by the nasal bone, laterally by the frontal process of the maxilla, and medially by the dorsal nasal septum.
  - As form and function are closely related in rhinoplasty, structurally sound middle nose anatomy is usually associated with ideal dorsal aesthetic lines (DALs).[2]
  - Confluence of the caudal upper lateral cartilage and dorsal nasal septum is most often a site of NAO as it forms the internal nasal valve.
  - The internal nasal valve is the area of greatest restriction in terms of nasal airflow (**FIG 1B**).

- The nasal septum provides crucial support for the external nose.
  - Seated firmly on the maxillary nasal spine, the septum provides support for the overlying upper and lower lateral nasal cartilages.
  - The dorsal septum is responsible for creation of the internal nasal valve.
  - The caudal septum extends beyond the maxillary nasal spine and provides structural support for the medial nasal base.
  - It is flanked by medial crura and intimately related to soft tissue structures of the columella.[1]
- The inferior turbinate extends from the lateral nasal wall into the lower nasal cavity.
  - Its proximity to the internal nasal valve makes hypertrophy problematic when present.
  - Although turbinate architecture is primarily a function of the bone, the overlying erectile tissue and surface mucosa contribute greatly to nasal function.
  - Erectile tissue fluctuates, thereby altering nasal resistance, and directly influences nasal airflow.
  - The respiratory mucosa provides immunologic benefit and mucociliary clearance.

DIFFERENTIAL DIAGNOSIS

- Stenosis/collapse of the external nasal valve
- Stenosis/collapse of the internal nasal valve
- Septal deviation
- Septal spur formation
- Inferior turbinate hypertrophy
- Nasal mass or polyp

PATHOGENESIS

- Intranasal deformity may result from congenital development, traumatic injury, or iatrogenic insult. Changes in nasal support and physiology may occur with aging resulting in NAO.
- Traumatic injury to the nasal septum may be classified by fracture patterns.[3]
  - High-impact trauma is associated with multiple septal fractures and displacement from the maxillary nasal spine.

PATIENT HISTORY AND PHYSICAL FINDINGS

- Relevant history in the obstructed patient includes laterality, timing and duration, worsening or alleviating factors, perennial or seasonal response, prior nasal surgery or trauma, and associated symptoms.

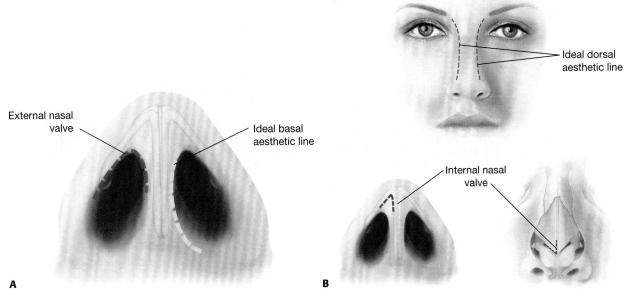

FIG 1 • A. Diagram of the external nasal valve. Nasal ala constitutes the lateral valve, whereas the columella creates the medial aspect. Note the ideal basal aesthetic line. **B.** Diagram of the internal nasal valve. Amalgamation of the caudal edge of the upper lateral cartilage to the dorsal septum creates the valve. Note the ideal dorsal aesthetic line.

- Progressively worsening symptoms and associated epistaxis should raise concern for neoplasm.
- Inspection of the nasal airway begins with study of the nasal base at rest and during respiration.
- The external valve is assessed initially.
  - Inspection should reveal a patent nostril, free of obstruction.
  - At rest, the lateral nostril (nasal ala) should demonstrate a stable, convex architecture.
  - The medial nostril (lateral columella) should exhibit ideal BALs.
  - External valve stenosis may be the result of obstruction from either of these directions.
  - Assessment during respiration is also performed to determine if collapse of the external valve is responsible for symptoms.
- Inspection of the internal nasal valve is accomplished with a nasal speculum. Care must be used to avoid widening of the valve on speculum insertion.
  - The upper lateral cartilage caudal margin can be readily appreciated through the nasal mucosa.
  - The angle created by the junction of this caudal margin and the dorsal septum is assessed.
    - A narrow angle at baseline suggests stenosis of the valve.
  - Collapse of the internal valve on respiration may also be identified as a cause for NAO. The Cottle test can confirm internal valve insufficiency.
- Evaluation of the septum also begins at the nasal base.
  - Deviation of the caudal septum to either side can obstruct the external valve.
  - Palpation and manipulation of the columella will clearly identify caudal septum position.
  - Examining the dorsal septum and septal body is performed with nasal speculum.
  - Deviation of the dorsal septum is determined as this may cause stenosis of the internal nasal valve.
  - The body of the nasal septum is surveyed for deviation and spur formation, either of which may cause NAO.

- The inferior turbinate is next examined also with use of a speculum.
  - Turbinate size, position, and tissue characteristics should be noted.
  - A large, boggy inferior turbinate with a bluish hue is associated with allergic response. These patients will likely have some degree of refractory symptom despite surgical reduction.
  - The location of turbinate hypertrophy guides surgical reduction and should be noted.
- Topical oxymetazoline is applied to determine the response to medical decongestant.
  - If topical treatment results in symptom resolution, a medical management trial is warranted. This often includes topical steroids and routine nasal toilet.
- Intranasal examination should also rule out less common etiologies of nasal obstruction such as nasal polyps and neoplasms.

IMAGING

- Although plain radiographs and computed topography can be used to evaluate nasal septum and turbinate position, they are not routinely required. NAO is a clinical diagnosis that results primarily from a focused history and physical examination.
- If concerns arise of other NAO causes, such as neoplasms or polyps, proper consultation and imaging are warranted.

NONOPERATIVE MANAGEMENT

- Patients who display any suggestion of an allergic component to their NAO should undergo a medical trial.
- Patients with allergic rhinitis are typically treated with reduced exposure to allergens, nasal irrigation with saline sprays, nasal steroids, and occasionally oral antihistamines.
  - Severe cases may benefit from immunotherapy.
  - Otolaryngology consult should be considered.

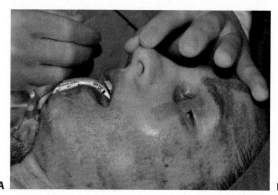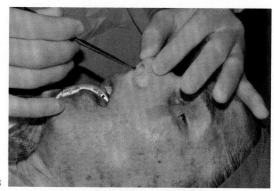

FIG 2 • A. Palpation and inspection of the nose can provide information on tip support. **B.** Help determine caudal septal position.

- Reassessment of these patients after 6 weeks of medical treatment should then be performed.
- If symptoms persist in the presence of obvious physical obstruction(s), surgical correction of the airway should be considered.

SURGICAL MANAGEMENT

- Surgeons should approach the nasal airway in a methodical manner.
- Preoperative assessment identifies the areas of concern as listed above.
- A detailed operative plan should be outlined to correct each of these problematic sites.
- Surgeons should be cognizant of the potential to create iatrogenic obstruction and avoid such sequelae.

Preoperative Planning

- Following proper diagnosis, patients are to be educated on anticipated outcomes.
  - Structural deformities of the nasal valves, septum, and turbinates are easily corrected with septorhinoplasty.
  - However, patients with any physiologic component to their NAO should be counseled about potentially persistent symptoms.
- Examination of the nose under anesthesia is performed prior to local injection and prepping of the patient.
  - Both visual and tactile examination of the tip and columella is completed (**FIG 2A**).
  - Palpation of the tip helps to determine support and cartilage integrity.
  - Gentle manipulation of the columella from side to side can help determine caudal septal position and soft tissue volume (**FIG 2B**).

Positioning

- Once in the operating room, the patient is intubated and positioned on the table.

- The most cephalic portion of the head extends just beyond the table.
- The stretcher may be placed head up to 15 degrees to minimize venous pooling in the operative field (**FIG 3**).
- A throat pack is gently placed and removed at surgery conclusion.
- Local anesthetic with epinephrine is injected into the planned incision sites.

Approach

- Treatment of the nasal airway can be accomplished through an open or closed rhinoplasty.
  - A closed approach is often used to improve alar support with grafts,[4] correct deviation of the septal body, and treat inferior turbinate hypertrophy.
  - The open approach rhinoplasty provides better visualization to the dorsal septum and internal nasal valve.
- The following techniques will be described as if all areas of the nasal airway are being corrected during an open approach septorhinoplasty.

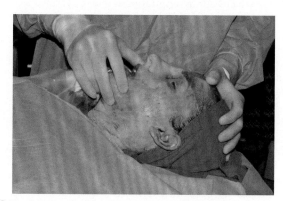

FIG 3 • Positioning of the patient for septorhinoplasty.

Septoplasty

- A transcolumellar incision is connected to bilateral infracartilaginous incisions to open the nasal envelope, exposing the nasal bones and cartilages.
- Dissection is continued to the anterior septal angle.
- Bilateral mucosal flaps are elevated away from septal cartilage and bone.
  - It is of the utmost importance to dissect directly on the surface of the septum as it is a bloodless plane.
- Once there is broad exposure of the septum, the upper lateral cartilages are separated from the dorsal septum.
- Prior to resecting the septal body, it is necessary to perform any planned reduction of dorsal or caudal septum.

- This sequence ensures that at least 1 to 1.5 cm of L strut can be preserved for nasal support.
- With preservation of adequate L strut, the deviated septum or spur can be resected (**TECH FIG 1A**).
- A Cottle elevator is used not only to elevate the septal flaps but to disarticulate the bony cartilaginous junction.
  - There is significant variation in bony cartilaginous junction patterns.[3]
- Using scalpel, the marked septum is resected.
  - This cartilage can be used to create spreader grafts and alar contour grafts.
- At the end of surgery, the mucosal flaps are placed together using a weaving transmural septal suture (**TECH FIG 1B**).

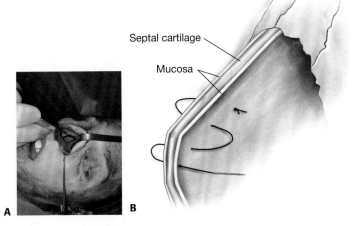

TECH FIG 1 • A. Preservation of adequate septal support is crucial. It is equally important to ensure preserved caudal septum rest sufficiently on the maxillary spine. **B.** Illustration of a weaving septal suture to approximate the septal mucosal flaps. Most commonly, a gut suture on a straight needle is used.

Internal Nasal Valve Repair

- Spreader grafts are an effective method of repair for internal nasal valve stenosis or collapse.
- Once the upper lateral cartilages are separated from the dorsal septum (**TECH FIG 2A**), grafts can be readily placed and secured.
- Graft length requires that they extend from underneath the nasal bones to the level of the internal valve. This can easily be measured when creating the grafts.

- Graft width is often 2 to 3 mm but may be balanced with aesthetic goals.
- If widening of the middle nose is to be avoided, grafts may be placed lower, thus allowing the upper lateral cartilages to advance over the grafts and join the dorsal septum (**TECH FIG 2B**).
- Once in position, the grafts are sutured with 6-0 polydioxanone suture.

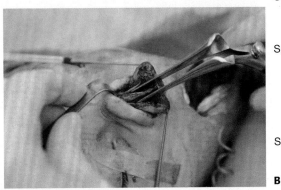
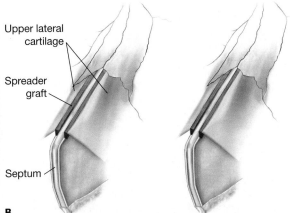

TECH FIG 2 • A. Separation of the upper lateral cartilages from the dorsal septum is required to place an internal nasal valve spreader graft. The overall goal is to widen the valve angle and increase support during respiration. **B.** Spreader grafts should extend from underneath the nasal bones to the internal nasal valve. They may be positioned lower if widening of the middle nose is of great concern.

■ External Nasal Valve Repair

- Repair of the lateral external valve involves fortification of the nasal ala.
  - Several different cartilage grafts have been described, but the alar contour graft [4] is suitable for most situations.
  - These grafts are typically created 2 mm wide and 8 to 10 mm in length.
- The ala is then carefully retracted with a double-prong skin hook.
  - Fine scissors are used to create a pocket just cephalic to the alar rim margin (**TECH FIG 3A**).
- Repair of the medial external nasal valve involves classifying the existing deformity.[5]
  - These deformities may be abnormal volume and/or position of the caudal septum, medial crura, and columellar soft tissue.[1]

- The caudal septum can be freed from adjacent soft tissue and inspected.
- Straightening of a deviated caudal septum may be accomplished with excision when appropriate.
  - If excision is not a viable option, scoring and repositioning to the midline with suture fixation are performed.
- Abnormal or premature medial crura footplate flare is corrected using the medical crura footplate approximation (MCFA).[6]
  - The MCFA includes making stab incisions at the site of footplate flare.
  - Then, the footplates are weaved together with polydioxanone suture, after which the incisions are closed (**TECH FIG 3B**).
- Understanding tissue dynamics of the lower lateral cartilages is important when influencing medial crura shape and position.[7]

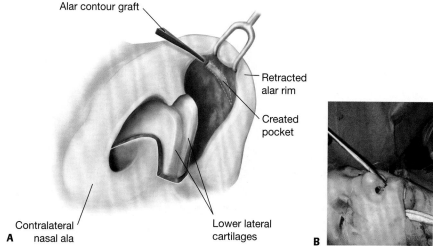

Alar contour graft

Retracted alar rim

Created pocket

Contralateral
A   nasal ala

Lower lateral cartilages

B

TECH FIG 3 • A. Alar contour grafts are a reliable way to improve structural support of the lateral external nasal valve. **B.** Treating a base deformity of the columella with the MCFA can help widen the nasal valve and create ideal BALs.

■ Turbinoplasty

- When treating hypertrophy of the inferior turbinate, the goals are tissue reduction and preservation of function.
- A scalpel is used to make an incision on the anterior surface of the inferior turbinate.
- The incision is carried posterior to the extent that allows introduction of bone-removing forceps.
- An elevator is used to dissect the overlying soft tissue away from turbinate bone.
- Bone and possibly erectile tissue in the location of obstruction are then removed.
- The wound is irrigated and the mucosa laid back into native position.
- The flap can be sutured back into place when needed.
- Submucosal resection (turbinoplasty) allows for bulk reduction to increase nasal airflow while preserving crucial mucosal function.
- An elevator is then used to lateralize both inferior turbinates (**TECH FIG 4**). This move should be highly controlled.

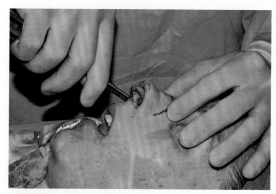

TECH FIG 4 • Following resection of excess bone and erectile tissue, the turbinate is outfractured in a controlled manner.

PEARLS AND PITFALLS

Relevant anatomy	▪ Understand the four common sites responsible for nasal obstruction: (1) external nasal valves, (2) internal nasal valves, (3) nasal septum, and (4) inferior turbinates.
Proper diagnosis	▪ Perform a focused history and physical to determine if NAO is a structural problem, physiologic problem, or combination.
Nasal valve physiology	▪ Repair of nasal valves (internal and internal) often involves structural strengthening with cartilage grafts.
Comprehensive septal assessment	▪ Evaluation of the septum requires attention to the (1) dorsal septum, (2) caudal septum, and (3) septal body.
Principles of turbinate technique	▪ Goals of turbinate hypertrophy treatment include reduction of tissue bulk with preservation of mucosal function.

POSTOPERATIVE CARE

▪ Functional reconstruction of the nasal airway typically requires placement of intranasal splints in addition to external splint.

▪ Splinting of the nasal airway provides additional support for the internal nasal valves and nasal septum. Moreover, the splints stabilize the lateralized turbinate and may circumvent adhesion formation between raw surfaces.

▪ The splints are removed at 1 week, and saline nasal sprays are continued for the next 4 weeks.

OUTCOMES

▪ Nasal valve reconstruction with spreader and alar grafts has been shown to be highly effective in treating nasal obstruction.

▪ Septoplasty, while effective for treatment of deviation in most patients, has been shown to be less satisfactory in those patients who also have allergic rhinitis.

▪ Turbinoplasty via submucosal resection has been shown to lower nasal resistance and preserve mucosal function.

COMPLICATIONS

▪ Nasal valve repair may be complicated by graft malposition and associated deformity.
  ▪ This may manifest as dorsal irregularity in the case of spreader grafts or alar/soft triangle deformity with alar contour grafts.

▪ Inferior malposition of spreader grafts may actually worsen nasal obstruction if they occlude the nasal valve.

▪ Septal surgery may be associated with perforation from injury to opposing mucosal surfaces.

▪ Adhesion formation may occur when two opposing raw surfaces are created.

▪ Epistaxis and recurrent symptoms are also potential complications of nasal airway surgery.

REFERENCES

1. Lee MR, Malafa M, Roostaeian J, et al. Soft tissue composition of the columella and potential relevance in rhinoplasty. *Plast Reconstr Surg.* 2014;134:621-625.
2. Roostaeian J, Unger JG, Lee MR, et al. Reconstitution of the nasal dorsum following component dorsal reduction in primary rhinoplasty. *Plast Reconstr Surg.* 2014;133:509-518.
3. Lee MR, Inman J, Callahan S, Ducic Y. Fracture patterns of the nasal septum. *Otolaryngol Head Neck Surg.* 2010;143:784.
4. Unger JG, Roostaeian J, Small KH, et al. Alar contour grafts in rhinoplasty: a safe and reproducible way to refine alar contour aesthetics. *Plast Reconstr Surg.* 2015;137:52-61.
5. Lee MR, Tabbal G, Kurkijan J, et al. Classifying columellar deformities in rhinoplasty. *Plast Reconstr Surg.* 2014;133:464e.
6. Geissler P, Lee MR, Unger J, et al. Reshaping the medial nostril and columellar base: five-step medial crural footplate approximation. *Plast Reconstr Surg.* 2013;132:553-557.
7. Lee MR, Geissmer P, Cochran S, et al. Decreasing nasal tip projection in rhinoplasty. *Plast Reconstr Surg.* 2014;134:41e-49e.

72
CHAPTER

Section XII: Facial Skeletal Augmentation with Implants

Chin Augmentation With Implant

Daniel A. Cuzzone and Barry M. Zide

DEFINITION

- Chin augmentation encompasses genioplasty with the use of mandibular osteotomies as well as placement of implants in the form of grafts or alloplastic materials. Herein we do not discuss osteotomies.
- The chin is a defining feature of the lower one-third of the face that connotes a sense of strength to the face.
- Correction of microgenia is desired in about 20% to 25% of patients undergoing rhinoplasty, with the goal of balanced facial symmetry.
- Implant-based augmentation of the chin may be performed with a variety of implant-based materials, each with its own set of benefits and perceived deficiencies (TABLE 1).
- Osteotomies to advance the lower border of the symphysis may accomplish the same thing, but the risks and benefits of each are not described herein.

ANATOMY

- The chin, as an anatomical subunit, is composed of the sublabial area and the pad.
- The mental nerve is the terminal branch of the inferior alveolar nerve. It is a branch of the third division of the trigeminal nerve and is responsible for sensation of the lower lip, portions of the chin pad, and menton (**FIG 1A**, blue area) except for a small area that is supplied by a sensory branch off the nerve to the mylohyoid (see **FIG 1A**, pink area; **FIG 1B**).
- The location of the mental foramen can be variable (**FIG 2**).
- Anatomical studies have demonstrated that the mental foramen is located inferior to the second mandibular premolar in about 50% of adults, between the first and second premolar in 25%, and posterior to the second premolar in 25% of the remaining population.
- It is located about halfway between the alveolar ridge and the inferior border of the mandible (8 to 10 mm from the inferior border) and is between 2 and 3 cm lateral to the midline.

- It may be lower in vertically short height mandibles.
- The mentalis muscles are paired mimetic muscles that elevate and compress the chin against the anterior mandible and indirectly raise the lower lip (**FIG 3**).

PATHOGENESIS

- Congenital and acquired factors may contribute the most to a hypoplastic mentum.
  - Aging
- Dentures that cause trauma to the mentalis origin may lead to soft tissue ptosis and poor projection.

PATIENT HISTORY AND PHYSICAL FINDINGS

- A pertinent history and physical exam are instrumental in optimal operative outcomes and should include an appreciation for the patient's aesthetic goals, history of prior facial surgery, or orthodontic/orthognathic treatment, and a comprehensive facial examination.
- Point by point assessment of the lower third of the face[1-3]
  - Lip eversion and position
  - Occlusion
  - Static chin pad thickness (normal 9 to 14 mm)
  - Labiomental fold depth and height
  - Dynamic chin pad motion while smiling (the pad may be effaced and in some cases may descend)
  - Symphyseal narrowness
- Assessment of lip position should be noted.
  - Normal interlabial gap is up to 3.5 mm.
  - Normal lower incisal show at rest is 2 to 3 mm.
  - Normal upper incisor show is up to 3.5 mm in males and up to 5.5 in females.
- Lower facial height should be noted. Sagittal implant projection will give the face a longer appearance; conversely, if the chin is deficient sagittally but long, an implant will not work well.
- Symmetry of the chin should be noted as well as skin irregularities.[4]

Table 1 Implant Subtypes and Characteristics

Material	Trade Name	Tissue Interface	Pros	Cons	Complications
Polydimethylsiloxane	Silastic (silicone rubber)	Fibrous capsule	Easily carved, easily placed and removed	Bone resorption (if too high), seroma, exposure	Malposition, extrusion, infection (may be salvaged)
High-density porous polyethylene	MEDPOR Su-Por	Limited tissue ingrowth	Versatile	Difficult to remove; requires hardware	Malposition, extrusion, infection (not salvageable)

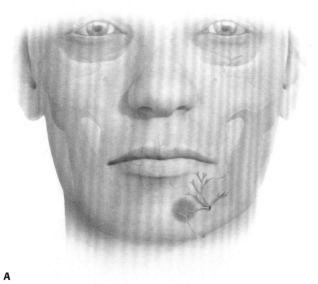 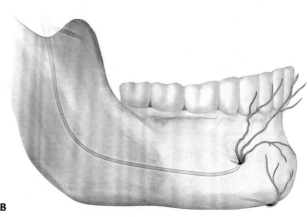

A   **B**

FIG 1 • **A.** Sensory distribution of the mental nerve seen in blue and the contribution of the sensory branch of the never to the mylohyoid in pink. **B.** Course of the sensory branch off the nerve to the mylohyoid (denoted by the *dotted white circle*).

- Dimpling may be seen after previous surgery, injury, or facial lesion such as Bell palsy.
- Assess in repose and during animation both from the frontal and profile view.
- When the chin symphysis is narrow, bony advancement may be inadvisable vs prosthetic augmentation.
- Dental occlusion
  - Prominent teeth may evert the lower lip, producing a more acute labiomental fold. A vertically high implant may worsen this. Also, a skeletally deep bite may seem to shorten the face with the occlusion, allowing the upper teeth to push the lower lip forward.

IMAGING

- High-definition preoperative photography is important for photo documentation and for perioperative planning.
- Views that should be obtained include frontal and lateral, with and without smile. The smile view shows how the chin pad moves dynamically.
- Radiographic evaluation is often reserved for secondary surgical procedures, with short mandibles where the mental foramina may be low, or to evaluate prior hardware.

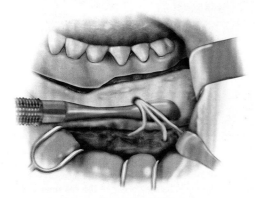

FIG 2 • Mental nerve as it exits from the mental foramen in the body of the mandible at about the level of the second premolar.

IMPLANT SELECTION

- Ideally, only small and medium silicone implants should be utilized because the larger ones tend to result in more erosion.

SURGICAL MANAGEMENT

Preoperative Planning

- Single oral or intravenous dose of antibiotic is provided as per the surgeon's preference.
- Implant-based chin augmentation can be performed under local anesthesia with oral sedation or with intravenous sedation with proper supervision.
- For intraoral placement, Peridex is prescribed starting 2 days prior to surgery, and a presurgical Betadine rinse with a few drops of peppermint oil may be helpful as a prep.

Positioning

- Supine with neck extension, which can be achieved with the use of a shoulder roll

Approach

- Chin augmentation can be performed either through an external submental incision or via an intraoral incision at the gingivolabial sulcus.
  - At least a 2.5- to 3.5-cm incision is needed for porous implants.
- External submental incisions allow more control regarding implant placement, and the incision can be used for cervical procedures.
- Intraoral incisions eliminate a visible scar, but the problem of asymmetric intraoral placement (especially with silicone) or improper placement level may lead to more resorption.
  - Implant placement is technically more difficult.
  - A 2-layered closure is required (muscle and mucosa).
  - The incision can be designed vertically or horizontally.
- Single or two-piece implants (usually porous) may be utilized. Two-piece implants have flexibility in design and accommodates to the shape of the patients. With intraoral placement of a porous implant, the incision must be larger and intraoral rinse prep is required.

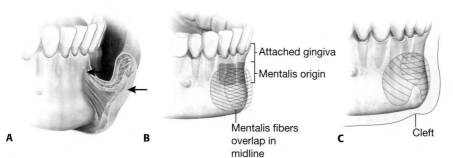

FIG 3 • **A.** The upper part of the mentalis muscle contains horizontally directed fibers that stabilize the lower lip (*arrow*). The oblique lower fibers allow the lip to pout. **B.** The mentalis muscle is a paired muscle that elevates and compresses the lip. **C.** It may have many configurations, ranging from complete overlap to divergence leading to a cleftlike appearance of the chin.

TECHNIQUES

■ External (Submental) Approach to Chin Augmentation

Markings

- The facial midline is marked extending from the chin pad to the submental area.
- A submental incision roughly 3.5 (for porous polyethylene) or 1.5 cm (for silicone) is marked near or in the submental crease (**TECH FIG 1**).
- Bilateral inferior alveolar nerve blocks are performed using 1% lidocaine with 1:100 000 of epinephrine, with or without bupivacaine.
- The submental incision and preperiosteal space are injected with a 50:50 mixture of 1% lidocaine and 0.5% bupivacaine with 1:100 000 epinephrine.

Porous Polyethylene Implant Precontouring

- While the local anesthetic takes effect, the implant is precontoured.
- The upper portion is pared down (30%–50%) using a bur or knife (**TECH FIG 2A,B**).
  - Note: Su-Por is softer and easier to carve.
- The lateral wings are reduced and tapered as necessary (**TECH FIG 2C**).
- The upper edge anteriorly is tapered at a 45-degree angle using a bur (**TECH FIG 2D**).
- The implant is divided in half, and a pilot hole is drilled in each side, 3 to 5 mm from midline (**TECH FIG 2E**).

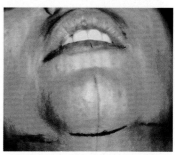

TECH FIG 1 • Marking the facial midline, from labiomental fold to hyoid, and the intended incision. (From Warren SM, Spector JA, Zide BM. Chin surgery VII: the textured secured implant—a recipe for success. *Plast Reconstr Surg.* 2007;120(5):1378-1385, with permission.)

- A second hole may or may not be necessary between the first hole and the end of the implant.

Incision and Exposure

- A no. 10 or 15 blade is used to incise and deepen the submental incision to the inferior border.
- Needle electrocautery dissection is usually employed down through the subcutaneous tissue to the periosteum. The soft tissue should be cleared from the mandibular border from canine to canine with cautery (**TECH FIG 3A**).
- A periosteal elevator is used to elevate the periosteum, and at the end of the dissection, the elevator is lifted to open the pocket farther (**TECH FIG 3B**).

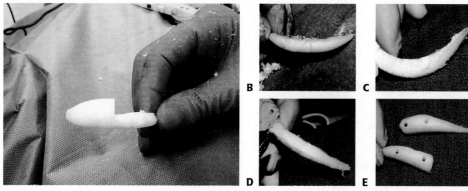

TECH FIG 2 • **A,B.** The upper 30% to 50% of the textured implant is removed so that the implant will provide projection only at the pogonion. **C.** The lateral projection of the textured implant is trimmed and then tapered. **D.** Returning to the upper portion of the implant, a bur is used to taper the upper edge at a 45-degree angle. **E.** The implant is divided in the midline, and two drill holes are placed in each half of the implant. The first drill hole is approximately 3 mm from the midline, and the second drill hole is halfway between the first hole and the end of the implant. (**B–E:** From Warren SM, Spector JA, Zide BM. Chin surgery VII: the textured secured implant—a recipe for success. *Plast Reconstr Surg.* (2007);120(5):1378-1385, with permission.)

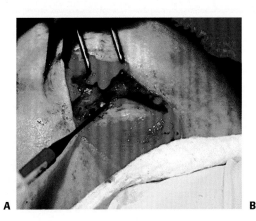
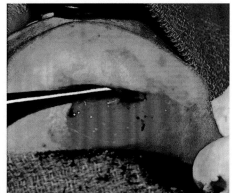
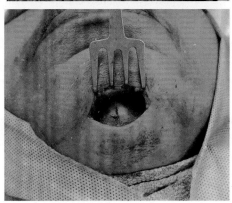

TECH FIG 3 • A. Electrocautery is used to clear the mandibular border from canine to canine, and then a periosteal elevator is used to complete the distal pocket. **B.** At the most distal extent of the dissection, the elevator is levered up to complete the pocket. **C.** A sterile no. 2 pencil is a good way to mark the midline. (**A,B:** From Warren SM, Spector JA, Zide BM. Chin surgery VII: the textured secured implant—a recipe for success. *Plast Reconstr Surg.* 2007;120(5): 1378-1385, with permission.)

- Subperiosteal dissection is continued laterally with care not to injure the mental neurovascular bundle that may be viewed. Lateral dissection as required from the midline is performed.
- This dissection is repeated on the contralateral side.
- The midline is marked on the menton using electrocautery, bur, drill, or a sterile pencil (**TECH FIG 3C**).

Implant Placement

- The left or right half of the implant is inserted into its respective pocket, and the central portion is aligned with the midline of the menton.
- According to implant thickness, titanium screws are used for fixation medially.
  - The medial screw is placed through the predrilled pilot hole and partially tightened to allow the lateral part to be positioned.

- The lateral screw placement holds the implant along the inferior border.
- Both screws are tightened and countersunk so that the screw head is below the surface of the implant (**TECH FIG 4A**).
- By only partially tightening the medial screw first, the implant position laterally can be decided perfectly.
- This procedure is repeated on the contralateral side (**TECH FIG 4B**).
- A dependent drain and a Canfield jaw bra are used for porous implants.
- Silicone implants can be placed as a single unit and secured to the periosteum with a suture.
  - Some operators use screws or pins for fixation, but trauma may cause the implant to split.
- The incision is closed in three layers: muscle, subcutaneous tissues, and skin.

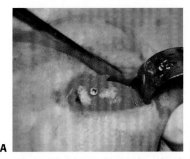
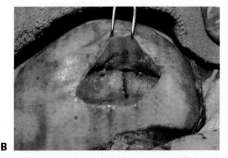

TECH FIG 4 • A. The central portion of the implant is aligned with the midline menton mark, and a screw is drilled and sunk through the medial pilot hole. This screw is partially tightened. Then, the lateral segment of the implant is exposed and held *exactly* along the inferior border. The second screw (lateral) is placed through the predrilled implant pilot hole. **B.** Both screws are tightened completely and countersunk so that the screw heads are below the implant surface to allow for further reduction of the anterior surface of the implant, if necessary (note that neither screw has yet to be satisfactorily countersunk in this image). (From Warren SM, Spector JA, Zide BM. Chin surgery VII: the textured secured implant—a recipe for success. *Plast Reconstr Surg.* 2007;120(5):1378-1385, with permission.)

■ Intraoral Approach to Chin Augmentation

- A midline marking is placed at the level of the pogonion.
- Further markings include the inferior margin of the mandible and the points where lateral undermining would be sufficient.
- Inferior alveolar nerve blocks are performed using 1% lidocaine with 1:100 000 epinephrine.
- Local anesthetic is instilled into the lip mucosa extending to the menton and laterally.
- A no. 15 blade or needle electrocautery is used to make a horizontal or 2 cm vertical or horizontal midline incision on the lip beyond the gingivobuccal sulcus.
  - It is paramount that at least 4 mm of a gingivomuscular cuff be left to facilitate two-layer closure.

- The incision is then carried down to the mandible ensuring that the mentalis muscle can be reattached.
- A subperiosteal pocket is developed using a periosteal elevator.
  - The pocket width is made slightly larger than the implant, but the midline should match the size of the implant correctly.
- The implant is marked in the midline to ensure central positioning.
  - The implant is then inserted into the pocket and placement is confirmed along the inferior border.
- The incision is closed in two layers to ensure independent closure of the muscle and then mucosa.
- An external jaw bra is placed.

PEARLS AND PITFALLS

Aesthetic considerations	■ The key is to bring balance to the lower one-third of the face
Assessment	■ Lip eversion ■ Occlusion ■ Static chin pad thickness ■ Labiomental fold depth and height ■ Dynamic chin pad motion while smiling
Dissection	■ Avoid damage to the mental nerves by understanding their anatomic position.
External submental approach	■ Minimize the length of the horizontal incision to what is needed.
Intraoral approach	■ Vertical or horizontal incisions can be used. ■ Resuspend the mentalis muscle.

POSTOPERATIVE CARE

- An elastic chin support is worn for 3 days.
- Drain removal (for porous implants) at day 1 or day 2 (if used).
- Soft diet, cool packs to the area, oral hygiene (eg, Peridex, for intraoral approach), and head elevation for 7 days. For an intraoral incision, liquids are continued for 36 hours postoperatively, followed by a transition to a regular diet.
- For intraoral placement, the patient continues the use of Peridex swish and spit for 5 days.
- Suture removal between 4 and 7 days postoperatively with the placement of Steri-Strips.
- Patients are seen within 1 week postoperatively and subsequently at 1, 3, 6 months, and 1 year.
- Patients should be questioned on the presence of numbness; if present, it should improve within 2 to 3 weeks of the operation.

OUTCOMES

- Improvement in chin projection and labiomental fold definition is expected following primary implant-based chin augmentation (**FIG 4**).
- The goal should be to provide lower pogonial projection and a labiomental fold that is not hyperacute.

COMPLICATIONS

- Surgical site infection has been reported between 5% and 7%.[3,5]
  - Silicone implants may be salvaged in the setting of infection, which is usually the result of unattended bleeding or poor closure.
- Hematoma—rare.
- Capsular contracture is more common with Silastic implants after removal compared to porous polyethylene implants because of tissue integration in the latter. Management may require removal, placement of a different type of implant, or osseous genioplasty.
- Nerve injury often manifests as lower lip numbness. This is often the result of stretch, compression by implant, or transection of the mental nerve.
  - Improvement is usually seen within 2 to 3 weeks. If symptoms persist beyond 3 weeks, trimming of the implant, implant pocket check, or direct nerve evaluation should be pursued.[6]
  - Paresthesias may occur if there is malposition of the implant leading to impingement of the mental nerve. As stated, management often necessitates repositioning or trimming of the implant.

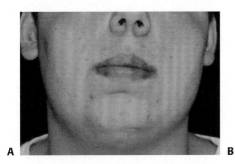
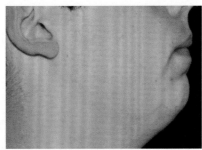
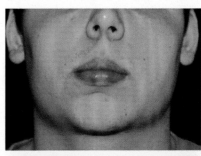
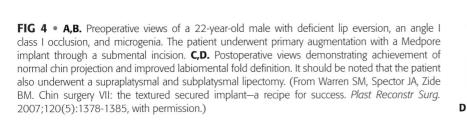
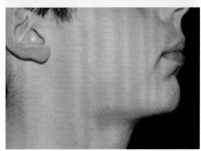

FIG 4 • **A,B.** Preoperative views of a 22-year-old male with deficient lip eversion, an angle I class I occlusion, and microgenia. The patient underwent primary augmentation with a Medpore implant through a submental incision. **C,D.** Postoperative views demonstrating achievement of normal chin projection and improved labiomental fold definition. It should be noted that the patient also underwent a supraplatysmal and subplatysmal lipectomy. (From Warren SM, Spector JA, Zide BM. Chin surgery VII: the textured secured implant—a recipe for success. *Plast Reconstr Surg.* 2007;120(5):1378-1385, with permission.)

- Chin ptosis may result from damage and insufficient repair of the mentalis muscle, thereby resulting in chin ptosis, lip ptosis, drooling, and increased incisor show. This is more likely with an intraoral approach. Chin pad ptosis may occur following implant removal, overly large pocket, or excessive burring. The capsule may contract and lead to a "balling" appearance. Removal of excess submental adipose and mentalis plication or repositioning may be necessary.[7]
- Mentalis dysfunction may manifest as either muscle spasm or dimpling of the skin of the chin. Botulinum toxin injections may address dimpling of the mentalis muscle.[3]
- Bone resorption may occur with implant placement.
  - Associated with more bone loss with implant placement above the thick inferior border
- Implant malposition

REFERENCES

1. Warren SM, Spector JA, Zide BM. Chin surgery VII: the textured secured implant—a recipe for success. *Plast Reconstr Surg.* 2007;120:1378-1385.
2. Zide BM, Pfeifer TM, Longaker MT. Chin surgery: I. Augmentation—the allures and the alerts. *Plast Reconstr Surg.* 1999;104:1843-1853.
3. Sinno S, Zide BM. Chin ups and downs: avoiding bad results in chin reoperation. *Aesthet Surg J.* 2017;37:257-263.
4. Aston SJ, Smith DM. Taking it on the chin: recognizing and accounting for lower face asymmetry in chin augmentation and genioplasty. *Plast Reconstr Surg.* 2015;135:1591-1595.
5. Strauss RA, Abubaker AO. Genioplasty: a case for advancement osteotomy. *J Oral Maxillofac Surg.* 2000;58:783-787.
6. Zide BM. The mentalis muscle: an essential component of chin and lower lip position. *Plast Reconstr Surg.* 2000;105:1213-1215.
7. Garfein ES, Zide BM. Chin ptosis: classification, anatomy, and correction. *Craniomaxillofac Trauma Reconstr.* 2008;1:1-14.

73

CHAPTER

Techniques for Placing Malar Implants

Erez Dayan, Dev Vibhakar, and Michael J. Yaremchuk

DEFINITION

- Prominent malar bones are considered attractive and youthful in most cultures.
- The malar area is a dynamic anatomic region of the face composed of underlying skeletal support, adipose tissue, and mimetic muscles of facial expression.[1]
- Characterization of the domelike shape of the malar area is largely subjective due to the lack of anthropometric and cephalometric landmarks. The inability to define "average" or "normal" for the malar area makes selection of implant shape, size, and position challenging.
- Malar augmentation using alloplastic implants yields an aesthetic benefit in select patients with relative malar hypoplasia.[2,3]

ANATOMY

- Skeleton
    - The malar eminence is the most projecting portion of the zygoma. Its convexity extends from lateral to the infraorbital foramen to the midaspect of the zygomatic arch.
    - It is perforated in its midaspect by the zygomaticofacial foramen for the passage of the zygomaticofacial nerve and vessels.
- Muscles
    - Muscles of the midface largely provide facial expression. Those that are freed from their origins during malar augmentation elevate the upper lip and include zygomaticus major, zygomaticus minor, levator labii superioris, and levator anguli oris (**FIG 1**).

- Nerves
    - The infraorbital nerve exits the maxilla through the infraorbital foramen and travels beneath the levator superioris and above the levator anguli oris. Its branches supply the skin of the lower lid, the side of the nose, most of the cheek, and the upper lip. This nerve must be identified and preserved.
    - The zygomaticofacial nerve exists through a small foramen located on the lateral aspect of the malar bone. It supplies a small portion of the skin of the upper cheek. It is routinely sacrificed during malar augmentation.

PATHOGENESIS

- Most frequently, patients who present for malar augmentation are within normal range and desire more definition, angularity, or balance to their facial contour.
- Studies have demonstrated retrusion of the midface and mandibular skeleton with aging, thus supporting alloplastic augmentation of the skeleton as a component of the facial rejuvenation armamentarium.
- Malar deficiency is often part of a generalized midface deficiency requiring soft tissue evaluation and treatment. As aging occurs, the retaining ligaments of the midface attenuate and soft tissues atrophy, leading to deflation and descent of the malar soft tissue complex.[3,4]
- Functionally, malar projection provides a platform to support overlaying the soft tissue as well as provide some protection against lower lid descent (**FIG 2**).
- Patients with craniofacial deformities often have functional and aesthetic consequences requiring more invasive

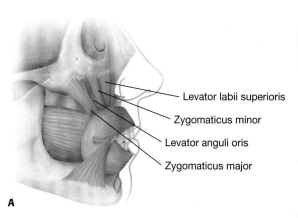

A

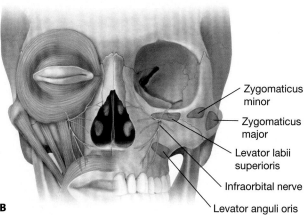

B

Levator labii superioris
Zygomaticus minor
Levator anguli oris
Zygomaticus major

Zygomaticus minor
Zygomaticus major
Levator labii superioris
Infraorbital nerve
Levator anguli oris

FIG 1 • **A,B.** Relevant facial musculature and intraorbital nerve in relation to malar implant placement.

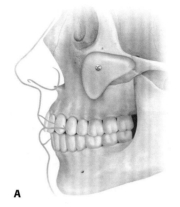
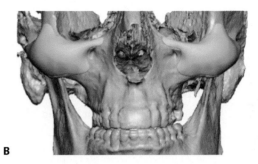

FIG 2 • A,B. Malar implant position on bony skeleton.   **A**   **B**

osteotomy and skeletal repositioning rather than malar alloplastic augmentation. However, in skeletally deficient patients with normal occlusion, alloplastic augmentation is often a more appealing option due to its less invasive surgery.[5]

PATIENT HISTORY AND PHYSICAL FINDINGS

- Physical examination should analyze both skeletal and soft tissue components, as well as overall facial balance. Asymmetries should be noted and demonstrated. It is helpful to review life-sized photos with the patient to define aesthetic concerns and goals.
- History should be obtained for any active or prior history of immunosuppression, connective tissue disorders, coagulopathy, facial trauma, and implanted facial hardware before surgery. Patients should also be asked regarding recent injections of neuromodulators or fillers (temporary or permanent).
- Patients with excessively thin skin, history of irradiation, or sinus disease are poor candidates for alloplastic malar augmentation.
- Patients may present with a desire to enhance aesthetics of other aspects of their face (ie, nose, periorbital region). The surgeon should be able to accurately diagnose malar deficiency and assess its contribution to the overall midface harmony to the patient.
- Malar skeletal augmentation is not a substitute for soft tissue augmentation or repositioning.

IMAGING

- In general, radiologic assessment is not needed. Size and position of malar implants are based on the aesthetic judgment of the surgeon.
- In patients with significant asymmetries, CT imaging may provide an advantage of multiplane views, three-dimensional reconstruction, life-sized models, and the manufacture of custom implants.

NONOPERATIVE MANAGEMENT

- Although fat grafting and synthetic filler injections are logical nonoperative techniques that may aid in restoration of soft tissue volume loss, they have a limited role in simulating the effect of increased skeletal projection.
- The aging process impacts both the soft tissue and skeletal components of the malar region. Depending on patient needs, either or both soft tissue and skeletal augmentation

may be appropriate to restore youthful facial contours. It is important for the clinician to be able to differentiate the two. For example, if skeletal augmentation is performed for a patient who requires soft tissue augmentation, it will result in an overly defined appearance. On the other hand, performing fat grafting or filler injections for a patient who requires skeletal augmentation will result in a spherical shape with inadequate definition.

SURGICAL MANAGEMENT

Preoperative Planning

- Informed consent should include risks of infection, extrusion, displacement, asymmetry, deformation, hematoma, seroma, and motor/sensory nerve injury, as well as the risks of anesthesia.
- Prior to the induction of anesthesia, the area desired for augmentation is determined with the patient in a sitting position. This is marked on the surface of the skin.
- The authors' preference is to use general endotracheal or nasotracheal anesthesia. This allows optimal preparation of the operative site and control of the airway. The use of local anesthesia and sedation is an alternative.
- Silicone rubber and porous polyethylene are the predominant implant materials.
  - The senior author prefers porous polyethylene implants (**FIG 3**). The implant material is semiflexible to conform to underlying bone when fixed with screws. Its porosity supports fibrovascular ingrowth, which avoids the potentially soft tissue distorting capsule formation inherent in smooth surface implants.
  - The preferred implants are designed to avoid impingement on the infraorbital nerve. Registration tabs aid in symmetric placement.

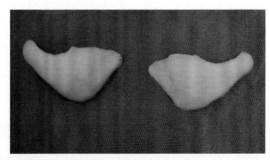

FIG 3 • Porous polyethylene malar implants.

Positioning

- Patients are placed supine on the operating room table at a 90-degree perpendicular position relative to the anesthesiologist to allow for maximal exposure.

Approach

- Malar augmentation may be performed through intraoral, coronal, or eyelid approaches.
- The operative approach depends on surgical preference, implant size, implant placement, and previous facial surgeries.

■ Preoperative Preparation

- Prior to antiseptic preparation and draping, a dilute solution of lidocaine and epinephrine (1:100,000) is infiltrated into the operative site for postoperative pain control and, most importantly, for intraoperative hemostasis.

- Intravenous cephalosporin or ciprofloxacin antibiotic prophylaxis is administered approximately 30 minutes preoperatively.
- 0.12% chlorhexidine gluconate oral rinse is prescribed for daily use beginning 3 days preoperatively and including the day of surgery.

■ Periorbital Approach

- The senior author prefers a transconjunctival retroseptal approach with lateral canthotomy (**TECH FIG 1A**).
- Wide subperiosteal dissection of the area to be augmented is performed, with identification and preservation of the infraorbital nerve.
- Implants are available with registration tabs that align with the lateral orbital rim and proximal zygomatic arch. This allows symmetric placement.

- Screw fixation immobilizes the implant and obliterates any gaps between implant and skeleton (**TECH FIG 1B**). Gaps between the implant and skeleton result in unanticipated increase in malar projection.
- The transconjunctival incision is realigned, the lateral commissure reconstructed, and the orbicularis and skin overlying the lateral orbital wall closed in layers.
- If chemosis is a concern, a temporary tarsorrhaphy stitch of 5-0 nylon is placed until the chemosis is resolved.

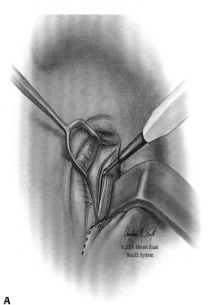

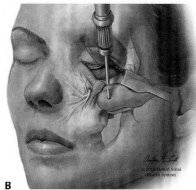

A   **B**

TECH FIG 1 • A. Transconjunctival approach to placement of malar implants. **B.** Screw fixation of malar implant via lower eyelid approach with care to avoid infraorbital nerve. (Printed with permission from ©Mount Sinai Health System.)

■ Intraoral Approach

Gingivobuccal Sulcus Incision and Dissection

- An upper sulcus incision is made far enough above its apex to allow sufficient tissue for a secure closure after implant placement.
- The dissection is carried to the maxillary bone where the periosteum is incised.
- With careful attention to and identification of the infraorbital nerve, subperiosteal dissection is performed over the malar eminence, up to the infraorbital rim, and onto the zygomatic arch nearly up to the zygomaticotemporal suture (**TECH FIG 2**).
- All efforts are made to avoid excessive bleeding and hematoma formation that predisposes to prolonged recovery and infection.

Pocket Formation

- Subperiosteal pocket dissection should allow for visualization of anatomic landmarks and proper placement of the implant.
- The surgeon should aim to create a pocket slightly larger than the implant itself.
- Of note, extending a malar implant onto the zygomatic arch has a significant impact on midfacial width.
- Implants can be trimmed and contoured with a scalpel or high-speed bur intraoperatively to suit the individual needs of the patient:

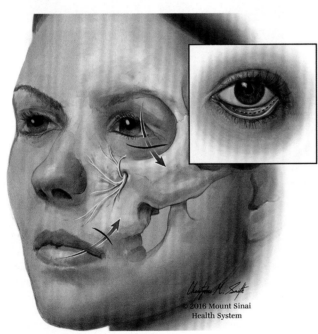

TECH FIG 2 • Upper gingivobuccal sulcus and lower eyelid approach to placement of malar implants. (Printed with permission from ©Mount Sinai Health System.)

- Hot sterile saline (70°C/106°F) can be used to soften the porous polyethylene implant for further contouring.

Fixation of Implants

- Once satisfactory implant position is achieved, position is ensured with screw fixation of the implant to the skeleton (**TECH FIG 3**):
  - Penetration of the sinus with the screw is of no clinical significance.
- The position of the implant relative to the infraorbital nerve is always visualized at the end of the procedure to be confident that any sensory deficit in the postoperative period reflects retraction-related trauma to the nerve, which is temporary, rather than implant impingement on the nerve, which will be permanent.
- The wound is irrigated with antibiotic solution prior to closure.
- The intraoral incision is closed with interrupted full-thickness resorbable sutures.

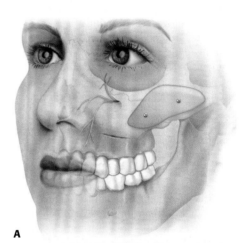

A

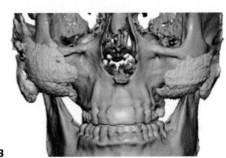

B

TECH FIG 3 • **A.** Screw fixation of malar implant via superior gingivobuccal sulcus approach. **B.** CT scan demonstrating unsatisfactory position of implant- asymmetry is not uncommmon.

PEARLS AND PITFALLS

Patient selection	■ Implant augmentation best corrects malar skeletal deficiency. Its effect on surface irregularities such as lower eyelid wrinkles or secondary bags is limited. ■ Skeletal augmentation is not a substitute for soft tissue augmentation or resuspension.
Surgical approach	■ Extended eyelid approach provides direct visualization of the skeleton and therefore optimal exposure for symmetric implant placement.
Implant selection and position	■ Extension of a malar implant onto the zygomatic arch impacts midface width. ■ Inadequate exposure of the three-dimensional midface skeleton is a common error predisposing to implant malposition, implant asymmetry, and infraorbital nerve impingement. ■ Registration tabs resting on the infraorbital rim and zygomatic arch assure symmetric implant placement.
Implant fixation	■ Screw fixation assures stable implant position. ■ Screw fixation applies the posterior surface of the implant to the surface of the bone, obliterating any gaps between the implant and the skeleton. Gaps result in unanticipated increases in projection of the implant.
Asymmetry	■ Direct visualization of the area to be augmented, incorporation of registration tabs into implant design, and screw fixation limit likelihood of asymmetry. ■ Minor asymmetries are often aesthetically inconsequential due to overlaying malar soft tissue.
Hematoma	■ All efforts are made to avoid hematoma predisposing to infection.

POSTOPERATIVE CARE

- Suction drains (round no. 10 French) if used are removed the morning after surgery. A supportive tape dressing is placed postoperatively and removed the morning after surgery.
- Oral antibiotics are prescribed for 7 days after surgery (cephalexin 500 mg q8h).
- When intraoral incisions are used, patients are asked to eat a soft diet for 72 hours postoperatively.
- Frequent mouthwashes are advised as well as careful tooth brushing.
- Patients are instructed to refrain from strenuous exercise for 2 to 3 weeks postoperatively.
- Significant edema, in the known absence of hematoma, may be treated with a standard steroid taper prescribed for 6 days.
- The patient is instructed to apply iced compresses to the area for 48 to 72 hours and to sleep with the head of bed elevated greater than 30 degrees or with three or four pillows.
- Follow up is at 1-, 2-, and 4-week intervals. Thereafter, long-term follow-up is at 6 months and 1 year.

OUTCOMES

- Appropriate patient selection and sound surgical technique provide most patients with satisfactory aesthetic outcomes (**FIGS 4** and **5**).

COMPLICATIONS

- Implant malposition, implant asymmetry, and sensory nerve dysfunction are avoided with wide subperiosteal exposure, direct visualization, registration tab implant design, and screw fixation. Although it is often cited that bone resorption underlying the implant is a complication, it is rarely clinically significant with malar implants.

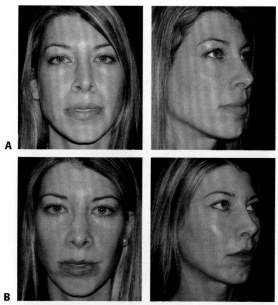

FIG 4 • Before **(A)** and 2 year after **(B)** placement of malar implants.

- Infection rates after facial implant surgery are low (less than 2%) when the techniques outlined in this chapter are employed. Acute infection is best managed by implant removal. Bacterial biofilm formation on the implant precludes antibiotic and host resistance efficacy. Antibiotic treatment will suppress the infection during treatment but will not cure it.
- Late infections (greater than 3 months post-op) have not been experienced in the senior author's experience. It is hypothesized that infections that are clinically manifested after 1 month reflect small bacterial contaminations at the time of surgery that are suppressed by host defenses and the postoperative antibiotic regimen.

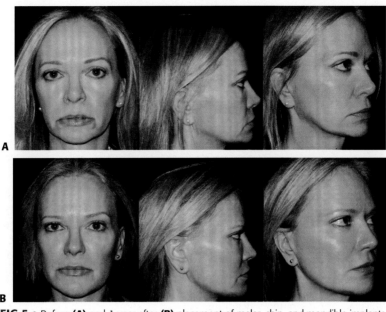

FIG 5 • Before **(A)** and 1 year after **(B)** placement of malar, chin, and mandible implants.

REFERENCES

1. Matros E, Momoh A, Yaremchuk MJ. The aging midfacial skeleton: Implications for rejuvenation and reconstruction using implants. Facial Plast Surg. 2009;25:252-259.
2. Raschke R, Hazani R, Yaremchuk MJ. Identifying a safe zone for midface augmentation using anatomic landmarks for the infraorbital foramen. Aesthet Surg J. 2013;33(1 suppl):13-18.
3. Yaremchuk MJ, Doumit G, Thomas MA. Alloplastic augmentation of the facial skeleton: an occasional adjunct or alternative to orthognathic surgery. Plast Reconstr Surg. 2011;127:2021-2030.
4. Shaw RB, Katzel EB, Koltz PF, et al. Aging facial skeleton: aesthetic implications and rejuvenation strategies. Plast Reconstr Surg. 2011;127:374-383.
5. Yaremchuk MJ. Secondary malar implant surgery. Plast Reconstr Surg. 2008;121:620.

Mandible Implants

Michael J. Yaremchuk, Dev Vibhakar, and Erez Dayan

DEFINITION

Patients with three types of skeletal morphology can benefit from implant augmentation of the mandibular body, angle, and ramus. These skeletal morphologies include those with:

- Normal dimensions. Most patients who desire mandible augmentation have lower face horizontal dimensions within normal range. These patients either desire a wider lower face (increased bigonial distance) or desire more definition and angularity to the mandibular border.[1]
- Skeletal deficiency. Approximately 5% of the population in the United States has skeletal mandibular deficiency leading to a class II occlusal problem. Most of these patients can have their dental relationships corrected by orthodontic treatment, which leaves their skeletal contours deficient. These patients can have their mandibular contours improved with implant augmentation.
- Surgically altered anatomy. Patients with mandibular deficiency who have had their class II malocclusion corrected by osteotomy and rearrangement remain deficient, but in another way.[2] Resultant displeasing postoperative contours include step-offs at the osteotomy sites and malposition of the aesthetically important angle and ramus. Alloplastic implants, particularly those designed and manufactured by computer imaging, can be used to improve contour in these cases.

ANATOMY

- All transverse facial dimensions are greater in men than in women with the greatest difference being the bigonial distance.[2]
- Skeletal anatomy
  - The aesthetically important portions of the mandible are the chin and ramus. The chin determines lower face height and projection in the midline, and the ramus determines lower face width (**FIG 1A**).
  - The mental foramen from which the mental nerve exits lies approximately at the interspace between the two premolars and about midway in the height of the dentulous adult mandible (**FIG 1B**).
- Muscular anatomy (**FIG 1C**)
  - The four muscles of mastication are predominantly responsible for movement of the mandible and include masseter, temporalis, medial pterygoid, and lateral pterygoid muscles. The only muscles of mastication encountered during mandibular augmentation are the masseter and indirectly the medial pterygoid which together form the pterygomasseteric sling.[3]

- The buccinator is also encountered during exposure for mandibular augmentation. It is principally a muscle of the cheek and forms the lateral wall of the oral cavity.[2,3]
- Nerve anatomy (see **FIG 1B,C**)
  - Inferior alveolar nerve is a branch of the mandibular nerve (V3). It enters the mandibular canal alongside the inferior alveolar vessels through the mandibular foramen, which is located in the lingual aspect of the ramus approximately halfway between its anterior and posterior borders. It is important to visualize the path of the inferior alveolar nerve when placing screws to immobilize mandibular implants.[3] This nerve (now termed the mental nerve) exits at the mental foramen. It provides sensation to the ipsilateral portion of the lower lip.

PATIENT HISTORY AND PHYSICAL FINDINGS

- Detailed history should include skeletal trauma, orthodontic therapy, or orthognathic procedures.
- Physical examination should explore occlusal relationships, skeletal contour, and relation of the mandible to other facial contours.
- Life-size posteroanterior and lateral photographs can be helpful when discussing aesthetic concerns and goals with the patient.
- Sample implants and model skulls are useful to demonstrate the application and visual impact of facial implant.

IMAGING

- Posteroanterior and lateral cephalograms provide useful data to aid in choosing an implant to best suit the patient.
- Three-dimensional computerized tomographic scans and the models obtained from their data can be invaluable in designing implants to correct asymmetries associated with congenital, posttraumatic, or postsurgical deformities (**FIG 2A,B**).

NONOPERATIVE MANAGEMENT

- Soft tissue augmentation in the form of autogenous fat grafts or synthetic fillers can simulate the visual effect of skeletal augmentation to camouflage limited skeletal deficiencies.[2–4]
- More aggressive soft tissue augmentation may expand the volume of the soft tissue envelope but at the expense of skeletal definition.[2]

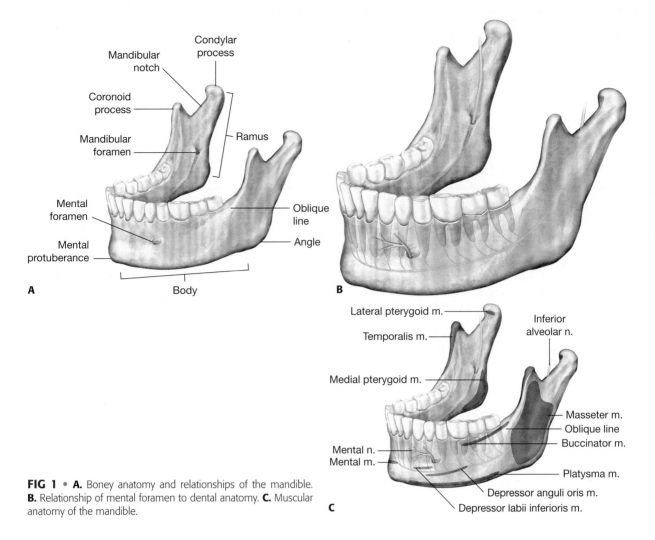

FIG 1 • **A.** Boney anatomy and relationships of the mandible. **B.** Relationship of mental foramen to dental anatomy. **C.** Muscular anatomy of the mandible.

SURGICAL MANAGEMENT

Preoperative Planning

- Patient history, physical examination, possible imaging, and review of patient photographs as well as pictures of others deemed attractive by the patient are all part of the preoperative planning.
- Numerous implant designs are available to change the shape of the mandible in three dimensions: bigonial width, ramus height, and body length, as well as the inclination of the mandibular border.
- Informed consent should include intrinsic risks and benefits of mandibular augmentation, such as the possibility of infection, extrusion, displacement, asymmetry, deformation, hematoma, seroma, motor/sensory nerve injury, as well as the risks of anesthesia.
- Prior to the induction of anesthesia, the area desired for augmentation is determined with the patient in a sitting position. This is marked on the surface of the skin.
- 0.12% chlorhexidine gluconate oral rinse is prescribed for daily use beginning 3 days preoperatively and including the day of surgery.

Positioning

- Patients are placed supine on the operating room table at a 90-degree perpendicular position relative to the anesthesiologist to allow for maximal exposure.

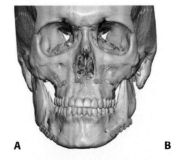
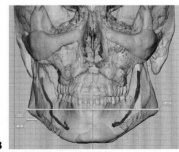

FIG 2 • **A,B.** Custom implants designed using CT scan data to correct irregularities and imbalance after orthognathic surgery.

■ Preoperative Preparation

- Prior to antiseptic preparation and draping, a dilute solution of lidocaine and epinephrine (1:100 000) is infiltrated into the operative site for postoperative pain control and intraoperative hemostasis.
- Intravenous antibiotic prophylaxis is administered approximately 30 minutes preoperatively. Oral equivalents are continued for 5 days after surgery.

- The authors' preference is to use general nasotracheal anesthesia. This allows optimal preparation of the operative site and control of the airway. However, skeletal augmentation can be performed with local anesthesia and sedation.
- The face and oral cavity are prepared with an iodine solution after placement of the throat pack.

■ Incision

- A generous intraoral incision is made at least 1 cm above the inferior gingivobuccal sulcus on its labial side to expose the ramus and body of the mandible (**TECH FIG 1A**).
- The anterior ramus and body of the mandible as well as their inferior borders are freed from their soft tissues in a subperiosteal plane. Care is taken to avoid minimal disruption of the pterygomasseteric sling. Disruption of the sling will result in roll-up of the masseter with an unsightly midramus bulge (**TECH FIG 1B**).

- If the mental area is also being augmented, a submental incision is made for access and exposure of the anterior mandible (**TECH FIG 1C**).
- The inferior alveolar nerve is visualized in its anticipated path to avoid its injury during screw fixation of the implant (**TECH FIG 1D**).
- As determined preoperatively, the implant can be trimmed with a scalpel or bur before its placement on the mandible.

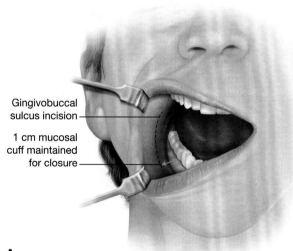

Gingivobuccal sulcus incision

1 cm mucosal cuff maintained for closure

A

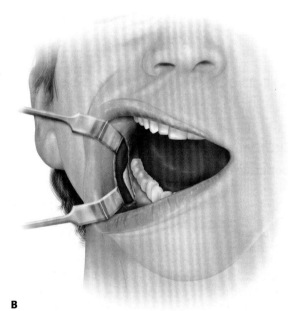

B

TECH FIG 1 • **A.** Placement of intraoral incision, at least 1 cm above the inferior gingivobuccal sulcus for optimal exposure. **B.** Soft tissues are elevated off the anterior ramous and body of the mandible in subperiosteal plane.

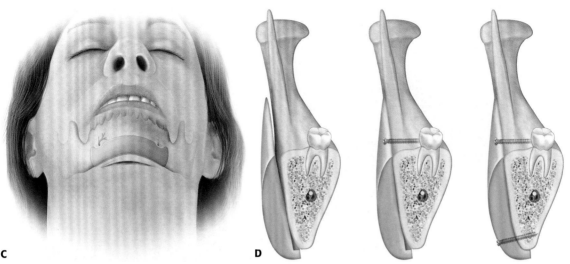

TECH FIG 1 (Continued) • **C.** Submental incision for genioplasty. **D.** Anatomic relationship of inferior alveolar nerve is anticipated to avoid injury during screw fixation of the implant.

■ Implant Positioning and Fixation

- Registration features at the inferior and lateral borders of the implant aid in appropriate implant positioning (**TECH FIG 2A**).
- Once satisfactory positioning of the implant is achieved, the implant is fixed to the mandible with titanium screws.
- A clamp designed to stabilize the implant to the mandible is useful in maintaining implant position during screw fixation (**TECH FIG 2B**).
- Intraoral screw fixation requires aggressive soft tissue retraction.
  - This limited access obligates the fixation screws to be placed obliquely. This oblique screw placement obligates screws to be from 8 to 14 mm in length.

- Screw placement should anticipate the expected path of the inferior alveolar nerve (**TECH FIG 2C**).
- When an external approach is preferred for screw fixation, access is obtained through stab wound incisions made in the neck skin.
- The one or two fixation screws not only immobilize the implant but also eliminate any gaps between the posterior surface of the implant and the anterior surface of the mandible (**TECH FIG 2D**):
  - Gaps result in unanticipated increases in effective implant augmentation.
  - Gaps may arise when there are prominences on the surface of the mandible. This is often the case at the oblique line of the mandible body. Reduction of these prominences allows for congruent application of the implant to the mandible.

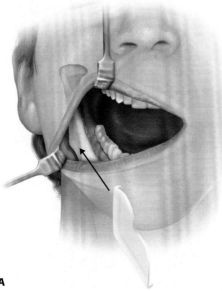

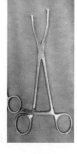

TECH FIG 2 • **A.** Registration tabs of inferior and lateral borders of implant aid in correct positioning. **B.** Clamp used to stabilize implant to the mandible during screw fixation.

TECHNIQUES

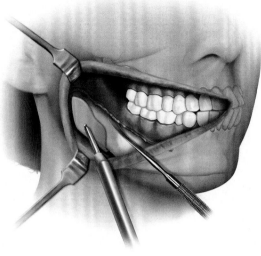
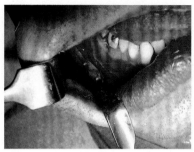

C

D

TECH FIG 2 (Continued) • **C.** Screw placement should anticipate the expected path of the inferior alveolar nerve. **D.** Close apposition of implant to the mandible is necessary with screws to avoid gaps leading to overprojection.

■ Assessment of Implant and Contour

- After implant fixation, mechanical contouring may be necessary to assure an imperceptible transition between the implant and mandible.

■ Closure

- The implant pocket is irrigated with antibiotic solution.
- A no. 10 French round suction drain is left in until the next morning:

- The drain skin exit is placed behind the ear lobule (**TECH FIG 3A,B**).
- The intraoral incision is closed in layers with absorbable sutures.

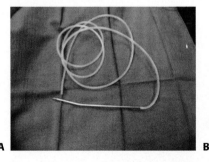
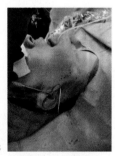

A

B

TECH FIG 3 • **A,B.** Placement of drain behind the ear lobule.

PEARLS AND PITFALLS

Surgical approach	■ Transoral approach provides rapid and precise placement of mandibular implants.
Implant fixation	■ Failure to fix the implant to the facial skeleton with a screw may lead to asymmetry or implant malposition. ■ Screw fixation applies the posterior surface of the implant to the surface of the bone, obliterating any gaps between the implant and the skeleton. Gaps result in unanticipated increases in projection of the implant.
Asymmetry	■ Asymmetry in the early postoperative phase may be related to asymmetric edema and tends to resolve within 1 to 2 mo. ■ Minor asymmetries are often aesthetically inconsequential due to overlaying thick masseter.
Secondary implant surgery	■ Expose both sides to compare implant position.

POSTOPERATIVE CARE

- A suction drain is routinely placed at the operative site and removed the morning after surgery. A supportive tape dressing is placed postoperatively and is usually removed the morning after surgery (**FIG 3**).
- Oral antibiotics are prescribed for 7 days after surgery (cephalexin 500 mg every 8 hours).
- Due to the intraoral incisions, patients are asked to eat a soft diet for 72 hours postoperatively. Patients are instructed to refrain from strenuous exercise for 2 to 3 weeks postoperatively.
- If there is significant edema the morning after surgery, then a standard steroid taper is prescribed for 6 days.
- The patient is instructed to apply ice for 48 to 72 hours and sleep with the head of the bed elevated greater than 30 degrees or with three or four pillows.
- Follow-up is at 1-, 2-, and 4-week intervals. Thereafter, long-term follow-up is at 6 months and 1 year.

OUTCOMES

- Appropriate patient selection and sound surgical technique provide a vast majority of patients with satisfactory aesthetic outcomes (**FIGS 4A–H, 5A–C,** and **6A,B**).

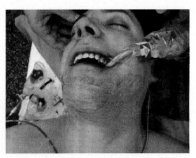

FIG 3 • Placement of supportive tape dressing.

COMPLICATIONS

- Postoperative complications are uncommon when the before-described protocol is adhered to.
- Sensory or motor dysfunctions are usually transient.
- Epinephrine injection, meticulous hemostasis, and suction drainage minimize the likelihood of hematoma.
- Good oral hygiene, meticulous hemostasis, and watertight wound closure minimize infection risk.
- The above complications may be minimized with wide subperiosteal exposure to the area that needs to be augmented and screw fixation to prevent implant movement.

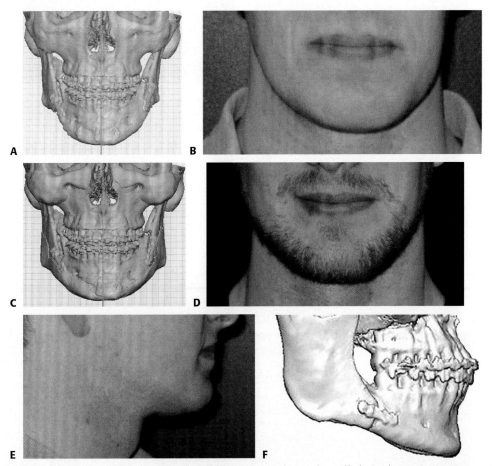

FIG 4 • **(A,B)** AP view of preoperative and **(C,D)** postoperative result of computer-designed mandibular implants to correct contour defect after orthognathic surgery (1 year postop). **(E,F)** Lateral view of preoperative and **(G,H)** postoperative result of computer-designed mandibular implants to correct contour defect after orthognathic surgery (1 year postop).

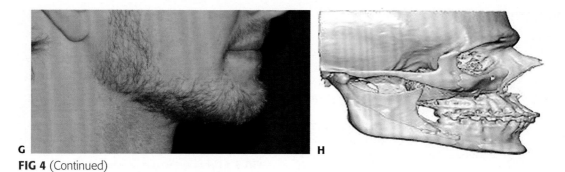

FIG 4 (Continued)

- In the senior author's overall experience with greater than 400 porous implants used for facial skeletal reconstruction, the infection rate was about 1.5%. If infection should occur, we recommend removal of the implant. Antibiotic therapy may temporarily suppress the infection, but the bacterial-induced biofilm prevents chemical eradication of the infection. Implant replacement 3 to 6 months after resolution of the infection has been effective.[2]

- Late implant infections (years after implant surgery) have been reported (eg, after dental surgery). To our knowledge, none of the senior author's patients have encountered this. We believe that infections that become apparent in the early months after surgery reflect small intraoperative bacterial contamination that was temporarily suppressed by perioperative antibiotics and host defenses.

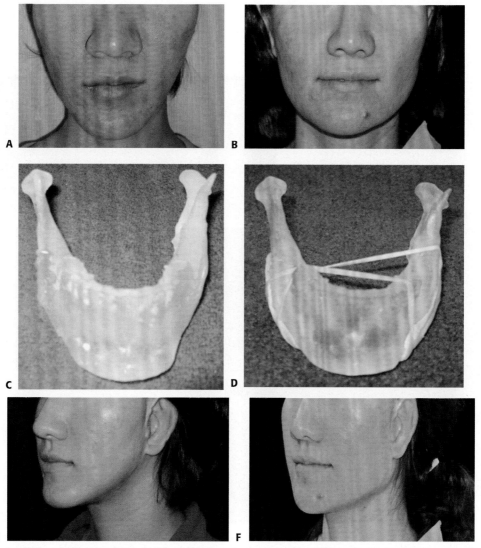

FIG 5 • **(A)** Preoperative (*left*) and **(B)** postoperative (*right*) results of a patient who underwent bilateral sagittal split osteotomy with resulting deformity and asymmetry at the osteotomy site (*left*) 1 year postop. **C,D.** Implants were customized to correct the resulting deformity (*right*). **E.** Preoperative (*left*) and **(F)** postoperative (*right*) results after custom implants to correct osteotomy site deformity after bilateral sagittal split osteotomy (1 year postop).

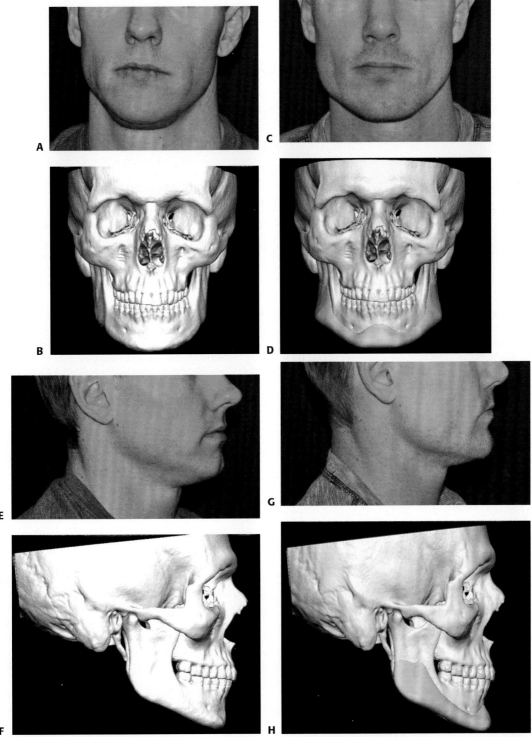

FIG 6 • **(A,B)** AP view of pre- (*left*) and **(C,D)** postoperative (*right*) results of aesthetic mandibular augmentation (1 year postop). **(E,F)** Lateral view of pre- (*left*) and **(G,H)** postoperative (*right*) results of aesthetic mandibular augmentation (12 months postop).

REFERENCES

1. Selber JC, Rosen HM. Aesthetics of facial skeletal surgery. *Clin Plast Surg.* 2007;34:437-445.
2. Yaremchuk MJ. Mandibular augmentation. *Plast Reconstr Surg.* 2000;106:697-706.
3. Yaremchuk MJ, Chen YC. Enlarging the deficient mandible. *Aesthet Surg J.* 2007;27:539-550.
4. Yaremchuk MJ. Making concave faces convex. *Aesthetic Plast Surg.* 2005;29:141-147.

75

CHAPTER

Technique for Chin Reduction

Jong-Woo Choi and Woo Shik Jeong

DEFINITION

- Facial contours can greatly affect a person's facial image. In particular, the shape of the chin is one of the most important parts in terms of facial image according to a recent consensus among facial plastic surgeons who perform facial contouring surgery.
- There are several ways to perform a chin reduction.
  - One is to reduce the whole mandible, including the chin, which is performed through mandibuloplasty.
  - The other is to reduce only the chin, which is performed with genioplasty.
- In terms of the surgical direction for chin reduction, there are two acceptable methods.
  - One is horizontal chin setback, which is associated with the mandible setback or chin setback procedure.
  - The other is vertical chin reduction, which is related to vertical reduction genioplasty. This method reduces the volume of the chin using narrowing genioplasty.
- This chapter describes how chin reduction can be properly achieved by selecting the best solution from among these various options according to the patient's status.

ANATOMY

- The mental nerve innervates the lower lip and chin region and passes through the mental foramen on the anterior surface of the mandible. The mental foramen is generally located in the apical region of the first and second premolars.[1]
- However, anatomical variation exists with respect to the mental foramen's location, and the anterior loop of the mental nerve should be considered with a safety zone left when the osteotomy line is planned.

PATIENT HISTORY AND PHYSICAL FINDINGS

- The chin reduction procedure can be applied to patients who complain of a prominent and wide chin or of protrusion of the mentum.
- Reduction with mandibuloplasty can improve aesthetic contouring of the chin and the appearance of a square face.

IMAGING

- The appearance of the chin is easily visualized on three-dimensional computed tomography.[2,3]
- Panoramic radiographs can also be helpful for locating the mental foramen.

SURGICAL MANAGEMENT

- Orthognathic surgery could be a good option for skeletal class III prognathism accompanied by chin protrusion. In contrast to reduction genioplasty, which is performed on the chin alone, mandibular setback resolves issues related to the whole mandible. Sometimes, simple reduction genioplasty cannot produce the desired results for patients with skeletal class III prognathism:
  - Regardless of the occlusion, the protruded mandible or chin should be corrected based on the whole facial profile. If the patient has a relative skeletal class III tendency, orthognathic surgery may be a better solution than simple chin reduction or mandibuloplasty would be. If the patient has a normal class I occlusion, clockwise rotational jaw/rotational mandibular setback could be a good alternative.
- In the past, mandible angle reduction was the common term for facial contouring surgery in Asia. However, this procedure should now be referred to as mandibuloplasty, as modern aesthetic facial contouring surgery primarily deals with the whole mandible, including the chin, body, and the mandibular angle:
  - To reduce the whole mandible, numerous modifications have been introduced, such as mandible angle resection, long curved mandibulectomy, and sagittal mandibular corticectomy.
  - Recent standards for mandibuloplasty include long-curved marginal mandibuloplasty with or without narrowing genioplasty. This method for one-piece mandibuloplasty should focus on the shape of the mandible as well as the amount of the marginal resection. Compared with traditional mandible angle resection or mandible reduction, one-piece mandibuloplasty affects the whole mandible.
- In contrast to mandibuloplasty, genioplasty techniques mostly affect just the chin. Various genioplasty techniques have been introduced. Advancing genioplasty is the most commonly used technique. For chin reduction, however, vertical reduction genioplasty is preferable.
  - Vertical reduction genioplasty can reduce the vertical chin dimension directly with an approximately 1:1 hard-to-soft tissue ratio, whereas the maxillary movement was not correspondent at hard-and-soft tissue ratio. This effect suggests that reduction genioplasty is a very effective and intuitive procedure.

- Whereas vertical reduction genioplasty primarily affects vertical control of the chin, narrowing genioplasty primarily affects horizontal control of the chin. There are various chin shapes, such as the broad chin, square chin, long chin, short chin, and trapezoidal chin, and the shape of the chin greatly influences the facial contour. Narrowing genioplasty has become one of the most popular procedures in facial contouring surgery.
- Narrowing genioplasty can be performed with mandibuloplasty of the chin, body, and angle. An alternative method is one-piece mandibuloplasty. There are few differences in these procedures, so surgeons can choose which to perform based on their personal preference.

Preoperative Planning

- The extent of chin correction should be determined individually according to the patient's chin width, the degree of mental protrusion, the course of the inferior alveolar nerve, and the patient's preference regarding the final chin shape.
- For fixation of bone segments, titanium miniplates, lag screws, or wires can be used and should be available.

Positioning

- The patient should be positioned supine on the operating table under general anesthesia via orotracheal or nasotracheal intubation.
- Horse-shaped supporting head table can be helpful for minimizing the head during the operation.

Approach

- The conventional intraoral vestibular incision is best performed after infiltration of hemostasis.
- Subperiosteal dissection is performed to expose the symphyseal region, except for the opening of the mental nerve with no. 15 blades or the cutting mode of Bovie coagulator.

■ Mandible Setback or Chin Setback

- Chin reduction related to the whole mandible could be achieved with mandibular setback based on sagittal split ramus osteotomy or intraoral vertical ramus osteotomy with a reciprocating saw.
- After the nasotracheal intubation, a 3- to 4-cm buccogingival incision is made from the 2 cm above the occlusal plane to the first molar, disclosing the subperiosteal plane for the sagittal split osteotomy of the mandible.
- Using the periosteal elevator, the periosteum on the mandible is elevated laterally and medially. The pterygomasseteric sling is detached with the round elevator, and the periosteum on the inferior border of the mandible is stripped from the mandible bone.
- Using the bur hole in the medial side made before, the reciprocating saw is used for the sagittal split osteotomy (**TECH FIG 1A**). Then, the osteotome is used to split the mandible.
- For fixation of mandibular setback (**TECH FIG 1B**), one rigid fixation with a titanium 6-mm-length miniplate on each side of Champy line can achieve stable fixation.
- When a buccogingival incision is used, the periosteum should be sutured with 3-0 or 4-0 Vicryl for preventing hematoma and infection.
- Then, the buccogingival incisions are closed with 4-0 Vicryl in continuous fashion.

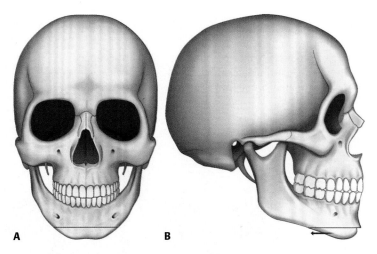

TECH FIG 1 • A. Sagittal split osteotomy. **B.** Chin setback.   A   B

■ Mandibuloplasty

- After the nasotracheal intubation, a 3- to 4-cm buccogingival incision is made from 2 cm above the occlusal plane to the first molar, and subperiosteal dissection is done using the curved round elevator while preserving the continuity of the periosteum:

- The whole mandible should be exposed, except for the mucosal attachment above the mental nerve.
- Next, the pterygomasseteric sling is released with the subperiosteal elevator without tearing:
  - A tear in the periosteum can harm the facial vessels or the marginal mandibular branch of the facial nerve.

- There are two ways to cut the lower jaw, depending on surgeon preference: from the angle to the chin and from the chin to the angle (**TECH FIG 2**):
  - Generally, an oscillating saw is used for mandibuloplasty, but a modified reciprocating saw, such a curved one, can also be used.
  - When an oscillating saw is used, the most posterior part of the ramus should be cut meticulously to avoid following the wrong direction to the condyle because direct visualization of the most posterior part of the ramus is not easy.

- In addition, surgeons should bear in mind the course of the mandibular nerve inside the mandible. A reduction that is too aggressive might cut the mandibular nerve, which results in the complete numbness of the lower lip.
- Finally, after removing the one-piece mandibular segments, the periosteum should be closed tightly to minimize soft tissue redundancy with 3-0 or 4-0 Vicryl.
- Of course, the mucosal closure should be both meticulous and watertight with 4-0 Vicryl in continuous fashion.

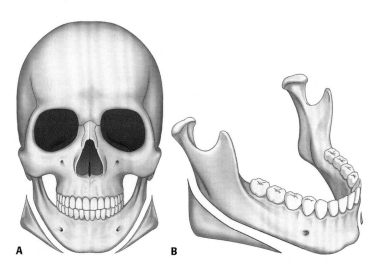

TECH FIG 2 • Mandibuloplasty.

■ Genioplasty

Vertical Reduction Genioplasty

- A 3-cm inverted-V-shaped buccomucosal incision is made from canine to canine, and subperiosteal dissection is performed, except for opening the mental nerve.
- Next, horizontal cutting can be performed with a reciprocating saw:
  - Leave at least 5 mm of bone just above the upper horizontal cutting line, as the mandibular nerve passes approximately 5 mm lower than the bony opening.

- Generally speaking, the chin setback or geniosetback procedure is not recommended, because the submental soft tissue might be redundant after the procedure.
- After osteotomy, bone segment designed for reduction is removed, and lower segment of the chin is fixed to the mandible with titanium miniplate (**TECH FIG 3**).
- The midline of the chin must correspond to the midline of the mandible but can be intentionally different to correct an asymmetry of the mandible.
- The periosteum is closed to minimize soft tissue redundancy with 3-0 or 4-0 Vicryl.

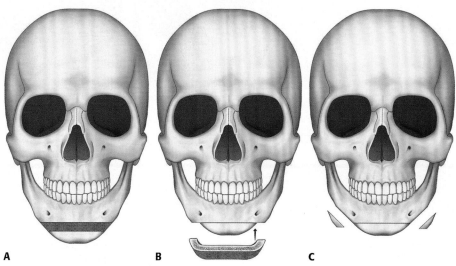

TECH FIG 3 • Vertical reduction genioplasty.

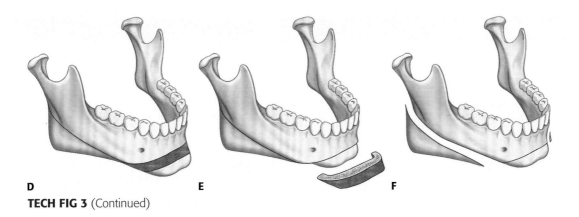

D **E** **F**

TECH FIG 3 (Continued)

Narrowing Genioplasty

- The overall procedure is similar to vertical reduction genioplasty.
- However, a π-shaped osteotomy is made using a reciprocating saw (**TECH FIG 4A**), and the central bony segments of the chin are removed to reduce the horizontal dimension of the chin (**TECH FIG 4**):
  - The horizontal dimension is controlled based on the amount of bone resected.

- A step deformity along the margin can be smoothed easily using marginal mandibuloplasty with a reciprocating saw.
- The two segments of the chin are secured together with wiring and fixed to the mandible with titanium miniplate.
- The periosteum and the mucosa are closed to minimize soft tissue redundancy with 4-0 Vicryl.
- Although mild submental redundancy can occasionally be a problem, the overall satisfaction is generally very high.

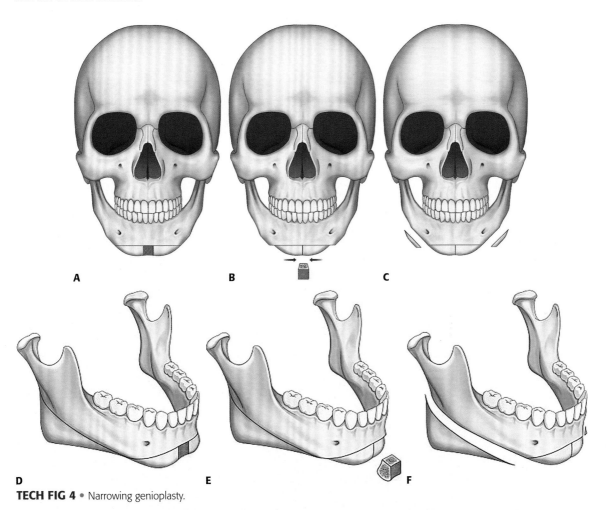

A **B** **C**

D **E** **F**

TECH FIG 4 • Narrowing genioplasty.

PEARLS AND PITFALLS

Approach	■ Subperiosteal dissection is performed except the opening of the mental nerve.
Osteotomy	■ When horizontal cutting is done with reciprocating saw, the important thing is to keep at least 5 mm bone just above the upper horizontal cutting line as the mandibular nerve passes the 5 mm lower than the bony opening.
	■ To avoid cutting submental soft tissue during osteotomy, which can result in submental hematoma, the fingertip of the contralateral hand can be used to perform slight palpation of the tip of the reciprocating saw during osteotomy.

POSTOPERATIVE CARE

■ To prevent submental hematomas, an elastic bandage on the chin area and a facial bandage can be applied 2 or 3 days postoperatively.

OUTCOMES

■ Lee and Ahn retrospectively reviewed 52 patients who underwent narrowing genioplasty.[4] All patients were satisfied with the more slender appearance of their chins:
  ■ The subjective grading was "much improved" in 67% of patients and "improved" in 33%.

COMPLICATIONS

■ Complications are uncommonly noted in Sykes and Suarez's study.[5]
■ Submental hematoma

■ Decreased sensation of the lower lip
■ Submental bulging and soft tissue sagging
■ Malunion or nonunion of bony segment
■ Infection

REFERENCES

1. Cutright B, Quillopa N, Schubert W. An anthropometric analysis of the key foramina for maxillofacial surgery. *J Oral Maxillofac Surg.* 2003;61(3):354-357.
2. Choi JW, Kim N. Clinical application of three-dimensional printing technology in craniofacial plastic surgery. *Arch Plast Surg.* 2015;42(3):267-277.
3. Jeong WS, Choi JW, Choi SH. Computer simulation surgery for mandibular reconstruction using a fibular osteotomy guide. *Arch Plast Surg.* 2014;41(5):584-587.
4. Lee SW, Ahn SH. Angloplasty revision: importance of genioplasty for narrowing of the lower face. *Plast Reconstr Surg.* 2013;132(2):435-442.
5. Sykes JM, Suárez GA. Chin advancement, augmentation, and reduction as adjuncts to rhinoplasty. *Clin Plast Surg.* 2016;43(1):295-306.

An Osseous Approach to Chin Deformities

76

CHAPTER

S. Anthony Wolfe and Saoussen Salhi

DEFINITION

- Osseous genioplasty was introduced in 1942, when Otto Hofer described a horizontal osteotomy of the mandibular symphysis through an external approach to correct the deficient chin on a cadaver.[1,2] However, we owe the first description of a genioplasty performed on a living patient to Gillies and Millard in 1957. They described a jumping genioplasty, through an external approach, where the lower border of the mandibular symphysis was osteotomized, advanced superiorly, and positioned on top of the upper mandibular segment.[2]
- In 1957, Richard Trauner and Hugo Obwegeser described the intraoral approach to the osseous genioplasty,[1-4] and later, in 1964, Converse and Wood-Smith expanded on the possible variations of the procedure.[1,2] In their description of the surgical technique, the osteotomized caudal segment of the mandibular symphysis was stripped of all of its muscular attachments before advancing it, thereby converting it to a free bone graft. This resulted in significant bone resorption, which prompted these surgeons to preserve the blood supply to the caudal segment.[4]
- Despite its description more than half a century ago, osseous genioplasty remains less frequently performed than alloplastic chin implants.[3] In 1950, Converse described the use of intraoral bone grafts for chin augmentation. These quickly fell out of favor because of their variable resorption, donor-site morbidity, and the successful introduction of alloplasts.[1] In 1953, Safian introduced the first silicone chin implant.[1]

ANATOMY

- When performing a genioplasty, pertinent anatomy relates to the mental nerve.
- The mental nerve is the terminal sensory branch of the inferior alveolar nerve, which is itself a branch of the mandibular division of the trigeminal nerve.
- The mental nerve provides sensory innervation to the lower lip and the chin.
- It exits the mandible through the mental foramen at the level of the second premolar.[3]
- The inferior alveolar nerve courses inferiorly prior to heading cephalad toward the mental foramen.[5] For this reason, the horizontal osteotomy of the mandibular symphysis performed during a genioplasty has to be placed 5 to 6 mm below the mental foramen.[5]

PATIENT HISTORY AND PHYSICAL FINDINGS

- Physical examination starts by dividing the face along the trichion, glabella, subnasale, and menton.[3] When these landmarks divide the face into equal thirds, the face is considered ideal.[2,3]
- The lower third of the face, delimitated superiorly by the subnasale and inferiorly by the menton, is further divided by the oral commissure into an upper third, the upper lip, and lower two-thirds: the lower lip, labiomental sulcus, and chin.[2] This allows assessment of the volume of the chin relative to the overall facial profile.
- The chin pogonion projection is assessed relative to the facial plane, the zero meridian, which is a line started at the nasion and dropped perpendicular to the Frankfurt horizontal. Ideally, the chin pogonion should be at or near the zero meridian, being more projected in men than in women. It should not be beyond the lower lip border.[3]
- Chin deformities are commonly divided into two categories: macrogenia and microgenia. Guyuron et al. distinguish seven different chin deformities based on the volume of the chin:
- Class I: macrogenia or chin excess
- Class II: microgenia or chin deficiency
- Class III: combined excess in one dimension and deficiency in another
- Class IV: asymmetric deformity
- Class V: witch's chin characterized by ptotic soft tissue and a deep labiomental groove
- Class VI: pseudomacrogenia or chin excess secondary to soft tissue excess overlying normal bony anatomy as evidenced by a normal cephalogram.[6]
- According to Guyuron et al., class II microgenia is the most commonly encountered chin deformity, followed by class II macrogenia and class III, a combination of both.[6] It is important to note that the microgenia or macrogenia can be present in a number of planes: vertical, horizontal, or both.[3]
- The chin can also be characterized by its spatial position. It can be positioned posterior to its ideal position at the zero meridian, which is referred to as retrogenia.
- When the retrogenia is secondary to mandibular retrognathia (class II malocclusion) or vertical maxillary excess leading to a clockwise rotation of the mandible, this is referred to as pseudoretrogenia.[3]
- Osseous genioplasty alone cannot address this issue, and the patient likely needs orthognathic surgery to correct the underlying malocclusion.
- Often, patients who present complaining of a deficient chin have mandibular hypoplasia with or without chin deficiency.
- For this reason, all patients should undergo an intraoral examination including an evaluation of the skeletal relationship of the maxilla and mandible to exclude any underlying malocclusion.[3]
- Finally, the experienced surgeon needs to rely on his or her eye and the patient's desired result.[3]

IMAGING

- In most patients, clinical examination and photographic analysis are sufficient to determine if the chin shows any abnormality in both its position and its volume.[3]
- A lateral cephalogram can provide quantitative confirmation of these abnormalities.[3]
- A frontal cephalogram can be helpful in planning the genioplasty osteotomy aimed at correcting an asymmetrical chin.[3]
- A panorex is used to identify the mental foramen and the dental roots and to plan the osteotomy and hardware placement to avoid injury to these structures.[3]

SURGICAL MANAGEMENT

- Many aesthetic surgeons favor alloplastic genioplasty[1,4] for its simplicity,[1,3,4] shorter operating time, ease of reversibility, decreased risk of injury to the mental nerve, and ability to perform under local anesthesia.[1] However, they are associated with higher infection rates, risk of extrusion,[1,7] erosion into the mandibular symphysis,[1,3,7] migration, capsular contracture, and unpredictable soft tissue response.[1]
- In contrast, osseous genioplasty eliminates the use of a foreign body, thereby avoiding the risk of infection, extrusion, migration, and bony resorption.[8] It also results in a more predictable soft tissue response[1] and improves the cervicomental contour[1] when the lower symphyseal fragment with its attached musculature is advanced, thereby tightening the submental region.[8] It is also a more versatile procedure[1,3,4,8] to correct chin deformities that an implant cannot, such as vertical macrogenia or microgenia,[3,4,7,8] chin asymmetry,[3,4,8] and significant sagittal microgenia.[3,7]
- We are not condemnatory of the use of alloplastic implants for the chin if they are used for the proper indication,

ie, mild sagittal deficiency[1,4] (generally less than 5 mm[3]) in a previously unoperated patient[3,4] and properly performed (placed through a submental incision and rigidly fixed to the underlying bone). Several contraindications to chin implants are cited in the literature, including systemic diseases such as cardiovascular diseases, diabetes, severe periodontal disease, and young age.[1]

- We do not however use them ourselves because we can do a genioplasty for every type of deformity, including mild retrogenia. Once a comfort level has been reached using power equipment to cut the mandibular symphysis, one can advance the chin, vertically shorten or lengthen the chin, and correct lateral deviations. This enables one to be able to treat the whole spectrum of chin deformities, not just the cases of mild retrogenia. A genioplasty has the added advantage of being a vascularized bone flap with its inferior attachments of geniohyoid, genioglossus, and anterior belly of the digastric muscle.[8,9] Therefore, the advanced segment does not undergo resorption,[8,9] and any postoperative buccal incision dehiscence maintains the potential to heal.

Positioning

- General anesthesia is preferred not because of pain issues but rather a concern that a good bit of blood and irrigating fluid in the mouth of a sedated patient might result in aspiration.
- If a patient is adamant about having the procedure performed under local anesthesia, good anesthesia can be obtained by mental nerve blocks and infiltration of the submental muscles.
- If general anesthesia is used, a nasal intubation is not essential because an oral tube does not interfere with access. The head should be extended, without a doughnut.

■ Osseous Genioplasty

- The lower labial sulcus is infiltrated with a vasoconstrictive solution.
- An incision is made with the needle-tip electrocautery, from to cuspid to cuspid, on the labial side of the gingivobuccal sulcus leaving a cuff of 3 to 4 mm superiorly containing mucosa and very little mentalis muscle and sparing the frenulum.
- Cutting through large amounts of mentalis muscle denervates the superior portion of the muscle and may lead to lower lip incompetence and incisive show, which is very difficult to correct.
- The periosteum is incised and a subperiosteal dissection is immediately begun. This dissection is intentionally limited at the level of the anterior surface of the symphysis, below the planned osteotomy line, to avoid ptosis of the chin pad.
- The dissection then proceeds laterally for identification and preservation of the mental nerves, located between the first and second bicuspids (**TECH FIG 1A**). Their vertical distance from the inferior border of the mandible can vary considerably. Dissection is carried beneath the nerves laterally and over the inferior border of the symphysis.

- The most important step is in marking for the cut. One must be able to see the patient's eyes. The midline is marked (a soft pencil is best), and then at right angles to this, a transverse line is drawn, being sure that it is parallel to the interlateral canthal line. This line must be at least 5 mm below the canine root and 6 mm below the mental foramen when extended laterally (**TECH FIG 1B**). This is to avoid injury to the inferior alveolar nerve, which dips down slightly before it exits the foramen. These lines are then scored using an oscillating saw (we prefer Aesculap, but the Stryker is also fine).
- The operator's left hand then holds the lower lip out of the way, and if possible, the entire full-thickness cut is made with the oscillating saw. Frequently, the bone laterally beneath the nerve may need to be cut with a reciprocating saw (the nerve should be gently shielded during the maneuver).
- The lower border should be cut free entirely with the saw; if one tries to wedge the basilar segment down with an osteotome, a fragment will remain on the basilar segment that interferes with proper movement.
- The basilar segment then can be moved as desired: forward, for retrogenia; upward, after removal of an appropriate strip of bone (remember the nerves), for

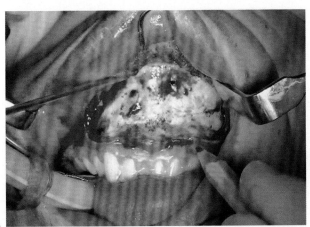 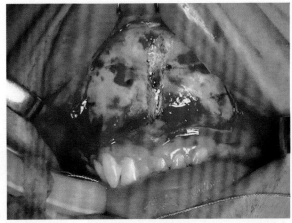

TECH FIG 1 • A. The right mental nerve can be seen just right of the pencil mark, exiting from the mental foramen. **B.** The superior horizontal pencil marks indicate the bilateral mental foramina. The inferior horizontal pencil mark indicates the level of the horizontal osteotomy, marked 6 mm below the level of the mental foramina. The vertical line marks the midline of the mandibular symphysis.

macrogenia; downward with an interpositional bone graft for microgenia; and laterally for chin point deviation. An advancement genioplasty can be fixed with wires or several long screws; other movements often require titanium miniplates and screws.

- The buccal incision is closed in one layer with 4-0 chromic catgut sutures, incorporating as much of the mentalis cuff as possible. If bone graft has been placed, a few deep sutures are placed in the mentalis muscle. Drains are not used.

▪ Variations

- Variations of the osseous genioplasty technique have been described to address all possible chin deformities.
- Sliding genioplasty: The basilar segment is moved anteriorly or posteriorly.[3,9]
- Jumping genioplasty: The basilar segment is used like an implant, placed anterior to the mandible. The muscular attachments to this segment are carefully maintained to maintain its vascularity and minimize postoperative resorption.
- Interpositional genioplasty: A bone graft is interposed at the osteotomy line to increase the height of the lower third of the face.[2,3,9] Converse et al. describe the use of iliac bone as bone graft.[9] However, we favor using the outer table of the cranium harvested in the parietal region as a bone graft in these procedures.
- Wedge genioplasty: Two osteotomy lines are performed below the mental foramen, and the intervening bone segment is removed.[2,3,9]
- Stepladder genioplasty: Two osteotomies create two bone segments. The most caudal of these segments is advanced over an already advanced more proximal segment.[3,9]
- Centering genioplasty allows correction of chin asymmetries.[3,9]

PEARLS AND PITFALLS

Occlusion	▪ Occlusion has to be assessed preoperatively to rule out pseudoretrogenia secondary to mandibular hypoplasia, which is better managed with orthognathic surgery.
Intraoral incision	▪ Incision has to be placed on the labial side of the gingivobuccal sulcus by leaving a mucosal cuff of 3–4 mm to facilitate closure.
Surgical technique	▪ Subperiosteal dissection is limited to the anterior surface of the mandibular symphysis to avoid postoperative ptosis of the chin pad.
Mental nerve identification	▪ The mental nerve is identified between the first and second bicuspid.
Mandibular osteotomy	▪ The midline of the symphysis should be marked and the osteotomy line is drawn perpendicular to the midline, 5 mm below the canine root, and at least 6 mm below the mental foramen.
Incision closure	▪ Closure of the incision can be done in one layer making sure to incorporate the mentalis muscle in the closure.

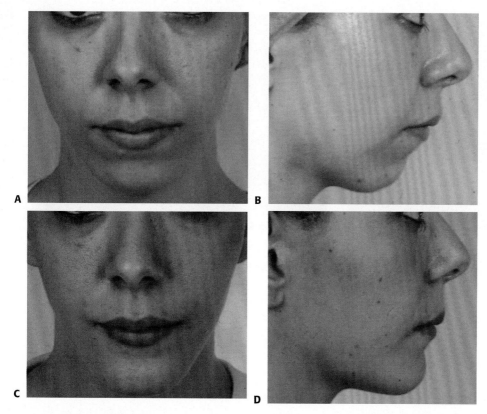

FIG 1 • Preoperative **(A,B)** and postoperative **(C,D)** photos of a patient who underwent jumping genioplasty for retrogenia.

POSTOPERATIVE CARE

- A light tape dressing is maintained for a few days.
- Patients may begin on a soft diet immediately.
- Patients are maintained on a soft diet for 3 weeks postoperatively.

OUTCOMES

- Before and after patient photos are shown in **FIGS 1** to **3**.

COMPLICATIONS

- Among the disadvantages cited for osseous genioplasty, when compared to alloplastic chin implants, need for general anesthesia, technical complexity, need to use power tools, risk of tooth root devitalization, and higher incidence of postoperative mental nerve paresthesias and postoperative discomfort were all cited.[1]

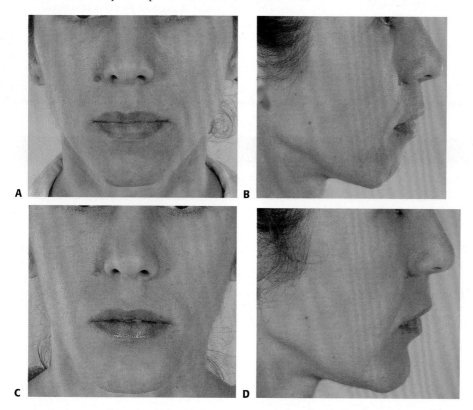

FIG 2 • Preoperative **(A,B)** and postoperative **(C,D)** photos of a patient who underwent removal of a chin implant and jumping genioplasty for long retrogenia.

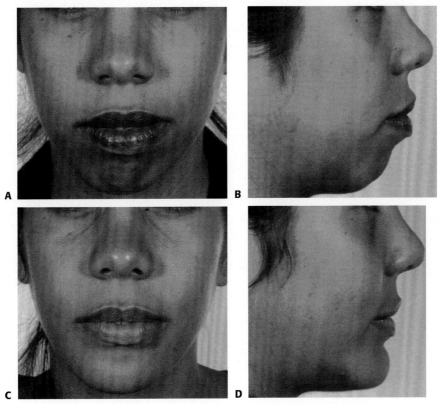

FIG 3 • Preoperative **(A,B)** and postoperative **(C,D)** photos of a patient who underwent wedge genioplasty and jumping genioplasty for long retrogenia.

- However, Guyuron et al. who compared osseous genioplasty and alloplastic chin implants, performed by a single surgeon, on two groups of patients, found no statistically significant difference in the amount of postoperative pain between the two groups of patients.[1]
- They did show a statistically significant higher incidence of temporary sensory loss over the mental nerve distribution in the osseous genioplasty group.[1]
- However, all patients experienced improvement over time, and this difference in incidence of nerve damage was no longer statistically significant over a long follow-up period.[1]

REFERENCES

1. Guyuron B, Raszewski RL. A critical comparison of osteoplastic and alloplastic augmentation genioplasty. *Aesthetic Plast Surg.* 1990;14(3):199-206.
2. Wolfe SA. Shortening and lengthening the chin. *J Craniomaxillofac Surg.* 1987;15(4):223-230.
3. Ward JL, Garri JI, Wolfe SA. The osseous genioplasty. *Clin Plast Surg.* 2007;34(3):485-500.
4. Wolfe SA, Rivas-Torres MT, Marshall D. The genioplasty and beyond: an end-game strategy for the multiply operated chin. *Plast Reconstr Surg.* 2006;117(5):1435-1446.
5. Kawamoto H. Osseous genioplasty. *Aesthet Surg J.* 2000;20(6):509-516.
6. Guyuron B, Michelow BJ, Willis L. Practical classification of chin deformities. *Aesthetic Plast Surg.* 1995;19(3):257-264.
7. Cohen SR, Mardach OL, Kawamoto HK Jr. Chin disfigurement following removal of alloplastic chin implants. *Plast Reconstr Surg.* 1991;88(1):62-66.
8. Wolfe SA. Chin advancement as an aid in correction of deformities of the mental and submental regions. *Plast Reconstr Surg.* 1981;67(5):624-629.
9. Converse JM, Wood-Smith D. Horizontal Osteotomy of the Mandible. *Plast Reconstr Surg.* 1964;34:464-471.

Section XV: Hair Transplantation

Indications and Techniques for Hair Transplantation

CHAPTER 77

Walter Unger and Robin Unger

DEFINITION

- Hair transplant surgery involves the transfer of hair from an area of anticipated lifelong permanence to an area of alopecia or evolving alopecia.
  - The principle of donor dominance, for this procedure, was established in 1959 by Dr. Norman Orentreich.
- Appropriate patients may include those with male pattern baldness (MPB), female pattern hair loss (FPHL), post-trauma and postsurgical areas of alopecia, as well as some cicatricial alopecias.
- Human scalp hairs grow naturally in individual bundles, called follicular units (FUs), composed of clusters of one to four follicles surrounded by layers of concentric collagen fibers.
  - Follicular unit transplantation (FUT), when performed properly, consistently results in a cosmetic appearance similar to natural scalp hair growth (**FIG 1**).
- The two primary methods of harvesting the donor hair are the strip excision method and follicular unit extraction (FUE).
  - The ratio of the donor/recipient area has expanded. Though it is 1:1 with large punch grafts, it is 1:2 to 4 with a strip excision and FUT, thus allowing surgeons to cover larger areas of alopecia with a natural appearance and good cosmetic density.
    - A 1 cm² section from the donor strip can cover 2 to 4 cm² of alopecia.
    - FUE in conjunction with strip harvest has further expanded the donor availability.
  - When FUE is used as the exclusive method for donor harvest, this decreases the number of relatively permanent scalp hairs that can be transplanted during a patient's lifetime, because each of the resultant punctuate scars (typically thousands) must be camouflaged by relatively permanent hairs.
- Good surgical planning in hair transplant surgery addresses current and future areas of alopecia. This principle is especially important when treating younger patients

(because of their long-term donor/recipient area ratios) and those with limited long-term donor hair availability.
- Preoperative evaluation and determination of candidacy should include a physical exam, review of relevant laboratory tests, and a review of the family history of hair loss.

ANATOMY

- The scalp is composed of five distinct layers: skin, subcutaneous layer, galea aponeurotica, loose connective tissue, and pericranium.
- The scalp has an excellent blood supply provided by a system of anastomoses between branches of the external and internal carotid arteries. The arteries run centripetally within the subcutaneous layer. This rich blood supply helps promote exceptional healing after scalp surgeries (**FIG 2A**).
- The sensory nerve supply is also centripetal and subcutaneous. If larger nerve trunks are injured in surgery, there can be significant hypoesthesia in the postoperative period (**FIG 2B**).
- The anatomy of the hair follicle has been described in many texts. The terminal hair is divided into an upper (infundibulum), middle (isthmus), and lower (inferior segment) region. A good harvest will remove intact follicles, and all segments will be transplanted (**FIG 2C**).

PATHOGENESIS

- Androgenetic alopecia
  - Androgenetic alopecia is the most common cause of hair loss in both men and women. It is also the most common reason for hair transplantation.
    - In unaffected scalp, the hair has a growing anagen phase of 2 to 6 years, an involution catagen phase of 2 to 3 weeks, and a resting telogen phase of 2 to 3 months.
    - In affected scalp, the anagen phase is significantly shortened, leading to the production of shorter and finer hairs.

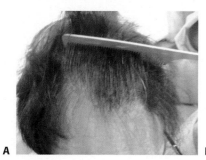
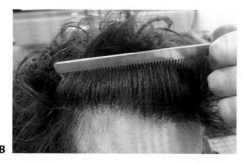

A   **B**

FIG 1 • A. Patient before surgery. **B.** Results after 1 year.

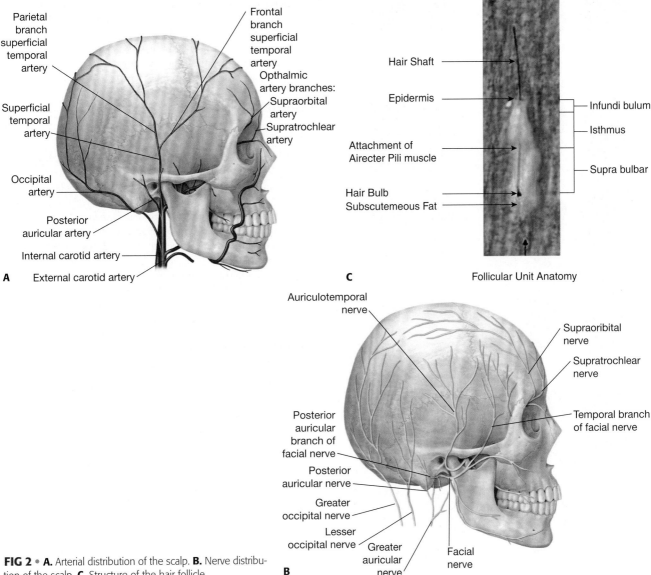

FIG 2 • **A.** Arterial distribution of the scalp. **B.** Nerve distribution of the scalp. **C.** Structure of the hair follicle.

- Androgens play a significant role in both MPB and FPHL, although FPHL has a more complex etiology involving multiple other potential sources, including inflammatory reactions and changes in estrogen and other hormone levels and the enzyme aromatase.
  - Genetic factors are important in determining the likelihood of developing MPB and FPHL—however, it is a polygenic mode of inheritance, with incomplete penetrance.
- Cicatricial alopecias
  - Cicatricial alopecias are, for unknown reasons, increasing in incidence in the population and therefore need to be considered in patients presenting with hair loss. The imposters of patterned hair loss to be wary of include frontal fibrosing alopecia (FFA), lichen planopilaris (LPP), and central centrifugal cicatricial alopecia (CCCA). Their pathogenesis is described in detail in other texts.[1]
  - Dermatoscopic exam and biopsy are helpful in diagnosis and evaluation of activity.
  - Surgery should ideally be avoided until the condition has become quiescent for at least 1 year.[2]

NATURAL HISTORY

- The natural history of male and female pattern alopecia is one of progressive hair loss over the patient's entire lifetime. Current treatments may slow the progression, but as yet, there is no known treatment to stop the evolution.[3]
- The Norwood pattern is shown in **FIG 3**.

PATIENT HISTORY AND PHYSICAL FINDINGS

- Patient history should focus on factors that may contribute to hair loss, including symptoms of hypo- or hyperthyroidism, adrenal imbalances, prolactinomas, nutritional deficiencies, and scalp symptoms noted by the patient (burning, itching, tenderness, flaking).[2]
- The history in female patients should also include questions that may indicate symptoms of androgen excess, such as those seen in women with polycystic ovarian syndrome (hirsutism, irregular menses, reproductive challenges, indicators of insulin resistance).[4]

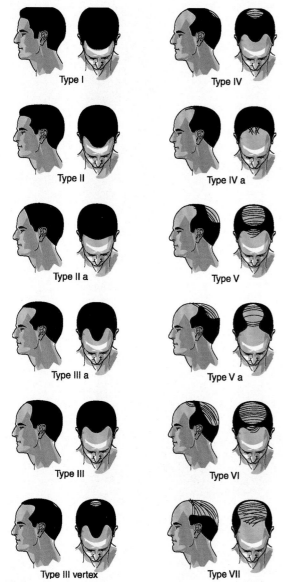

FIG 3 • Norwood classification. (From Landeck L, Otberg N. Hair loss. In: Schalock PC, Hsu JTS, Arndt KE, eds. *Lippincott's Primary Care Dermatology.* Philadelphia, PA: Wolters Kluwer; 2010:410-436, with permission.)

- Events or conditions that cause telogen effluvium should be ruled out; these most often include major physical or emotional stresses, post–severe febrile illness, postsurgery, and postpregnancy. Hair transplant surgery should not be performed until at least 6 months after the resolution of the effluvium—this allows the donor hair to start regeneration and helps identify major areas of concern.

- The history should also clarify the pace of the hair loss and unusual accelerations—a very rapid onset of shedding raises suspicion for etiologies other than androgenetic alopecia.
- The family history of hair loss is pertinent as a guide to determine the eventual degree of patterned loss but is not accurately predictive in many patients.

IMAGING

- Dermoscopy has become a very useful tool in evaluating patients for hair transplant surgery (**FIG 4**).
  - A thorough dermatoscopic exam may reveal more subtle signs of diseases more appropriately treated with a medical rather than surgical approach—including frontal FFA, LPP, CCCA, and alopecia areata patchy or diffuse type.
  - Dermoscopy can also help to determine the degree of miniaturization in the hair-bearing rim. This may inform the surgeon as to how conservative or aggressive the surgical plan should be.[5]
- Biopsy and dermatopathological evaluation may be useful to confirm the underlying condition responsible for the alopecia. Again, dermoscopy guidance may be helpful in this process to guide the surgeon in the area most appropriate for biopsy.

DIFFERENTIAL DIAGNOSIS

- Patterned hair loss may be difficult to distinguish from these entities, especially in their less active periods.
- There also may be some coexistence with MPB/FPHL:
  - Alopecia areata and diffuse alopecia areata ("incognito")
  - Telogen effluvium
  - FFA
  - LPP
  - Tinea capitis
  - CCCA
  - Discoid lupus erythematosus
  - Folliculitis decalvans
  - Syphilis

NONOPERATIVE MANAGEMENT

- Medical therapy
  - FDA-approved treatments with proven efficacy for MPB include minoxidil and finasteride (**FIG 5A,B**).
  - FDA-approved treatment with proven efficacy for FPHL is topical minoxidil 2% twice daily or 5% once daily. Off-label treatments include antiandrogens such as finasteride, spironolactone, and cyproterone acetate.[2]
  - Dutasteride 0.5 mg daily may also be used (off-label) in patients who fail to show response to finasteride.
- Prostaglandin analogs: Studies thus far have been limited and have failed to show a significant positive effect.

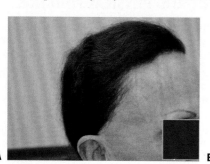
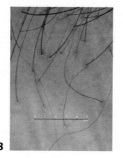

FIG 4 • **A.** Distribution of hair loss in a patient with frontal fibrosing alopecia (FFA). **B.** Dermatoscopic photo showing the periphery of FFA. Characteristics include alopecic area devoid of follicular ostia, slightly white in color; hair in the periphery shows perifollicular casts and relative absence of vellus hair.

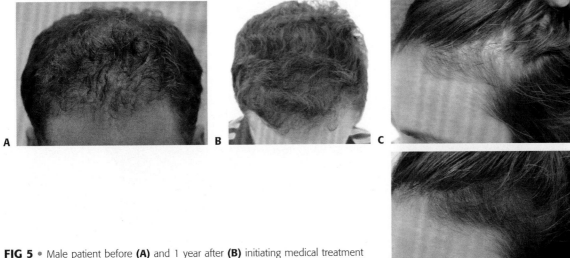

FIG 5 • Male patient before **(A)** and 1 year after **(B)** initiating medical treatment with finasteride 1 mg daily. Female patient with typical hair loss in the frontotemporal regions before **(C)** and 4.5 months after **(D)** one treatment with PRP/ACell/microroller.

- Low-level laser and light devices for hair loss have been shown in limited studies to produce some benefit as compared to sham devices—proposed mechanism of action is mediated by absorption of cytochrome oxidase, resulting in increased oxygen consumption and adenosine 5′-triphosphate (ATP) production. In some patients, it may also produce and anti-inflammatory effect.[2]
- Mesotherapy: Superficial scalp injections of pharmaceuticals and vitamin compounds. Compounds used include minoxidil, biotin, pantethol, finasteride, dutasteride, tretinoin, and other vitamins and minerals. Further studies are necessary to determine efficacy and which compounds at which concentrations are optimal.
- Platelet-rich plasma (PRP): Very few controlled studies have been completed to provide evidence-based data on this modality for hair loss treatment. Nevertheless, anecdotal reports and the experience of credible hair restoration surgeons (HRS) are encouraging.[6]
  - There are many approaches being used by HRS for this procedure. Standardization is necessary and will enable more meaningful evaluation of the procedure's efficacy.
  - Typically in our practice, 60 mL of blood is drawn from the patient and centrifuged to produce PRP. This is then mixed with 25 mg of ACell (an extracellular matrix derived from a porcine bladder) and injected into the area of hair loss. It may be used as a stand-alone procedure or to enhance the results in hair transplant surgery (in the latter scenario, it is also used to bathe grafts prior to implantation).[7]
  - When done as a stand-alone procedure for hair loss by one of the authors, microneedling with a 2.5-mm microneedle is performed prior to injection of the PRP/ACell.
  - PRP has been demonstrated to increase overall hair counts and hair diameter, while microscopic findings reveal thickened epithelium, proliferation of collagen fibers and fibroblasts, as well as greater numbers of blood vessels around hair follicles in areas that have been treated with PRP (**FIG 5C,D**).[7]
  - More studies are needed to confirm the efficacy of this treatment, the ideal approach to be utilized, and frequency of treatments required.

- Micropigmentation is a technique that utilizes tattoos to simulate short hairs on the scalp.
  - It can be used to hide scars and create the illusion of greater hair density in hair-bearing areas. The type of pigment, color chosen, and depth of ink placement can impact the long-term appearance of this type of camouflage.
- Other camouflage techniques include
  - Small hairpieces
  - Powders or hair fibers that camouflage the color contrast between hair and scalp, thereby making hair appear fuller
  - Alternative hair styling

SURGICAL MANAGEMENT

- Donor area evaluation is undertaken to determine the area from which hair is most likely to be permanent and thus will ostensibly persist in the recipient area long after transplantation.
  - The senior author conducted a study of 328 men aged 65 years or older in whom areas containing at least 8 hairs per 4-mm diameter circle were measured.[3] The dimensions established from this study represent the region of harvest that would be "safe" (ie, the hairs would persist) in approximately 80% of patients under the age of 80 years. This persisting region of the donor scalp was termed the "safe" donor area (SDA) and later the safest donor area to denote that no area is perfectly "safe" (**FIG 6A**).
  - These boundaries have since been modified for FUE. Because of the less visible resultant punctate scarring from this alternative technique, Cole's FUE SDA is somewhat expanded (203 cm²) and includes 14 subdivisions based on hair density but importantly was based on only 94 patients, nearly all of whom were in their 30s or 40s—and for both reasons, it is therefore most probably a less reliable guide regarding long-term planning (**FIG 6B**).
- Donor harvest approach
  - As previously mentioned, there are two main donor harvest approaches: strip harvest and FUE.
    - TABLE 1 summarizes the benefits and disadvantages of each method.

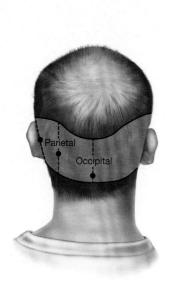

A Alt's safe donor area

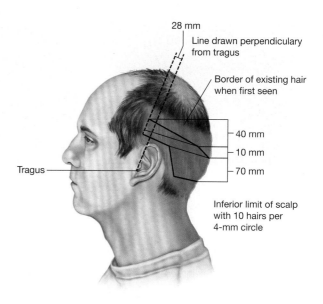

B Unger's safe donor area

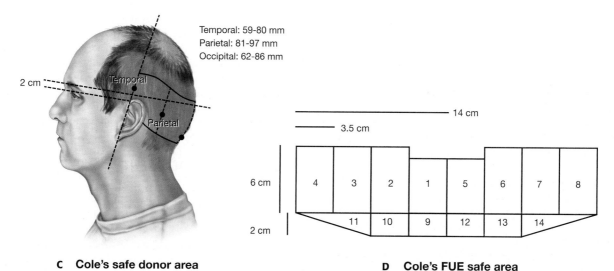

C Cole's safe donor area

D Cole's FUE safe area

FIG 6 • Unger and Cole safe donor area.

Table 1 Benefits and Disadvantages of Follicular Harvest Techniques

Method	Pros	Cons
Strip harvest	• Higher FU yield • Narrow donor area • Higher follicle survival • More protective tissue surrounding hair follicles and predictable graft quality • Harvest stays within the confines of the safe donor area • Ability to choose the size of the grafts • Donor not visible under hair from day 1 postop	• Long linear scar that may be visible when the hair is cut short • More painful postop period • Longer postop healing period with some exercise restriction • Potential for loss of dormant follicles—greater in unrecognized cases of telogen effluvium
FUE	• Shorter postop healing • Less painful postop period • Minute punctuate scars that are less visible even with the hair worn short especially with less contrast between hair and scalp color • A good complement technique when scalp laxity is limited or for repairs • Less tissue discarded with potential dormant follicles	• Lesser FU yield • Wider donor area harvested (some HRS extend past the safe donor area to achieve higher graft yield) • Less tissue around hair follicles (skinny grafts) and less predictable quality, contributing to lower follicle survival • Usually requires shaving the donor area for larger sessions • Lowers the density in the donor area perceptibly after larger harvests or multiple procedures

- Ideally, HRS should have all tools available to tailor the procedure to each patient's individual needs.
- Both methods of harvest primarily use follicular unit (FU) grafts almost exclusively in the recipient area.
  - One of the authors sometimes uses double follicular units (DFU) when a strip harvest is use and the area to be treated has pre-existing permanent hair. This very frequently pertains to women with thinning behind the hairline zone and older males with minimal hair/skin color contrast.
- Donor strip harvest
  - Goals
    - Minimize the amount of hair follicle transection as the strip is excised and dissected.
    - Extract donor strip widths with prudent caution in order to minimize closing tension.
    - Produce only a single scar regardless of the number of sessions performed on a single patient.
  - Assessment of scalp laxity prior to surgery is of tantamount importance; this can be done with calipers or manually.
  - The donor strip should be removed from the densest zone of the fringe hair. Any subsequent strip excision should include the previous scar so only one thin linear scar remains.
- FUE
  - Goals
    - Maximize the amount of hair removed from the most permanent hair-bearing fringe while minimally altering the architecture of the donor area. Keep in mind also that the fringe hair will continue to decrease in density somewhat over the patient's lifetime.
    - Minimize transection during extraction, yet try to harvest with some protective tissue; this should be a goal even if the technique involves fractional harvesting of follicular groups.
    - Minimize the amount of scar tissue within the donor area by varying punch diameters to keep it as small as possible (without increasing transection rates) and try to evenly disperse the harvest sites.
  - FUE grafts may be removed from the Unger's traditional SDA and should ideally have a tapering zone superior and inferior to make the density change more subtle. The temporal regions may also be harvested more extensively with this technique than with strip harvesting.
  - FUE may be used to harvest hairs from the beard area on the neck and inferior to the lower mandible.[3] These grafts can be used to camouflage scars and to thicken regions that already have been transplanted. Other body hair survival is much more unpredictable.

- Recipient area approach
  - The authors strongly believe in planning that includes treating current areas of hair loss simultaneously with future areas of loss in the zone of the recipient area being addressed (front, midscalp, or vertex).
    - Although patients may intend to return to "complete things," they may be unable to do so because of life events. A well-planned hair transplant should look natural over the patient's entire lifetime.
    - On average, 25% to 30% of grafts may be placed in future areas of loss—this number is obviously higher in patients treating their MPB very proactively and is lower in those who present with more advanced hair loss.
  - Other physicians believe that transplanting a maximum portion of currently noticeable hair loss is more important than concomitantly treating the less noticeable future areas of loss. As long as the patient is fully informed, this policy is reasonable: it gives the patient more immediate satisfaction, and the future areas of loss can be treated when needed.
  - The authors do not ask patients to change their hairstyle or usual length of hair for the procedure. This hair serves as a guide for the placement of hair to be transplanted and also provides postoperative camouflage.
  - Some surgeons shave the recipient area to facilitate the completion of larger surgeries with greater ease and within a more reasonable time frame.

Preoperative Planning

- Preoperative instructions include the discontinuation of medications or substances that may increase bleeding.
  - In particular, 10 days before surgery, acetylsalicylic acid (ASA), or any drugs containing it that influence platelet activity, should be discontinued—this instruction is suspended in patients taking ASA or anticoagulation for therapeutic purposes. The patient is also asked to abstain from alcohol consumption for 1 week preoperatively.
  - Twice-daily application of topical minoxidil to the recipient area is started 1 week prior to surgery due to the theoretical increase in blood flow that may decrease the likelihood or severity of temporary hair loss.
  - Patients with limited scalp laxity having strip surgery are instructed on how to massage their scalp during the 4 weeks prior to surgery in order to increase the laxity within the donor area, thus enabling a wider strip harvest and a greater FU yield.
- Prophylactic perioperative antibiotics are given to patients 1 hour prior to surgery and 6 hours later as a precaution.
- The surgical design is drawn the morning of surgery and discussed again with the patient (**FIG 7A**).

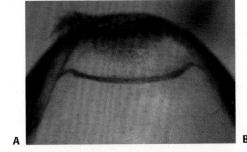 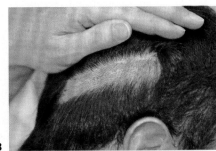

FIG 7 • **A.** Markings for hairline and borders for surgery. **B.** Preoperative period after donor area hair has been trimmed. A scar from the previous surgery is visible in the center of the trimmed region.   **A**   **B**

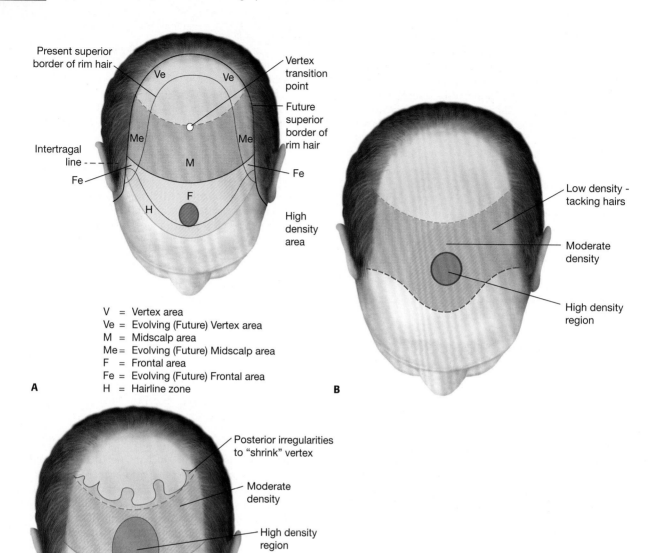

V = Vertex area
Ve = Evolving (Future) Vertex area
M = Midscalp area
Me = Evolving (Future) Midscalp area
F = Frontal area
Fe = Evolving (Future) Frontal area
H = Hairline zone

FIG 8 • Zones of treatment regions, including current and future areas of alopecia.

- Many photographs are taken on the morning of surgery, an even greater number if the recipient area contains pre-existing hair.
  - Results are optimal and reproducible when photos are standardized. A ceiling or photographer's light immediately behind the photographer and a uniformly bright background color enhance the viewing of the scalp by creating contrast, thus outlining the peripheral boundaries of progressing alopecia and hair.
- The laxity in the donor area is evaluated carefully with the neck in a neutral position.
  - The donor area hairs to be harvested are trimmed to 2 to 3 mm in length to facilitate implantation and orientation of the hair at that time (**FIG 7B**).

Hairline Design

- The hairline design is arguably the most important step. There are no firm rules.
  - The contour should be consistent with a natural aging hairline (different among ethnic groups). In most male patients, this involves incorporation of temporal recessions.
- The major anatomic landmarks, borders, and zones of normal hair-bearing scalp need to be well understood and effectively reproduced (**FIG 8**).
  - With the increased demand for HRS among young adults in the early stages of MPB, one of the most important principles of hairline placement is "do not place a hairline too low."

- A guideline for locating the anterior midpoint of a hairline is to look somewhere in the zone between the vertical and horizontal planes of the scalp. Discuss with the patients their wishes and desired hairstyle as this may influence somewhat the position of the superior "frame" of the face.
  - To create the illusion of a slightly lower hairline without expending too many FU, surgeons may construct a "widow's peak."
- From the anterior midpoint, the frontal hairline should run more or less parallel to the ground or slope slightly upward when viewed from the side until it meets the temporal hairline at a point drawn from the lateral epicanthus to a point where it meets the remaining temporal hair.
- Throughout the hairline, the transition zone (the anterior 0.5- to 1-cm region) should contain both microirregularities (intermittent density clusters more noticeable under close examination than from a distance) and macroirregularities (protrusions along the path of the hairline that cause it to appear less linear when viewed from a distance).
  - It is important to note that the macroirregularities may change the contour of the hairline and thus need to be chosen carefully.
- It is generally not advisable to advance temporal points in young male patients who may experience a progressive posterior recession of their temples that their limited donor reserve may not be able to sufficiently address once the transplanted hair is placed too far anterior to the progressively receding temporal hairline (thus leaving an unnatural "island" of transplanted hair).
  - When the donor-to-recipient ratio allows, however, temporal points should be advanced no farther than to an intersection of two lines: one drawn from the tip of the nose, over the pupil to the anterior tip of the temporal point, and a second line drawn from the most anterior midpoint to the tragus.
- In addition to hairline design varying with degree of hair loss, ethnic considerations should be made when creating this anterior-most pattern.
  - Caucasians generally have dolichocephalic, or ovoid, skulls; East Asians tend to have brachycephalic, or rounded, skulls.
  - The hairline design in East Asians is comparatively wider and flatter, with curved (rather than sharp) frontotemporal angles. The relatively higher caliber of East Asian vs Caucasian hair may make multihair FU more noticeable. It is therefore important to camouflage these higher-caliber haired FUs with additional rows of single-haired grafts anteriorly.
  - Patients of African descent tend to have mesocephalic skull shapes of intermediate length and width that support hairlines that are flatter than Caucasian patients, but not as flat as those found in most East Asians. Unlike East Asian patients, however, a natural hairline appearance is more easily achieved in patients of African descent due to not only the hair curl and the finer caliber hair but also the minimal contrast between the color of the hair and skin and the frizz, which creates an illusion of density and any tendency for grafts to be noticeable.
- Appropriate facial framing in female patients often entails a more rounded hairline design that incorporates observations derived from examination of 360 female volunteers (**FIG 9**).

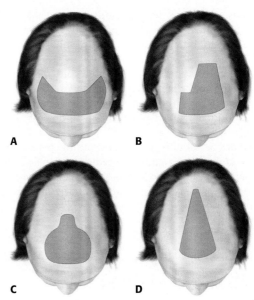

FIG 9 • Most advantageous patterns for graft distribution in female patients.

- A widow's peak (observed in 81% of female hairlines)
- An anterior midpoint placed a mean distance of 5.5 cm superior to the glabella
- Lateral mounds with an apex of 3.75 to 4 cm from the frontal midpoint (98% of females)
- Temporal mounds 3.5 to 3.75 cm lateral to the apex of lateral mounds
- Temporal recessions in a concave oval contour that contain fine hairs (87% of females)
- More often with females than with their male counterparts, native residual vellus hairs can be followed to recreate their hairline pattern.

Positioning

- During the donor removal in a strip harvest, the patient begins in a prone position, using a prone pillow to access the occipital donor area (**FIG 10**).
  - The head can be turned from side to side to access the lateral regions of the donor area.
- During longer FUE procedures, the patient's position is changed multiple times, including prone position, lateral positions, and even supine positions with the head turned from side to side. This alleviates discomfort during the FUE harvest.
  - Positioning in FUE procedures is very individual among surgeons and their teams. It has become apparent that the FUE grafts are very fragile and even short periods

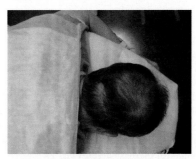

FIG 10 • Positioning of patient in the prone pillow for donor excision.

of desiccation or long periods without blood flow may be detrimental.[3] Thus, positioning is optimized to allow overlap of excision, removal, and implantation phases.

- In most cases, the sites are created and the grafts are implanted with the patients in a supine position.
  - If the vertex is the recipient area, however, the optimal position will be prone for a portion of sites and implantation.
- Some HRS perform the procedure with the patient in a sitting position for the entire procedure—often in a special chair with a head rest to stabilize the head. In the authors' experience, patients tend to find this fairly uncomfortable for long periods.
- Anesthesia

- All patients are given long-acting oral medication to start the day, including an antianxiolytic (lorazepam 2 mg), a sedative (diazepam 10 to 20 mg), and an analgesic (hydrocodone/acetaminophen 5/500 mg).
- Just prior to injecting the local anesthesia, the patient is given fentanyl and midazolam intravenously for immediate effect.
- Anesthesia is typically performed as a field block with lidocaine 2% with 1/50 000 epinephrine. First wheals are placed at 2.5-cm intervals, and then the block is completed by injecting laterally from within the anesthetized areas. Occasionally, stronger anesthetics are used.

T E C H N I Q U E S

■ Donor Strip Harvest

- Magnification is used to assist in excision and dissection under direct visualization.
  - The transection rate in strip harvest varies depending on the surgeons' and technicians' experience and is generally less than 1%.
- The area to be harvested is tumesced in the subcutaneous layer with saline. This helps separate the follicles, thus minimizing follicle transection. It also lifts the tissue above the deeper and larger vasculature and nerves.
- A single no. 15 blade is used to incise along the inferior edge of the donor area followed by the superior edge.
  - The lateral ends of the strip are tapered before the tissue is removed.
  - Some HRS superficially score the surface with a blade to a depth of mid-dermis and use skin hooks to allow for greater visualization or tissue spreaders to bluntly separate the tissue and reduce transection rates further.
- The strip is removed from the bed using a single blade, again under direct visualization, to ensure dissection occurs in the relatively avascular plane just deep to the follicular bulbs (**TECH FIG 1**).

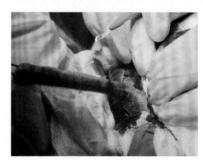

TECH FIG 1 • Excision has been started. Note the intact follicles and limited depth of incision.

- Any significant bleeding vessels are cauterized, excepting those that are immediately adjacent to follicular bulbs.
- One very helpful pearl is to remove a strip from the occipital region first and close that area with sutures before reassessing the scalp laxity in the adjacent parietal and temporal regions and excising those strips. This is especially beneficial when the donor area tension is somewhat unpredictable.

■ Donor Site Closure

- Choosing the strip width and closing the donor wound in sections, as described above, is helpful to avoid any unexpected areas of tension.
  - One region of the scalp can "borrow" laxity from another area and lead to otherwise unanticipated increased tension.
- Over the mastoid region, where tension is more often higher than expected, wedge-shaped sutures may also help relieve tension.[2]
  - This technique eases the work (W) required for closure more effectively than sutures placed perpendicular to the wound edge by increasing the distribution of force (F) along the wound edge. With F and wound edge displacement (d) being constant in the formula for work ($W = Fd\cos\theta$), the magnitude of work is reduced as the angle (θ) increases (**TECH FIG 2A**).

- The donor area may be closed in a single layer or double layer, depending on the surgeon's preference.
  - The double layer helps to decrease tension on the more superficial epidermal layer, but it also carries the risk of worsening the scar in individuals with hyper-reactive healing.
  - If the patient is undergoing a second surgery, the healing from the first surgery can be a guide. If the scar spread after suture removal and there was no hypertrophic healing, a double-layer closure nearly always results in a finer scar compared to a single-layer closure.
- If a double layer is used, the authors prefer PDSII 3-0 or Maxon 3-0.
  - Depending on the wound length, four to eight buried interrupted sutures are placed deep to the level of the follicles, to approximate the base of the wound (**TECH FIG 2C**).

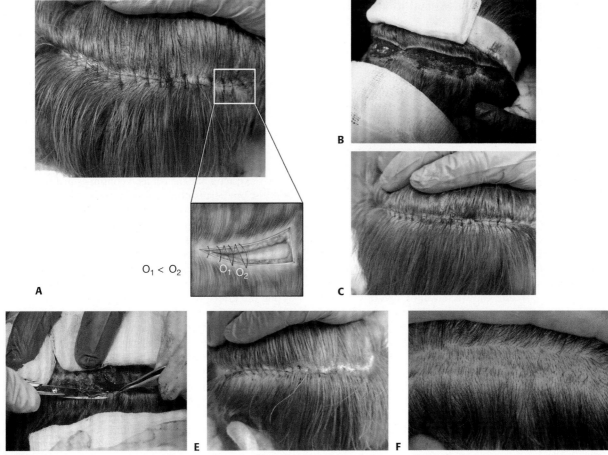

$O_1 < O_2$ $O_1\ O_2$

TECH FIG 2 • **A.** Suture pattern in a wedge shape to decrease tension on closure over the mastoid regions. **B.** Deep sutures in place in double-layer closure. **C.** Donor area after closure of the superficial layer. **D.** In trichophytic closure, the epidermal layer being trimmed is approximately 1 mm wide and 1 mm deep. If the hair follicles are slightly further apart from one another, the width may need to also be slightly larger. **E.** Partially completed trichophytic closure. **F.** Final appearance of scar in donor area.

- The superficial epidermal layer is closed with 3-0 Supramid or 3-0 Prolene. Usually, a running suture is utilized with stitches placed approximately 4 to 5 mm apart from one another, ensuring good approximation of the epidermal edges.
  - The needle should pass through the dermis and exit just below the level of the bulbs.
  - Beware sutures that are too close or too far from the wound edge.

- Trichophytic closure can be used to help further camouflage the resultant scar.
  - In this technique, prior to closure, a 1-mm section of epidermis is carefully removed from the superior or inferior ledge of the wound, maintaining a level superficial to the sebaceous gland (**TECH FIG 2D**).
  - The epidermal edges are then approximated and the wound is closed (**TECH FIG 2E,F**).

FUE Harvest

- FUE harvest can be accomplished by several methods: manual punch, oscillating or rotating motorized punch (dull or sharp or even a modified sharp punch), suction-assisted device, or robotic device.
  - Each of these methods has unique detailed requirements to produce ideal results.
- Originally involving the use of a sharp 1-mm "cookie cutter"–like punch, hair follicles trimmed to 2 mm in

length were extracted manually in a random distribution so as to avoid overharvesting any particular area, which might result in a "moth eaten" appearance.[1]
- Gradually, powered instruments for FUE largely replaced manual punches by demonstrating increased extraction speed and efficiency.[6] Increased speed, however, requires heightened attention to avoiding follicle transection or follicle "decapitation" that may occur when a sharp punch is introduced at the improper angle.[8]

TECHNIQUES

- Variable tissue and hair characteristics such as follicle curvature, angle of exit from the skin, or splaying arrangement beneath the skin surface may further increase the challenge of avoiding follicle transection.
- To minimize follicle transection, nonsharp motorized punches have been developed to perform "blunt" dissection of FUs from the skin. Rather than cutting the deep segment of a follicle with an unforeseen curvature, a dull punch can push the follicle within the cylinder and thereby reduce transection rates.
  - Alternatively, a two-step manual process involving an initial "scoring incision" at a 0.3- to 0.5-mm depth around the follicle followed by the insertion of a blunt dissecting cylinder that reaches the full depth of the follicle (approximately 4 to 5 mm) enables full separation of the intact follicle from its native tissue prior to manual extraction using forceps.
- A newer technique involves an oscillating motorized unit and a modified blunted thin-walled punch. Limited reports indicate this may lower transection rates dependably (below 3%) and allow removal of a graft with limited mechanical traction and more tissue surrounding the FU, regardless of patient's tissue characteristics.
- Larger punches alter the architecture of the donor area and may leave more perceptible scars. In most cases, the punch should be smaller than 0.95 mm in its external diameter.
- A surgeon's ability to properly position the punch according to the follicle's angle of exit from the skin surface requires proper (5× to 6.5×) magnification.
- The following step-by-step description applies to most techniques:
  - For large FUE cases, the donor areas are shaved.
  - Sterile saline tumescence injected at both a superficial and deeper depth helps to increase the space between FU, increases the predictability of hair follicle angle deep to the skin surface by making the follicles more erect, and separates the follicle bulb from the underlying vascular and nerve plexus.
    - The tumescence can dissipate fairly quickly and therefore needs to be repeated frequently as the surgeon progresses to subsequent areas.
  - The punch is centered over the FU and advanced.

- There is a tactile sensation that can be appreciated when the FU has been "released."
- Initially, several of the grafts should be extracted to check if the depth is sufficient to minimize trauma during the extraction phase.
  - Once a depth has been determined, most physicians will incise up to a hundred grafts or more and then extract using a two-handed method to pull the grafts while simultaneously depressing the surrounding tissue to assist in release.
  - Depending on the position and region of harvest, occasionally, an assistant can follow along and extract while the surgeon continues incisions.
- Most physicians now employ a method of creating sites prior to the extraction phase and alternating graft extraction and graft implantation throughout the surgical day; thus, the more fragile FUE grafts do not remain outside the body for long periods.
- As noted earlier, the patient needs to be positioned and repositioned throughout the day to facilitate harvesting the grafts and maintaining good ergonomics for the surgeon.
  - Certain positions also enable the technicians to implant the grafts simultaneously while the harvest continues.
- It is worth repeating that the grafts need to be kept moist from the time of extraction to implantation.
- The robotic technique of harvesting FUE does make the process faster and also has a faster "learning curve" for the physician. Nevertheless, some patients complain of the discomfort of the positioning chair and prolonged immobility.
  - The smallest punch size used with the robot has an internal diameter of 0.9 mm, but external diameter of 1.1 mm, so the punctuate scars are larger than ideal.
  - The trend of "fractional harvesting of follicular groups"—removing only some hairs within a follicular group—helps preserve donor architecture and is not possible with the robotic punch.
- Many physicians, including the authors, pack the donor sites with PRP and ACell after the harvest is complete, to potentially minimize the visibility of the scars and alteration of the subcutaneous tissue during healing. Theoretically, this should facilitate a second FUE procedure.

■ Graft Preparation

- Once a strip is removed (**TECH FIG 3A**), it is immediately transferred to a dish with a chilled holding solution. The authors use HypoThermosol with liposomal ATP (10:1 mL proportion). This solution has been shown to improve survival of the grafts while outside the body, as compared to saline or other solutions.
  - Akin to organ transplantation, factors of negative influence include ischemia-induced hypoxemia and subsequent ATP depletion (resulting in subsequent apoptosis) as well as ischemia-reperfusion injury.

- Graft preparation takes place on ClearVue boards (translucent horizontal cutting surfaces made of polyurethane), which allow backlighting to project through the tissue. Lighting from above is provided by Meiji lights with adjustable intensity.
  - Magnification requirements vary between technicians; some prefer magnifying loupes, while others use microscopes.
- The strip is initially "slivered" into "slices" that are one FU in width (**TECH FIG 3B**).
  - The strip needs to be kept moist during this entire process with frequent spraying of chilled saline.

- One end of the strip is anchored with a 20-G needle, and countertension is provided with Adson forceps. A single Personna blade held on a small blade handle is gently pulled toward the technician to carefully dissect the tissue between the follicles.
- The slices thus produced are then turned on their sides and divided into the individual grafts.
  - The grafts are sorted according to number of hairs and hair texture and stored again in the chilled holding solution (**TECH FIG 3C**).
- FUs are kept intact: they are not subdivided unless there is an insufficient number of single hair grafts for the hairline.
- The ideal "pear-shaped" graft (**TECH FIG 3D**) possesses little or no surplus epidermis and retains an appropriate amount of protective dermis and subcutaneous adipose tissue around the follicle, the intact sebaceous glands, and the dermal papilla so as to reduce sensitivity to traumatic handling, temperature changes, and graft desiccation (the main cause of poor graft survival).
  - These characteristics are rarely achieved with FUE grafts, which are mechanically pulled out of the skin with a combination of traction and perifollicular pressure after a shallow circumferential incision and so are more fragile. Some of the newer developments in blunt dissection with a very thin-walled punch appear to improve the amount of surrounding tissue in the FUE grafts.
- FUE grafts rarely require much "preparation." They are sorted according to number and caliber of hairs.

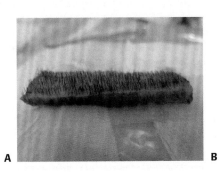
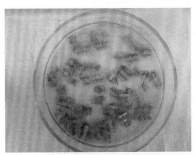
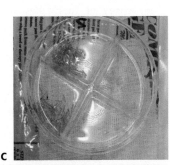
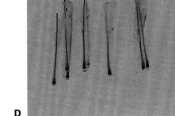
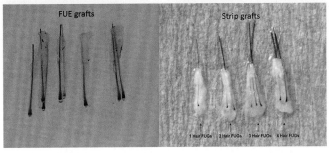

TECH FIG 3 • **A.** A strip harvest after removal. **B.** A "sliver" removed from the strip. **C.** FU grafts sorted in the dishes filled with a storage solution (HypoThermosol and liposomal ATP) and kept chilled. **D.** FUE grafts on the left and FU grafts from strip on the right.

■ Creation of Recipient Sites

- The recipient site creation is arguably the most important step in producing excellent cosmetic results.
  - The surgical plan should already include an estimate of how large an area needs to be addressed, including current and future areas of alopecia.
  - Then, the physician needs to determine approximately how many grafts will likely be harvested; this then guides the determination of the density of sites to be created.
  - There should be micro- as well as macroirregularity to create a very natural appearance. The density of the hairline should be lower than the density created posterior to the hairline to produce a feathered effect.
  - The lateral hairline is formed by the anterior "temporal humps." These areas are re-created (at an angle very acute to the scalp) in patients who are severely receded in these regions.
- The angle and direction of recipient site incisions should in almost all cases mimic those of any significant amount of pre-existing hair, regardless of its location.
  - To do otherwise results in transection of those hairs, and every study on follicle transection has demonstrated decreased number and/or hair caliber of transected follicles.
  - Generally, the authors make sites parallel to the direction of the hair (**TECH FIG 4**).
  - In the temporal regions and eyebrows or other areas requiring a very acute angle, sites are made perpendicular to the hair direction.
  - If there is any movement of the FU within the site, it will not result in the hair direction being less flush with the scalp.
- The hairline zone should be completed with only single-hair FU, with the finer one-haired and some two-haired FU placed anterior to the higher-caliber ones.
  - The sites are made using a 20-G needle and follow the angle and direction of existing hair.
  - The density of sites may vary between 25 and 35 FU/cm² depending on the effect being sought.
- Behind the hairline zone, the sites are created using a 19-G needle for two-haired and some three-haired FU,

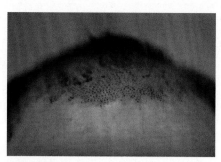

TECH FIG 4 • Recipient site pattern.

and the three- or four-haired FUs are placed posterior to that in sites made with an 18-G needle or 1.3-mm blade that is cut to size.

- The density of these sites varies between 20 and 35 hairs, depending on the distribution of the graft size, the area needing coverage, and the overall density availability.
- The three-haired FU and follicular families are concentrated in regions where higher density is desired.
  - This includes a region behind the hairline transition zone and within a larger oval-shaped region in the frontal forelock.

- There is much debate regarding the ideal density of sites within the field of hair restoration surgery.
  - The authors believe the ideal density depends on many factors, including hair characteristics, final expected pattern of alopecia, donor availability, and patient objectives.
  - The ideal density achieves the greatest cosmetic impact over the largest area of the future pattern of alopecia; it is not a predetermined number.
- Creation of recipient sites in the midscalp and vertex follows a similar surgical plan, in that, nearly always, current and future areas are treated.
  - The site density again depends on the size of area that has to be treated and the donor hair available over the patient's lifetime.
- The vertex should ideally not be surgically treated until the frontal two-thirds of the area of MPB are satisfactorily completed.
  - This area responds best to medical treatment and is generally least cosmetically important to patients.
- Pre-existing hair should be protected during site creation, and grafts should be placed in the future areas of loss to be certain that the transplanted area remains "connected" to the fringe hair.

Hair Transplantation in Women

- The most important aspect in hair transplantation in women is the planning stage.
  - **FIG 9** shows the most important cosmetic regions to treat in women to make the greatest impact in a single surgery.
  - Unlike male patients, who are totally alopecic in the areas of concern, most females' scalp hair is getting progressively sparser.
  - The recipient area is fairly diffuse and the donor area is generally smaller and more inferior in females. Density needs to be created very strategically.
  - The hairline zone should be more feathered in women than in men. If preauricular hair is being transplanted, the patient should be instructed that trimming the hair to make it more wisplike after surgery may be helpful.

- Sites for FU are usually made with 20-G or 19-G needles, depending on the size and caliber of the grafts following the exact angle and direction of the existing hair.
  - In women, the coarser hairs are more likely to be terminal hairs that will last over many years; these should be considered when choosing exactly where to place a transplanted hair.
- One of the authors makes some sites with a blade cut to size for DFU; grafts that contain two FUs.
  - After several samples of DFU are produced, the grafts are tested in the sites to ensure a good fit. The size is usually between 1.2 and 1.3 mm.
  - These grafts seem to produce more volume in the area in which they are placed and potentially reduce the postoperative telogen effluvium frequently seen in women.

Hair Transplantation into Scars From Cicatricial Alopecia, Trauma, or Postrhytidoplasty

- The major pearl for hair transplantation into scar tissue is related to the real-time evaluation of the vascular supply. No epinephrine should be used in the area prior to starting. This allows the surgeon to evaluate blood flow throughout the area.
- Sites are created using either a 20-G or 19-G needle, and the site should be made deeper than usual, to try to access the vascular bed beneath the scar tissue.

- Site density should be between 10 and 20 FU/cm² in the first pass.
  - If the blood supply seems quite good, density can be used adjacent to the scar (eg, anterior to a postrhytidoplasty scar).
- Patients should expect that at least a second surgery will be necessary to create acceptable hair density. Often, neovascularization after the first surgery has occurred and the density of sites can be higher.
- Sometimes, the tissue has poor recoil and the grafts tend to slide out.
  - In such cases, tissue glue can help hold the grafts in place.

■ Facial Hair Transplantation

- Scalp hair can be transplanted into the eyebrow, beard, mustache, and eyelash areas.
  - The techniques involved in these procedures are very similar to those used to treat areas of patterned hair loss with a few exceptions.
- The sites are created almost exclusively with the 20-G needle, and almost all grafts are one- or two-haired grafts.
- The grafts should be cherry-picked from regions of the donor area with matching texture.
- The angles of the sites need to be particularly acute on the face, and the hair needs to be oriented so it does not curl in the wrong direction.

- Eyelash transplantation is particularly difficult to perform and produce natural results. The hairs at the nape of the neck are well suited for this purpose.
  - A curved needle is used to make sites in the lid margin and the hair is threaded through and directed to follow natural lash curvature.
  - Some surgeons used scalp hairs threaded onto a crescent needle, which is then threaded through the lid.
  - Trichiasis (misdirection of the eyelash) can be a significant complication.

■ Implantation of Grafts

- Graft implantation requires very skilled technicians with excellent hand-eye coordination and a gentle touch.[9,10]
- In our office, the grafts are bathed in PRP + ACell in small dental rings prior to implantation. The dental rings allow the grafts to remain moist while limiting the need for constant change of field of focus to retrieve more grafts.

- The graft is grasped by the fat at the proximal portion of the follicle and gently placed with jeweler's forceps into the recipient site.
- Implanters have been gaining in popularity, especially in FUE cases. They reduce graft handling and potential damage. They also reduce the need for highly trained technicians.
  - The graft is threaded onto an implanter by holding it by the hair.
  - The implanter is then inserted into the site and atraumatically delivered.

PEARLS AND PITFALLS

Planning	■ The surgical plan should take into consideration the long-term pattern. ■ The patient should be well informed and well educated about the probable outcome and the possible complications accompanying each technique. ■ Unrealistic long-term goals should be discouraged during the consult and the day of surgery.
Anesthesia	■ A thorough evaluation of the patient's overall health status should be obtained by good history and P.E. and coordinating with the patient's primary care physician for other health issues. ■ The physician should be knowledgeable of the medication's pharmacodynamics, side effects, toxic levels, and drug interaction and their corresponding management. ■ When indicated, it is best to get an anesthesiologist for the patient's overall safety.
Donor harvest	■ The surgeon should only take an optimally sized donor area to permit closure without tension to avoid the development of wide scars. ■ Using monofilament absorbable sutures in the subcutaneous layer helps eliminate "dead space" and lessen tension for good wound closure. ■ Hemostasis should always be employed to avoid blood clot formation in the donor area. ■ A solution of 3.33 mg/mL of triamcinolone (10 mg/mL) + 0.5% Marcaine can be injected into the donor area to lessen postoperative swelling.
Grafts	■ Avoid transections by making one follicle wide slivers to easily divide the grafts into its natural groupings. ■ Leave enough tissue around the grafts for protection during placement. ■ Eliminate the epidermis during graft cutting leaving a tear-shaped graft. ■ Always keep the grafts moist by frequently spraying with normal saline during cutting and storing them into normal saline solution or HypoThermosol + ATP solution.
Recipient sites	■ Create irregularities along the hairline to provide a natural look. ■ Meticulously follow the hair direction to minimize trauma and shock loss to the surrounding follicles. ■ The hair transplant surgeon should address the "future areas" of loss when making the recipient sites. ■ The surgeon should always balance between "dense packing" especially the hairline and frontal area and doing a lower number of FU/cm² for wider recipient areas especially for patients with limited donors. ■ The angle of the recipient site should be determined before attempting to plant a graft.

PEARLS AND PITFALLS *(Continued)*

Graft implantation	
	■ Avoid overhandling and unnecessary manipulation of the grafts to minimize traumatic injury.
	■ Keep the grafts moist and store them in appropriate storage solutions such as normal saline or Hypo-Thermosol with or without ATP. PRP can also be used to store the grafts right before implantation.
	■ Always use "ring containers" when placing grafts to avoid drying and graft death.
	■ In experienced hands, the use of implanters can be a safe and fast method of planting the grafts.
	■ The grafts should ideally be at the same level of the original hairs. Buried grafts can cause ingrown hairs and skin dimpling of the recipient sites when healed.

■ Elevated grafts can be prone to getting dislodged during the postop period and hair washing.
■ Assistants should be comfortably positioned when planting the grafts. This would improve their technique and would minimize traumatic handling of the grafts.
■ The recipient area should be thoroughly cleaned and the implanted grafts checked one more time before bandaging.

POSTOPERATIVE CARE

■ Immediately after the procedure is finished, an antibiotic ointment is applied to the recipient and donor areas, and the head is bandaged overnight.
  ■ This practice has been continued by the authors because the occlusion provides a moist environment that is beneficial for healing and also acts as a physical barrier to microbial invasion.
■ The bandage is removed the first day after surgery and nurses wash the recipient and donor areas.
  ■ Our patients are encouraged to continue soaking and cleaning twice daily to help dissolve any crusts that have formed and keep the surgical areas clean.
■ Patients also apply lubricant to the surgical areas to keep them moist and use minoxidil 3.5% for its vasodilatory effect and potential for decreasing telogen effluvium.
■ Postoperative pain after strip harvest is usually minimal.
  ■ Patients complain of a "tight" feeling in the donor area.
  ■ After FUE, patients report very little discomfort, likened sometimes to a bad razor burn (**FIG 11**).
■ In addition to analgesic use (acetaminophen or narcotics), patients are instructed to apply ice for 10- to 15-minute intervals along the nape of the neck to help decrease edema, which may add to the tension along the suture line.
■ The authors generally remove sutures between 8 and 10 days after surgery.
  ■ In cases of an increased risk of wound dehiscence (eg, multiple donor area scars and marked tension upon donor wound closure) or instances of excessive scalp laxity upon donor site closure, sutures should be left in place for a longer period of time, usually 10 to 14 days.
■ 4 to 5 weeks after surgery, patients are encouraged to return for evaluation.

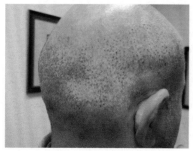

FIG 11 • Donor area after FUE harvest.

■ On occasion, there is excessive erythema or hyperesthesia in the donor area; this may be treated with intralesional triamcinolone acetonide (3.33 mg/mL).
■ Patients should be alerted to possible postoperative sequelae:
  ■ Tissue edema may become most evident 3 to 5 days postoperatively in the forehead and temple areas.
    • Patients are encouraged to ice these areas and maintain a supine or lateral position as much as possible for the initial 72-hour postoperative period. It is generally mild, but in 1 out of approximately 50 patients, it may be severe enough to cause ecchymosis around the eyes.
  ■ Scalp hypoesthesia resulting from severed sensory nerves during the processes of both donor harvest and recipient site creation
    • This generally resolves in 3 to 6 months however, depending on the size and location of the nerve, may take up to 18 months to return to normal.
  ■ Telogen effluvium, or temporary hair loss sometimes referred to as "shock loss," may be experienced by approximately 10% to 20% of male patients and 40% to 50% of females.
    • The temporary nature of this effluvium, which may affect 10% to 25% of the pre-existing recipient area hair, is emphasized during the consultation. It resolves in 2 to 3 months, but if a patient is not emotionally prepared for this likelihood, he or she should not undergo HRS.

OUTCOMES

■ Although patients may vary considerably, the general timeline for hair growth after a session is as follows:
  ■ Newly transplanted vellus hairs begin to appear around the 3rd or 4th postoperative month, although the addition of PRP to our surgical procedures seems to result in some hairs being retained and growing without a dormant phase.
  ■ The number and caliber of transplanted hairs continue to increase until full growth can be appreciated approximately 18 to 24 months after a session.
■ One surgery can create a cosmetically excellent result in any one region of the recipient area (**FIGS 12 to 14**).
  ■ The hair transplanted will last as long in its new area as it would have lasted in the donor area.
■ The results become less dense over time because pre-existing hair is lost over time and some donor area hair, even in the SDA, is lost with the passage of time.

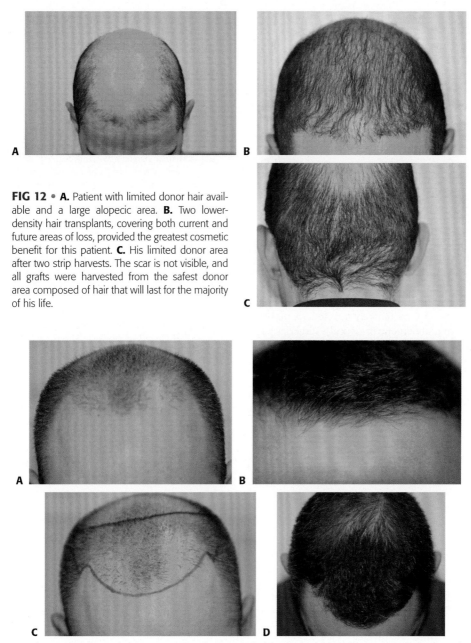

FIG 12 • A. Patient with limited donor hair available and a large alopecic area. **B.** Two lower-density hair transplants, covering both current and future areas of loss, provided the greatest cosmetic benefit for this patient. **C.** His limited donor area after two strip harvests. The scar is not visible, and all grafts were harvested from the safest donor area composed of hair that will last for the majority of his life.

FIG 13 • A,B. This patient has a very dense donor region. Given his age and objectives, a higher-density surgical plan was chosen. **C,D.** Appearance after one surgery.

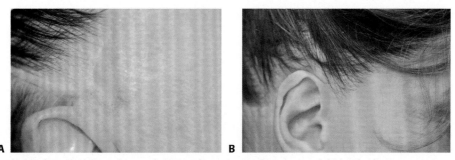

FIG 14 • A. Patient postrhytidoplasty. **B.** Patient after one hair transplant to camouflage scars and thicken hairline.

- ▪ Medical therapy in conjunction with surgery will help mitigate this effect.
- ▪ One of the most important questions regarding FUE is whether the graft survival is comparable to the survival of grafts obtained from a strip harvest.
  - ▪ Limited studies performed to date suggest that survival is considerably lower.
  - ▪ One study involving four patients and 3560 hairs/follicles, which was presented at the ISHRS annual meeting 2015, showed at 14 months only 61.4% of the FUE grafts had regrown, while 86% of the strip harvest–derived FU had regrown. More studies are required.

COMPLICATIONS

- ▪ Beyond focal neuralgia, uncommon donor area complications include wound dehiscence and arteriovenous fistulas as well as aesthetic complications of visible scarring, keloid or hypertrophic scarring, or donor hair effluvium.
- ▪ Within the recipient area, the uncommon, but most serious complication of central recipient area necrosis results from vascular compromise and is more likely in smokers, diabetics, and patients having undergone prior scalp surgeries.
- ▪ Folliculitis or ingrown hairs. These are uncommon and less severe complications that can occur in up to 20% of patients in a very mild form or a much smaller percentage in a more severe presentation. This may be treated with either warm compresses or a course of a first-generation cephalosporin, such as cephalexin, depending on the severity.

REFERENCES

1. Rogers N. Imposters of androgenetic alopecia: diagnostic pearls for the hair restoration surgeon. *Facial Plast Surg Clin North Am.* 2013;21(3):325-335.
2. Unger R, Wesley C. Technical insights from a former hair restoration surgery technician. *Dermatol Surg.* 2010;36:679-682.
3. Varothai S, Bergfeld W. Androgenetic alopecia: an evidence-based treatment update. *Am J Clin Dermatol.* 2014;15(3):217-230
4. Herskovitz I, Tosti A. Female pattern hair loss. *Int J Endocrinol Metab.* 2013;11(4):1-8.
5. Rose PT. Hair restoration surgery: challenges and solutions. *Clin Cosmet Investig Dermatol.* 2015;8:361-370.
6. Alves R, Grimalt R. Randomized placebo-controlled, double-blind, half-head study to assess the efficacy of platelet-rich plasma on the treatment of androgenetic alopecia. *Dermatol Surg.* 2016;42(4):491-497.
7. Uebel CO, da Silva JB, Cantarelli D, Martins P. The role of platelet plasma growth factors in male pattern baldness surgery. *Plast Reconstr Surg.* 2006;118(6):1458-1466.
8. Cooley J. Bio-enhanced hair restoration. *Hair Transpl Forum Int.* 2014;24(4):128–130.
9. Speranzini M. FUE graft placement with dull needle implanters into premade sites. *Hair Transplant Forum Int.* 2016;26:2.
10. Unger R. Female hair restoration. *Facial Plast Surg Clin North Am.* 2013;21(3):407-419.

Index